Mohs Micrographic Surgery

Mohs Micrographic Surgery

George R. Mikhail, M.D.

Director, Mohs Micrographic Surgery Section
Department of Dermatology
Henry Ford Hospital
Detroit, Michigan

1991
W.B. SAUNDERS COMPANY
Harcourt Brace Jovanovich, Inc.
Philadelphia ■ London ■ Toronto ■ Montreal ■ Sydney ■ Tokyo

W. B. Saunders Company
Harcourt Brace Jovanovich, Inc.

The Curtis Center
Independence Square West
Philadelphia, PA 19106

Library of Congress Cataloging-in-Publication Data

Mohs micrographic surgery / [edited by] George R. Mikhail.
p. cm.
ISBN 0-7216-3415-X
1. Microsurgery. I. Mohs, Frederic E. (Frederic Edward).
II. Mikhail, George R.
[DNLM: 1. Microsurgery—methods. 2. Skin
Neoplasms—surgery. WR 500 M6992]
RD33.6.M64 1991
617′.05—dc20
DNLM/DLC 90-8941

Editor: W. B. Saunders Staff
Designer: Paul Fry
Production Manager: Ken Neimeister
Manuscript Editor: David Prout
Illustration Coordinator: Walt Verbitski
Indexer: Nancy Newman
Cover Designer: Michelle Maloney

Mohs Micrographic Surgery ISBN 0-7216-3415-X

Printed in the United States of America.

Last digit is the print number: 9 8 7 6 5 4 3 2 1

To Elizabeth,
Michael, and Marianne,
with love.

Contributors

Dennis E. Babel, Ph.D.
Director of Microbiology, Department of Dermatology, Henry Ford Hospital, Detroit, Michigan.

Mark R. Balle, M.D.
Department of Dermatology, Mohs Surgery Section, Henry Ford Hospital, Detroit, Michigan.

Gerald Bernstein, M.D.
Clinical Professor of Medicine (Dermatology), University of Washington School of Medicine, Seattle, Washington.

Eric A. Breisch, Ph.D.
Professor of Anatomy, United States International University, San Diego, California.

Daniel W. Collison, M.D.
Fellow, Mohs Micrographic Surgery, Department of Dermatology, Iowa Methodist Medical Center, Des Moines, Iowa; Fellow, University of Iowa, Iowa City, Iowa.

Hubert T. Greenway, M.D.
Head, Mohs Surgery Unit, Division of Dermatology and Cutaneous Surgery, Scripps Clinic and Research Foundation, La Jolla, California.

William C. Hanke, M.D.
Professor of Dermatology, Pathology and Otolaryngology; Indiana University School of Medicine; Indianapolis, Indiana.

Paul O. Larson, M.D.
Assistant Professor, Department of Surgery, University of Wisconsin, Madison, Wisconsin.

Melissa W. Lee, B.S.
Research Associate, Department of Dermatology, Indiana School of Medicine, Indianapolis, Indiana.

David Levin, M.A.
Manager, Department of Photography, Henry Ford Hospital, Detroit, Michigan.

George R. Mikhail, M.D., M.S.
Clinical Associate Professor of Dermatology, University of Michigan Medical School, Ann Arbor, Michigan; Senior Staff Physician, Department of Dermatology, Henry Ford Hospital, Detroit, Michigan; Director, Mohs Micrographic Surgery Section, Henry Ford Hospital, Detroit, Michigan.

Robert A. Mohr, B.A.
Head of Department of Medical Art and Prosthetics, Henry Ford Hospital, Detroit, Michigan.

Frederic E. Mohs, M.D.
Emeritus Professor of Surgery, University of Wisconsin, Madison, Wisconsin.

John M. Pelachyk, M.D.
Senior Staff Physician and Director of Dermatopathology, Henry Ford Hospital, Detroit, Michigan; Clinical Assistant Professor of Dermatology, University of Michigan Medical School, Ann Arbor, Michigan.

Steven A. Proper, M.D.
Assistant Clinical Professor, Department of Medicine, Division of Dermatology, University of South Florida, College of Medicine, Tampa, Florida.

Paul T. Rose, M.D.
Assistant Professor, Department of Medicine, Division of Dermatology, University of South Florida College of Medicine, Tampa, Florida.

Gary B. Rosen, M.D.
Resident, Department of Dermatology, Henry Ford Hospital, Detroit, Michigan.

Linda S. Selak, H.T. (A.S.C.P.)
Histotechnologist and Coordinator of Mohs Micrographic Surgery, Department of Dermatology, Henry Ford Hospital, Detroit, Michigan.

Stephen N. Snow, M.D.
Assistant Professor, Department of Surgery, University of Wisconsin, Madison, Wisconsin.

George B. Winton, M.D.
Clinical Assistant Professor, Department of Internal Medicine, Division of Dermatology, James Quillan College of Medicine, East Tennessee State University, Johnson City, Tennessee.

John A. Zitelli, M.D.
Staff Physician, Montefiore Hospital, University Health Center of Pittsburgh, Pittsburgh, Pennsylvania.

Foreword

The need for a new book on Mohs micrographic surgery is obvious to those of us who try to keep up with the innovations in the technique and the new uses for the method. I tried to update current knowledge with books published in 1956 and 1978, but with increasing numbers of micrographic surgeons and the resulting plethora of information in the various specialty journals, it is again time to bring the current data together in book form.

Having known and esteemed George Mikhail for more than 20 years, and having followed his steady progress in our specialty since his training with me, I feel that he is in a superb position not only to write about his own experiences but also to know to whom to delegate the writing of chapters on subjects in which they have special expertise. He has been active in the field since 1968 and has attended and actively participated in the scientific meetings of the American College of Chemosurgery as well as the newly named American College of Mohs Micrographic Surgery and Cutaneous Oncology. He has held positions as secretary-treasurer and president of the American College of Chemosurgery, and, through these activities, he became acquainted with everyone who is active in the development of the field.

At Henry Ford Hospital, George has had access not only to experts in various surgical fields for consultation and cooperation in the care of patients but also to Edward Krull, M.D., the pioneer in the teaching of dermatologic surgery at the meetings of the American Academy of Dermatology. From these contacts, he fully appreciates the need for interspecialty cooperation for the maximum benefit of his patients.

FREDERIC E. MOHS, M.D.

Preface

The approaches to the management of cutaneous neoplasms are diverse. They include electrosurgery, cryosurgery, laser surgery, cold knife excisions, and radiotherapy. The success of any of these methods depends on the proficiency of the physician administering the particular treatment.

Frederic E. Mohs, M.D., originated the microscopically controlled excision of cancers in the late 1930s. The technique is at present universally recognized as a standard surgical procedure. Dermatologists and surgical specialists acknowledge and appreciate the value of Mohs surgery because it assures complete ablation of neoplasms with maximal preservation of normal tissues.

The practice of Mohs surgery is an art that requires proficiency in clinical and surgical skills, pathology, and anatomy. An entire chapter, arranged in an atlas-like format, is devoted to the pathology of tumors commonly encountered in a Mohs surgery practice. Familiarity with the clinicopathologic features of tumors is integral to the successful application of this type of surgery.

The book has been planned to be comprehensive in scope when scrutinized from a practical perspective. It is designed to serve as a guide to physicians who may be called upon to advise or treat cutaneous lesions that are suspected of being or proved to be malignancies. This comprises many medical professionals including dermatologists, plastic surgeons, general surgeons, otolaryngologists, ophthalmologists, urologists, oncologists, and general and family practitioners. Physicians-in-training in Mohs surgery should find it useful in acquiring basic knowledge of the important facets of this art. This book may also serve as a guide to histotechnologists and nurses who are, or who plan to become, members of a Mohs surgery team.

With the increasing awareness of Mohs surgery on the part of medical professionals and the public and the continuing increase in incidence of skin cancers, this modality is bound to reach higher stature and to become wider in scope. This work has been assembled with the above considerations in mind.

GEORGE R. MIKHAIL, M.D.

Acknowledgments

The material contained in this book represents the practical knowledge and expertise of physicians who are outstanding in the field of Mohs surgery. Sincere thanks and gratitude are expressed to the gracious contributors who have given time and effort to make this publication possible.

While chairman of the Department of Dermatology at Henry Ford Hospital, Dr. Clarence S. Livingood was instrumental in sending me to Madison, Wisconsin, in 1968 to train in Mohs surgery. His support and attention are greatly appreciated. When Dr. Edward A. Krull succeeded Dr. Livingood as chairman of the department, he established the Mohs Surgery Section. His encouragement and valuable advice during the preparation of this book deserve special thanks.

Special mention is due to a great teacher and a dear friend, Dr. Frederic E. Mohs. Heartfelt thanks are addressed to him for his genuine encouragement and kindness to the editor during the last 22 years.

Sincere appreciation is extended to Deborah A. Chesney for typing the great majority of the manuscript and to Julie Lelo, Monica Y. Murphy, Paula Minter, Irene A. Golasa, and Leo Bernardo for their assistance in preparing and entering follow-up data of patients into the computer and for their suggestions to render the recording of the data easier.

Table of Contents

CHAPTER 1

Origin and Progress of Mohs Micrographic Surgery

Frederic E. Mohs, M.D.

Innovation—change in the established way of doing things—often does not come as an immediate, complete solution to a problem, but it may evolve in a series of halting steps. The latter process was operative in the origin and development of Mohs micrographic surgery, a method that provides complete microscopic control of the excision of accessible forms of cancer.

ORIGIN OF THE IDEA

The circumstance that initiated the thought process that led to the new method occurred in the early 1930s while I was a Brittingham Research Assistant to Professor Michael F. Guyer, geneticist and chairman of the Department of Zoology of the University of Wisconsin. In a study of the effect of intratumoral injection of colloidal platinum, we had observed a dense infiltration of leukocytes in the tissues around implanted cancers but almost none within the neoplasms. During experiments with various other irritants, zinc chloride was injected in a 20% solution, a concentration that inadvertently caused tissue necrosis. Microscopic examination revealed the usual disparity of the leukocytic infiltrate around and within the tumor, but an incidental observation was that the microscopic structure of the killed tissue was retained the same as if the tissue had been excised and immersed in a fixative solution. This observation of in situ fixation might have been unrecorded and forgotten had it not suggested the idea that it might be the basis for a method by which cancers could be excised under complete microscopic control.

Just how this microscopic control would be achieved was not clear at first. Vertically cut serial sections would not be practical because of the excessively large number of sections that would have to be prepared and examined. Either step sections or representative sections from random locations would leave gaps between the sectioned areas. Finally, the idea was conceived of excising the tissues layer by layer and microscopically examining the entire undersurface of each horizontally-cut layer by the systematic use of frozen sections.

DEVELOPMENT OF THE FIXED TISSUE TECHNIQUE

Although the general concept was quite simple, numerous questions had to be answered in the laboratory before the method would be ready for clinical trials.[1] For example, if in situ fixation of the tissues were to precede the excision of the layers, how could precise control of fixation be achieved? Injection of zinc chloride solution into the tumor produced erratic tissue fixation, and if the solution entered a blood vessel, the rat convulsed and died in a minute or two. Applying the solution to the surface produced erratic and insufficient penetration. Finally, incorporating the zinc chloride in a specially designed paste vehicle made possible the desired accurate control of fixation over a wide range of depth.

Choice of in Situ Fixatives

Before settling on zinc chloride as an in situ fixative, a number of other chemicals were tested. Some were ruled out because of excessive systemic toxicity when used on large tumors; these included arsenic trioxide, phenol, and mercuric chloride. Antimony trichloride distorted tissue structures and penetrated intact skin, and necessitated special care in its use. Alkalis, such as sodium and potassium hydroxide, were rejected because they liquified the tissues with significant loss of tissue structure. Silver nitrate was ruled out because of the danger of argyria.

Advantages of Zinc Chloride

The most satisfactory in situ fixative proved to be zinc chloride, a chemical discovered in 1815 by Sir Humphry Davy of Bristol, United Kingdom, and first extensively used for destruction of cancer a decade later by Canquoin of Paris[2] and by Bougard of Brussels.[3] The favorable characteristics of zinc chloride are:

1. *Good in situ fixation* not only for preservation of the histological features of the tissues but also for making the tissue firm for easy excision and handling of the specimens and for producing a bloodless, white surface on which the source of each specimen can be precisely indicated by dye marks with a 20% solution of merbromin (Mercurochrome).
2. *Good penetration* into the tissues with precise control of the depth of fixation by varying the thickness and extent of area of the applied fixative preparation, and the time it is permitted to act.
3. *Abrupt cessation of fixation* after approximately 18 hours.
4. *Lack of damage to the healing qualities* of the underlying tissues; this contrasts with necrosis caused by heat which damages the tissues beyond the limits of the burn necrosis.
5. *Lack of systemic toxicity* in the doses ordinarily used.
6. *Safety in handling* because the chemical does not readily penetrate the skin's keratin layer unless a keratolytic such as dichloroacetic acid is applied.
7. *Lack of odor.*
8. *Lack of any tendency to increase metastasis.*

The last advantage was demonstrated by dividing a total of 144 rats bearing implants of metastasizing Flexner-Jobling carcinoma into treated and control groups.[1] The treated rats were purposely subjected to prolonged, subcurative doses in an attempt to demonstrate possible increased metastasis, but there were only 28% with metastases in that group, whereas there were 42% in the controls. Clinical experience with many thousands of patients has confirmed the conclusion that in situ fixation with zinc chloride has no tendency to increase the incidence of metastasis.

Vehicles to Carry and Release the Fixative

In developing a vehicle to carry and release the fixative, it seemed logical to emphasize the use of an inert granular material to provide a matrix to permit the zinc chloride solution to percolate down between the particles like water permeates through sand. However, to prevent the solution from settling to the bottom of the container and also to provide a consistency that would keep the material in place when applied to a lesion, a binder would be needed. Not finding the desired substances in our chemical storeroom, I visited an old-fashioned pharmacy where the 85-year-old proprietor pulled out drawers containing a black granular antimony ore, stibnite, and a number of plant extracts including bloodroot powder, *Sanguinaria canadensis.* The stibnite, after passing through an 80-mesh sieve, provided the best granular matrix of any of the numerous materials tested. For the binder, *Sanguinaria canadensis* was selected from all the other plant extracts. The pharmacist suggested this material, and he demonstrated how he mixed zinc chloride in the powder to make a paste for application to his customers' skin cancers. The paste was too soft, and it was obvious that a thick layer would not stay in place on a lesion.

After many trials, a 4 to 1 proportion of stibnite and *Sanguinaria canadensis* was found to hold and release the zinc chloride solution in a controlled manner. A satisfactory formula containing approximately 45% zinc chloride by weight was formula Z-108A:

Stibnite (80-mesh sieve)	40 gm
Sanguinaria canadensis	10 gm
Zinc chloride, saturated solution	34.5 ml

The fixative preparation had sufficient body to prevent the solution from settling to the bottom of the container and to enable it to stay in place on the lesion to which it was applied. It was held in place by a thin layer of absorbent cotton which, in turn, was covered by a petrolatum-spread, gauze-backed cotton dressing to provide occlusion. Occlusion was needed to prevent variations in the consistency of the fixative with changes in the atmospheric humidity.

The paste vehicle was determined by the patent office to be original enough to be patented, and I signed all rights over to the Wisconsin Alumni Research Foundation for one dollar in 1944. The purpose of patenting was to prevent others from doing so and selling it indiscriminately to persons not trained to use it with complete microscopic control. Arrangements were made with the Department of Pharmacy of the University of Wisconsin, Madison, to supply the fixative at approximate cost to physicians certified to use it properly.

OTHER TECHNICAL INNOVATIONS

Frozen Section Technique

Improvement of the frozen section technique was an early necessity because the large, flat, horizontally cut specimens had to be complete to avoid gaps in the sectioning. The orientation of the specimens in relation to the microtome knife, the mounting, and the staining were all designed to produce complete sections.[4]

Because of the large number of sections, every step in the processing was examined to cut minutes or seconds from the time needed to prepare and examine the sections. If the sections were obviously complete, the technician could put three or four different sections on a slide. This saved time for both the technician and for the physician examining the sections. If the specimens were of tissues that might have missing parts, however, three or four cuts of the same specimen could be placed on the same slide. If the physician noticed any gaps in the section, he or she could request a recut.

Our technician developed great skill in mounting the specimens on the microtome stage so that after only a few passes of the knife the sections were complete, including the skin that often is on one edge. The staining with hematoxylin and eosin produced excellent, easy-to-diagnose sections. In recent years, cryostats are replacing the microtomes because the thinner sections provide more cytologic detail that is especially useful in diagnosing the peripheral margins of melanomas.

Color Coding

Color-coding the edges of the horizontally cut specimens was needed for precise orientation as the sections are scanned in the microscope. For greatest accuracy, it is advisable that the micrographic surgeon excise and mark the two edges of each specimen himself or herself, rather than excising the entire layer and letting the technician divide it into specimens, mark the edges, and draw the map. Three dyes that persist through the processing of the sections are all that are needed: red (20% merbromin solution [Mercurochrome is supplied as a powder by Humco Laboratory, 1008 Whitaker St., P.O. Drawer 2550, Texarkana, TX 75501]), blue (Prussian blue, as in concentrated laundry bluing), and black (India ink). On the maps showing the source of each specimen, the red edge is designated by a solid line, the blue by a dotted line and the black by a wavy line (see Chapter 2).

PRESENT USES FOR FIXED TISSUE TECHNIQUE

Melanoma

Melanoma is currently considered the most important indication for Mohs micrographic surgery, fixed tissue technique (MMS-fixed) by the staff of the Mohs Surgery Clinic at the University of Wisconsin Hospital and Clinics. The reasons for this preference are twofold: First, MMS-fixed provides a safe means to selectively follow out the clinically unpredictable contiguous outgrowths that may extend a considerable distance beyond the clinically observed melanomatous mass. Because the incisions are only through fixed (killed) tissues, the danger of spilling and disseminating the highly transplantable melanoma cells is obviated. Second,

TABLE 1–1. Five-Year End Results for Three Types of Melanoma

Type of Melanoma	Total Number*	Indeterminate Cases†	Determinate Cases		
			Total	*Successful*	*Cure Rate*
Nodular	91†	18	73	38	52%
Superficial spreading	66	14	52	40	77%
Lentigo maligna	43	13	30	23	77%
Total, all types	200	45	155	101	65%

*Series of consecutive patients with Stage I melanomas
†Patients without evidence of melanoma when they died or were lost track of before completion of the five-year follow-up. Note the unusually high proportion of nodular melanomas.

MMS-fixed also provides a relatively safe means of managing satellites which are embolically-produced, noncontiguous foci that are more common with melanoma than with any other neoplasm. Any visible satellites are removed along with the primary melanoma. Microsatellites, which are too small to be seen clinically, are not moved or disturbed. The wound is allowed to heal by granulation, and if any satellites appear, they can be relatively safely removed with MMS-fixed.

Transection of silent contiguous outgrowths or of noncontiguous satellites with conventional surgery can be hazardous. The danger is the ease with which the highly transplantable melanoma cells can be spilled and disseminated during undermining to permit wound closure or be concealed for a long time under a graft or flap.

The sparing of normal tissues that is possible and safe with MMS-fixed is an especially important advantage in the treatment of melanomas of facial areas such as the eyes,[5] ears,[6] and nose.[7] In other areas where the saving of normal tissue may not be so important and the melanoma has microscopic features that suggest there might be microsatellites, the removal of an extra margin of apparently normal tissue is advised.

The five-year cure rates achieved with MMS-fixed compare favorably with surgical results in each of the levels of invasion from Clark's levels 2 to 5.[8,9] Currently, the five-year cure rate for 200 patients with Stage I melanoma is 65.2%, even though an unusually high proportion were of the nodular type and had invaded the subcutaneous tissues (Table 1–1).

A melanoma registry, directed by Stephen Snow, M.D., and Paul Larson, M.D., at the Mohs Surgery Clinic at the University of Wisconsin Hospital and Clinics records the results of others as well as our own. We expect that these data and the publications of others will establish MMS-fixed as a viable alternative to wide conventional surgical excision of melanoma.

Extensive Neoplasms

Large neoplasms, especially those involving bone, often are best managed with MMS-fixed.[9] The successive layers of bone can be removed with a chisel or rongeur, and their sources can be mapped the same as nonosseous tissues. After decalcification in a decalcifying solution, frozen sections are cut, processed, and examined. The residual layer of fixed bone demarcates cleanly in about three weeks, permitting removal in large sheets exposing healthy, well-vascularized granulations. The wound can be allowed to heal by second intention, or it can be covered with a graft or flap.

Penile Carcinoma

Carcinoma of the penis with invasion of the erectile tissue often is more easily removed with MMS-fixed because of the lack of difficulty in achieving hemostasis during removal of the layers. Moreover, there is no problem of bleeding during separation of the final layer of fixed tissue. Excision with complete microscopic control not only ensures eradication of the cancer, but it avoids partial or complete amputation that is usual with conventional surgery unless the cancer is limited to the prepuce.[10]

Cancer and AIDS

Cancer in patients with AIDS can be safely treated with MMS-fixed as reported for the first time by Hruza and Snow.[11] The fixation with zinc chloride inactivates the human immunodeficiency virus (HIV) and, with other routine universal barrier precautions, minimizes the danger of infection of surgical and laboratory personnel. A recurrent, highly invasive, morpheaform basal cell carcinoma in the right nasal alar groove was removed in four microscopically controlled stages and the defect was repaired with a graft."

Gangrene

Gangrene in patients with diseases that impair the circulation and healing potential of the tissues was considered a possible use of the fixed tissue technique after we observed the excellent healing by second intention after removal of cancers.[12] More than 600 patients with diabetes or arteriosclerosis causing gangrene have been treated with the zinc chloride fixative, with 72% healing at the conservation level of amputation.[13,14] A large majority of these patients would otherwise have required more extensive surgical amputations.

Similar results were achieved in patients with gangrene associated with thromboangiitis obliterans, Raynaud's disease, frostbite, and arterial embolism or thrombosis.[9] Thermal burns can produce eschars that are slow to separate because of damage to the reactive and healing capabilities of the tissues just beyond the actual necrosis. Thus, in some burns chemical fixation of the tissues to a level of a few millimeters beyond the burn necrosis can produce well-vascularized granulation tissue in 7 to 10 days, whereas the burn slough may require 2 or 3 weeks to separate and the granulations would be less well vascularized.

Osteomyelitis

Osteomyelitis occurring in connection with diabetic gangrene in metatarsal bones has responded well to conservative amputation with the zinc chloride fixative.[9] Even recalcitrant osteomyelitis of larger bones such as the tibia can be successfully treated with the fixative, as reported by Bennett and Goldman.[15] X-rays are useful to determine the extent of osteomyelitis.

Tetanus

Tetanus with serious, generalized spasticity was successfully treated by in situ fixation in two patients with lesions on the lower leg[13] and knee,[16] respectively. In the first patient, the infected lesion was in a pus-filled tract under a varicose ulcer traumatized by thorns of a raspberry bush; in the second patient, the infection was in a puncture wound made by a nail in a board in a farmyard. Both patients promptly recovered as the causative organisms were killed and as diffusion of the soluble toxin was stopped.

The microscopic control of MMS-fixed was useful in determining the depth of the tetanus lesions, but in the treatment of gangrene and osteomyelitis, the gross appearance of the abnormal tissue suffices to determine the level of amputation.

DEVELOPMENT OF THE FRESH TISSUE TECHNIQUE

From the beginning, I maintained that the unique and important feature of chemosurgery was the complete microscopic control of excision rather than the in situ chemical fixation.[17] For that reason I would have preferred the term *microsurgery,* but after the pioneering work of Alexis Carrel in the 1920s, the term was used to designate dissection of minute structures under the microscope. Therefore, my associates and I thought another term was needed. Hence, the name *chemosurgery* was chosen because, at that time, the tissues were being chemically fixed in situ prior to excision. As we had hoped, the term eventually came to be synonymous with *microscopically controlled surgery.* Actually, even when the fixed tissue technique was being used for all cancers, there were situations where layers were removed without in situ fixation. For example, if the cartilages of the helix of the ear or the nasal ala were being closely approached, the final layer was excised in the fresh, unfixed state in order to avoid an unsightly defect from the loss of cartilaginous framework.

The impetus for wider use of the fresh tissue technique came in a circuitous way. In 1951, when R. R. Allington, M.D., returned for his second period of training with me, he demonstrated his technique for excising or curetting the bulk of the cancer and then achieving prompt hemostasis by wiping off the blood with a cotton-tipped applicator and quickly following with an applicator soaked in dichloroacetic acid. I previously had occasionally used a debulking procedure, but the time lost securing hemostasis often didn't justify the procedure. His innovation was immediately adopted, and in 1953, I began to make movies of the procedure. During removal of a pigmented basal cell carcinoma on a lower eyelid, I removed the main mass and then applied dichloroacetic acid and the zinc chloride fixative for removal with the fixed tissue technique. However, because a silent outgrowth extending laterally on the lid margin was holding up the filming, I injected a local anesthetic and excised the next two layers with the fresh tissue technique. It worked so well that thereafter I used the fresh tissue technique for most eyelid cancers and for some small- or medium-sized cancers elsewhere. Later in 1953, a basal cell carcinoma on the lower eyelid and adjacent cheek was removed with the fresh tissue technique, and sutures were placed but not tied until the sections were examined. The scar was invisible, and there was no recurrence in 10 year.

The fresh tissue technique was described and illustrated in my chapter in Epstein's first edition of *Skin Surgery*[18] in 1956 and in 10 articles during the following decade, but there seemed to be reticence among others in the field to omit the in situ fixation. At a San Francisco meeting hosted by plastic surgeon Richard Shepard, M.D., and dermatologist Theodore Tromovitch, M.D., along with 12 chemosurgeons from the Bay area, I asked if any had tried the fresh tissue technique. None said they had, although several had employed Allington's debulking procedure.

At the 1969 meeting of the American College of Chemosurgery, I reported the use of the fresh tissue technique for 66 basal cell carcinomas (14 indeterminate) and four squamous cell carcinomas (one indeterminate) of the eyelid with five-year cure rates of 100% for both. These results were reported in the Bulletin of the American College of Chemosurgery.[19]

COMPARISON OF FRESH AND FIXED TISSUE TECHNIQUES

Acceleration of interest in the fresh tissue technique began in 1970. In October, a paper on chemosurgery for periorbital cancer by Robins, Henkind, and Menn was presented at the annual meeting of the American Academy of Ophthalmology and Otolaryngology.[20] Henry Menn described my results with the 70 patients treated with the fresh tissue technique, and I discussed the subject on invitation by the program chairman. In December, Theodore Tromovitch, M.D., presented a significant series of 75 patients treated with the fresh tissue technique at the annual meeting of the American College of Chemosurgery. At that time, I had treated 127 patients with the fresh tissue technique (103 periorbital and 24 other sites). With the evident interest of other chemosurgeons, I decided it was time to initiate a large series of patients treated with the fresh tissue technique to delineate the indications and limitations for the method and to determine whether the five-year cure rates would be as high as with the fixed tissue technique.

Preliminary reports (not five-year end results) for basal cell carcinoma (BCC) by Tromovitch and Stegman in 1974 indicated successful results in 99 of 102 patients (97%),[21] and by me in 1976 indicated successful results in 3,450 of 3,466 patients (99.8%).[22] Presently, after many thousands of patients have been treated with the Mohs micrographic surgery, fresh tissue technique (MMS-fresh), there is no doubt that the five-year end results are essentially the same for the fixed and fresh techniques. Therefore, MMS-fresh now is used for most BCCs and squamous cell carcinomas (SCCs), but as pointed out above, MMS-fixed is usually preferred for melanoma,[23] extensive cancers involving bone, and carcinomas invading the penile erectile tissue.

The reliability of MMS for BCC is well established. An extensive analysis of the recurrence rates with the various therapeutic modalities for both primary (previously untreated) BCCs[24] and recurrent (previously treated) BCCs by Rowe, Carroll, and Day[25] show strikingly lower recurrence rates with MMS as compared with surgical excision, radiotherapy, cryosurgery, or electrodesiccation and curettage (Table 1–2). Comparisons could be made for SCC if a similarly careful search of the literature were made for that neoplasm.

WOUND REPAIRS

Immediate repairs following MMS-fresh includes simple closures,[26] partial closures,[27] use of guiding sutures to prevent deformities,[28,29] and a wide variety of flaps and grafts.[30] Many of the repairs are done by micrographic surgeons, but for the more complicated repairs, the services of plastic surgeons, head and neck surgeons, oculoplastic surgeons, and microsurgeons are often employed. Healing by second intention is still a much used option, especially

TABLE 1–2. Comparison of Five-Year Recurrence Rates with Various Treatment Modalities

	Primary Basal Cell Carcinoma	Recurrent Basal Cell Carcinoma
Mohs micrographic surgery	1.0%	5.6%
Surgical excisions	10.1%	17.4%
Radiotherapy	8.7%	9.8%
Cryosurgery	7.5%	13.0%*
Electrodesiccation and curettage	7.7%	40.0%

*Less than five years—no statistics for five-year follow-up of cryosurgery cases.

when the cancer has recurred after previous therapy and there is a chance for outlying, noncontiguous foci that might be disseminated during undermining to permit closure or might be concealed for a long time under grafts or flaps.[23,29,30]

ORGANIZATION AND ACCREDITATION

Forming an organization for our specialty was first considered during the aforementioned meeting with 12 chemosurgeons in San Francisco. We decided that our numbers were sufficient to justify looking into the proposal. The American Medical Association had no objection, and a planning session was held at the 1967 meeting of the International Congress of Dermatology in Munich. In attendance were dermatologists William Bush, Roger Laubenheimer, Roy Leeper, Perry Robins, George Vavruska, and myself. Dr. Vavruska of Montreal was especially helpful in drawing up the constitution, and he convinced us that *American* rather than *International* in the name was preferable because national organizations tend to be more successful. The first annual meeting of the American College of Chemosurgery was held in 1967 before the December meeting of the American Academy of Dermatology in Chicago, with 23 chemosurgeons in attendance. Because of the advent of the fresh tissue technique, the name was changed in 1986 to the American College of Mohs Micrographic Surgery and Cutaneous Oncology. *Micro* indicated the use of the microscope, *graphic* the drawings of maps, and *Mohs* was voted to avoid ambiguity as to how the procedure is carried out. Cutaneous oncology was added to express our interest in oncology as it pertains to the skin. The initials are not an acronym, but this may be an advantage because one has to think of each word in order to remember ACMMSCO.

Accreditation for the first several years of the American College of Chemosurgery was quite informal because to join and maintain membership one had only to provide evidence of persistent activity in the specialty by submitting a list of cancers that had been excised. Now we have a Fellowship Training Committee and rules to ensure at least a year of training in the method. I have always maintained that one should resolve to go into the specialty seriously and not just dabble in it, but I hope restrictions will not be so stringent that otolaryngologists, head and neck surgeons, oculoplastic surgeons, plastic surgeons, and other surgical specialists will be discouraged from being involved in the field. I think we can all learn from each other, and this would be to the benefit of our patients.

INTERSPECIALTY INTEREST

Dermatologists' interest in MMS was inevitable because most of its indications are for skin cancer. I originally thought surgeons would be most interested. Therefore, my first five clinical articles on the method and its use for cancers of the skin, lip, nose, and ear, and for gangrene were published in surgical journals. About 50 surgeons expressed interest over the years, but only six entered the field sufficiently to have articles published describing their work.[31–37] Dermatologists, on the other hand, came in hundreds as visitors, observers, or trainees for periods up to a year, and their publications in dermatologic journals were so numerous that they cannot be listed here. Following my one-hour special lecture at the 1946 meeting of the American Academy of Dermatology, the publication of an article in the *Archives of Dermatology*[38] and, particularly, the presentation of a lecture to the Dermatology Section of the California Medical Association in 1948,[39] I was convinced that the most enthusiastic interest would be among dermatologists.

Being a skin disease, skin cancers usually are seen first by dermatologists who are familiar with their clinical and microscopic appearance and the differential diagnosis from similar appearing noncancerous lesions. Moreover, from their experience with treatments lacking total microscopic control of excision, they realize that, despite the sacrifice of a margin of normal-appearing tissue, there is a substantial number of recurrences, especially with cancers that have already recurred after previous treatment.[40]

I think William Middleton, M.D., internist and dean of the University of Wisconsin School of Medicine, was more perceptive than I when he suggested that I begin the clinical trial in the dermatology division of internal medicine. I spent four years with Otto Foerster, M.D., who came from Milwaukee once a week as Chairman of Dermatology, and with Roscoe McIntosh, M.D., who managed the daily operation of the dermatology clinic from 1936 to 1940. Both promptly recognized the value of the microscopic control in following the silent outgrowths that skin cancers frequently exhibit. This value was strikingly demonstrated by models of cancers made by a medical student whose doctoral thesis led to an article on the modes of spread of skin cancer.[41]

When Dr. McIntosh died in 1940, Dr. Erwin Schmidt, Chief of Surgery, invited me to transfer to the surgery department where more spacious facilities were available. This turned out to be a wise move. I had firm support from the various surgical specialists and worked closely with Dr. Schmidt for many years. He wrote a wonderfully perceptive foreword to my first clinical article.[42] The plastic surgeons did many complicated repairs after I removed far advanced, recurrent cancers, of which there was a tremendous backlog. Close cooperation with our chief otolaryngologist, Wellwood Nesbit, M.D., demonstrated the potential of the method in the treatment of laryngeal cancer, for which the tissue-sparing advantage and the reliability of the procedure were demonstrated in eight cases.[9,13] Also, the treatment of oral cancers with microscopic control permitted saving of a strut of mandible in cases in which "commando" surgery would have resulted in a total hemimandibulectomy. Parotid carcinoma also could be removed safely at a relatively conservative level, as demonstrated by my first case of a carcinoma that was considered inoperable by four midwest specialists; it was removed without facial paralysis and the doctor-patient is still living over 50 years later.[43,44] Carcinoma of the maxillary sinus also proved to be amenable,[13] as did cancers of the lips.[45,46] Cooperation with gynecology for vulvar carcinomas[13] and extramammary Paget's disease[47] demonstrated excellent results. Cooperation with an oculoplastic surgeon, Richard Dorzbach, M.D., on difficult periorbital cancers was mutually helpful.[48–50] Urology consultation during treatment of patients with carcinomas of the penis was beneficial.[10] Neurosurgical consultation can be helpful when extensive intranasal cancers extend through the cribriform plate into the cranial cavity. Avoidance of possible dangerous consequences by the neurosurgeon placing a flap of temporal fascia and muscle under the dura to protect the cerebrum was successful in a case of Mikhail's.[51] I have had instances of cancerous invasion of the frontal lobe, with problems of cerebral protrusion because of increased intracranial pressure. The use of intravenous urea, as developed by our chief neurosurgeon, Manucher Javid, M.D., was a welcome innovation that could prevent this complication.[9,52]

MMS involves the spheres of so many specialists that close, cordial interspecialty cooperation is essential. The interchange between micrographic surgeons and other surgical specialists should be a two-way street. Probably one reason why otolaryngologists, plastic surgeons, oculoplastic surgeons, and general surgeons have not progressed as well as dermatologists in MMS has been their unwillingness to insist on having their own facilities for preparing and examining the frozen sections. They are used to sending their specimens to the pathology laboratory for processing and examination. With a few notable exceptions, pathologists do not exactly follow our precepts of how to cut and examine the specimens, and the surgeons often do not appreciate the need to remove and precisely mark the origin of each specimen on the lesion and on a map.

Mohs micrographic surgery is a developing field in which there are opportunities for technical improvement and for extension of the total microscopic control to the management of diseases that have previously been explored inadequately or not at all. These challenges are what make MMS an exciting specialty for those with a pioneering spirit. One such person

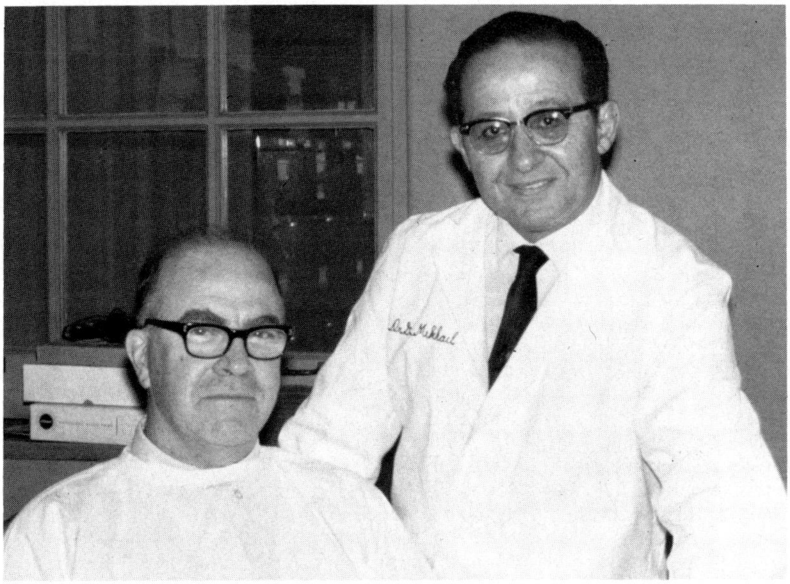

FIGURE 1–1. F. E. Mohs with his trainee George Mikhail in 1968.

is our editor, George Mikhail, M.D., who was standing by me when he was a trainee 21 years ago (Fig. 1–1).

REFERENCES

1. Mohs FE, Guyer MF: Pre-excisional fixation of tissues in the treatment of cancer in rats. Cancer Res 1:49–51, 1941.
2. Caquoin C: cited in Wolff J: Die Lehre von der Krebskrankheit. Jena: Fischer 3:107, 1913.
3. Bougard C: cited in Wolff J: Die Lehre von der Krebskrankheit. Jena: Fischer 3:107, 1913.
4. Mohs FE: The preparation of frozen sections for use in the chemosurgical technique for the microscopically controlled excision of cancer. J Lab Clinic Med, 33:392, 1948.
5. Mohs FE: Microscopically controlled surgery for periorbital melanoma: Fixed-tissue and fresh-tissue techniques. J Dermatol Surg Oncol 11:284–291, 1985.
6. Mohs FE: Fixed-tissue micrographic surgery for melanoma of the ear. Arch Otolaryngol Head Neck Surg 114:625–631, 1988.
7. Mohs FE: Mohs micrographic surgery fixed-tissue technique for melanoma of the nose. J Dermatol Surg Oncol 16:1111–1120, 1990.
8. Mohs FE: Chemosurgery for melanoma. Arch Dermatol 113:285–291, 1977.
9. Mohs FE: Chemosurgery: Microscopically Controlled Surgery for Skin Cancer. Springfield, IL: Charles C Thomas, 1978.
10. Mohs FE, Snow SN, Messing EM, Kuglitch ME: Microscopically controlled surgery in the treatment of carcinoma of the penis. J Urol 133:961–966, 1985.
11. Hruza GJ, Snow SN: Basal cell carcinoma in a patient with acquired immunodeficiency syndrome: Treatment with Mohs micrographic surgery fixed-tissue technique. J Dermatol Surg Oncol 15:545–551, 1989.
12. Mohs FE, Severinghaus EL, Schmidt ER: Conservative amputation of gangrenous parts by chemosurgery. Ann Surg 114:172–281, 1941.
13. Mohs FE: Chemosurgery in Cancer, Gangrene and Infections; Featuring a New Method for the Microscopically Controlled Excision of Cancer. Springfield, IL: Charles C Thomas, 1956.
14. Mohs FE: Chemosurgical amputation for gangrene. Surgery 57:247–253, 1963.
15. Bennett RG, Goldman MP: Chemosurgical debridement of osteomyelitic bone by zinc chloride fixative. J Dermatol Surg Oncol 13:771–775, 1987.
16. Davila de Pedro R, Mohs FE: Extirpation of a nidus of infection with tetanus bacilli by chemosurgery. J Dermatol Surg Oncol 7:629–631, 1981.
17. Mohs FE: Chemosurgery, a microscopically controlled method of cancer excision. Arch Surg 42:279–295, 1941.
18. Mohs FE: The chemosurgical method for the microscopically controlled excision of cutaneous cancer. In Epstein E (ed): Skin Surgery. Philadelphia: Lea & Febiger, 1956.
19. Mohs FE: Cancer of eyelids. Bull Am Col Chemosurgery 3:10–11, 1970.
20. Robins P, Henkind P, Menn H: Chemosurgery in treatment of cancers of the periorbital area. Trans Am Acad Ophthalmol Otolaryngol 70:1,228–1,235, 1971.
21. Tromovitch TA, Stegman SJ: Microscopically controlled excision of skin tumors: Chemosurgery (Mohs) fresh tissue technique. Arch Dermatol 110:231–232, 1974.
22. Mohs FE: Chemosurgery for skin cancer. Fixed tissue and fresh tissue techniques. Arch Dermatol 112:211–215, 1976.
23. Mohs FE: The width and depth of the spread of melanoma as observed by a chemosurgeon. Am J Dermatopathol (suppl) 6:123–126, 1984.
24. Rowe DE, Carroll RJ, Day CL: Long-term recurrence

rates in previously untreated (primary) basal cell carcinoma: Implications for patient follow-up. J Dermatol Surg Oncol 15:315–328, 1989.
25. Rowe DE, Carroll RJ, Day CL: Mohs surgery is the treatment of choice for recurrent (previously treated) basal cell carcinoma. J Dermatol Surg Oncol 15:424–431, 1989.
26. Mohs FE: Chemosurgery. In Mandel MA (ed): Clinics in Plastic Surgery. Philadelphia: W. B. Saunders, 1980.
27. Lang PG: The partial closure. J Dermatol Surg Oncol 11:966–969, 1985.
28. Albright SD: Surgical gem: Placement of "guiding sutures" to counteract undesirable retraction of tissues in and around functionally and cosmetically important structures. J Dermatol Surg Oncol 7:446–449, 1981.
29. Mohs FE: Chemosurgery: Microscopically controlled surgery for skin cancer—past, present and future. J Dermatol Surg Oncol 4:41–54, 1978.
30. Mohs FE: Micrographically controlled surgery for skin cancer. In Stark RB (ed): Plastic Surgery of the Head and Neck. New York, Churchill Livingstone, 1986.
31. Szujewski HA: Microscopic guidance in the treatment of skin cancer. Plast Reconstr Surgery 5:524–531, 1950.
32. Phelan JT, Milgrom H: The use of Mohs chemosurgery technique in the treatment of skin cancers. Surg Gynecol Obstet 125:549–560, 1967.
33. Phelan JT: The use of the Mohs chemosurgery technique in the treatment of basal cell carcinoma. Ann Surg 168:1,023–1,029, 1968.
34. Shepard RA, Wood DA: Chemosurgery. Stanford Med Bull 8:193–201, 1950.
35. Shepard RA: Chemosurgery in the treatment of carcinoma of the skin. J Int Col Surg 30:220–228, 1958.
36. Moles JB, Ghosh BC: Chemosurgery for basal cell carcinoma. JAMA 210:1,959–1,961, 1969.
37. Benteen FH, Arminosco JA, Fredell CH, Blau MH, Eisenstein MW: Is chemosurgery advisable for superficial skin cancers of the face? Modern Med 30:16–22, 1969.
38. Mohs FE: Chemosurgical treatment of carcinoma of the face. Arch Dermatol 56:143–156, 1947.
39. Mohs FE: Chemosurgery in cutaneous malignancy. Calif Med 71:173–176, 1949.
40. Menn H, Robins P, Kopf A, Bart R: The recurrent basal cell carcinomas. Arch Dermatol 103:628–631, 1971.
41. Mohs FE, Lathrop TG: Modes of spread of cancer of skin. Arch Dermatol 66:427–439, 1952.
42. Mohs FE: Chemosurgery, a microscopically controlled method of cancer excision. Arch Surg 42:279–295, 1941.
43. Mohs FE: Chemosurgical treatment of tumors of the parotid gland: A microscopically controlled method of excision. Ann Surg 129:381–393, 1949.
44. Mohs FE: The chemosurgical treatment of tumors of the parotid gland. A microscopically controlled method of excision. Acta Union Internat Contre Cancer 9:105–108, 1953.
45. Mohs FE: Chemosurgical treatment of cancer of the lip. A microscopically controlled method of excision. Arch Surg 48:478–488, 1944.
46. Mohs FE, Snow SN: Microscopically controlled surgical treatment for squamous cell carcinoma of the lower lip. Surg Gynecol Obstet 160:37–41, 1985.
47. Mohs FE, Blanchard L: Microscopically controlled surgery for extramammary Paget's disease. Arch Dermatol 115:706–708, 1979.
48. Mohs FE: Micrographic surgery for the microscopically controlled excision of eyelid cancers. Arch Ophthalmol 104:901–909, 1986.
49. Mohs FE: Micrographic surgery for the microscopically controlled excision of eyelid cancer: History and development. Adv Ophthal Plast Reconstruct Surg 5:381–408, 1986.
50. Mohs FE: Microscopically controlled excision of medial canthal carcinoma. Ann Plast Surg 7:308–311, 1981.
51. Mikhail GR, Roushdy SB, Knighton RS, et al: Cranial invasion by basal cell carcinoma. J Dermatol Surg Oncol 12:459–464, 1986.
52. Javid M: Urea in intracranial surgery. J Neurosurg 18:51–57, 1961.

CHAPTER 2

Techniques and Indications for Mohs Micrographic Surgery

Stephen N. Snow, M.D.

In the mid-1930s, Frederic E. Mohs developed a new type of excisional surgery that used the microscope to determine the complete margin of skin cancers in three dimensions.[1,2] The original term "Mohs chemosurgery" was officially changed in 1985 to "Mohs micrographic surgery." The *micro* is from microscope, and *graph* refers to a layer-by-layer pictorial representation of the tumor configuration (Fig. 2–1).

Micrographic surgery is based on the observation that skin cancers often grow contiguously (Fig. 2–2A) and send out microscopic tentacles of tumor cells for considerable distance beyond the clinically visible and palpable margins of the neoplasm (Fig. 2–2). By excising the tissue layer by layer and by examining the entire deep surface of each layer under the microscope, the tumor can be followed to its termination. The construction of a map or graph to guide surgery allows these silent outgrowths to be accurately located and selectively excised (Fig. 2–3). This method provides substantial assurance of eradicating the cancer while obviating the need to remove arbitrarily a wide margin of normal tissue. Micrographic surgery is therefore particularly useful for managing facial skin cancers, where the preservation of as much normal tissue as possible is important for maintaining the functional and esthetic integrity of facial structures. Except for very large cancers, micrographic surgery is usually performed on an outpatient basis with a local anesthetic.[3–11]

Traditional methods of determining tumor margins include a clinical assessment of the lesion and a microscopic examination of vertical

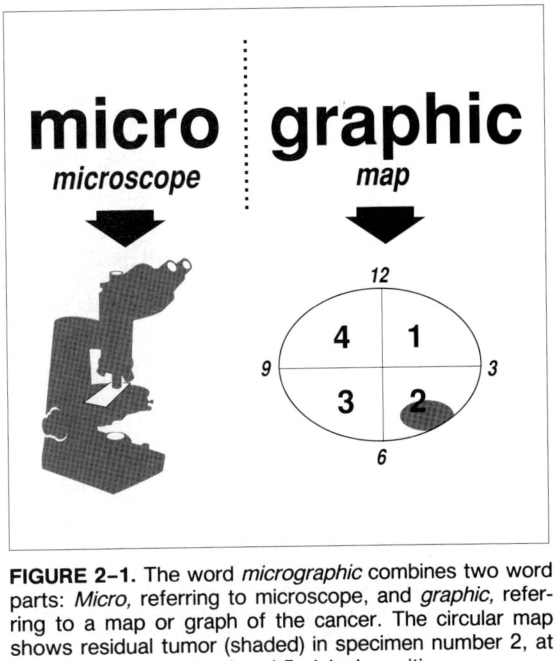

FIGURE 2–1. The word *micrographic* combines two word parts: *Micro,* referring to microscope, and *graphic,* referring to a map or graph of the cancer. The circular map shows residual tumor (shaded) in specimen number 2, at the edge between the 4 and 5 o'clock positions.

I thank Betsy True for her illustrations, Amy Hatfield for word processing, William Welch for medical editing, and Eric Alvin for photographic reproductions.

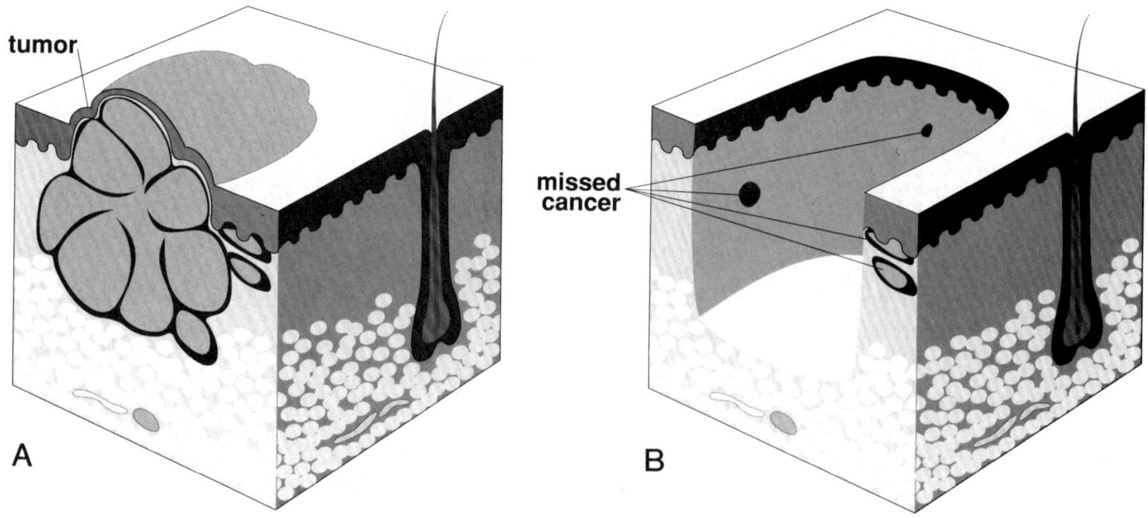

FIGURE 2–2. *A,* Skin cancer may be likened to an iceberg; there is often more tumor below the skin than there is above it. *B,* Traditional surgery may not always completely remove the tumor.

frozen sections of excised tissue. If a tumor is well localized, a 2 mm margin is generally recommended, especially if the tumor is near a vital facial structure. But Burg and colleagues[12] showed that, even for clinically well-localized basal cell carcinomas, an average margin of 5 mm is necessary to eradicate the cancer. With morphea-like cancers and lesions greater than

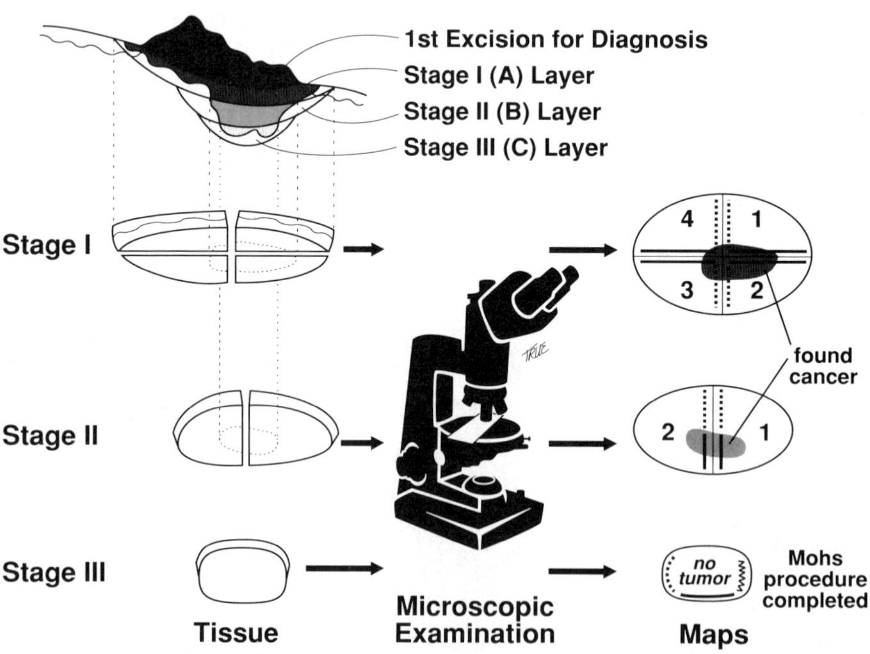

FIGURE 2–3. This schematic illustrates how the Mohs technique assures complete tumor removal. Obvious cancer (black) is obtained for diagnosis (upper left). Cancer visible only by microscopic examination is outlined by dots in each layer. In Stage I, a layer was removed and divided into four specimens (as viewed from the bottom); after microscopic examination, residual tumor was found only in the central area of all four specimens. In Stage II, a central layer was excised and bisected; after microscopic examination, residual tumor was found only in the center of specimens 1 and 2. In Stage III, another small block specimen was removed; after microscopic examination no residual tumor was found. In this case, the Mohs procedure consisted of three stages of excision and the microscopic examination of seven specimens.

2 cm in diameter, an average normal tissue margin of 9 to 10 mm is needed to completely remove the cancer. Using arbitrary surgical margins erroneously assumes that tumor growth is symmetrical in all directions and for all cancers, regardless of whether or not they have been treated previously.

Conventional microscopic methods of examining the excisional margins have also proved inaccurate. Two examples are the bread-loaf method (Fig. 2–4A) and the quadrant method[13–15] (Fig. 2–4B). Both of these methods rely on an examination of vertical sections taken at random intervals. When a tissue sample is microscopically seen to have clear margins, the standard assumption is that the entire margin from which the sample was taken is also tumor-free. The failure of these methods to identify residual tumor between the sampled areas is often responsible for local recurrence despite a pathology report indicating clear margins.

With Mohs surgery (Fig. 2–4C & D), 100% of tumor margins are microscopically examined, in contrast to the 0.01% examined with standard excisional and histologic methods.[16] The Mohs technique is also an improved method of tissue sampling. The five-year cure rate for primary cancers treated by Mohs surgery is greater than 99%,[17] compared with 93% for tumors treated by conventional surgical excision. For recurrent cancers, Mohs surgery provides a greater than 95% cure rate, compared with 80% for all other methods.[18]

Mohs micrographic surgery can maximize the effectiveness of an operation, minimize the removal of normal tissue, and deliver safe and reasonably cost-effective care for patients with skin cancer. In principle, Mohs surgery can be divided into four phases: (a) the saucerized sur-

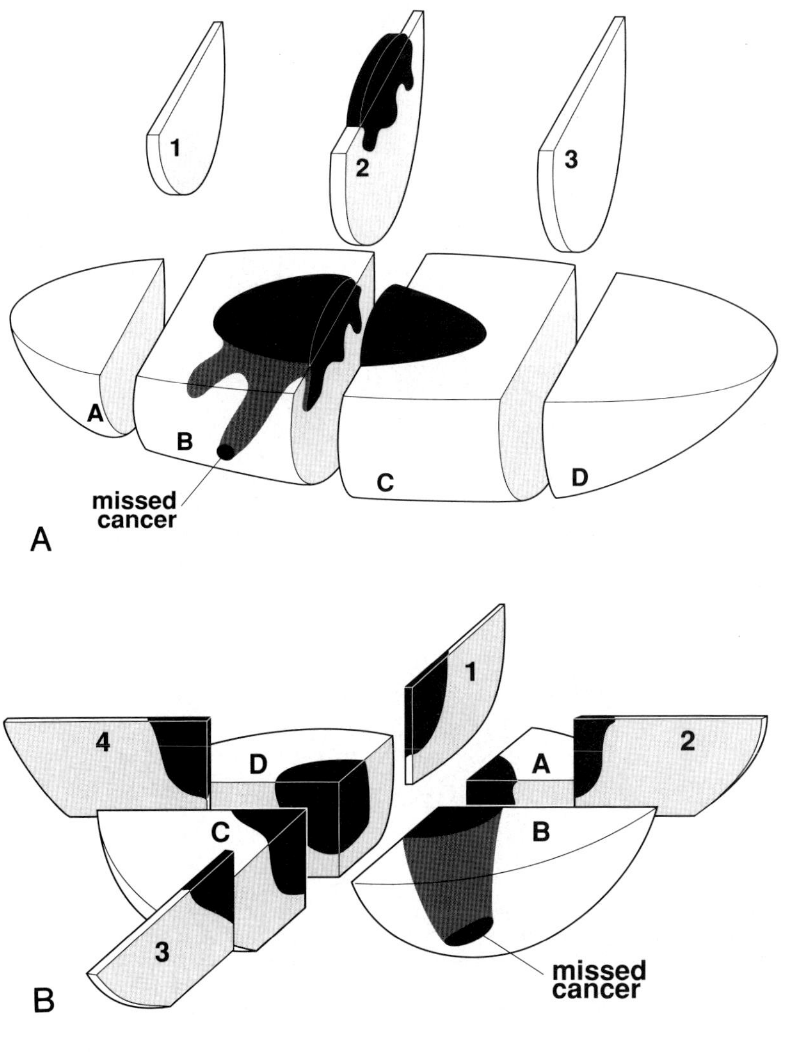

FIGURE 2–4. *A*, Bread-loaf sections for checking tissue margins: In this method, vertical sections 1, 2, and 3 were taken from the middle and at both ends of tissue blocks (A, B, C, and D). All three sections appeared clear of tumor; however, there was residual cancer in block B that was missed and may recur. *B*, Four-quadrant sections: In this method, vertical section numbers 1 to 4 were taken from the 3, 6, 9, and 12 o'clock positions. All four sections were clear of tumor; however, there was residual cancer in block B that was not found and may recur. *Illustration continued on following page*

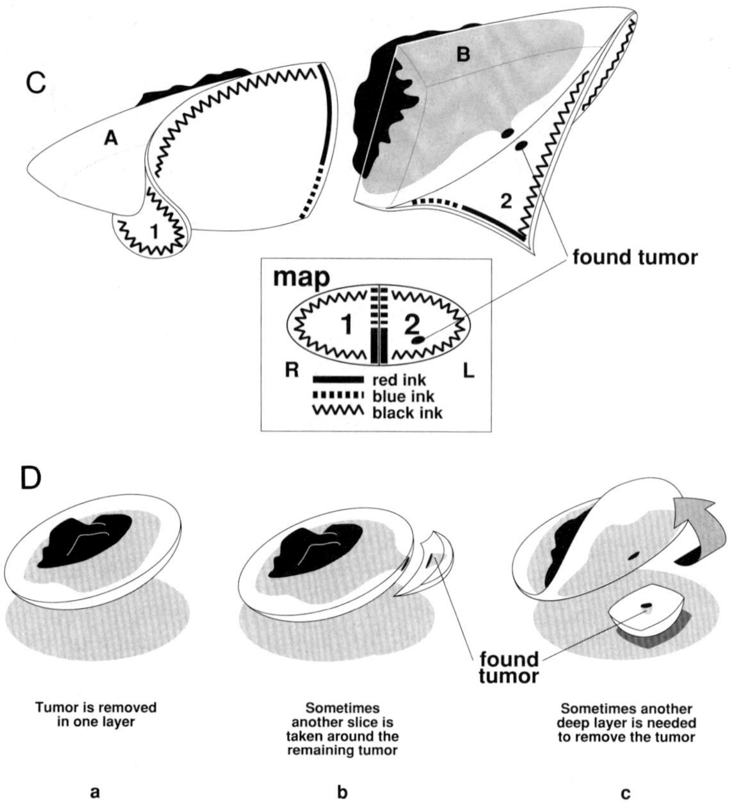

FIGURE 2–4. *Continued C*, Mohs sections: In this method, horizontal sections were taken from the bottom surface and sides of each tissue block. Cancer was found toward the center of specimen number 2. *D*, Schematic showing how Mohs surgery finds superficial and deep cancers. The size of the excised layer is tailored to the size of the residual tumor focus. Frequently, the tumor is removed in the first layer (a). Sometimes it is necessary to take a wider margin to remove the tumor (black *in* (b). Sometimes it is necessary to take a deeper layer to remove the tumor (c).

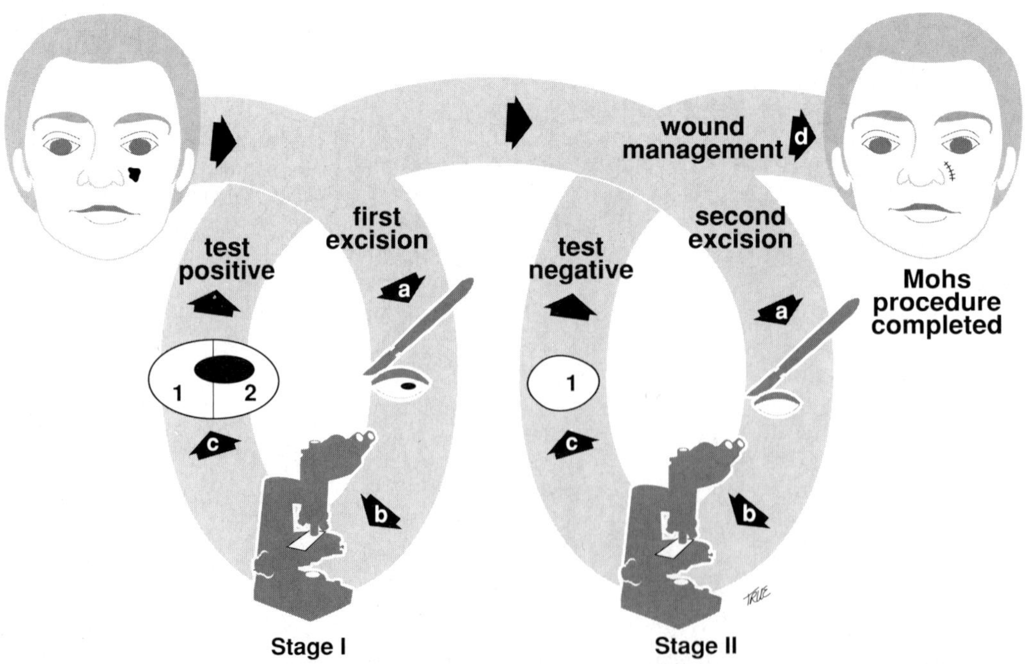

FIGURE 2–5. This schematic illustrates the cyclic nature of Mohs surgery. The four main components are the excision of a disc of tissue (a), microscopic examination (b), the appropriate marking of the map when residual cancer is found (c), and wound management (d). In Stage I, the tumor was removed, examined with the microscope. Some residual tumor (black) was found mostly in specimen number 2. In Stage II, a deeper layer was removed and examined microscopically. In the second layer, no remaining cancer could be found. The defect was then closed with stitches (d).

gical excision of a disc of tissue, (b) the microscopic examination of frozen sections, (c) mapping or graphing of found tumor, and (d) wound management (Fig. 2–5). In practice, Mohs surgery provides a logical method of tumor excision and wound management that optimizes healing and esthetic results while not compromising the early recognition of tumor in difficult or recurrent cancers.

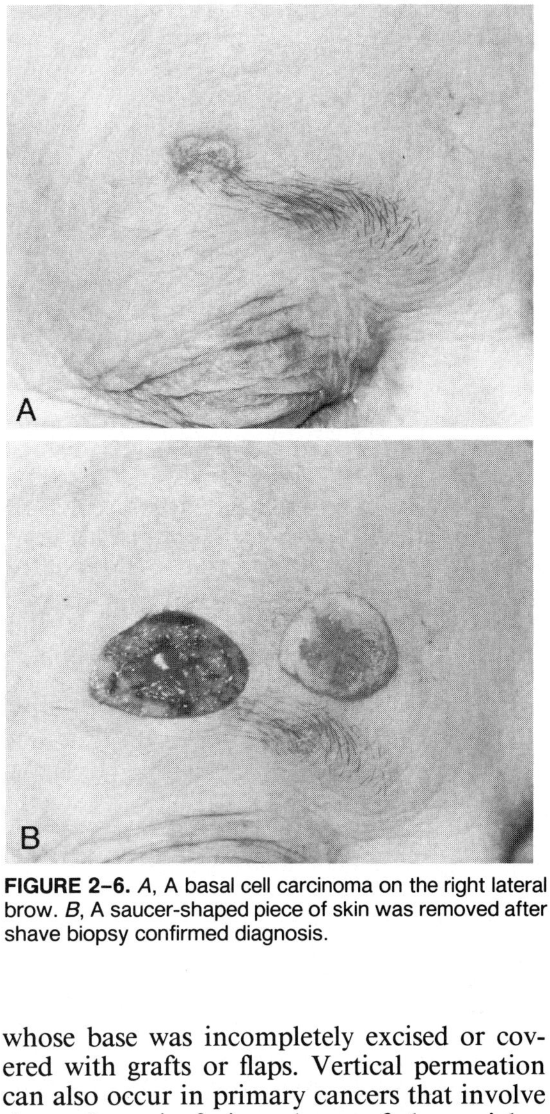

FIGURE 2–6. *A*, A basal cell carcinoma on the right lateral brow. *B*, A saucer-shaped piece of skin was removed after shave biopsy confirmed diagnosis.

TECHNIQUES IN MOHS SURGERY

Saucerized Excision of a Disc of Tissue

A skin cancer is removed in a series of layers, one layer at a time. The first layer, a saucer-shaped specimen removed by debulking, permits microscopic diagnosis; it also reduces the number of layers needed to reach a tumor-free plane. Depending on the location and size of the original tumor, the margin and thickness of the surgical layer vary from 2 to 4 mm. On a patient's face, where most skin cancers occur, thin layers are removed to conserve as much tissue as possible and to preserve the functional and esthetic integrity of the eyelids, nose, lips, and ears (Fig. 2–6). Saucer-shaped specimens naturally have beveled edges; this shape permits the cryostat operator to flatten the specimen so that its bottom and all its margins can be sliced as a single unit and examined in the same plane under the microscope.

Mohs surgery incorporates a technique by which the horizontal (radial) and vertical growth patterns of skin cancers are delineated, recorded, and statistically evaluated. The preoperative and postoperative dimensions of the tumor help evaluate the accuracy of assessing clinical surface margins, and a microscopic examination of the tumor base defines the depth of invasion. The number of stages of excision reflects the number of individual horizontal layers that must be excised and microscopically examined to reach a tumor-free plane. These stages can be divided into predominantly vertical and horizontal stages as a function of the overall direction of tumor extension. Most skin cancers can be completely treated after the first layer is removed; others may require that additional deeper or wider layers be removed (Fig. 2–4D). Deep, vertical penetration signals the possibly serious involvement of nerves, vessels, glands, cartilage, or bone. Vertical invasion most often occurs in recurrent tumors whose base was incompletely excised or covered with grafts or flaps. Vertical permeation can also occur in primary cancers that involve the embryonic fusion planes of the perialar, preauricular, and postauricular areas. Horizontal spread suggests less aggressive tumor behavior, except when the tumor involves the eyelids, cornea, lips, nose, or ear. Horizontal growth most often occurs in tumors on the trunk and the extremities where the thick dermis impedes tumor penetration. In reality, most tumors spread in three dimensions, and complete excision signifies the removal of both vertical and horizontal components.

The Excised Tissue Layer

The histographic and pathologic processing of tissue for micrographic surgery begins with the division of the excised layer into smaller units that allow the entire deep surface to be easily and completely sectioned with the microtome. Usually, the exact orientation of the layer relative to anatomic landmarks of the face is mapped before the tissue is divided. A Polaroid photograph can be useful for orienting specimens from large or complex tumors.[19] Other steps to maintain specimen orientation include color-coding (inking) the specimen edges and drawing a map of the defect with the numeric origin of each specimen.

Division of Excised Tissue Layer

Immediately after a thin layer of tissue is excised, it is divided for frozen section processing (Fig. 2–7A). Subunits of the tissue also can be created during the excision by using skin nicks to mark the origin of the cut edges (see Fig. 2–36). The division of the tissue into subunits serves two purposes: (1) it makes the size of the specimen suitable for mounting on the cryostat object disc and the histology slide (Fig. 2–7E), and (2) it allows the specimen to be appropriately flattened so the lateral and deep margins can be sectioned in the same plane (Fig. 2–7G & H).

The number of specimens is the number of tissue subunits whose undersurfaces are microscopically examined in search of a tumor-free plane. This number is usually directly proportional to the degree of complexity of the overall excision and the degree of horizontal and vertical penetration of the tumor.

The size of individual specimens ranges from 0.5 to 1.5 cm. Ideally, a specimen should easily fit on the cryostat object disc. Cartilaginous or spherical tissue that is variously convex or concave cannot be uniformly flattened unless it is divided at the curvature apex, partially bisected at the top surface, or trimmed of cartilage before being processed. Similarly, specimens that contain large amounts of soft tissue, such as fat or muscle, necessitate disproportionately longer freezing times before they can be sectioned. Thin sections devoid of nicking, folding, and freezing artifacts are usually difficult to obtain if the temperatures of the microtome blade and the tissue significantly differ. Also, specimens of fibrotic scar tissue often contract unpredictably and thereby make it difficult to obtain a flat section of their undersurface. The tissue layer should be divided so that the fewest number of sections can be processed without compromising the ability of the histotechnician to obtain a complete horizontal section of each specimen. Sometimes a very small specimen disc may be sectioned without being subdivided.

Color-Coding Tissue Edges

The edges of thin specimens are marked with colored dyes (Fig. 2–7B to D). Three colors are readily available: red (20% merbromin in water), blue (concentrated laundry bluing, or soluble Prussian blue or ferrous ferrocyanide), and black (India ink). Often, however, only two colors (red and blue) are needed because the epidermal edge of the specimen can be identified by the presence of stratified squamous epithelium and hair follicles. If the specimen is rectangular, three margins are colored, with red used between (inferior or superior) the blue- and black-colored margins. The fourth unmarked edge also serves as a marker. By convention, the sequence of coloring is red, blue, and black. This sequence allows for corrections of mismarkings because blue can cover red, and black can cover both blue and red. Commercial products such as the Davidson Marking System (Bradley Products Inc. P.O. Box 201405, Bloomington, MN 55420) are also available.

The process of coloring the tissue margins is a little tricky for novices because the dyes tend to run into each other if not properly used. The skin edge of the tissue is grasped with forceps and the other edges are colored. The applicator is picked up and excess dye is absorbed with cotton gauze; holding the applicator upside down prevents dye from dripping. Both applicator and tissue specimen can be steadied by apposing the tips of the small fingers as the tissue edge is inked. After the margins of the specimen are colored, the specimen is placed right-side up on a saline-soaked gauze pad to prevent the bottom of the tissue from drying. Subsequent specimens are grasped, colored, and set on the gauze in numerical sequence until all of the specimens of that layer are marked. The entire tissue edge is colored, unless the specimen is so small that the dyes unavoidably bleed into one another. If the specimen is very small, only one edge is marked, or no marking is done at all. An alternative technique is to color all free edges of the tissue; this makes the edges more apparent when the technician and surgeon view the slide. Coloring all the edges is helpful during the training of new histotechnicians because it makes the terminal margin of the specimen apparent. The dyes stay on during tissue processing and can be easily seen

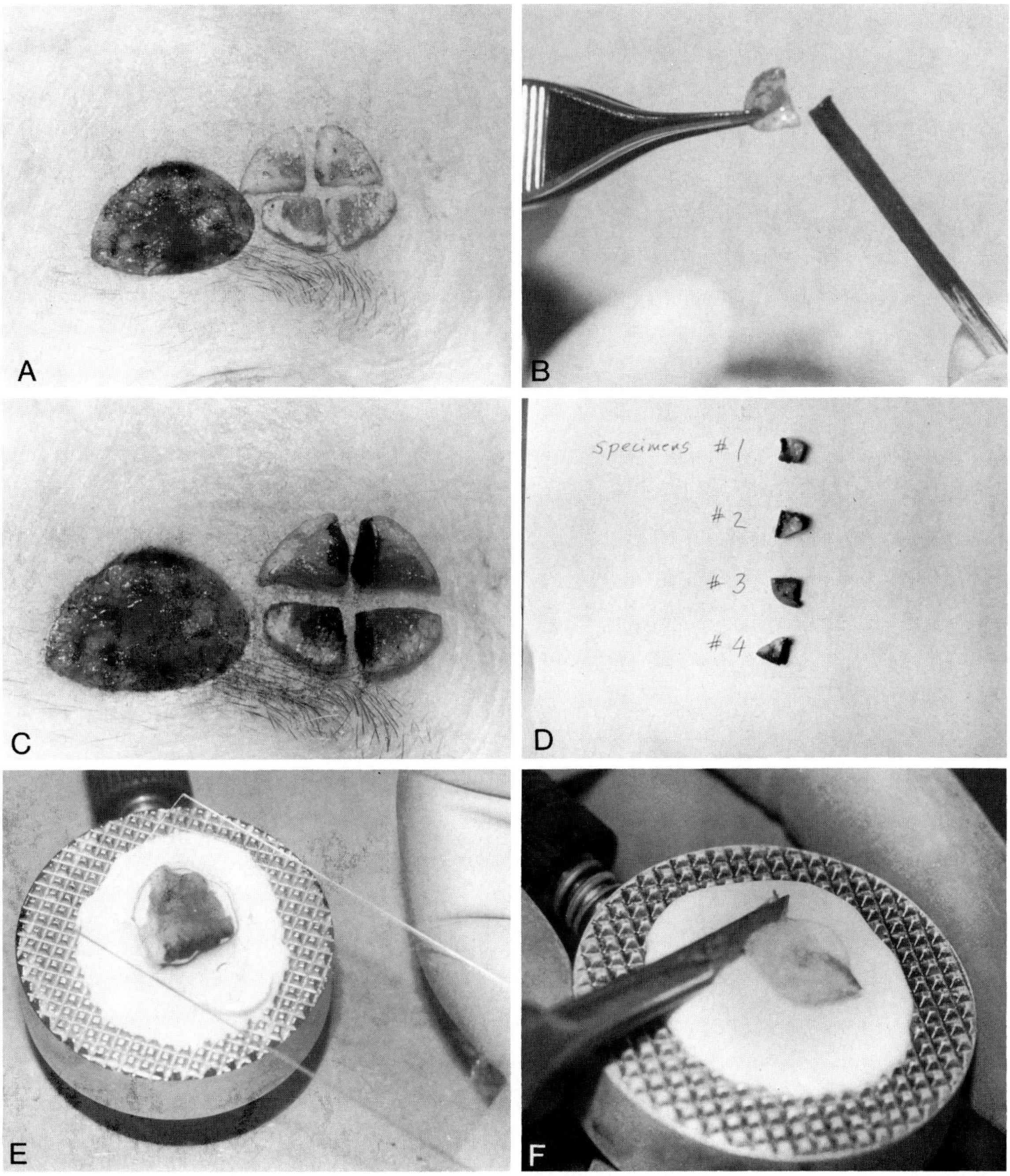

FIGURE 2–7. *A*, The disc of tissue was divided into quarters. *B*, The edge of each quarter piece was colored with a different color ink to show the different sides. *C*, The appearance of the specimens after they were colored and placed adjacent to the defect from which they were taken. *D*, Arrangement of the four specimens in the sequential order in which they will be processed. *E*, The deep surface of the tissue was prepared for sectioning. Using a glass slide, the tissue was mounted bottom-face-up in optimum cutting temperature (OCT) embedding compound (white). *F*, The scalpel was used to pry up the skin edge. The tissue was then reflattened so that the edges and bottom were at the same plane.

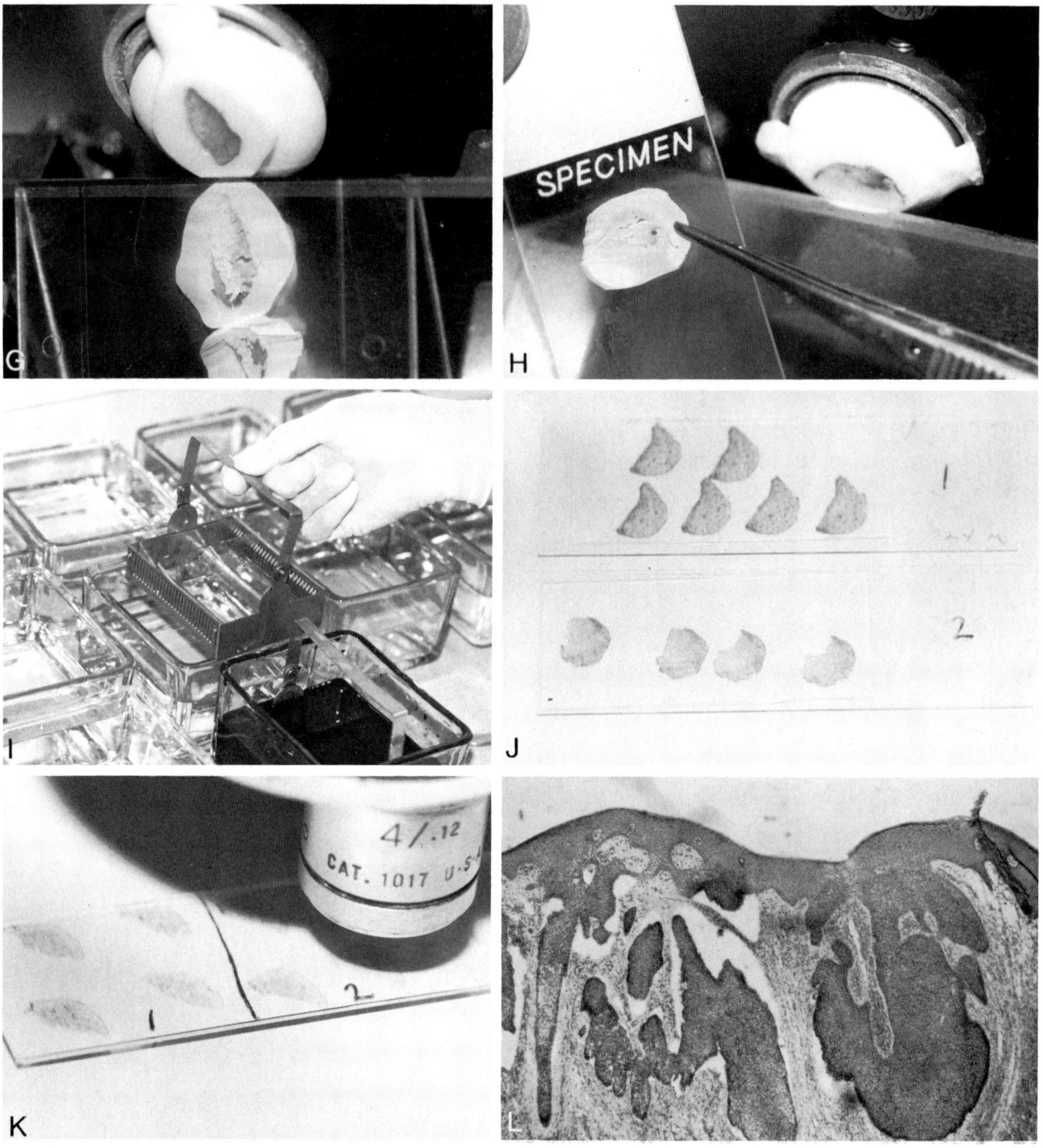

FIGURE 2–7. *Continued G*, Thin tissue sections were cut by the freezing microtome (cold knife). *H*, Individual sections were mounted onto a glass slide. *I*, The tissue slides were stained in hematoxylin and eosin. *J*, Stained tissue specimens as they appear before microscopic examination. Sometimes dark areas may be seen, which are suspected for cancer (see Fig. 2–8). *K*, Microscopic examination of the slide at 40× magnification. *L*, Microscopic appearance of typical basal cell carcinoma at the skin edge.

Illustration continued on following page

when the specimen is mounted on the cryostat specimen holder and in frozen sections before and after staining.

The dyes unavoidably blend into one another at the intersection of the colored edges, but this is of little consequence because the area of re-excision is often greater than the total area of intersection (1 to 2 mm). Care must be taken to avoid excessively coloring the edges more than 1 mm across the deep surface of the specimen. Excess ink may obscure tumor recognition. To the cryostat operator,

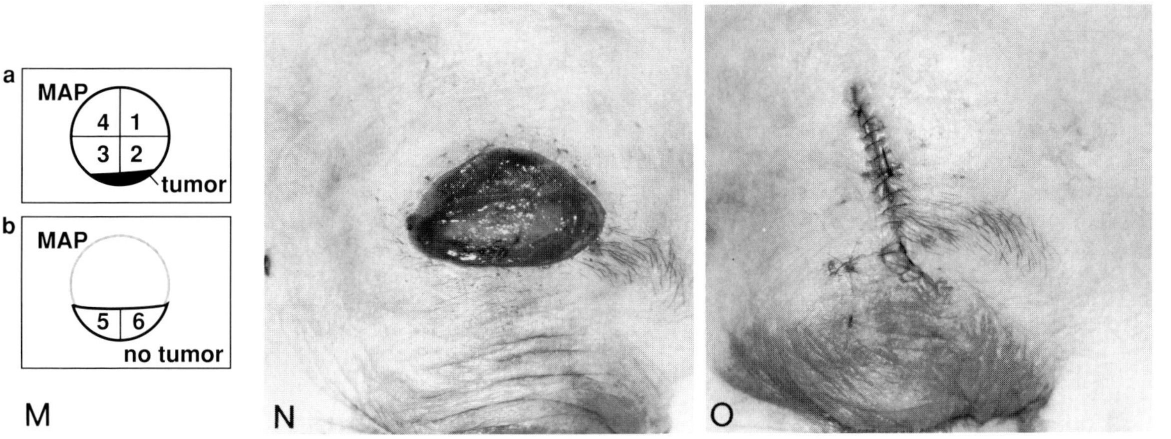

FIGURE 2–7. *Continued M,* Map indicating there was residual cancer found in specimen numbers 2 and 3 (a). The patient was recalled for re-excision of only the lower portion of the defect, represented by specimen numbers 5 and 6 (b). *N,* Appearance of midbrow defect after excision of specimen numbers 5 and 6. Microscopic examination of these specimens showed no residual tumor. The defect may now be repaired. *O,* Appearance of defect after O-to-T closure. Mohs treatment is now complete.

the colored edge also serves as the terminal margin of the tissue, and too much dye creates a pseudomargin. As a consequence, the technician cuts a smaller microsection extending to the pseudomargin but falsely thinks that the total bottom surface area of the specimen was sectioned. Any residual cancer at the real margin, beyond the pseudomargin, is missed. The appropriate size of the microsection can be double-checked by superimposing the stained final microsection on the map; the fit should be without significant defect. If all inked edges are identified microscopically, it is concluded that a complete section was obtained by the histotechnician.

The steps taken to ink the edges of specimens are summarized thus:

1. The anatomic orientation of the layer is maintained by holding the 12 o'clock position of the layer and matching it with the 12 o'clock top position of the gauze (usually marked with a red dot) on which it is placed. The top surface of the layer is faceup. The bottom surface of the layer is facedown against a firm surface on which the specimen is divided.
2. The layer is divided into halves or quadrants without disturbing the orientation of the individual subdivided specimens.
3. The specimens are picked up and inked one at a time in numeric order; the forceps in the nondominant hand determines the first specimen.
4. The right, left, and non-inked edges of each specimen are the patient's right, left, and cephalic directions and are determined before the specimen is picked up and inked.
5. As a recall aid, the relative position of the edges are made reliably consistent by using one's natural hand position and oneself as reference points as the specimen is grasped.
6. The specimen is held by the noncolored edge and the other edges are inked.
7. Red ink is used to color the first edge.
8. The edge is inked by holding the applicator upside-down.
9. The vertical side and bottom of each edge is inked. After the vertical side has been inked, the specimen is flipped over to check if the bottom edge has also been inked. When the tissue is flipped over, there is no mix-up in inking the correct edge because it has already been partially inked.
10. Steps 8 and 9 are repeated for each different color of ink; steps 4 to 9 are repeated for each specimen inked.
11. The inked specimen is placed right-side up on a different gauze in numeric order.
12. When the specimens are cut on the microtome, each specimen is flipped over bottom-side up so that the deep surface of the specimen is cut with the microtome.

Tissue Map or Graph

A map of the defect is drawn after the layer of tissue is excised and divided into subunits (Fig. 2–7C & D). In small or complicated layers, drawing the map about twice the actual size of the defect makes it easier to read. The map includes an outline of the defect in relation to surrounding anatomic structures, how the excised layer was divided, the origin of each subunit within the defect, the appropriate color codes for each subunit, and the sequential order in which the subunits are to be processed by the histotechnician (Fig. 2–7D).

Because Mohs surgical defects are usually circular or oval, the conventional numbering sequence begins at the 1 o'clock position and proceeds clockwise until all the specimens are numbered. This numbering sequence can be confusing when large specimens have central specimens. To counter this problem, Picoto and Picoto[20] suggested numbering from left to right or from top to bottom. The crucial point is that each specimen should match its corresponding numbered map position (Fig. 2–8A & B).

The location of colored edges is shown on the map with the symbols: solid lines for red dye, dotted lines for blue, and zigzag lines for black. Each microscopically examined specimen is matched with the corresponding subunit specimen on the map of the defect. When residual tumor is identified in a specimen, the specific location of a tumor is matched to the closest color. A red pencil is used to identify residual tumor on the map. Mapping and coloring excised tissue provides a more systematic method of examining excised tissue for residual cancer than the traditional use of suture ligatures at the apices of a fusiform excision and the random sampling of the defect margin.[13,14,21] If there are areas of questionable malignancy or precancerous changes that are not excised, these areas can be indicated with a different colored pencil (green or blue). These suspect areas are removed or may be observed for changes on follow-up examinations.

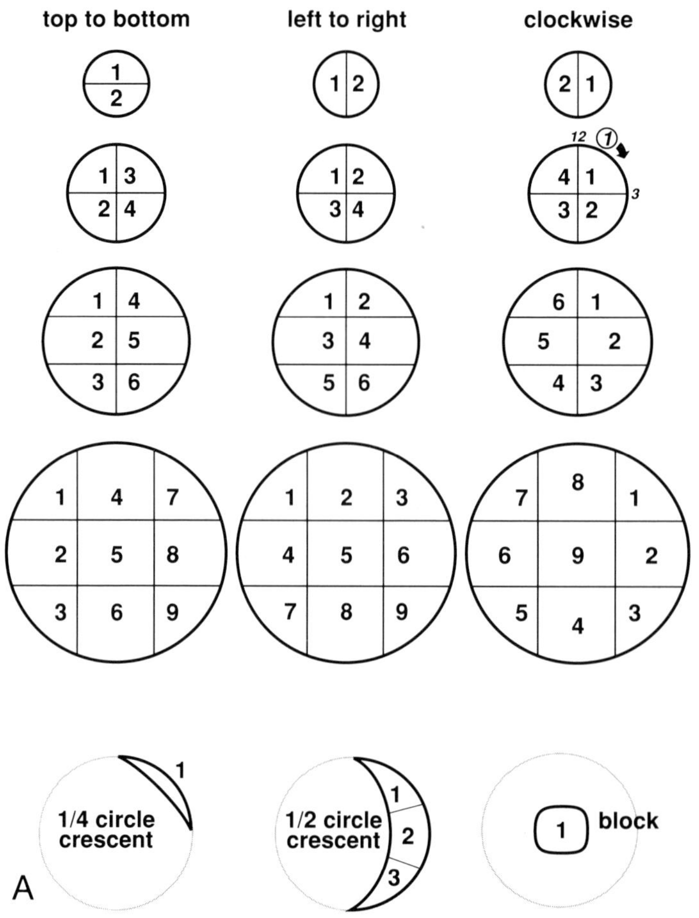

FIGURE 2–8. *A*, Examples of different kinds of Mohs maps and numbering sequences of the tissue specimens. The basic map is circular. The circle may be divided into halves or quadrants. The number of specimens depends on the size of the tumor. Examples of numbering include: left to right, top to bottom, or clockwise (the most common). Parts of layers may be donut-shaped (not shown), crescent-shaped, semicircular or block-shaped, depending on the outline of the residual cancer. Left and right sides are viewed from the reader's perspective.

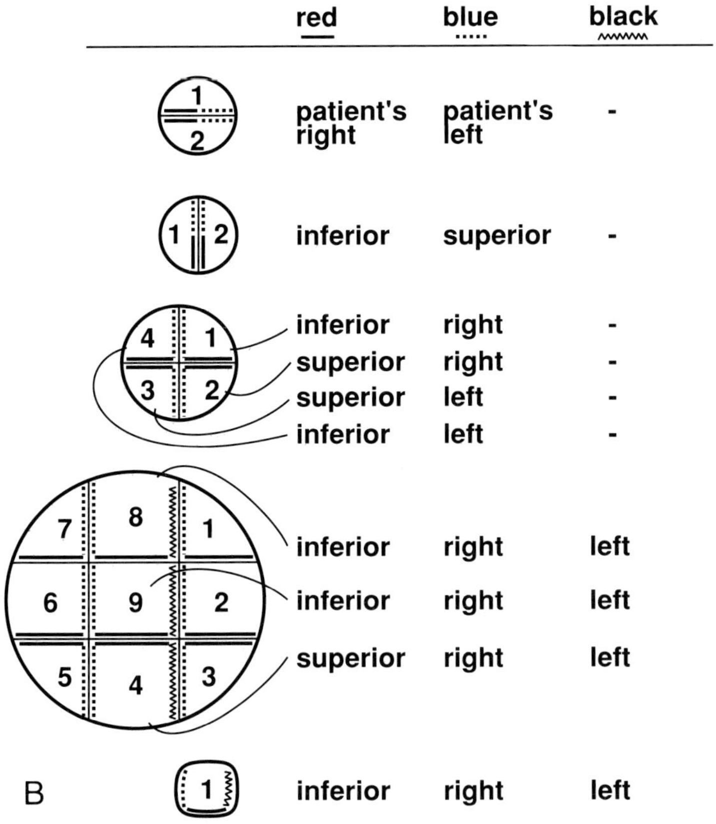

FIGURE 2–8. *Continued B,* Schematic showing some variations of coloring (inking) the tissue edges. As an aid to memory, in the first example, red (solid straight line) is right and blue (broken line) is left, and in the second example, red is inferior (hell) and blue is superior (heaven). In the other examples, the apposing specimen edges are inked identically where possible.

Horizontal Sectioning of Specimen Undersurfaces

Rather than being cut vertically, each quadrant of the divided layer is placed bottom-side up on the microtome stage so that horizontal microsections can be taken from its undersurface (deep surface). Complete horizontal sections are obtained by (1) flattening the specimen, (2) raising the peripheral margins, and (3) shaving down several microlayers of tissue with the microtome blade to level it before representative microsections (usually two to four complete microsections per tissue quadrant) are taken for microscopic examination (Fig. 2–7E to H). See Chapter 16 for details of tissue processing.

Microscopic Examination of Frozen Sections

Specimens can be microscopically examined under low (×40) and high (×100) magnification (Figs. 2–7J to L and 2–9A & B). If the microscopic examination reveals cancer at any point, it is assumed that the corresponding point in the immediately subadjacent tissue on the patient also contains cancer. The sections are scanned systematically so that no cancerous area is missed. The usual procedure is to begin at one edge of the specimen and sweep back and forth in lines parallel to the edge until the entire specimen has been examined. Ordinarily the low-power objective is used, and if the section is intact, a thorough examination takes only a few moments. Sometimes, a part of the section will be missing, in which case the technician usually places several tissue slices on the slide so that the operator can piece together a complete picture of the section by examining and comparing all of the specimens together.

Although the tissue can be scanned at low magnification, tiny clusters of cancer cells are more easily identified at higher magnification. Morpheaform basal cell carcinoma, microcystic adnexal carcinoma, dermatofibrosarcomas, Merkel cell tumors, and perineural squamous cell carcinoma are also easier to identify at higher magnification. When cancer is detected,

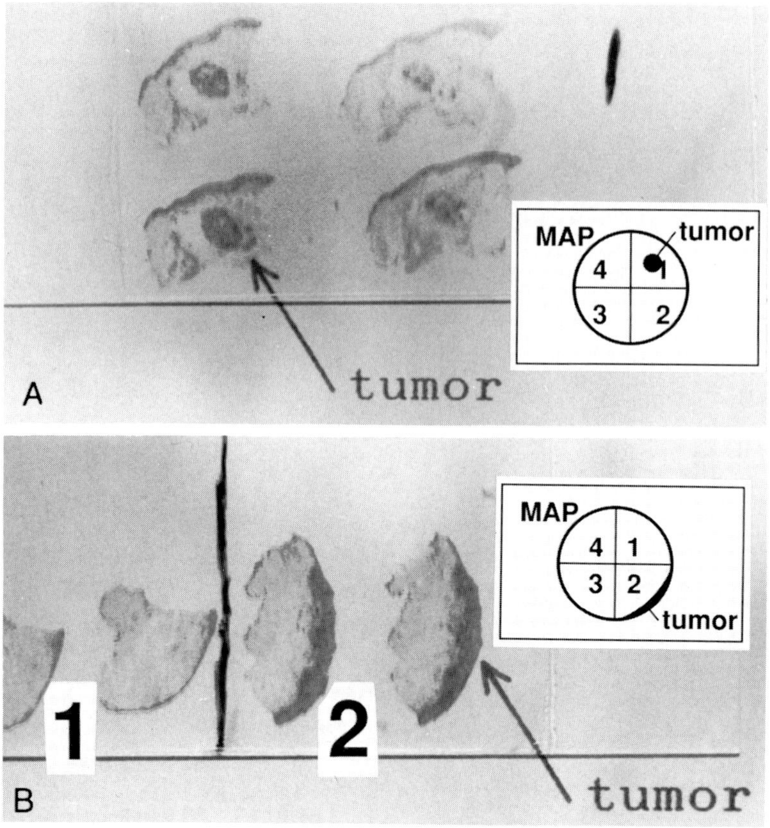

FIGURE 2–9. *A*, Histology slide shows hypothetical case of how residual cancer may appear grossly within a sample of tissue after sectioning and staining. The dark spot in specimen number 1 was confirmed microscopically to be cancer. *Inset:* The corresponding map was marked positive (black) for cancer; only this area was removed and microscopically re-checked. *B*, Histologic slides show hypothetical case of how residual cancer may appear grossly at the edges. The dark thickened line (at the edge of specimen number 2) microscopically was confirmed to be cancer. *Inset:* The corresponding map was marked positive (black) for cancer; only this area was removed and microscopically re-checked.

the exact location of the residual tumor is indicated on the map by matching it to the numbered specimens and the color markings on the sections. If the microscopic examination shows gaps or areas of incomplete horizontal sectioning, the specimens should be reprocessed, or an additional layer that incorporates the deficient area be excised to ensure a continuous layer for microscopic examination. Anatomic structures that are observed, such as nerve, cartilage, muscle, tendon, bone, and glandular material, should always be indicated on the map to help avoid any mix-up of tissue specimens. Also, a thorough microscopic examination of clinically observed tissue planes may provide information about avenues of microscopic extension (e.g., 2.4% to 4.6% of squamous cell carcinomas[2,22] and about 0.1% of basal cell carcinomas show perineural involvement[23]).

The microscopic anatomy of cancer is important for understanding regional variations in the biological behavior of tumors and for planning proper management. Probably the two most important observations to determine whether the skin margin is positive or negative for residual cancer are (1) nuances of tumor differentiation or dedifferentiation that are microscopically evident in the transition of nodular to morpheaform basal cell carcinoma and the transition from a Broders' grade 1 squamous cell carcinoma to grade 4 and (2) the microscopic involvement of nerves, lymph nodes, and other structures. The transition of the primary cancer to a more aggressive one is often apparent at the deeper margins of the excision rather than in the primary lesion.[24] Currently, there are more than 15 different types of basal cell carcinoma that can be identified histologically. Morpheaform, adenocystic, microadnexal, and carcinomas with squamous cell differentiation are variants associated with a high incidence of local recurrence and with the development of metastasis. Similarly, high-grade squamous cell carcinoma may be associated with perineural invasion and regional metastases, even in a relatively small primary lesion. Patients with this carcinoma may benefit from postoperative adjunctive radiation[22] or node dissection. Sometimes the invasion of lymph nodes by basal cell carcinoma can be detected microscopically even in the absence of any clinical evidence of lymphadenopathy.[25] This potential perineural invasion and regional metastasis emphasize the importance of examining all areas of the excision for changes in histologic features and of assuming the least favorable pathology when considering repairs.

An inexperienced operator may confuse the terminal extensions of a cancer with non-neoplastic structures. For example, collections of leukocytes, capillary vessels, and the glandular portions of eccrine glands may be mistaken for cancer, but when compared with the original histology of the neoplasm, proper identification can be achieved. Tangentially cut or obliquely cut rete ridges, hair follicles, and sebaceous glands sometimes resemble cancer on casual viewing. But comparison with other areas of the section that obviously contain these normal structures usually will serve as clues. Also, review of specimens from earlier stages of excision will help resolve doubts.

Continuity of excision, specimen mapping, and the microscopic interpretation of pathology are the essence of Mohs micrographic surgery and render the method efficient. Pathologists should be consulted when the histopathology is uncertain and when there is need for special stains or immunoperoxidase studies.[21,26] The competence of appropriately trained Mohs surgeons to read histopathology slides of skin cancer prepared by frozen sections is demonstrated by an extremely low recurrence rate of primary cancers.[17,18,27,28]

Wound Management

In simple cases, after a cancer-free plane of excision is reached, the wound can be closed in a side-to-side manner or permitted to heal by granulation. Mohs surgery is often complete after one or two layers of excision, and the defect may be immediately repaired by primary closure (Fig. 2–7M to O).

For complicated or recurrent cancers, much consideration is given to how best to manage the wound. If a complex closure is contemplated, the complexity of the repair should be balanced with the difficulty of tumor excision and the potential for recurrence. Often the type of repair performed depends on many factors, including the location, size, and type of cancer; the complexity of the excision; the possibility of recurrence; the likely esthetic and functional results; and the expectations of the patient.

Wounds from tumors excised by Mohs surgery are often smaller than wounds created by traditional surgery because the Mohs method does not unnecessarily remove normal, uninvolved skin. In fact, most wounds can be closed simply or allowed to heal by second intention without major reconstructive surgery. Second intention is preferred for recurrent cancers and cancers of the nasal labial fold, temple, and postauricular sulcus where the esthetic results after Mohs surgery are often superior to results with grafts or flaps.[29] Because healing by second intention is relatively slow, especially on the lower extremities, primary closure of extremity defects may be considered. Second intention scars are usually homogeneous with the surrounding tissue and are softer and more esthetic than scars produced by grafts from distant donor sites.

Wounds that expose cartilage, tendon, nerve, and bone demand special care and dressing to prevent desiccation necrosis. Oxycel or Gelfoam placed directly over exposed bone or cartilage may inhibit granulation tissue formation.

Repair by partial closure in selected anatomic areas also promotes rapid healing with excellent cosmetic results and few complications.[30] In principle, the wound edges are brought together so as to reduce the size of the defect while trying to get the wound "going in the right direction." The residual defect is packed with Oxycel cotton for hemostasis. Sutures are removed about 1 week later. The residual defect heals soon and without complication. Experience and judgment are necessary to properly select and execute partial closures in order to produce good cosmesis and preserve function.

Coverage with a thin skin graft is preferred if recurrence is possible and the cosmetic and functional results are acceptable. The use of skin flaps to repair defects is indicated to preserve the functional integrity of major facial structures such as the nose, eyes, lips, and ears.[31,32]

Flaps are useful for rebuilding the rima of the ala nasi, for preventing ptosis or eversion of the eyelid or lip, for covering exposed bone and cartilage, and for replacing deep defects of the face and extremities. For recurrent or difficult cancers, flaps should be used judiciously.[33,34]

Fresh and Fixed Tissue Techniques

There are two Mohs methods of excising skin cancer, the fresh tissue technique and the fixed tissue technique. It is important to keep in mind, however, that both of these methods are performed along the same principles already outlined.

The fresh tissue technique is most often used, and the name is now synonymous with Mohs micrographic surgery. The fixed tissue technique (or chemosurgery) continues to be an appropriate way of designating the alternative procedure by which layers of tissue are removed after the tissues have been pretreated with the zinc chloride fixative paste.

In the fresh tissue technique, a local anesthetic is infiltrated around the tumor, then a thin layer of tissue is excised. Hemostasis is generally controlled by pressure and electrocoagulation. Most cancers can be treated by this technique in a few hours. Large and complex tumors may necessitate several stages before a tumor-free plane is reached.

If the cancer involves bone, the paranasal sinuses, or penile erectile tissue, the fixed tissue technique may be preferred for removing cancerous bone or for controlling bleeding in the corpus cavernosum. The fixed tissue technique is also preferred for recalcitrant skin cancer and melanoma; in situ fixation minimizes the inadvertent seeding of highly malignant cancerous tissue on the excisional surface during surgery. In addition, the fixed tissue technique is appropriate for patients with the acquired immunodeficiency syndrome (AIDS) because the fixed tissue technique is a bloodless procedure. (Table 2–1).

Fixed tissue is excised by first applying two chemicals to the tumor. Full-strength dichloroacetic acid (DCA) is applied to the treatment area, 2 to 3 mm beyond the clinical margins of the lesion. A cotton-tipped applicator is used to apply the keratolytic acid until the area is dead white, indicating that the acid has penetrated through the keratin, which would otherwise bar the penetration of zinc chloride. To aid in acid penetration, loose keratin scale may be gently scraped off with a dull scalpel and DCA reapplied. A 2- to 3-mm layer of paste, consisting of 40% zinc chloride, is then applied and held in place with a thin layer of cotton. The cotton is covered by more cotton on which petrolatum has been spread to provide an occlusive dressing. The dressing is held in place with strips of adhesive tape, which should not overlap and should allow for swelling. Duoderm or Microfoam tape is applied circumferentially around the surgical site to protect the skin and provide a secure base on which to tape.

TABLE 2–1. Indications for Fixed Tissue Technique

Invasive, satellite, and in-transit melanoma
Skin cancer in patients with AIDS
Invasive penile carcinoma
Carcinoma involving bone and sinuses
Refractory tumors
Gangrene, chronic osteomyelitis, tetanus and chronic radiodermatitis

Depending on the tumor and the preference of the surgeon, a local anesthetic may be subcutaneously injected 1 to 2 cm around the area to be treated without significantly affecting the penetration of the fixative. An analgesic such as 300 mg of acetaminophen with 30 mg of codeine phosphate is prescribed as needed. Between 2 to 24 hours later, a thin layer of tissue is excised for microscopic examination from a bloodless field without the use of a local anesthetic. The fixed tissue layer is taken 2 to 3 mm within the border of the fixed skin to avoid cutting into nonfixed living tissue. Gauze soaked with normal saline or a 4% boric acid solution is placed over the wound to keep the area moist while the tissue is processed. Fixed tissue is processed exactly the same as fresh tissue.

Fixed tissue has a dense, firm consistency that is different from unfixed tissue. Fixed epidermis is white and readily incised. Fixed dermis is characteristically off-white in color peppered with zinc chloride particles (black) and has the consistency of soft leather. Fixed fat lobules have a greenish-gray hue and is softer to cut. Fixed blood vessels have an intraluminal thrombi (black). Fixed tissue is removed sharply with scalpel and scissor excision. The thickness of the excised layer of fixed tissue is about ⅛ inch. Care must be taken to maintain a uniform plane of excision devoid of scalpel nicks. In large cancers, a fresh surgical blade may need to be changed because the zinc chloride and the DCA tend to dull blades. Partially fixed tissue is softer, more hydrated, and may have a blush or red color. Unfixed tissue is painful and bleeds easily when cut. Bleeding may be controlled with pressure, Oxycel, 100% DCA, or gauze impregnated with a thin layer of the zinc chloride fixative. Rarely, electrocautery or suture ligatures are needed.

If there is residual tumor, the patient is recalled, the dichloroacetic acid and the zinc chloride fixative paste are reapplied on the areas positive for residual cancer, and the cancerous area is re-excised, usually the following day. The procedure is repeated until no microscopically visible tumor is identified. After a cancer-free plane is achieved, an occlusive dressing consisting of Polysporin ointment at the skin margin, a double layer of vaseline gauze and several layers of cotton gauze are placed over the fixed tissue to absorb the drainage and to stimulate fixed tissue separation. The bandage is changed every 2 to 3 days or when it becomes saturated.

The separation of fixed tissue is caused by an exudative process. A leukocytic infiltration circumferentially around the fixed tissue results in a sterile purulent-colored drainage that collects at the base and margins of the fixed tissue layer. This is a tissue reaction phenomenon in which normal tissue attempts to separate the dead (fixed) layer. It is not due to infection. At the skin margin, subepidermal vesicles appear that coalesce to form a circumferential bullous halo around the fixed tissue. The vesicles rupture spontaneously leaving a raw open skin edge. Incisions made into the vesicles do not accelerate fixed tissue separation but may encourage spontaneous bleeding from the nonfixed skin margin. Some parts of the fixed tissue separate faster than others. The thickness of the final layer of fixed tissue may range from 2 to 5 mm. Loose fragments of fixed tissue may be cut with a blunt curved scissors at 7 to 10 days. Alternatively, the fixed tissue will completely spontaneously sequestrate at approximately 2 weeks after the last treatment and is often found attached to the bandage when it is removed. The spontaneous separation of fixed tissue is usually without complications leaving a remarkably clean wound consisting of a bed of granulation tissue. Subsequently, the defect can be repaired with a graft or allowed to heal by second intention. To save time and to speed wound healing in the management of very early melanomas and other special situations, one may excise the fixed tissue layer by standard surgery immediately after reaching a tumor-free plane and close the wound with stitches. For difficult or recurrent tumors, healing by second intention is preferred to skin grafts or skin flaps because it prevents the delayed recognition of recurrent tumor.

INDICATIONS AND LIMITATIONS

Indications for Mohs surgery center around the method's distinct advantages: a high cure rate and the conservation of normal tissue (Table 2–2). On the face, where most skin cancers occur, Mohs surgery usually produces smaller defects and scars than other methods of treatment. As a consequence, reconstructive surgery is unnecessary in most cases. Mohs surgery is indicated for skin tumors that primarily spread by direct extension. This growth pattern is typical of most basal and squamous cell skin cancers and the early stages of superficial spreading melanoma and lentigo malignant melanoma.

TABLE 2–2. Main Indications for Mohs Micrographic Surgery

Primary cancers near the eyes, nose, lips, and ears
Recurrent tumors
Morphea-like tumors, microcystic adnexal tumors, dermatofibrosarcoma, Merkel cell carcinoma, malignant fibrohistiocytoma
Young patients with skin cancer
Tumors greater than 2 cm in diameter
Immunocompromised patients
Previous history of x-ray or ultraviolet light treatment for acne
Basal cell nevus syndrome

Indications for Mohs surgery depend on several considerations. The main ones are:

1. Whether the cancer is primary or recurrent
2. The location of the tumor
3. The histologic type of the tumor
4. Special situations, such as perineural involvement and deeply penetrating tumors.

An understanding of the propensity for skin cancer to invade local structures is essential for successful micrographic surgery. The highest cure rate is for the treatment of primary cancers that have not been previously treated by other methods (Table 2–3).

Recurrent Cancer

Mohs surgery is recommended in all recurrent tumors.[18,27] Even when a single, isolated recurrent focus at the edge of a treatment scar is detected, experience shows that retreatment by conventional methods is often inferior to Mohs surgery. The problem with recurrent tumors is the inability to reliably predict the number and extent of outlying foci of cancer cells within a

TABLE 2–3. Advantages of Mohs Micrographic Surgery

Cost-effective outpatient surgery
Precise control of tumor margins
Conservation of the maximum amount of healthy tissue
Better than 98% cure rate for tumors not treated previously
Better than 93% cure rate for recurrent tumors

previously treated scar. In the case of surgical excision and closure, the area of potential recurrence also includes the entire area of undermining. Furthermore, there is considerable variability in the effectiveness of different methods of treatment and the proficiency with which they are performed.

Before recurrent cancer is treated by Mohs surgery, a diagram is drawn to show the relationship between the focus of the recurrent tumor and the scar over the previously treated area. If there are several suspect areas, each is numbered before a biopsy is performed. Areas that are positive for recurrent tumor are treated individually, removed one layer at a time, and mapped as described above. If the individual foci merge or are close together, the lesions can be removed together as a single layer while maintaining proper orientation to the scarred area. If the recurrent tumor involves a major portion of the scarred area or there is reason to suspect the presence of outlying foci in the remaining scar, the scar can be excised as a layer and microscopically examined as described above. Alternatively, if the scarred area does not appear to contain cancer, it can be simply observed if the patient can be trusted to return for periodic evaluation.

For recurrent tumors, wound healing by second intention is generally preferred, or the wound can be partially closed from side-to-side. Simple wound management often takes longer but does not disturb tissue planes manipulated by previous treatment. Alternatively, wounds covered by skin grafts heal faster, and they allow observation and palpation through

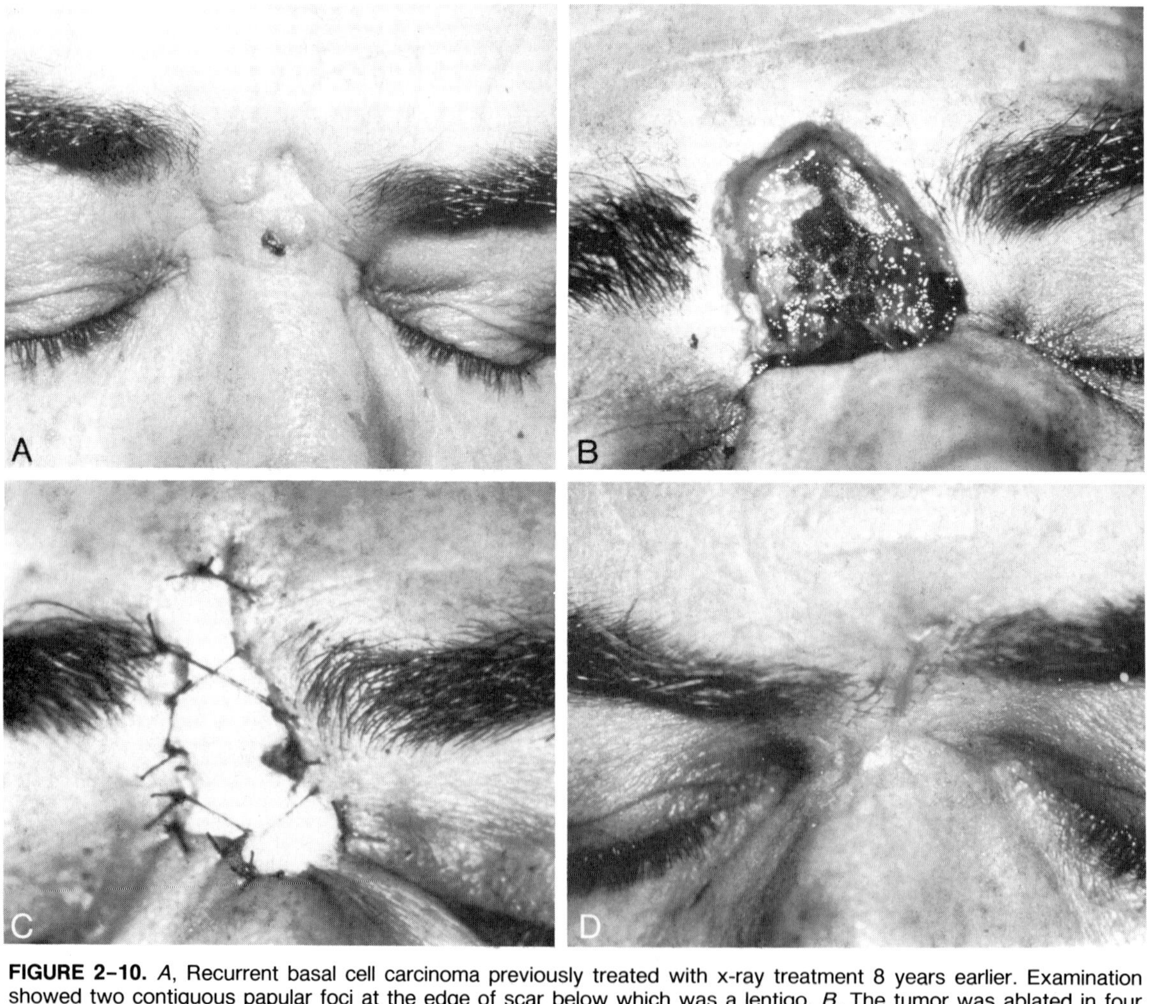

FIGURE 2–10. *A*, Recurrent basal cell carcinoma previously treated with x-ray treatment 8 years earlier. Examination showed two contiguous papular foci at the edge of scar below which was a lentigo. *B*, The tumor was ablated in four layers of Mohs surgery with exposure of underlying bone. *C*, The wound was closed partially with 4-0 silk and the residual defect covered with a layer of Polysporin ointment and packed with oxidized cellulose (Oxycel) cotton for hemostasis. *D*, Appearance of wound at 6 months; no evidence of disease after 6 years of observation.

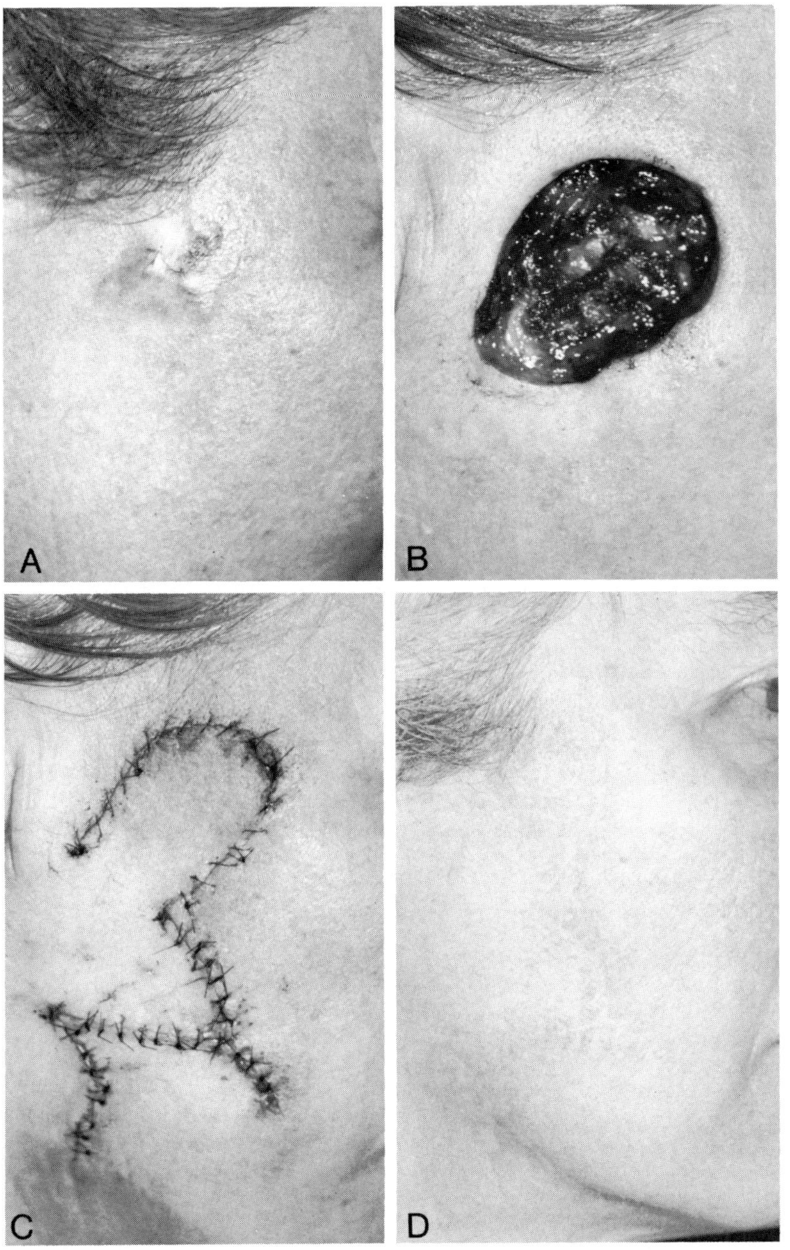

FIGURE 2–11. *A*, Morphea-like basal cell carcinoma of the right cheek. The patient gave a history of previous x-ray treatment for acne at age 17. The tumor had already been excised twice. *B*, Defect after three stages of Mohs surgery. The depth of penetration involved the periosteum overlying the zygomatic arch. The patient experienced temporary lower lid paralysis for approximately 6 months. *C*, The defect was repaired with a bilobed flap harvested from the lower cheek. *D*, Follow-up photo at 10 months; no evidence of disease after 5½ years of observation.

the thin grafted skin to detect foci that may be trapped beneath the graft. Local skin flaps can also be used to repair deep defects or to maintain the functional competence of the nose, eyes, lips, and cheeks, as long as one understands the risk of transposing skin that may contain tumor or of burying tumor beyond the reach of palpation and inspection. The normal appearance of a graft, however, is no guarantee against the presence of underlying incipient carcinoma. Because of these considerations, the safest course consists of minimal surgical repair followed by an appropriate period of observation. If after 6 months to 2 years there is no evidence of recurrent disease, definitive plastic repair can be considered. Most patients will opt for second intention healing when the risks and benefits are properly explained to them. Figures 2–10 and 2–11 show examples of recurrent cancers treated by Mohs surgery.

Anatomic Location

Mohs surgery is ideal for skin cancers of the eyelids,[32] nose,[2] lips,[35] ears,[36] scalp,[37] and genitalia.[38] Local anatomy and exogenous factors in these regions often modify the growth pattern of skin cancer. Soft tissues such as dermis, fat, and muscle do not offer substantial resistance to tumor penetration. As a consequence, even relatively small cancers can invade deeply and cause significant cosmetic deformity and functional disability before they are recognized and treated. The deep penetration of tumor is less likely where bone and cartilage are present, but the tumor may spread radially by skimming along the hard surface of the tissue and eventually invade deep structures through natural cleavage planes from which extirpation is difficult. With conventional treatments, the complete excision of a facial tumor is hampered by the natural tendency to remove less tissue than necessary in an effort to maximize esthetic results.

Periorbital Region

Tumors that arise in the periorbital skin, except those at the inner canthus and lid margin, tend to penetrate vertically. Periorbital skin, muscle, and the orbital septum offer little resistance to tumor penetration. In the inner canthus, there is only a thin layer of skin covering the bone, and tumors are diverted horizontally.

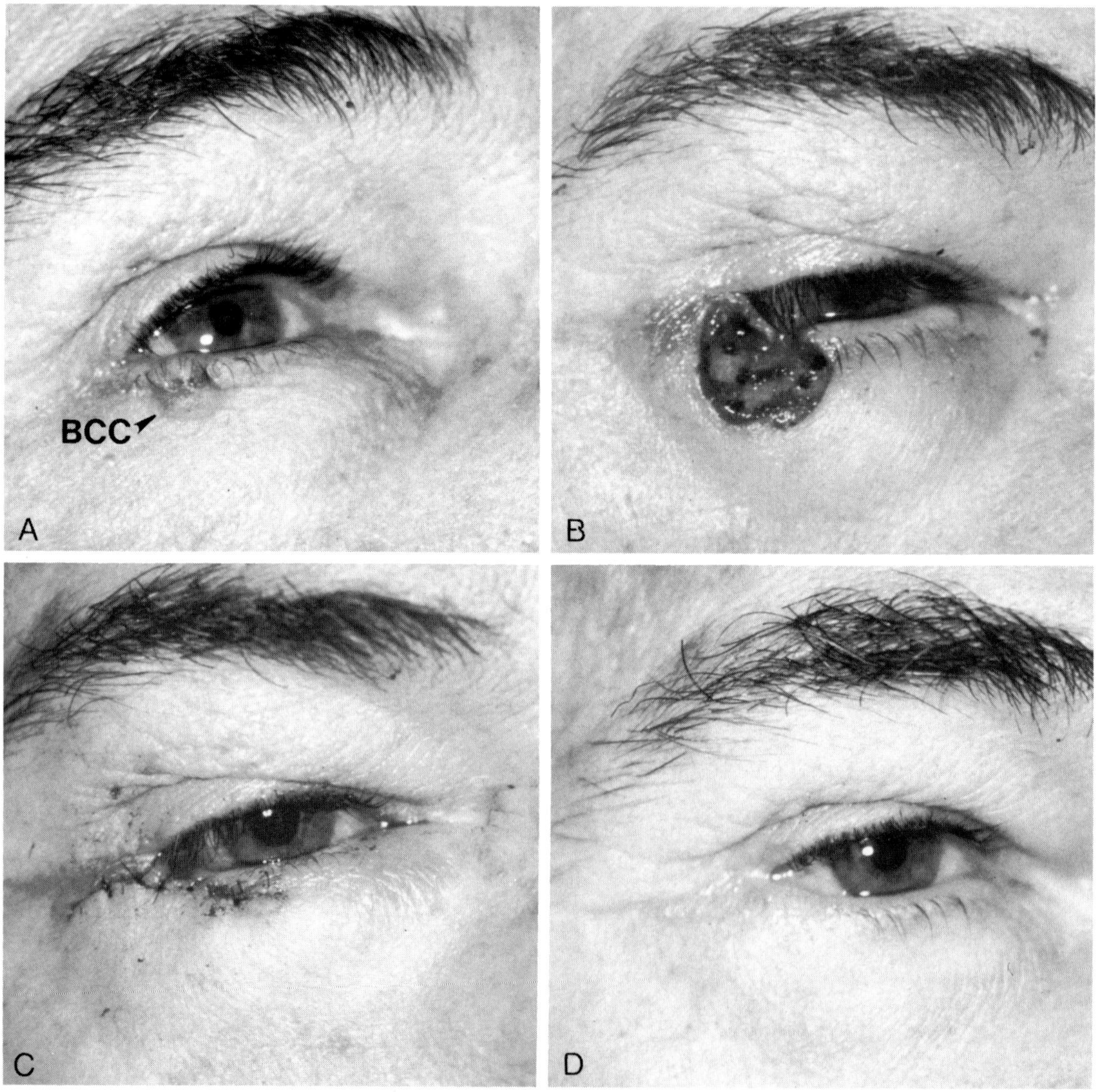

FIGURE 2–12. *A*, Basal cell carcinoma of the lateral lower lid and margin of the right eye. *B*, Defect after two stages of Mohs surgery; a small microscopic focus was found to extend through the commissure to the upper lateral lid margin. *C*, Horizontal closure of defect; a small lateral dog ear was revised. *D*, Follow-up photo at 3 months; no evidence of disease after 5 years of observation.

The medial canthal tendons provide some resistance, but penetration between the relatively softer muscle fibers can occur. Nasal and lacrimal bones are thin, and eventually tumor erosion occurs at the suture lines and bone cortex. The nasolacrimal duct may also be invaded, with eventual extension to the intranasal and sinus areas. Tumors arising on the lid margins may spread both radially along the conjunctival mucosa and vertically into the soft tissue. The tarsal plate, however, is a barrier to tumor penetration. The upper tarsal plate is wider and thicker than the lower one. Tumors of the lower lid margin may encircle the lower tarsal plate. In elderly patients who suffer from poor vision, cancers in the periorbital area are often difficult to discern. Growths behind eyeglass frames and nose rests are often obscured, and when patients remove their eyeglasses they may find it difficult to see those growths (Fig. 2–12).

Nasal Region

On the basis of tumor biology, most cancers of the nose can be divided into four anatomic regions: midline (bridge and tip), lateral bridge, ala nasi, and nasolabial fold. Cancers that involve the midline of the nose may spread laterally along the nasal bone and lateral cartilage, or vertically through the midline between the medial articulating surfaces of the nasal bone, and lateral and alar cartilages. Nasal tip tumors involve the columella by superficial extension along the skin or by direct extension between the alar cartilages (Fig. 2–13). On the upper

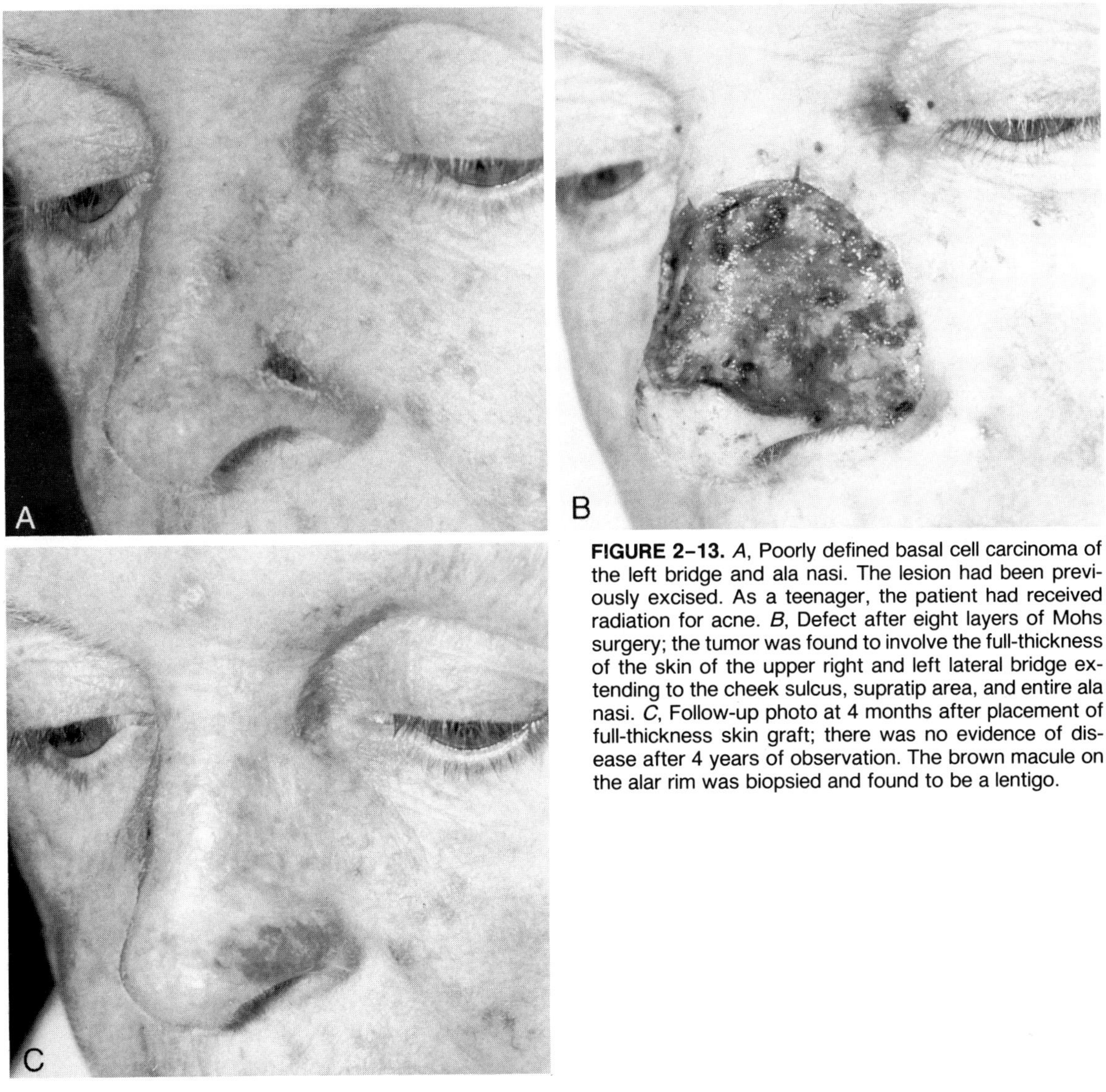

FIGURE 2–13. *A*, Poorly defined basal cell carcinoma of the left bridge and ala nasi. The lesion had been previously excised. As a teenager, the patient had received radiation for acne. *B*, Defect after eight layers of Mohs surgery; the tumor was found to involve the full-thickness of the skin of the upper right and left lateral bridge extending to the cheek sulcus, supratip area, and entire ala nasi. *C*, Follow-up photo at 4 months after placement of full-thickness skin graft; there was no evidence of disease after 4 years of observation. The brown macule on the alar rim was biopsied and found to be a lentigo.

bridge, direct invasion into the nasal cavity is impeded by the nasal bone. However, the tumor may indirectly enter the nasal cavity by traveling in the connective tissue of the upper lateral cartilage to its superior tip, which is normally overridden by the nasal bone. Perforation into the nasal cavity may occur anywhere, but a very susceptible area is the alar groove. In this region the inferior lateral margin of the alar cartilage dovetails with the superior border of the fibrous ala nasi. The surrounding firmer tissues serve to direct tumor cells into this triangular groove of soft tissue and into the nasal cavity. Tumors that arise from the nasolabial fold invade deep tissue by traveling along the embryonic fusion plane between the cheek, nose, and the skin of the upper lip.[2,6]

Lip Region

Cancers on the upper and lower lips may exhibit exophytic, endophytic, or combination growth patterns. Most cancers of the upper lip are basal cell carcinomas that originate on the glabrous skin of the upper lip and involve the vermilion border and lip proper by direct extension. Lower-lip cancers tend to be squamous cell carcinomas that tend to remain localized to the mucosa of the lip.[35] Early cancers extend radially along the mucous membrane. Except for aggressive cancers, the thick lip shelf of the orbicularis oris muscle is a barrier to deep tumor invasion (Fig. 2–14). If the tumor penetrates muscle, it spreads in between the mucosal glands. Occasional perineural extension along the mental and inferior alveolar

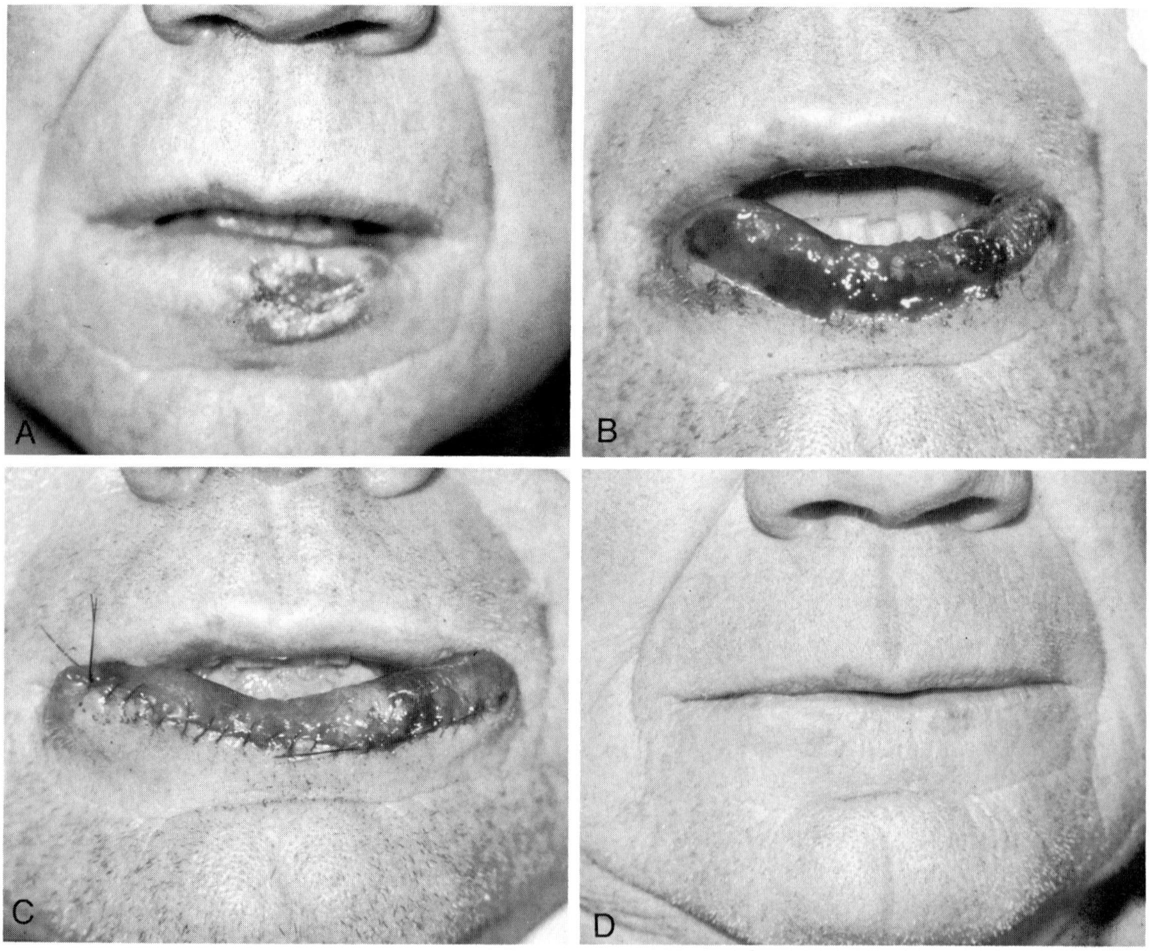

FIGURE 2–14. *A*, Squamous cell carcinoma of the lower lip. *B*, Defect of lower lip after complete tumor excision was accomplished in two layers. *C*, Anteroposterior closure using 4-0 nylon running sutures after dog ears were excised at both ends. *D*, Follow-up photo at 2 weeks; there was no evidence of disease after 7 years of observation.

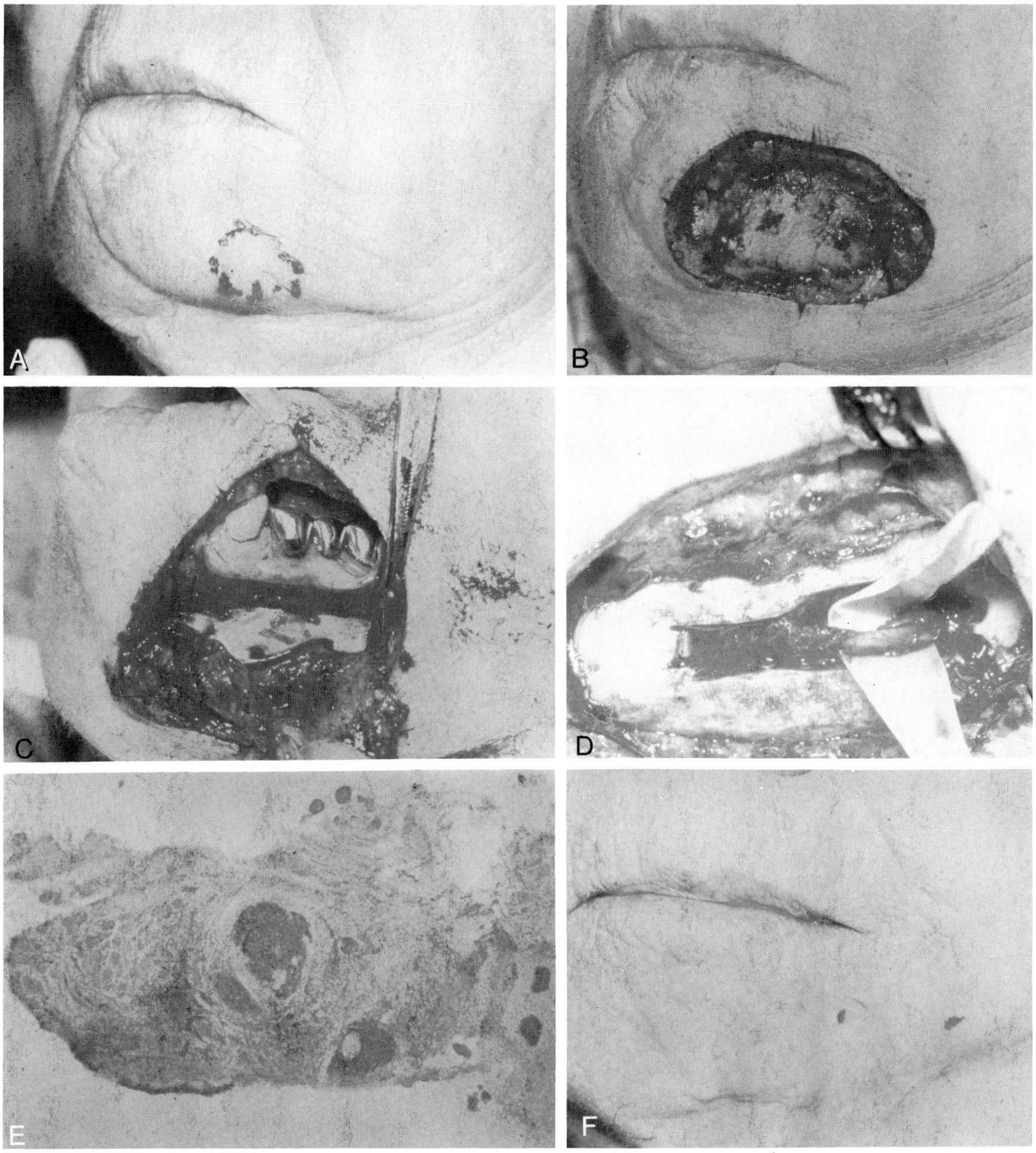

FIGURE 2–15. *A*, Recurrent basal cell carcinoma of left chin: The patient had been experiencing pain in left jaw area for about 1 year. *B*, Defect after three stages of Mohs surgery; microsection taken from the mental nerve was positive for perineural tumor. Single, double, and triple nicks were cut in the specimen and skin edge simultaneously to indicate the origin of specimens. *C*, Thru-and-thru defect into mouth. Periosteum of mandible being removed to expose the mental foramen. *D*, Partial inferior alveolar canalectomy. Inferior alveolar nerve isolated by Penrose drain. Approximately 2 cm of inferior alveolar nerve had to be resected to complete the excision of the tumor. *E*, Photomicrograph of basal cell carcinoma extending along the inferior alveolar neurovascular bundle. *F*, Follow-up photo at one year after wound was closed with a transposition flap from upper neck; there was no evidence of disease after 3 years of observation.

nerves occurs in large and aggressive cancers (Fig. 2–15).

Ear Region

From a surgical perspective, cancers of the ear can be divided into those arising from the anterior surface, the posterior surface, and the retroauricular sulcus.[36] Radial extension is the usual mode of tumor spread. On the anterior surface, the skin is closely attached to the cartilage. Often only one deep layer can be removed before cartilage is exposed (Fig. 2–16).

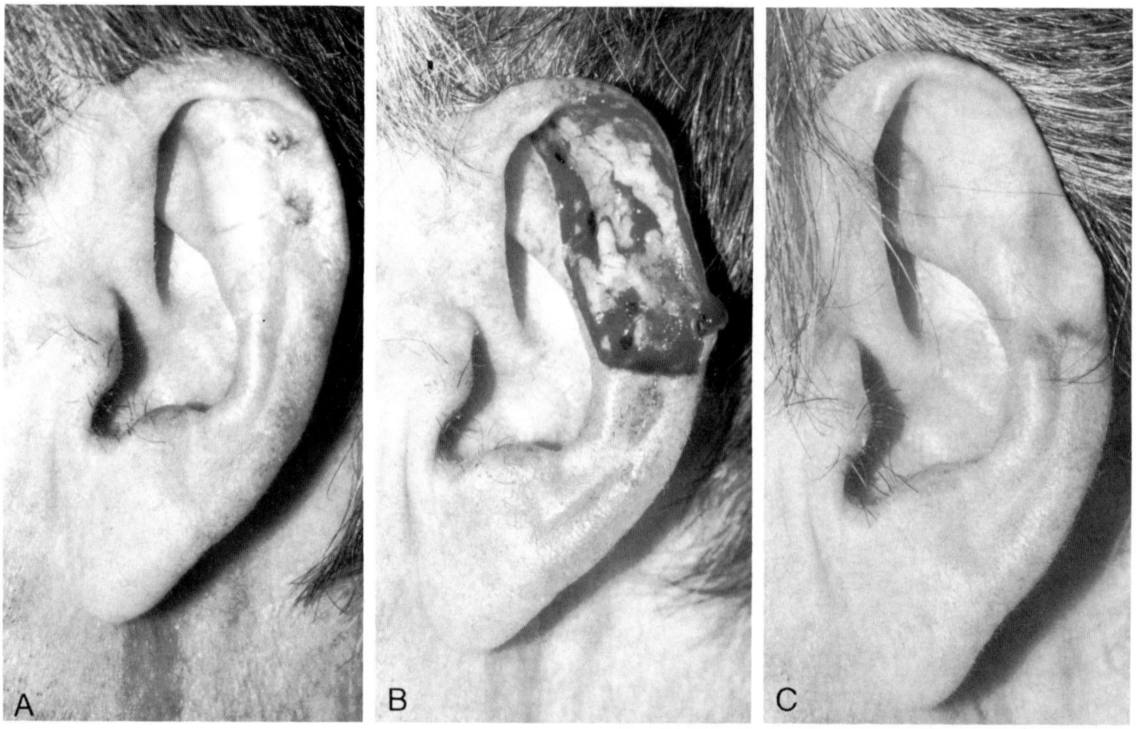

FIGURE 2–16. *A*, Basal cell carcinoma of the left superior helix. *B*, Defect after three layers of Mohs surgery; the tumor skimmed along the anterior cartilage to the posterior surface. The helical and antihelical cartilage was removed in some areas. The remainder of the viable cartilage was fenestrated to permit rapid granulations to cover the exposed cartilage. *C*, Follow-up photo at 4 months after placement of split-thickness skin graft; no evidence of disease after 2 years of observation.

In the conchal area, tumor may spread medially to involve the external auditory canal and pass through the spaces in the cartilage (valves of Santorini) to involve the parotid gland. On the posterior pinna, the skin is a little thicker and permits the excision of at least two deep layers before the cartilage is reached. The postauricular sulcus is an embryonic fusion plane between the ear, scalp, and neck skin. Deep extension exposes the parotid gland inferiorly and the mastoid bone posteriorly (Fig. 2–17).

Ear surgery is complicated by cartilaginous concavities and convexities that even inhibit the micrographic treatment of skin cancers. In the conchal area, angled (60-degree) Beaver or No. 15C Bard-Parker blades and handles often aid the excision of tissue layers. Hemostasis is achieved with pressure and with pinpoint electrocoagulation to minimize the production of necrotic tissue, which may lead to bacterial colonization, infection, and chondritis. An occlusive dressing of Polysporin ointment with Gelfoam or Instat for hemostasis is used to protect the cartilage from desiccation necrosis.

Genital Region

Mohs surgery provides a high local cure rate for penile cancer [38–42] that is comparable to the cure rate for penectomy, but without the associated psychological and functional disability (Fig. 2–18). Patients with stage I (glans and prepuce) lesions should be observed. Stage II (sulcus and shaft) lesions may be considered for prophylactic lymph node biopsy or superficial lymph node dissection. Bilateral lymph node biopsy or dissection may be appropriate in patients with recurrent tumors, tumors larger than 3 cm in diameter, deep tumors that invade the corpora cavernosa, and in obese patients in whom detection of lymphadenopathy is difficult. The use of magnetic resonance imaging or computed tomography can help identify patients who have genital disease that may benefit from early-intervention node dissection.

Mohs surgery is also indicated for early vulvar cancer (Fig. 2–19) because it can provide complete tumor excision without complete

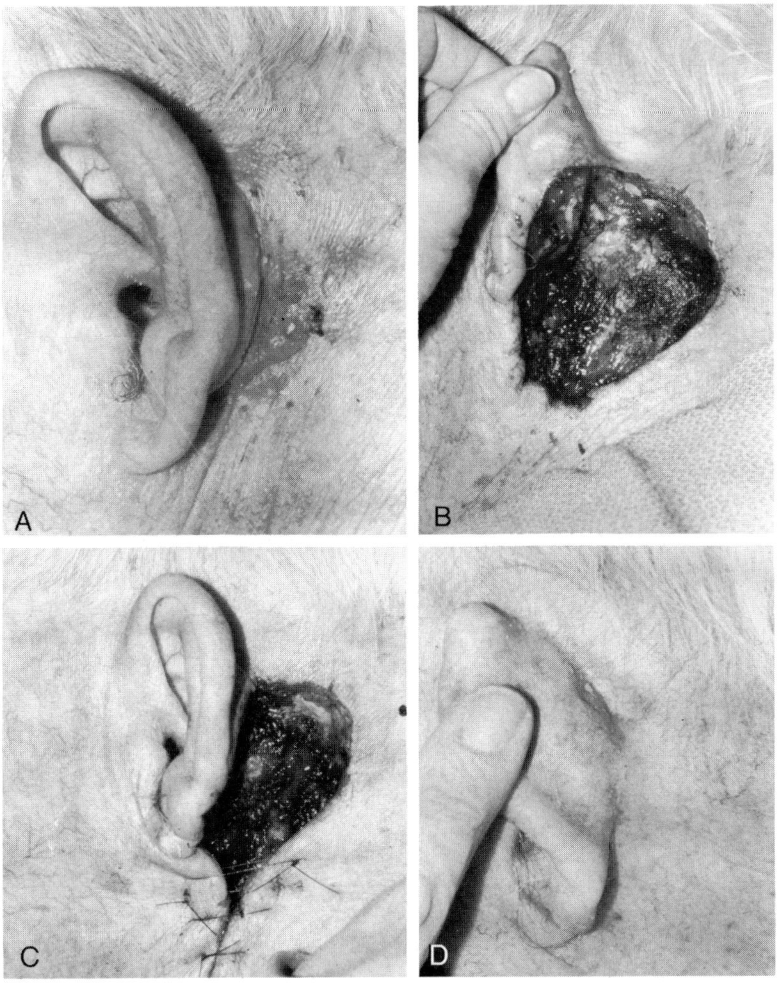

FIGURE 2–17. *A*, Basal-squamous cell carcinoma of the postauricular sulcus of 3 years' duration. *B*, Defect after four layers of Mohs surgery. The radial component of the tumor involved almost the entire lower posterior pinna and extended posteriorly into the sternocleidomastoid muscle and mastoid bone. Ablation of the tumor required excision of part of the parotid gland. *C*, Residual postauricular defect after the wound was partially closed. *D*, Wound healed in 2 months without complications; follow-up photo at 5 years; no evidence of disease after 6 years of observation.

vulvectomy.[43] There is a tendency for vulvar carcinomas, especially midline tumors, to be bilateral. Thin vulvar carcinomas (less than 5 mm thick) may metastasize to inguinal nodes. About 25% of invasive vulvar cancers have micrometastases in nonpalpable nodes; thus, groin dissection is indicated and careful follow-up is mandatory.

Other Anatomic Areas

Mohs surgery is indicated for the preservation of normal structures of the hands and feet. Squamous cell carcinomas of the nailbed (Fig. 2–20) and plantar surface (Fig. 2–21) can be successfully managed with the Mohs technique (see Chapter 21). In large or complex cancers, a multidisciplinary approach is needed (Fig. 2–22).

Cancer Histology

The key feature of the Mohs technique for ensuring high cure rates is the correct interpretation of histologic slides. Tumor growth actually occurs in three dimensions, but as the tumor is followed to its termination, a single plane of invasion usually predominates.

Epidermal Invasion

Carcinoma in situ comprises a group of cancers ranging from squamous cell carcinoma (Bowen's disease or erythroplasia of Queyrat) to extramammary Paget's disease, sebaceous carcinoma, superficial spreading melanoma, and lentigo maligna melanoma. Although each of these cancers has its own characteristic histology, tumor invasion is usually radially along the epidermis. Frequently, a focus may break

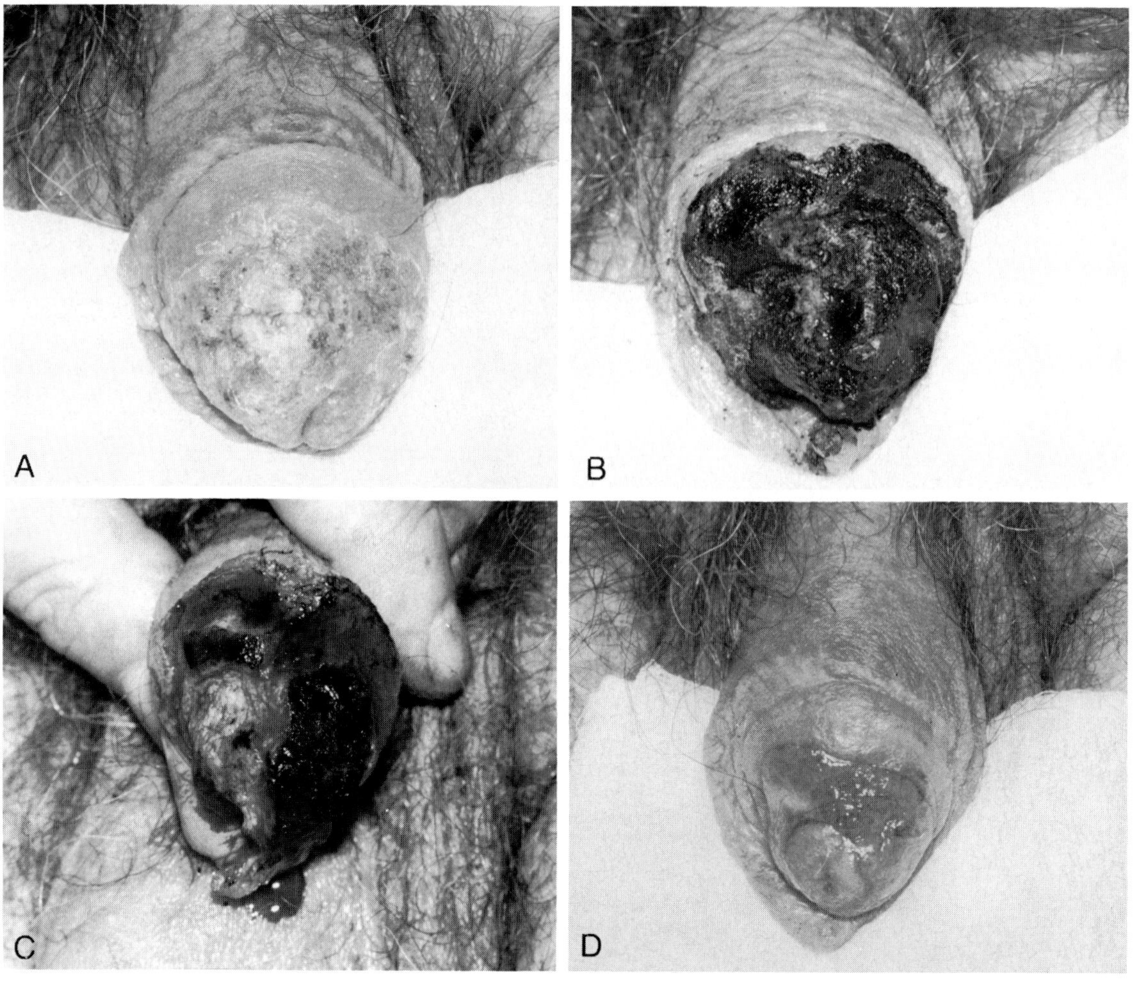

FIGURE 2–18. *A*, Verrucous squamous cell carcinoma of the glans penis. *B*, Tumor excised with thermocautery knife at 170°C. Blackened area consists of oxidized cellulose Oxycel cotton cellulose and Monsel's solution, applied to control erectile tissue bleeding. *C*, Defect at completion of four stages of Mohs surgery. *D*, Follow-up photo at 1 month. Wound almost healed by second intention; urinary and sexual functions were normal. No evidence of disease after 4 years of follow-up.

through the basement membrane or may involve adnexal structures and, from there, invade the deeper dermis. In these cases, a full thickness of skin including hair follicles and appendages should be excised (Fig. 2–23). Intraepithelial spread may involve the full thickness of the epidermis, as in Bowen's disease (Fig. 2–23) or the "buckshot" distribution of superficial spreading melanoma (Fig. 2-24), or only the basal layer of the epidermis as in atypical melanocytic hyperplasia, lentigo maligna melanoma, and extramammary Paget's disease (Fig. 2–25).

Intradermal Carcinoma

Intradermal carcinoma comprises a group of neoplasms such as morphea-like basal cell carcinoma (Fig. 2–26), dermatofibrosarcoma (Fig. 2–27), and microadnexal carcinoma that characteristically spread through the dermis.

Subcutaneous Tissue Invasion

Tumors that invade the subcutaneous tissue—with perineural, perilymphatic, parotid, muscle, tendon, nasal lacrimal duct, or bone in-

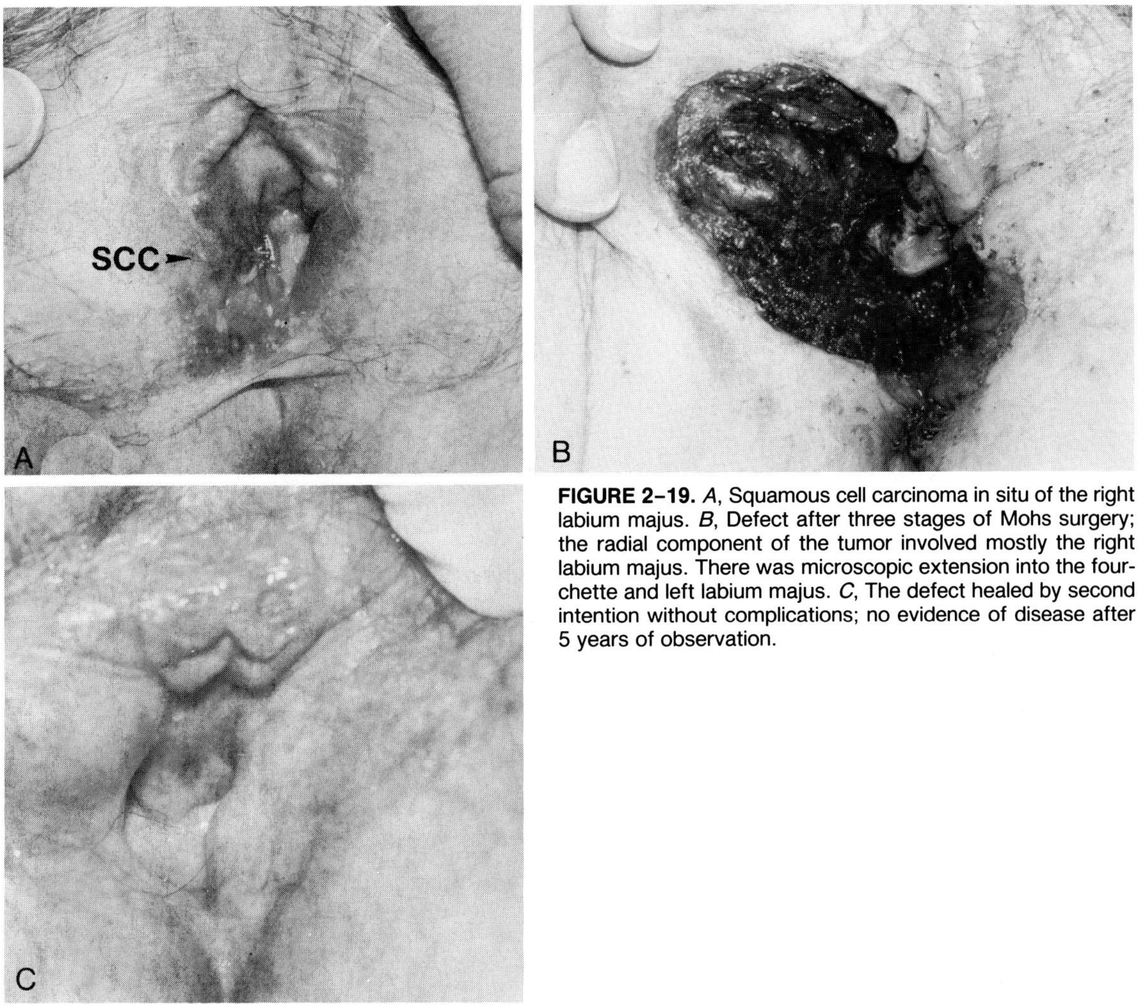

FIGURE 2–19. *A*, Squamous cell carcinoma in situ of the right labium majus. *B*, Defect after three stages of Mohs surgery; the radial component of the tumor involved mostly the right labium majus. There was microscopic extension into the fourchette and left labium majus. *C*, The defect healed by second intention without complications; no evidence of disease after 5 years of observation.

volvement—include basal cell carcinoma (Fig. 2–28) and squamous cell carcinoma. Outlying foci of melanoma and lymph node invasion by cancer may be microscopically evident (Fig. 2–29).

With training and daily practice, one can readily use the Mohs technique to microscopically recognize and map most skin cancers. Although the interpretation of some sections is difficult because of tangential sectioning and inflammation, a review of the primary biopsy slide often helps to recreate a mental image of the cancer and to distinguish tiny foci of cancer cells from normal tissues. Alternatively, the use of paraffin-embedded permanent sections, special stains, and immunoperoxidase techniques may help identify histopathologically unusual cancers.

Special Situations

Mohs surgery is indicated for cancer that persists after excision and for lesions larger than 2 cm in diameter. It is also appropriate for young patients and patients with the nevoid basal cell carcinoma syndrome when maximal conservation of normal tissue is important.

Indications for Fixed Tissue Technique

Malignant Melanoma

Malignant melanoma, especially superficial spreading melanoma and lentigo maligna melanoma, often sends out finger-like projections

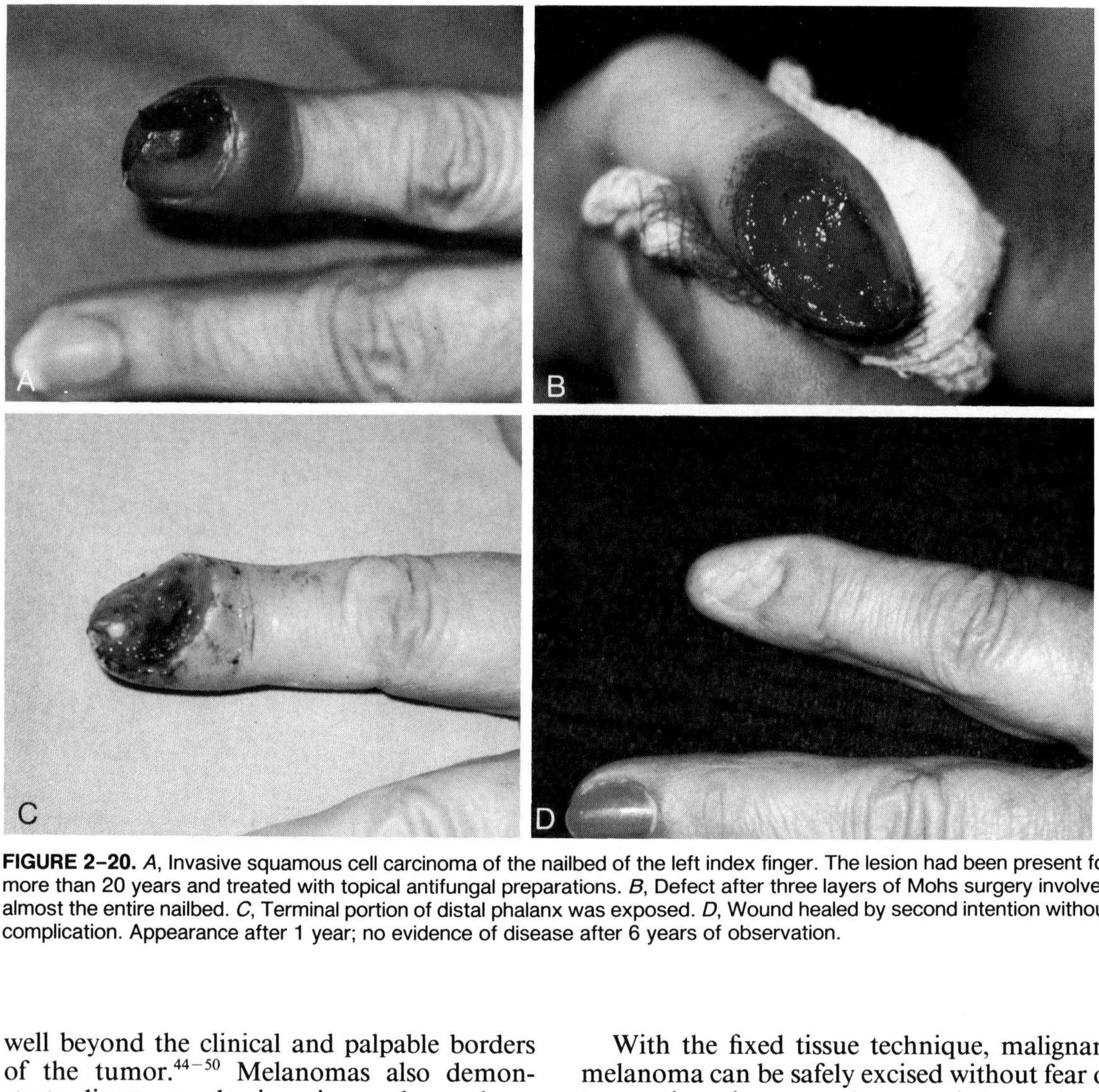

FIGURE 2–20. *A*, Invasive squamous cell carcinoma of the nailbed of the left index finger. The lesion had been present for more than 20 years and treated with topical antifungal preparations. *B*, Defect after three layers of Mohs surgery involved almost the entire nailbed. *C*, Terminal portion of distal phalanx was exposed. *D*, Wound healed by second intention without complication. Appearance after 1 year; no evidence of disease after 6 years of observation.

well beyond the clinical and palpable borders of the tumor.[44–50] Melanomas also demonstrate direct vascular invasion and may hang precariously within the vessel lumen. The degree of vascular invasion seems to be related to Clark's level: 0% for Clark's level 1, 12% for Clark's level 2, 25% for Clark's level 3, 40% for Clark's level 4,[51] and 63% for Clark's level 5. In one publication, the incidence of intraspecimen metastasis was reported to be 5.2% (13/249) and appeared to be independent of depth or level of penetration.[52] Although it is rarely observed, the inadvertent transection of these satellites during excision of nonfixed tissue can potentially spread the tumor and compromise survival. Only 36% of patients who have malignant melanomas with local satellites survive for 5 years, compared with 89% of patients who have similar melanomas but without local satellites.[47,50]

With the fixed tissue technique, malignant melanoma can be safely excised without fear of transecting intravascular or intraspecimen melanomatous deposits because all incisions are through fixed, i.e., dead, tissue. If satellite deposits appear later, they can be removed safely with the fixed tissue method. The average duration of treatment is 3 days (Fig. 2–30). The 5-year survival rates in a series of 200 patients treated with the fixed tissue technique were 89% for Clark's level 2, 88% for Clark's level 3, 63% for Clark's level 4, and 38% for Clark's level 5.[50] These results compare favorably with results for standard wide surgical excision. A preliminary report by Zitelli and colleagues[50] supports the use of the fresh tissue technique in a small series of melanoma patients (see Chapter 14).

The fixed tissue technique has the disadvantage of not allowing an accurate Breslow thick-

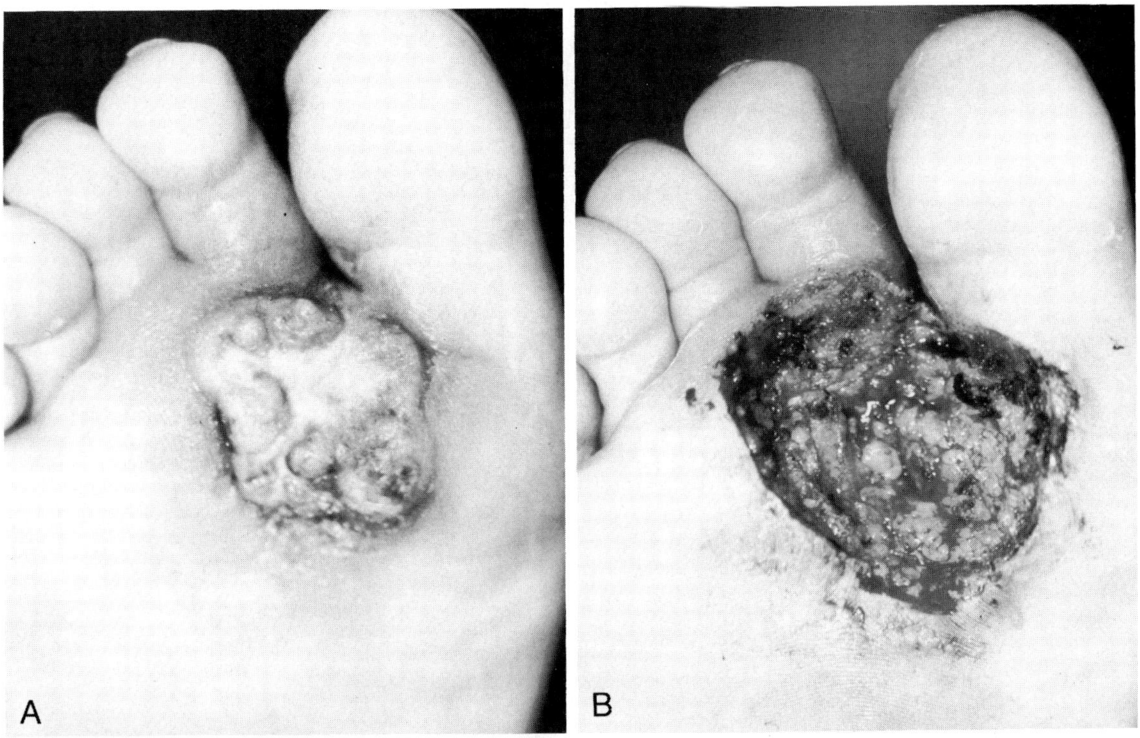

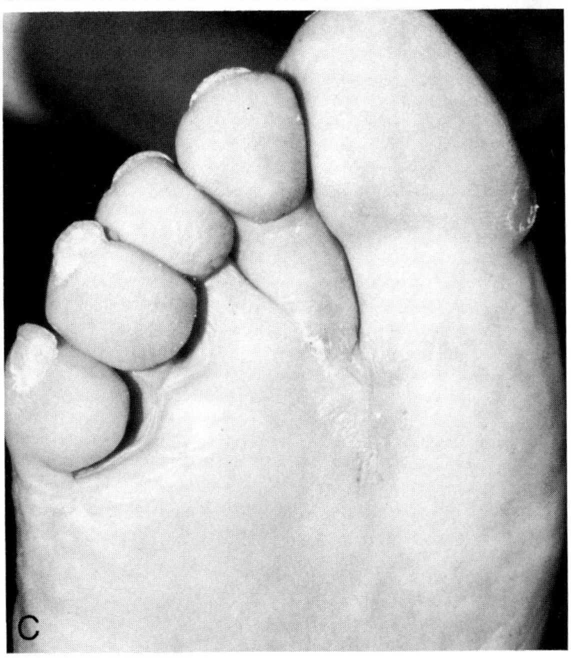

FIGURE 2–21. *A*, Verrucous squamous cell carcinoma of the plantar surface of the right foot, which had been treated as a wart for 20 years. *B*, Defect after two stages of Mohs surgery. *C*, The wound healed by second intention without complications. Follow-up photo at 10 months; no evidence of disease after 6 years of observation.

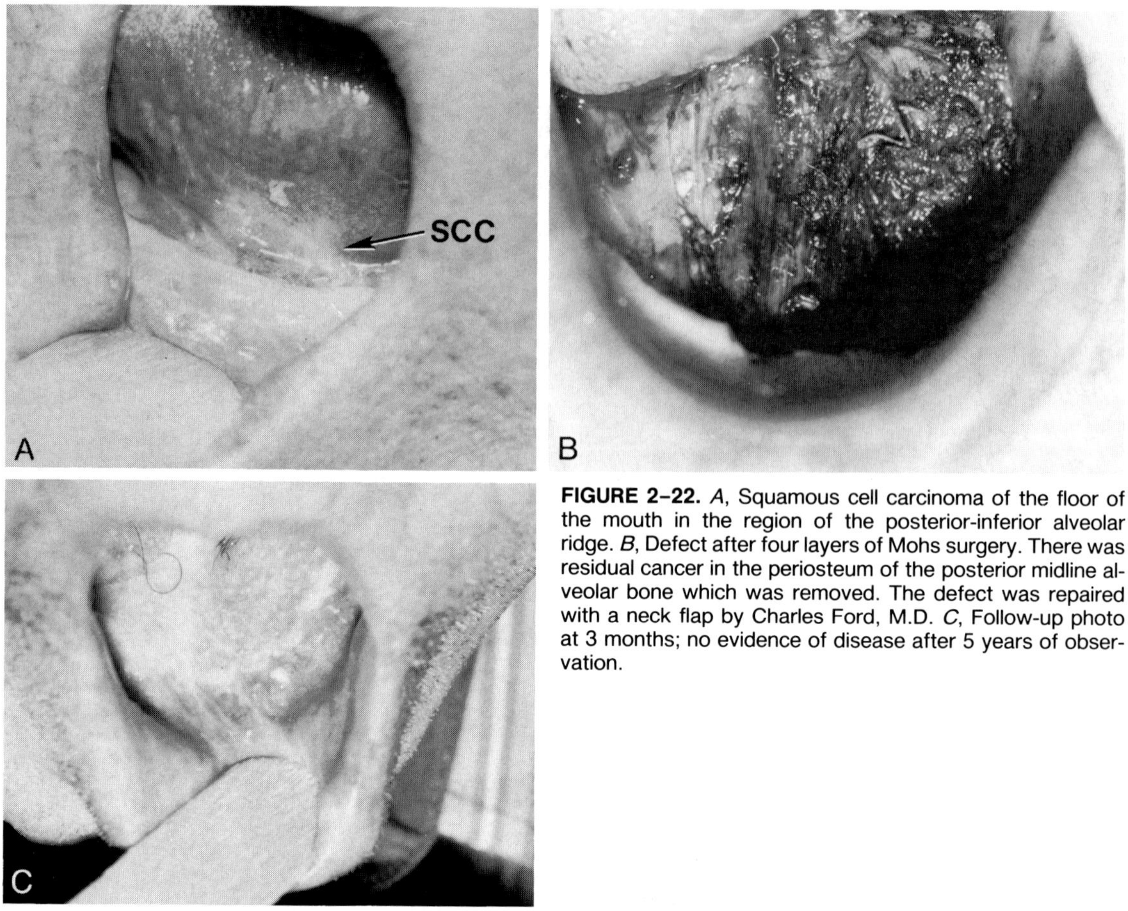

FIGURE 2–22. *A*, Squamous cell carcinoma of the floor of the mouth in the region of the posterior-inferior alveolar ridge. *B*, Defect after four layers of Mohs surgery. There was residual cancer in the periosteum of the posterior midline alveolar bone which was removed. The defect was repaired with a neck flap by Charles Ford, M.D. *C*, Follow-up photo at 3 months; no evidence of disease after 5 years of observation.

ness measurement to be performed. Most histopatholgists are unaccustomed to reading tissue fixed with zinc chloride, and the dehydration artifact of the paste is different from formalin-fixed, paraffin-embedded tissue. Amelanotic melanomas are rare and not easily recognized. In these cases, and in melanoma patients with previous fresh tissue biopsies, fixed tissue treatment is an acceptable alternative treatment. With the combined fresh and fixed tissue method, the melanoma can be excised to determine histologic type, Clark's level, and Breslow's thickness, while the base of the lesion is safely evaluated and treated by the fixed tissue technique (Fig. 2–31).

AIDS and Skin Cancer

Metastatic basal cell carcinoma has been reported in patients with AIDS or AIDS-related complex (ARC), probably as a result of their impaired immune system.[53] The fixed tissue technique can be used to treat these patients because it allows the tumor to be excised from a bloodless field, sterilizes the tissue, and permits the cancers to be mapped in order to ensure a high local cure rate (Fig. 2–32).[54]

Penile Carcinoma

Superficial squamous cell carcinoma of the penis can be excised using the fresh tissue technique and local anesthesia.[40,41] But if the tumor involves erectile tissue, the fixed tissue technique[38,39] also can be used to control bleeding from the noncontractile vascular spaces of the erectile tissue (Fig. 2–33).

The tumor is first infiltrated on the operative site blockhead with local anesthetic. If epinephrine is diluted with the local anesthetic, only the smallest amount needed to produce analgesia is injected. This precaution is warranted

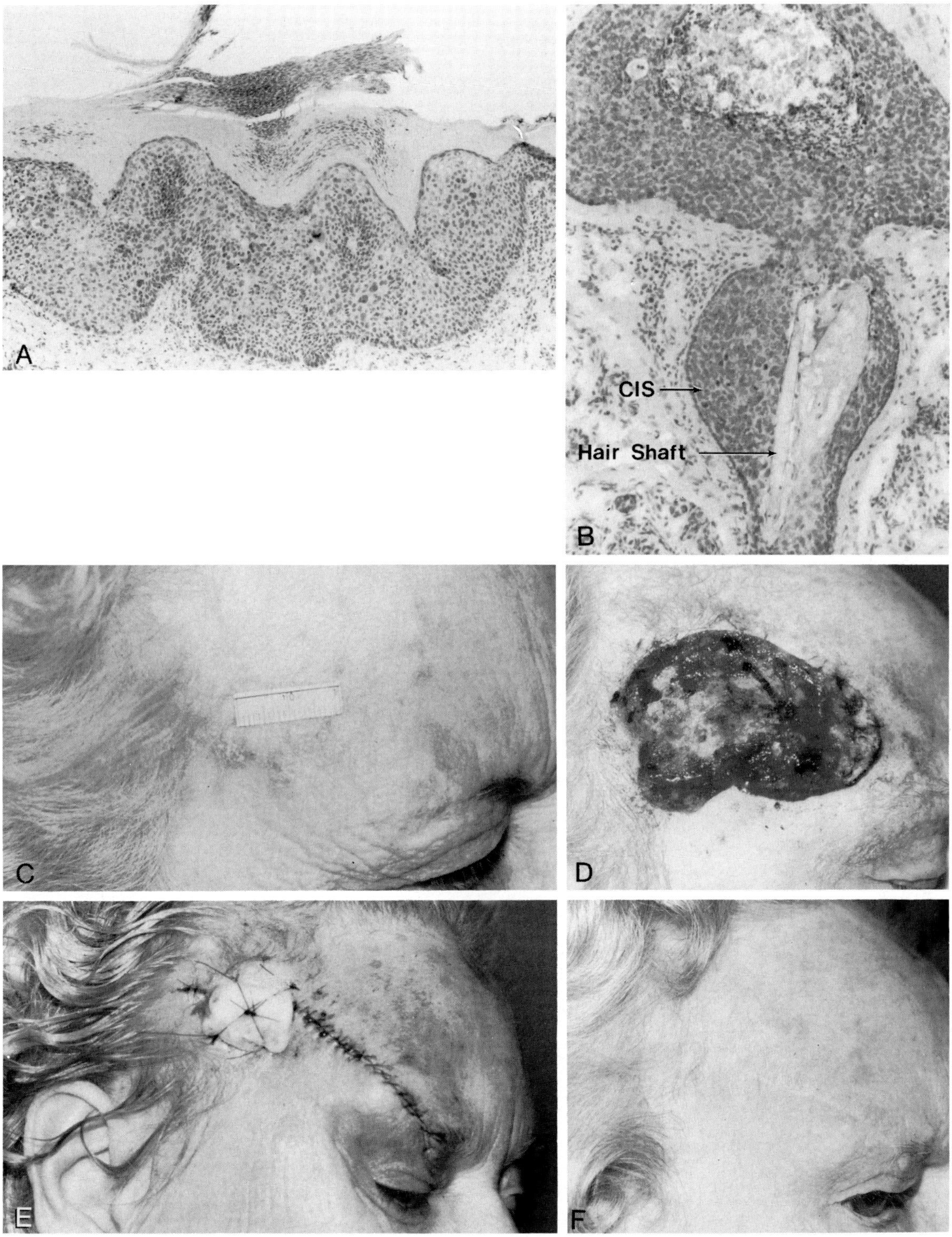

FIGURE 2-23. *A*, Squamous cell carcinoma in situ. *B*, Intraepidermal and intrafollicular epithelium involved by carcinoma in situ. *C*, Clinical appearance of squamous cell carcinoma in situ on the right temple and hairline. *D*, Defect after four layers of Mohs surgery. Full-thickness skin was excised because of tumor extension into hair follicles. *E*, Partial side-to-side closure of the defect combined with a full-thickness skin graft. *F*, Healed wound at 6 months; no evidence of disease after 2½ years.

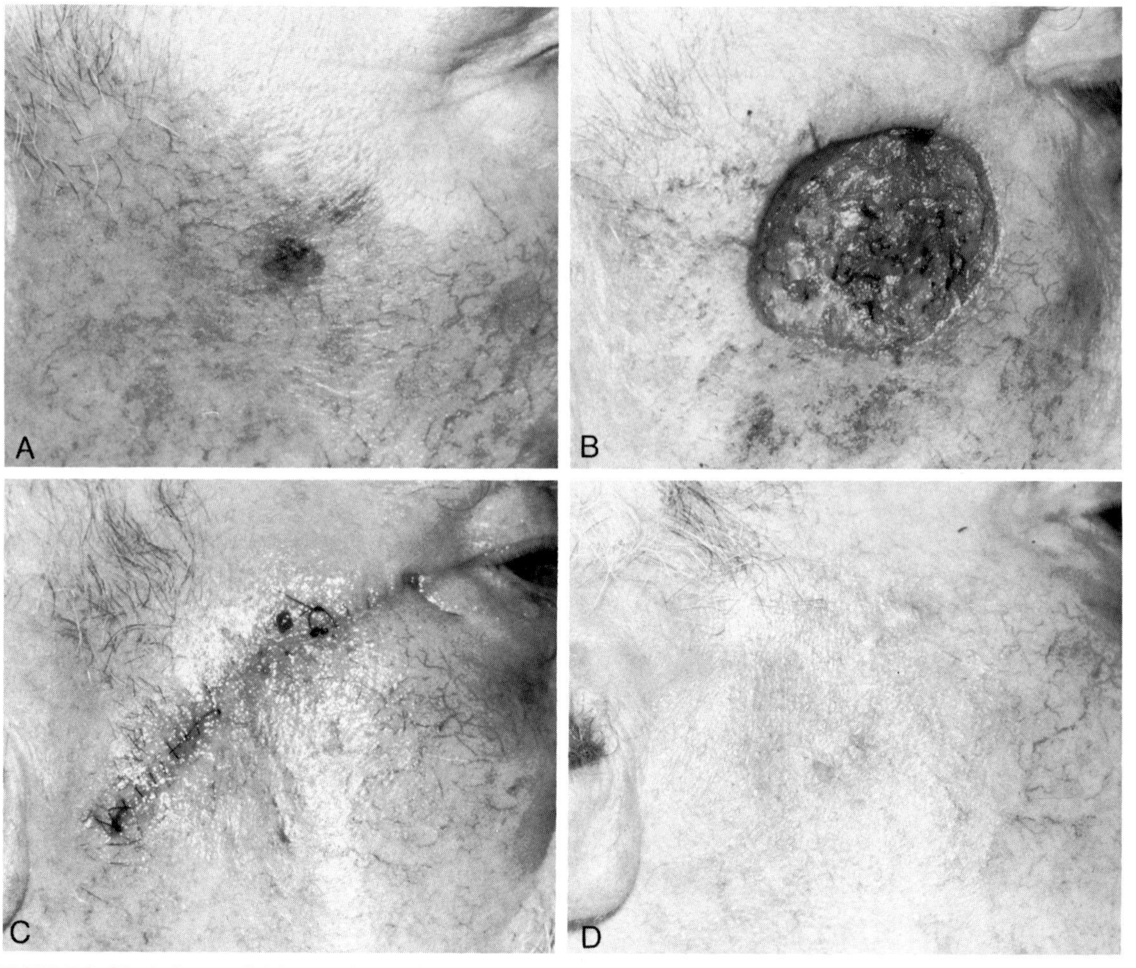

FIGURE 2–24. *A*, A superficial spreading melanoma in situ on the right cheek. *B*, Defect after two layers of Mohs surgery, fresh tissue technique. *C*, Appearance of wound after side-to-side closure. *D*, Healed wound at one month; no evidence of disease after 2 years of observation. Superficial spreading milanoma is a recognized pathological subtype of malignant melanoma.

because excess epinephrine could cause necrosis, although we have not encountered this complication in 29 cases of squamous cell carcinoma of the penis. The solution is injected 2 cm proximal to the cancer, to avoid implanting malignant cells along the needle tracts, or in a fan-like pattern at the base of the penis.

After the debulking procedure is complete, excess blood is wiped away with a cotton-tipped applicator. Then the wound is wiped with an applicator that has been dipped in full-strength dichloroacetic acid (or a saturated solution of trichloroacetic acid). The acid is also applied to a 2 mm zone of skin at the periphery. After the skin becomes white, the zinc chloride fixative paste is applied and an occlusive dressing is added. If the lesion is close to the urethral meatus, a waxy emollient (Orabase) that is insoluble in urine can be applied to the edge adjacent to the meatus. This emollient prevents the dressing from becoming wet and thus prevents the fixative paste from being diluted. The use of the fixative paste may cause a moderate degree of soft-tissue swelling. But any resulting urethral obstruction usually is not severe enough to necessitate catheterization, unless the patient has a preexisting meatal stricture or the spongy urethra is cancerous (Fig. 2–33D). (See Chapter 12.)

Cancerous Bone

When cancer involves facial bones and sinuses, selected areas of bone can be removed by chis-

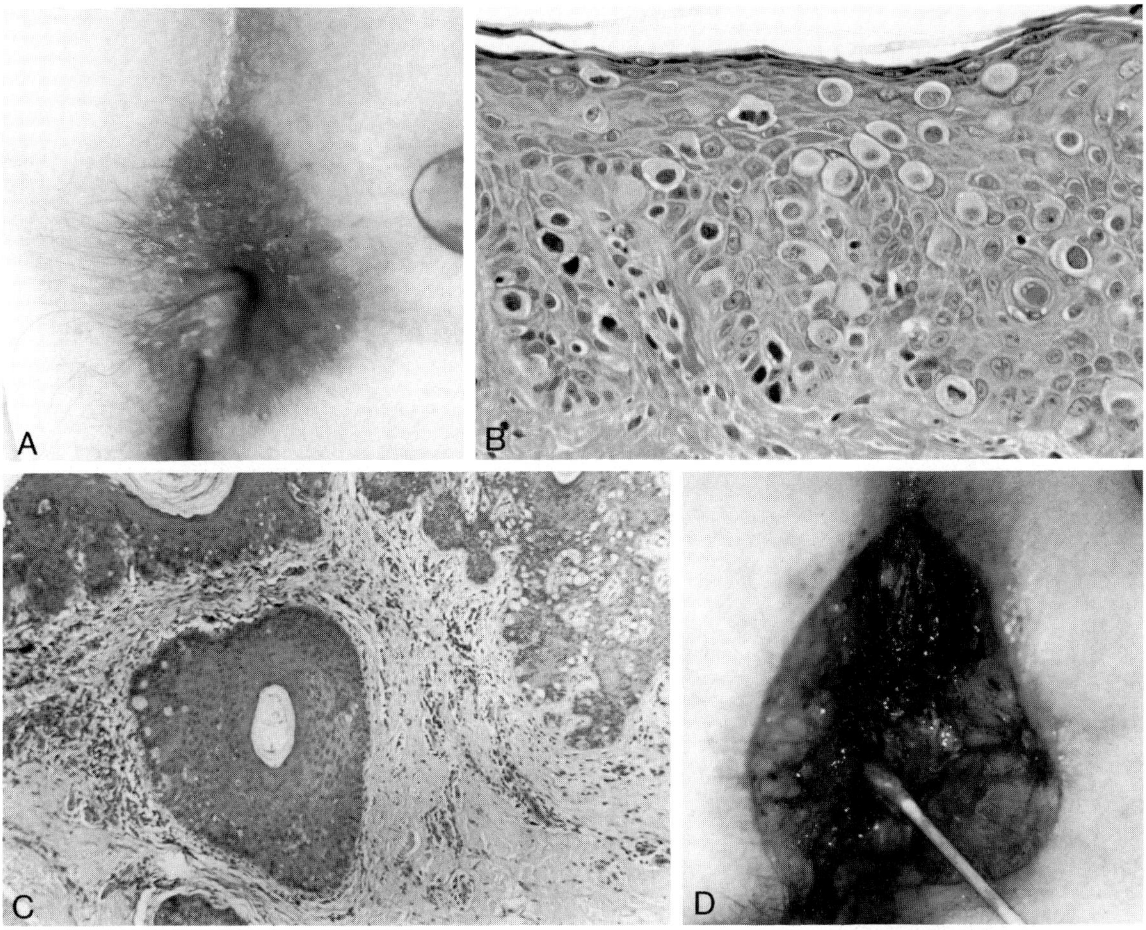

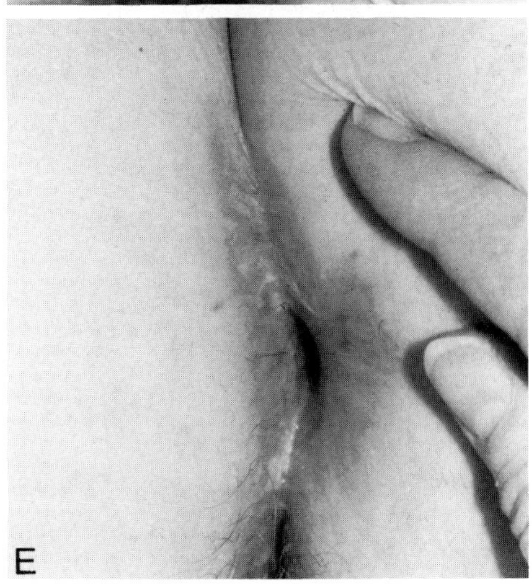

FIGURE 2–25. *A*, Appearance of recurrent extramammary Paget's disease of the perianal area. *B*, Photomicrograph shows extramammary Paget's cells throughout the full thickness of the epidermis. *C*, Extramammary Paget's cells with follicular involvement. *D*, Appearance of wound after five layers of Mohs surgery; the tumor extended 3 cm into the anal canal. *E*, Wound healed by second intention without complications. Seen here at one year; no evidence of disease after 5 years of observation.

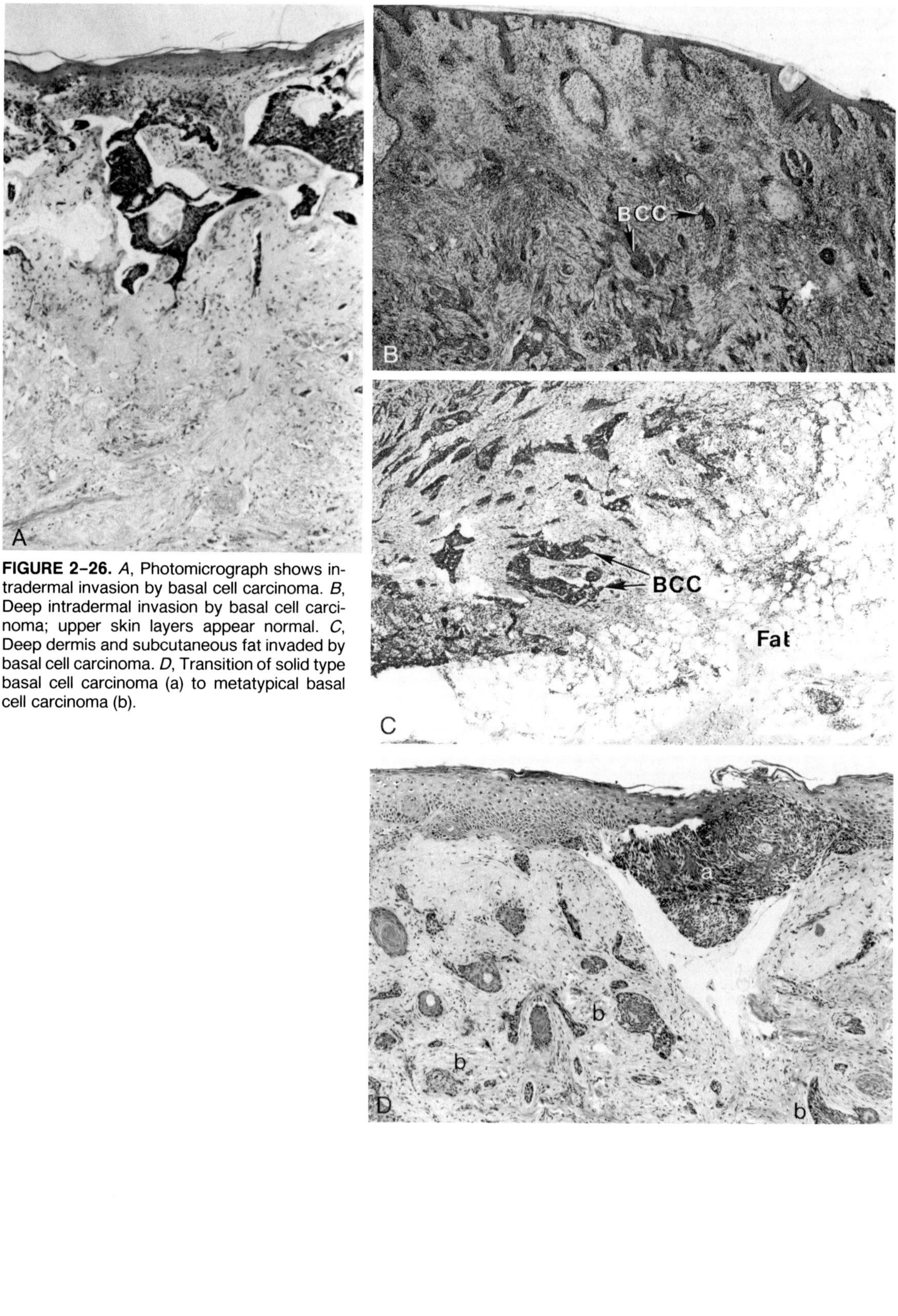

FIGURE 2–26. *A*, Photomicrograph shows intradermal invasion by basal cell carcinoma. *B*, Deep intradermal invasion by basal cell carcinoma; upper skin layers appear normal. *C*, Deep dermis and subcutaneous fat invaded by basal cell carcinoma. *D*, Transition of solid type basal cell carcinoma (a) to metatypical basal cell carcinoma (b).

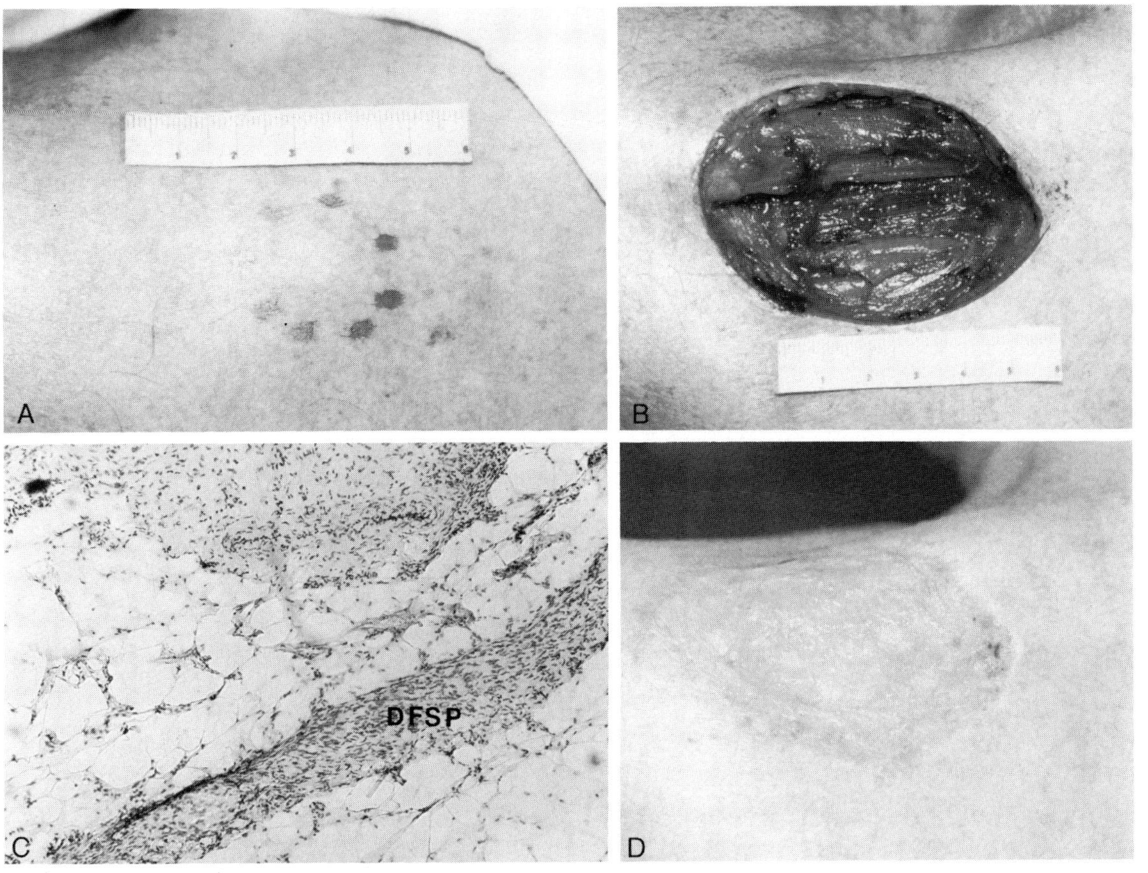

FIGURE 2–27. *A*, Dermatofibrosarcoma protuberans overlying the left posterior trapezius muscle of 3 months' duration. Patient's occupation is a telephone dispatcher, and this site is where the telephone rested. *B*, Defect after three layers of Mohs surgery; the vertical depth of penetration involved the fascia overlying the trapezius muscle which was also excised. *C*, Subcutaneous fibrous septum invaded by dermatofibrosarcoma protuberans. *D*, The defect was covered with a split-thickness skin graft; no evidence of disease after 3½ years.

eling or after they have been fixed with zinc chloride paste (Fig. 2–34). Decalcification and microscopic examination are then done to ensure that the tumor has been completely excised.[2] The excision of bone is accomplished using the standard procedure of applying zinc chloride fixative paste directly to the bone. (It is not necessary to pretreat the area with dichloroacetic acid, unless the tumor is a keratinizing basal cell carcinoma or a squamous cell carcinoma.) The paste is removed the next day, and bone samples are excised using rongeurs or a chisel; no anesthetic is needed because there is no pain in the fixed tissue. Alternatively, the bone can be allowed to spontaneously sequestrate from a bed of granulation tissue in 2 to 3 weeks. Bone specimens are usually decalcified in ethylenediaminetetraacetic acid (EDTA) overnight before they are sectioned on the cryostat.

The management of exposed bone by second intention healing consists of, first, applying an occlusive dressing that prevents the desiccation necrosis of cortical bone, then periodically chiseling away desiccated bone[55,56] until the exposed bone is covered by granulation tissue.

The bone is cleaned with mild soap and sterile saline solution every 1 to 2 days. Then it is covered with a layer of antibacterial ointment (Polysporin), or boric acid ophthalmic ointment, and a nonstick pad. Hydrogen peroxide can be used to clean the soft-tissue margins, but prolonged, direct application may desiccate the bone. Despite these measures, the central superficial layers of bone may become dry and thus prevent the migration of granulation tissue from the tissue margins. Desiccated bone proximal to the advancing margin of granulation tissue is gently chiseled away weekly until

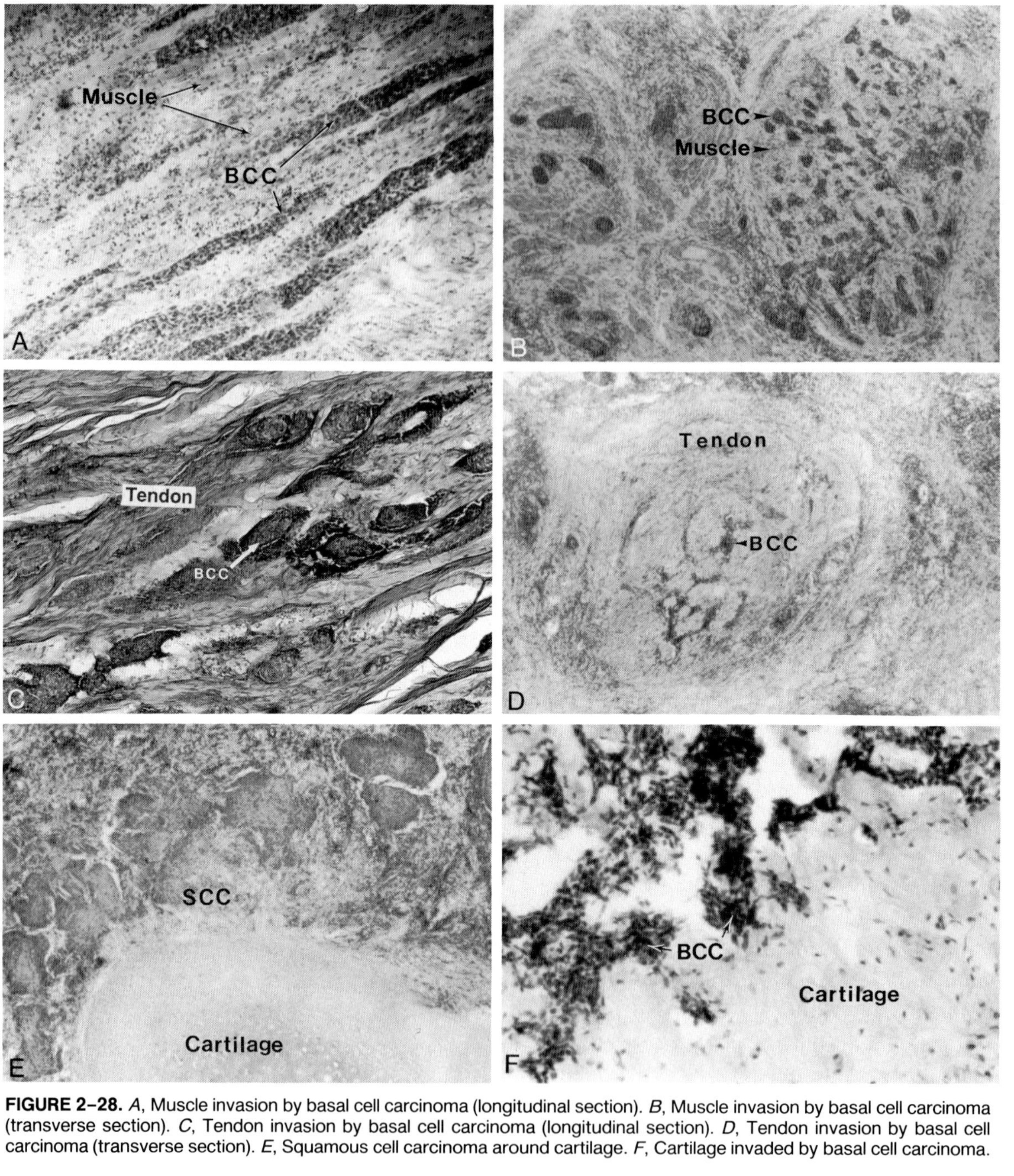

FIGURE 2–28. *A*, Muscle invasion by basal cell carcinoma (longitudinal section). *B*, Muscle invasion by basal cell carcinoma (transverse section). *C*, Tendon invasion by basal cell carcinoma (longitudinal section). *D*, Tendon invasion by basal cell carcinoma (transverse section). *E*, Squamous cell carcinoma around cartilage. *F*, Cartilage invaded by basal cell carcinoma.

the bone is covered by granulation tissue. Alternatively, granulations can be stimulated centrally by partially decorticating the bone using the power drill or chisel until spontaneous bleeding occurs.[56] Complete decortication into the spongy bone yields granulations within 1 week.

After the bone is covered by granulation tissue, it can be covered with a skin graft or allowed to reepithelialize from the periphery. Healing by granulation tissue is time-consuming. It may take 4 to 6 weeks for a 2 cm diameter wound to heal by second intention.[56] Skin grafts may be preferred for large defects be-

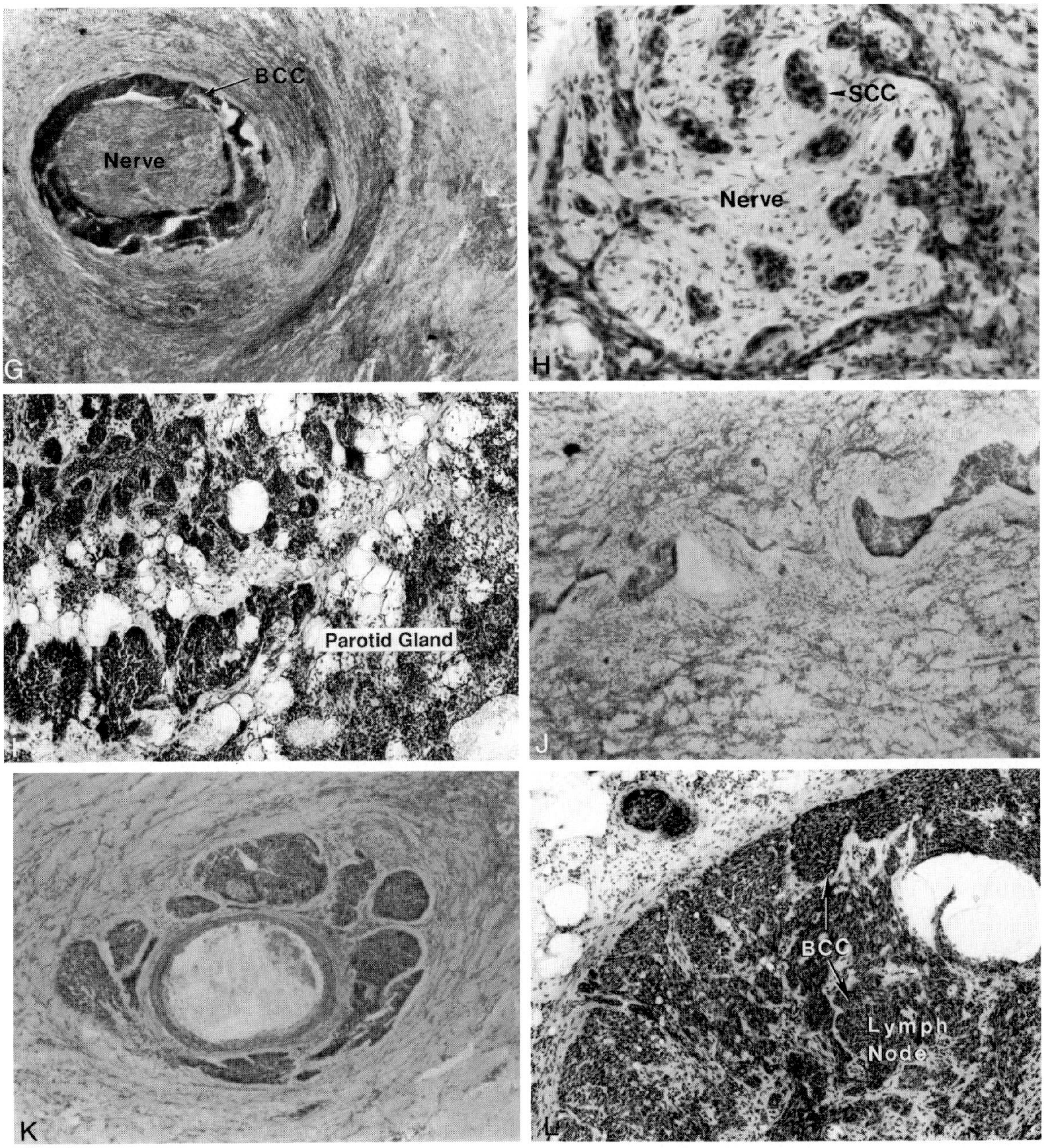

FIGURE 2–28. *Continued G*, Perineural extension of basal cell carcinoma (transverse section). *H*, Intraneural extension of squamous cell carcinoma (transverse section). *I*, Parotid gland invasion by basal cell carcinoma. *J*, Intralymphatic vessel extension of basal cell carcinoma within subcutaneous tissue (courtesy of Thomas Myers, M.D.). *K*, Basal cell carcinoma in perivascular lymphatics (courtesy of Thomas Myers, M.D.). *L*, Lymph node invaded by basal cell carcinoma.

Illustration continued on following page

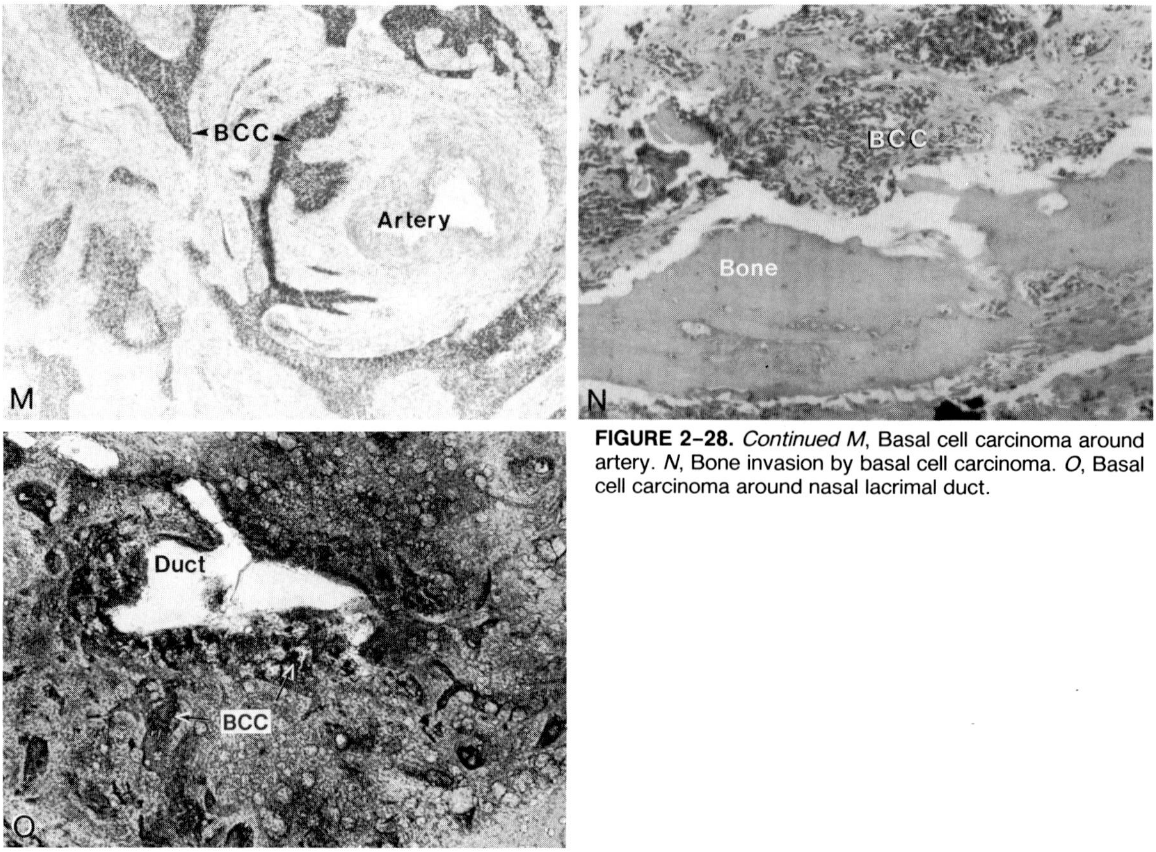

FIGURE 2–28. *Continued M*, Basal cell carcinoma around artery. *N*, Bone invasion by basal cell carcinoma. *O*, Basal cell carcinoma around nasal lacrimal duct.

cause the spontaneously reepithelialized epidermal layer is unstable and readily breaks down with minor trauma. When dealing with recurrent tumors, healing by second intention may be preferred to local skin flaps.

The thickness of cortical bone varies with its anatomic location and with the patient's age and sex. Decortication in the temple region may be performed after appropriate consultation. Care should be taken not to inadvertently perforate the spongy bone and inner table of the temple region, where the bone may be no more than 3 mm thick. Bone that has been previously irradiated is sclerotic and contains few fibroblasts; it will not heal readily by granulation. Such exposed bone should be covered with either a local skin flap or a free flap.

Exposed bone is kept moist with a layer of antibacterial ointment and a double layer of petrolatum gauze, iodoform gauze, or Adaptic dressing. A bulky dressing consisting of fluffed cotton balls or gauze is added to provide a cushion, to level the defect with the surrounding skin margin, and to absorb tissue fluids, excess ointment, and perspiration. On large areas of exposed bone, the dressing is changed every 2 to 3 days. The bandage is removed, and the wound is cleaned with sterile water or saline and washed with diluted povidone (greater than 1:100) soap or baby shampoo. Antibacterial ointment and dressing are then reapplied. Microfoam tape protects the underlying skin from injury caused by frequently applying and removing tape. On the scalp, Band-net netting will hold the dressing in place without tape.

Recurrent Neoplasms

Tumors that recur after Mohs micrographic surgery (fresh tissue technique), radiation, chemotherapy, or cryosurgery can be successfully treated with the fixed tissue technique. The advantages are (1) the need for local anesthesia, which may implant malignant cells along the needle tracts, is obviated, and (2) it

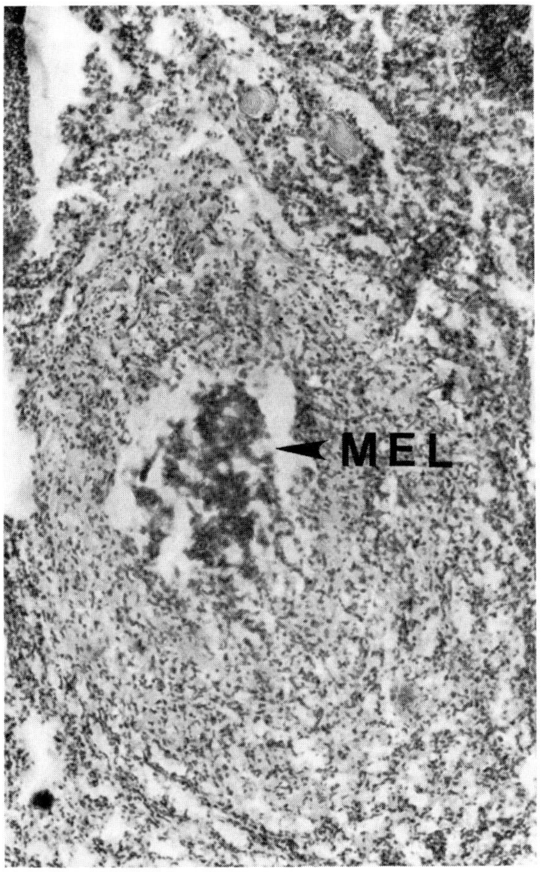

FIGURE 2–29. Local melanoma satellitosis in a patient with a nodular melanoma of the nasal bridge removed by the fixed-tissue technique.

avoids seeding malignant cells because the excision is done in nonviable, fixed tissue.

Limitations

Mohs surgery is an excellent means of treating some cancers, but there are situations in which other methods can provide similar cure rates and similar cosmetic results. Several extenuating circumstances should also be considered in the overall evaluation of a patient's treatment. These factors include the patient's general health, anticoagulant medication, tumor size, cost and duration of treatment, and transportation problems (Table 2–4).

For small lesions, the removal of layered specimens sometimes necessitates the excision of more tissue than is needed to cure the cancer. For superficial and nodular basal cell tumors, treatment by curettage and desiccation often provides comparable cure rates and sometimes better esthetic results. For cancers of the trunk and extremities, the advantages of the Mohs technique are not as obvious as for facial cancers.

TABLE 2–4. Disadvantages of Mohs Micrographic Surgery

Labor intensive and time-consuming procedure (requires an average of 3 hours to treat a cancer)
Limited number of qualified Mohs surgeons (physicians need training in skin surgery, pathology, and oncology)
More expensive than traditional outpatient surgery because of special laboratory processing and microscopic examination (requires specialized histologic laboratory and high-quality binocular microscope)

Noncancerous Conditions

The fixed tissue technique also may be used for gangrenous digits,[57] chronic osteomyelitis,[58] and radiodermatitis.[59] Among diabetics, about 75% of appendages are saved through treatment with the fixed tissue technique rather than with limb amputation. The cause of the beneficial effects of the zinc chloride paste have not been thoroughly studied, but such effects may be due to the stimulation of inflammation, the angiogenesis of granulation tissue, or a bactericidal effect on infected tissue.[60] Diabetic patients who are also organ-transplant recipients have very poor peripheral circulation and may not benefit from the application of zinc chloride paste to gangrenous tissue.

OVERALL PERSPECTIVE

Ideally, facial skin cancers should be entirely excised while as much normal tissue as possible is preserved. The method should be simple, painless, curative, cost-effective, and widely available. No one method of excision meets all these criteria, but micrographic surgery comes very close. For small cancers, and for patients who refuse surgery and local anesthesia, radiation therapy and topical chemotherapy are reasonable alternatives. Good results also can be obtained with electrocautery and cryosurgery. When the total excision of the cancer and the maximum preservation of normal facial struc-

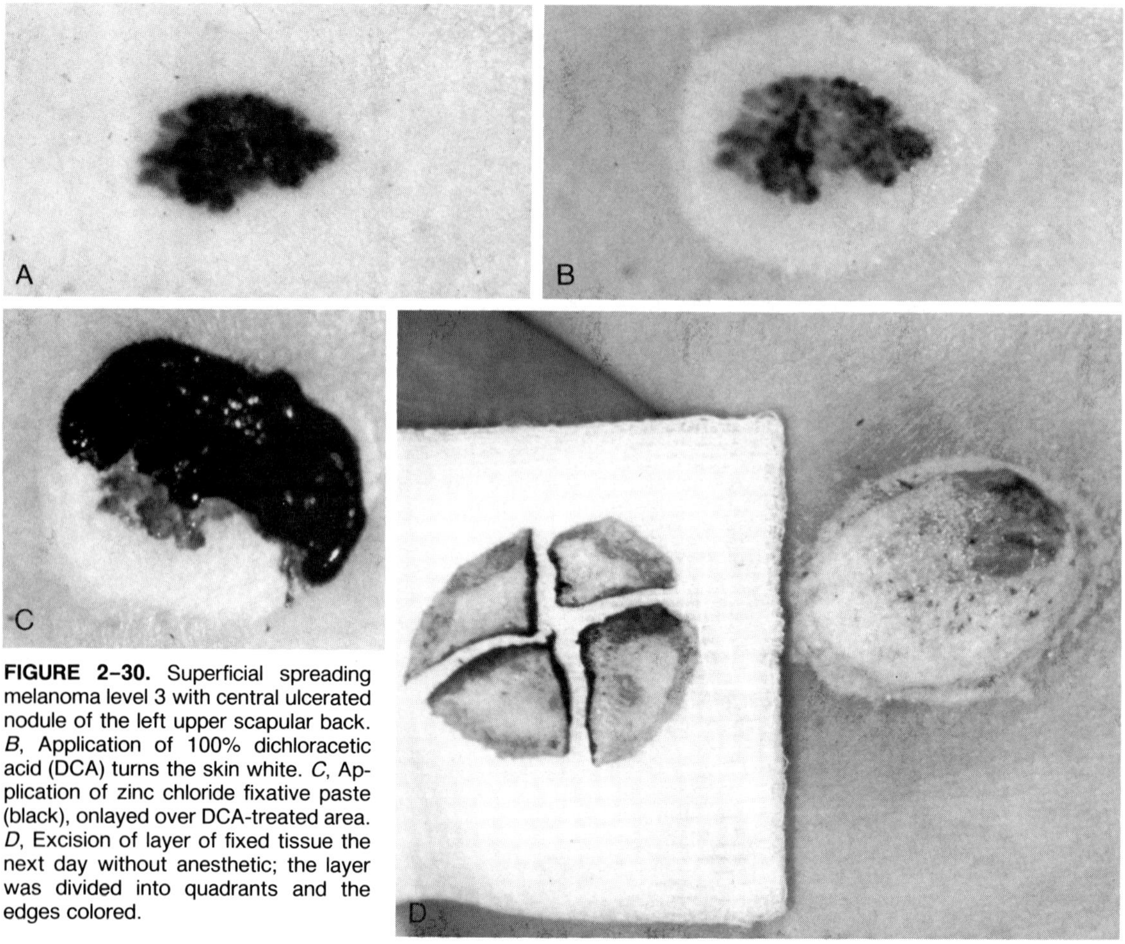

FIGURE 2–30. Superficial spreading melanoma level 3 with central ulcerated nodule of the left upper scapular back. *B*, Application of 100% dichloracetic acid (DCA) turns the skin white. *C*, Application of zinc chloride fixative paste (black), onlayed over DCA-treated area. *D*, Excision of layer of fixed tissue the next day without anesthetic; the layer was divided into quadrants and the edges colored.

tures is desired, Mohs micrographic excision gives the best results.

SCALPEL TECHNIQUE

Mohs surgery is performed with the scalpel held in the pencil grip. This grip naturally offsets the angle of the scalpel blade and provides a beveled incision 30 to 45 degress from the vertical plane (Fig. 2–35). The exact angle is not important as long as a complete, intact cutaneous edge is included on the peripheral specimens. It is, however, easier for the technician to bring up the cutaneous edge of the specimen when the angle is 45 degress rather than 90 degrees. A No. 10 scalpel blade can be used with large tumors to provide a larger, layered excision.

The lateral palm of the hand holding the scalpel is gently rested on the patient to stabilize the scalpel. Precise control of the scalpel is provided by the action of the interosseous muscles of the hand and the forearm muscles. Firm, steady traction is provided by the assistant and surgeon. The initial, circumferential incision establishes a smooth outline of the intradermal excision necessary for the scalpel exit during the horizontal excision of the first layer of tissue. An even skin contour devoid of intracutaneous nicks creates an unblemished tissue margin that, when sectioned, provides a complete layer of tissue without tissue voids.

For convenience, the incision is divided into thirds, which may be unequal arcs of a circle or an ellipse, depending on the outline of the tumor. For right-handed surgeons, the positional limits are from 12 to 5 o'clock for the first third, from 9 to 5 o'clock for the second, and from 12 to 9 o'clock for the third. The first third is cut with the forehand position, the second with the backhand position, and the third is cut with a sidestroke incision. Each incision intersects the preceding one at precisely the

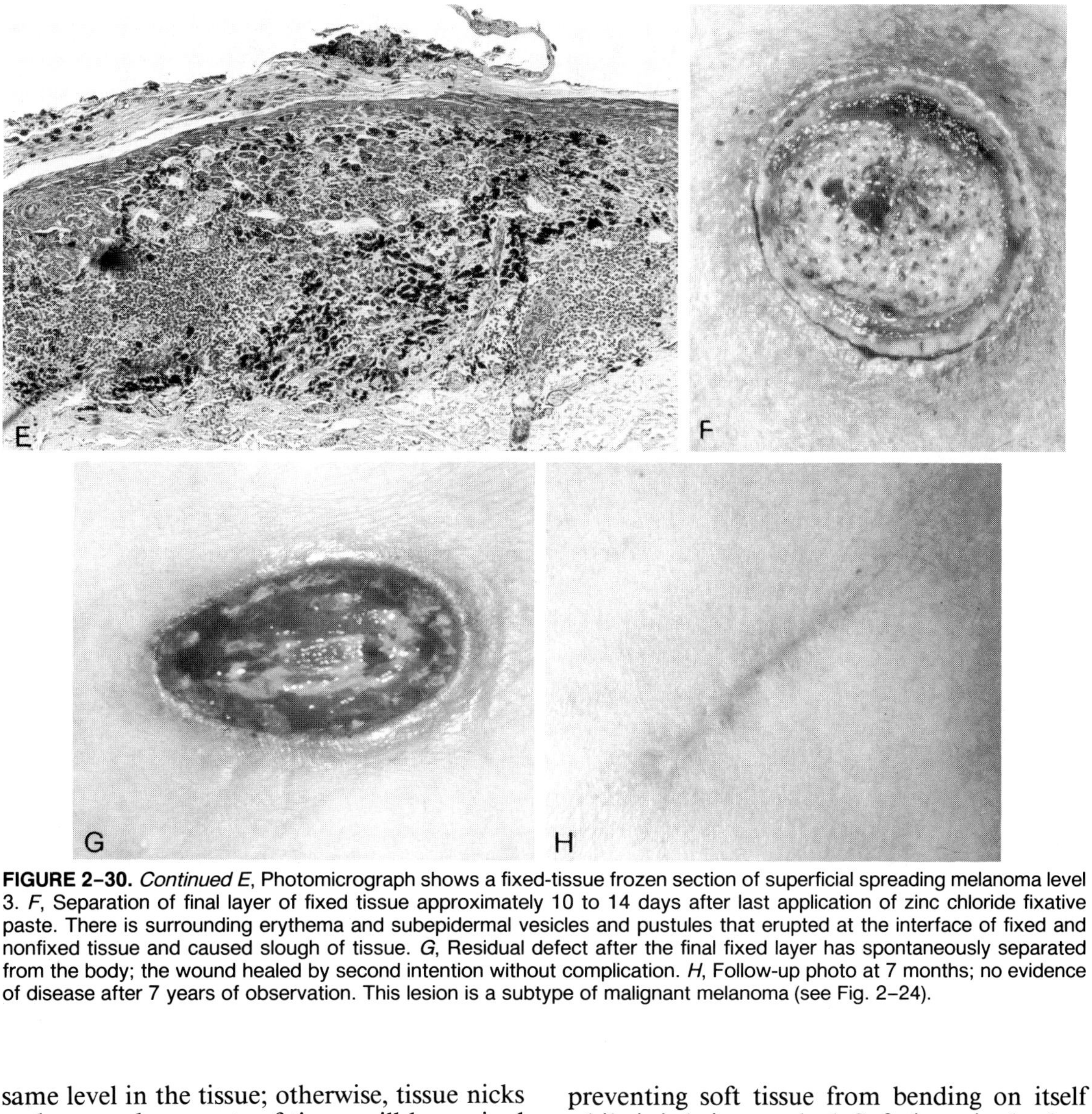

FIGURE 2–30. *Continued E*, Photomicrograph shows a fixed-tissue frozen section of superficial spreading melanoma level 3. *F*, Separation of final layer of fixed tissue approximately 10 to 14 days after last application of zinc chloride fixative paste. There is surrounding erythema and subepidermal vesicles and pustules that erupted at the interface of fixed and nonfixed tissue and caused slough of tissue. *G*, Residual defect after the final fixed layer has spontaneously separated from the body; the wound healed by second intention without complication. *H*, Follow-up photo at 7 months; no evidence of disease after 7 years of observation. This lesion is a subtype of malignant melanoma (see Fig. 2–24).

same level in the tissue; otherwise, tissue nicks and unequal amounts of tissue will be excised and will diminish the likelihood of complete tissue excision and uniform tissue freezing.

Individual variations, the use or nonuse of circumferential incisions, and the sequence of incisions vary among surgeons. The sub-bursting pressure of the scalpel is generally reserved for superficial cancers and cancers of the nose, ears, and eyelids, where a single intradermal stage of excision may be sufficient to completely remove the tumor. Bursting pressure through dermis into fat is done for deeper cancers that overlay fatty tissue and where closure is anticipated.

Plain forceps provide the advantage of a relatively broad platform for grasping tissue and preventing soft tissue from bending on itself while it is being marked. Soft tissue is also less likely to be torn or punctured with plain forceps than with toothed forceps. Toothed forceps allow eyelid skin to be precisely handled, but their narrow tips also cause soft tissues to fold, which sometimes interferes with the proper marking of individual tissue margins. The use of platform toothed or spatulated Russian forceps may prevent tissue folding of the flats. Mohs surgery is easier if sharp serrated scissors are used to excise layers of soft fatty tissue from eyelids, cheeks, and extremities. Serrated scissors grip the tissue and prevent it from sliding away as the cutting blades are brought together. Scissors are also useful for dividing large layers into smaller specimens. If a

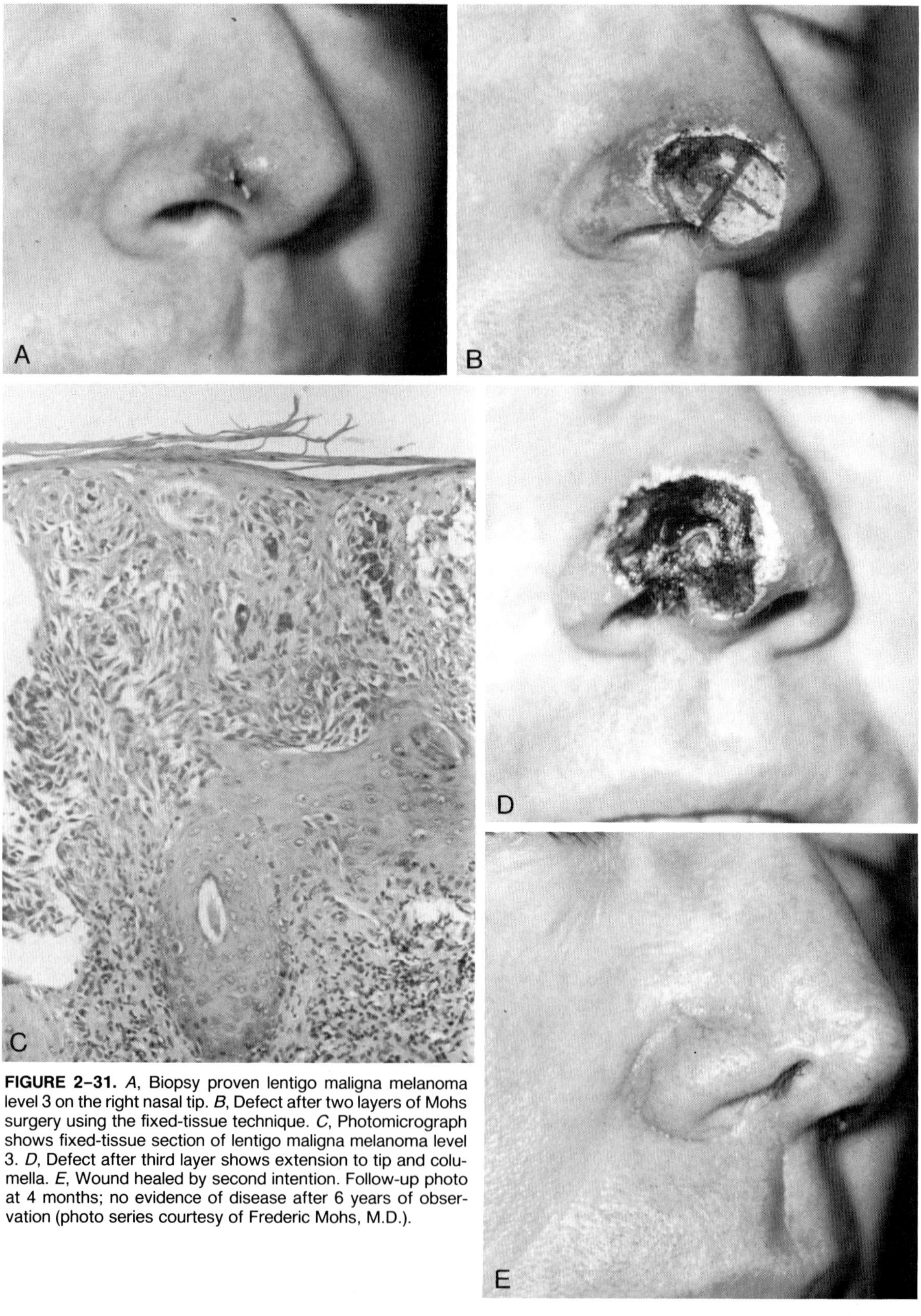

FIGURE 2–31. *A*, Biopsy proven lentigo maligna melanoma level 3 on the right nasal tip. *B*, Defect after two layers of Mohs surgery using the fixed-tissue technique. *C*, Photomicrograph shows fixed-tissue section of lentigo maligna melanoma level 3. *D*, Defect after third layer shows extension to tip and columella. *E*, Wound healed by second intention. Follow-up photo at 4 months; no evidence of disease after 6 years of observation (photo series courtesy of Frederic Mohs, M.D.).

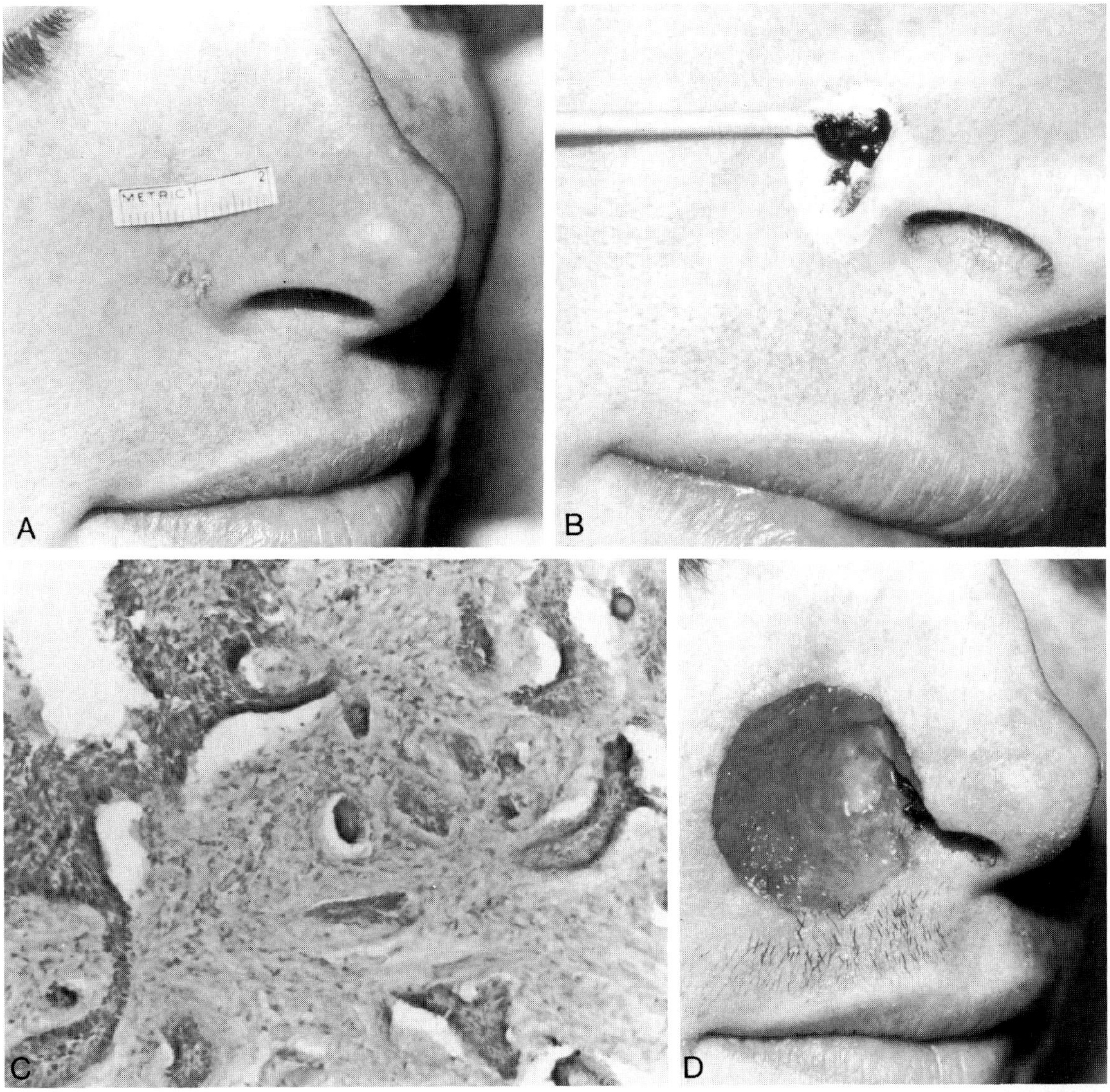

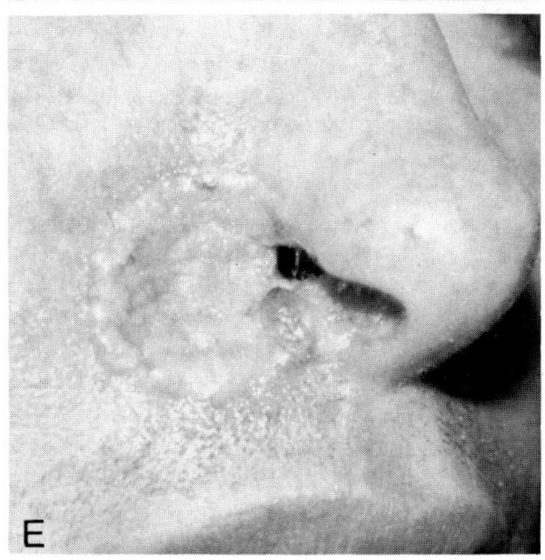

FIGURE 2–32. *A*, Biopsy proven morphea-like basal cell carcinoma of the right nasal labial fold in a patient with acquired immunodeficiency syndrome (AIDS). The tumor was recurrent after previous surgical excision. The fixed-tissue technique was used to kill the tissue and avoid blood exposure. *B*, Application of zinc chloride fixative paste. *C*, Microscopic examination of the fixed tissue showed obvious basal cell carcinoma deep in the dermis of the nose and cheek. *D*, Defect before repair with split-thickness skin graft. *E*, Follow-up photo at 2½ months; no evidence of disease after 3 years of observation.

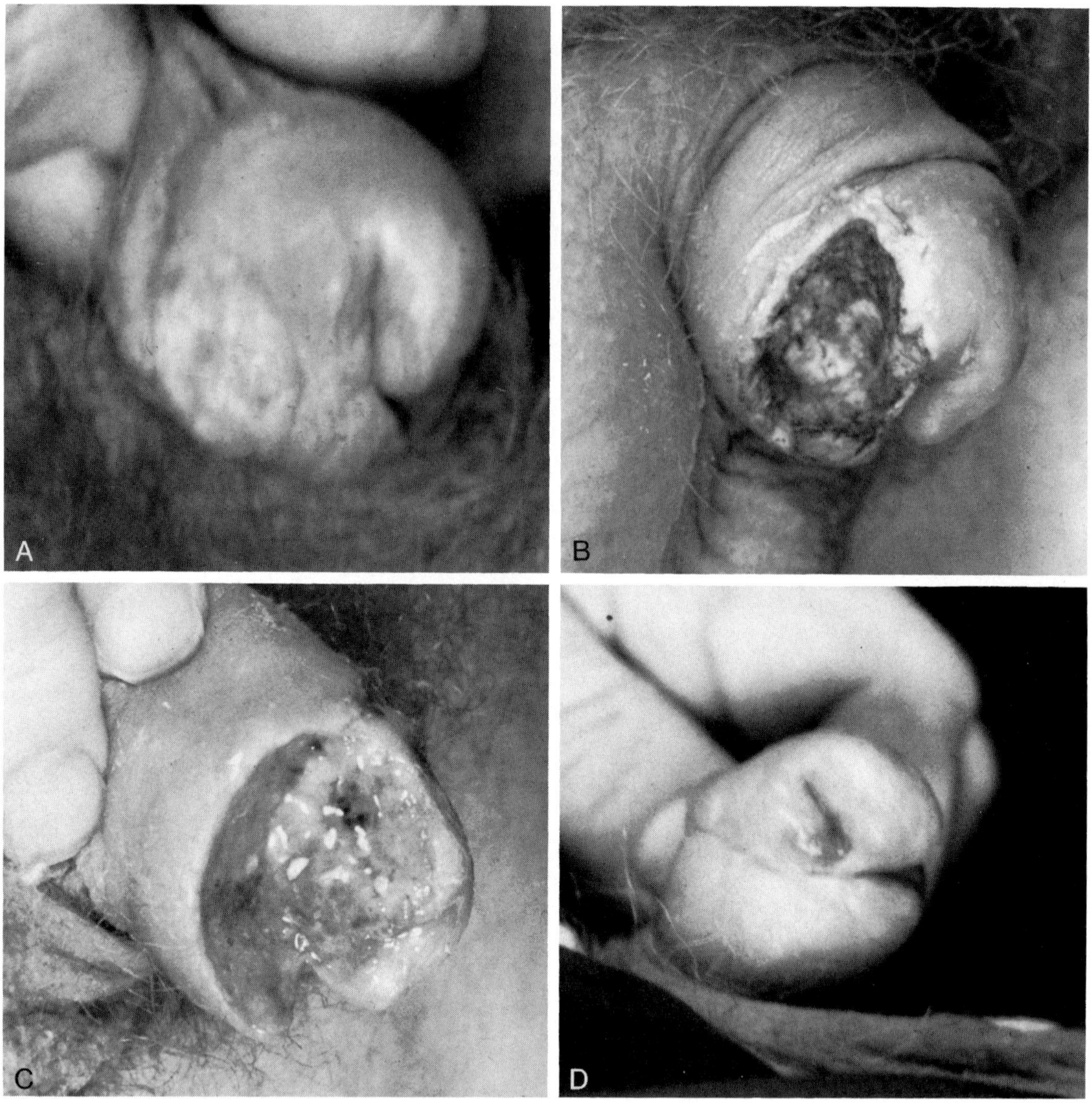

FIGURE 2–33. *A*, A recurrent squamous cell carcinoma of the right glans penis; the tumor had been previously treated by radiation, surgery, and curettage. *B*, Wound after five layers Mohs surgery—fixed-tissue techinque. *C*, Wound after separation of final layer of fixed tissue. *D*, Healed lesion: There was slight deviation of urine flow; however, sexual function was normal. No evidence of disease after 7 years of observation (photo series courtesy of Frederic Mohs, M.D.).

scalpel is used to subdivide tissue, a small plastic cutting board provides a firm surface to cut against.

Mohs layers can be scored in situ (Fig. 2–36) to provide an accurate method of determining the origins of tissue specimens. With this technique, a partial layer is taken from beyond the area where the tissue is to be scored. Both the specimen and the adjacent skin margin are nicked as the scalpel is drawn across the layer. The free margin of the remaining tissue is thereby undercut, so the scalpel can be reintroduced to completely cut the layer. Staples, sutures, or ink markers are more durable. Other means for locating the origin of specimens include sutures, staples, colored inks, photographs, and anatomic landmarks.

SEMISTERILE PROCEDURE

Even though Mohs surgery is generally conducted under semisterile conditions, infections have been extremely rare because of general

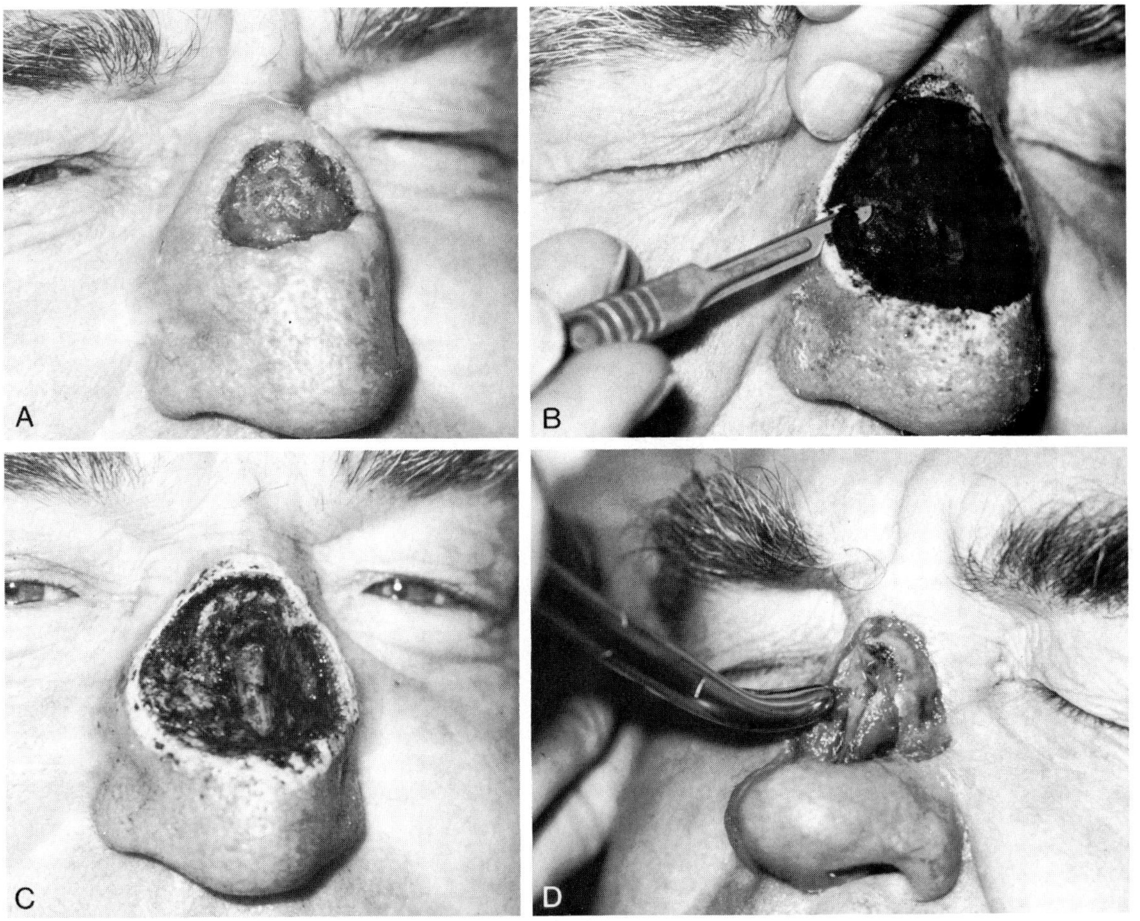

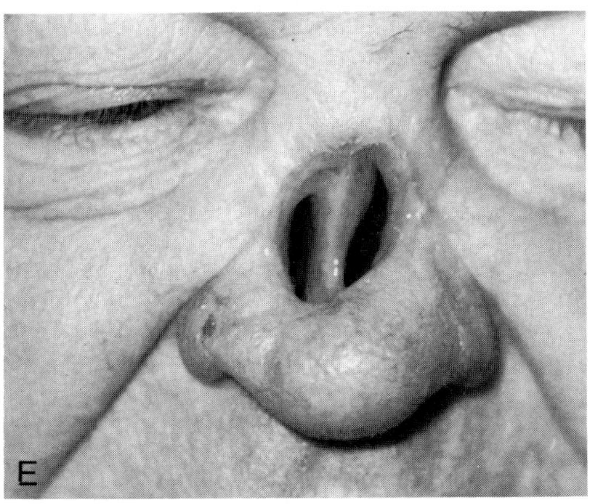

FIGURE 2–34. *A*, Recurrent squamous cell carcinoma of the bridge of nose, previously treated by excision and cryosurgery. *B*, Excision by fixed-tissue technique. *C*, Defect at completion of three layers of treatment. *D*, Appearance of granulations after separation of final layer of fixed tissue; excision of nasal bone with rongeur. *E*, Follow-up photo at 6 months; no evidence of disease after 7 years of observation.

precautions and good surgical technique. Proper disinfection (the chemical killing of bacteria) and sterilization (the chemical and physical killing of all forms of microbial life, including spores) are essential for both Mohs surgery and dermatologic surgery.[61] The proper selection of patients and the maintenance of clean work habits help ensure a germ-free environment and guard against self- and cross-contamination and the development of surgical complications. Patients and personnel with obvious pustular acne or herpetic lesions, for example, carry potentially contagious bacteria and viruses.

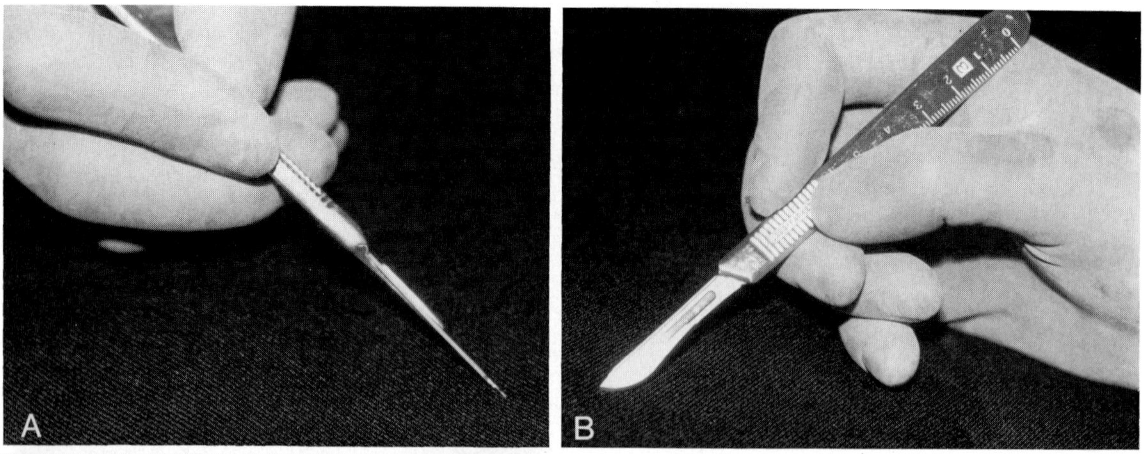

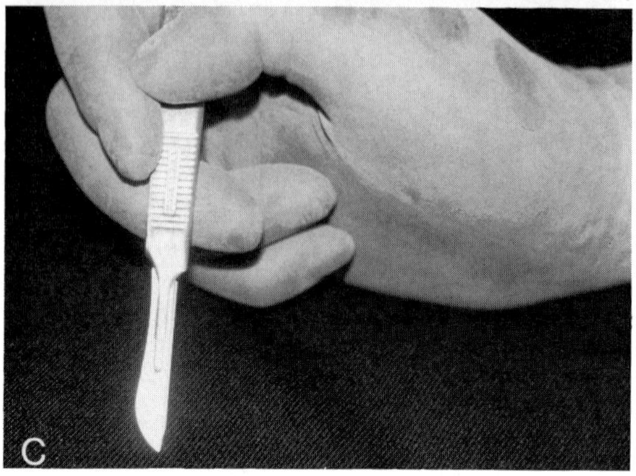

FIGURE 2–35. *A*, Scalpel position showing 45-degree beveled incision (frontal view). *B*, Forehand position of scalpel; the scalpel moves in the direction of the blade, toward the body. *C*, Backhand position of scalpel; the scalpel moves in direction of blade, away from the body.

Protective Wear

Sterile gloves are mandatory. A surgical cap and face mask are cumbersome, but they prevent hair and oral and nasal droplets from contaminating the surgical site. The need for protective wear is especially true if the surgeon or assistant has a head cold. A recent study found that about 4% of commercial latex gloves have invisible puncture holes.[62] In lengthy procedures, excessive sweating in gloves washes luminal bacteria to the skin surface and these may discharge into the operative field if the gloves are defective. Used gloves should not be washed and reused. Surfactants may cause "wicking" through undetected holes. Disinfectants may cause glove deterioration.

Disinfectants

Isopropyl alcohol (70%) is used to disinfect all surgical areas, including the scalp, except the genital area, perianal area, and the lower legs and feet—for which povidone-iodine (Betadine) is recommended. Iodoform is an excellent surgical scrub that kills a broad range of bacteria and viruses and produces few adverse

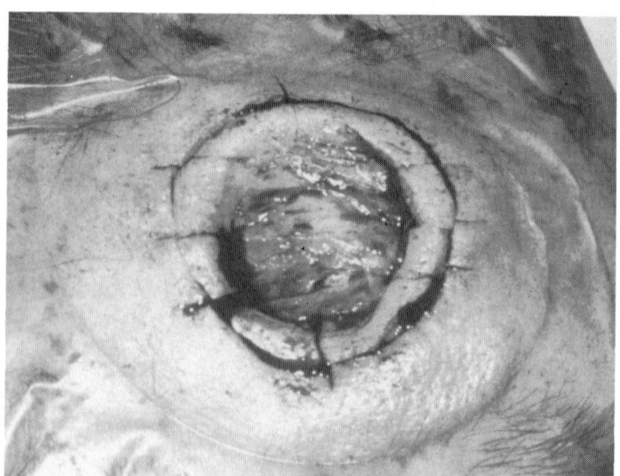

FIGURE 2–36. Photograph shows the division and origin of eight specimens after the layer of tissue was scored and the matching skin margins nicked (courtesy of George Mikhail, M.D.).

reactions. Povidone-iodine is also toxic to dividing cells, even in low concentrations, and should not be used inside open wounds unless followed by irrigation. Chlorhexidine (Hibiclens or Bactoshield 2) is also excellent; it causes very little contact dermatitis and photosensitivity but, in high concentrations, irritates the eyes. Deafness has been reported when chlorhexidine was introduced into the middle ear through perforated ear drums.

Drapes

Sterile surgical drapes are used to protect the surgical field against contamination from adjacent nonsterile skin. Cloth or disposable fenestrated drapes should be wider than the length of the suture to prevent any contamination of the suture tail, which often extends beyond the site of the operation. In small or brief operations, additional holes in plastic drapes may be made to improve ventilation of the nose and mouth to lessen patient anxiety and feelings of claustrophobia. Use cloth drapes for hairy areas and adhesive drapes for predominantly non–hair-bearing areas. In complex repairs of the face, drapes are preferably placed pericranially to expose the entire face, so that repairs may be readily assessed from all angles.

Postoperative Washing

Both sutured and open wounds of the soft tissues are treated similarly. Except for contaminated wounds or defects exposing ear cartilage, the postsurgical site is generally not disturbed until the second postoperative day. Ear wounds are cleaned after the first day to reduce the possibility of chondritis by covering them with a layer of antibiotic ointment and bandage. If cartilage is exposed during the excision of a layer, to save time, the remaining cartilage is usually carefully fenestrated in the same operative session, and the patient is asked to return one week later. Desiccated cartilage is excised, and the patient is asked to return in 3 weeks if wound healing is not progressing at a satisfactory pace. Wounds about the eyes are gently irrigated with tepid water only, followed by a thin layer of antibacterial ointment. In other noncritical areas, the wound is gently washed twice a day with soap and water, followed by hydrogen peroxide for irrigation and to remove dead tissue. Hydrogen peroxide may be used alone if washing with soap and water is inconvenient. An adhesive bandage is placed over a sutured wound for appearances, or it may be exposed to the air. Dry open wounds are kept reasonably moist with antibacterial ointment and a thick bandage. Overly moist open wounds are made dry by applying merbromine and using a hair dryer. The amount of ointment and bandage used to cover the wound should be no more than necessary to encourage the wound to form a very thin flaky crust.

Mohs surgery is practiced under as sterile conditions as possible within the limitations of working around the nose, lips, and ears, which normally contain a variety of organisms. Moreover, the pilosebaceous units contain many bacteria and other flora that make it impossible to completely eliminate them with normal surgical scrubbing. Because 20% of the resident skin flora is beyond the reach of scrubbing and antiseptics, the skin cannot be sterilized. Open wounds are often colonized, but they are not necessarily infected if necrotic tissue is removed daily. Periodic cleaning with soap and water or hydrogen peroxide is a simple measure that removes bacteria-laden organic debris and minimizes the amount of resident flora until granulation tissue is stimulated. There are many resident bacteria on the face, but good blood circulation and strict sterile procedures minimize wound contamination.

Bleeding should be controlled with pinpoint electrocoagulation to minimize the amount of necrotic tissue and to reduce the chance of bacteria colonizing the necrotic tissue. The accumulation of more than 10^6 bacteria/mm^3 forebodes infection.

Antibiotic Prophylaxis

There is some justification for using prophylactic antibiotics for clean wounds in the axilla and groin.[61] These areas are more prone to the development of incipient infections after dermatologic surgery.

OUTPATIENT SURGERY

Same-day outpatient surgery is a safe, efficient, cost-effective means of providing good health care that has been practiced by dermatologists and other surgical specialists (otolaryngologists, ophthalmologists, gynecologists, and plastic surgeons) for decades. Outpatient sur-

TABLE 2–5. Advantages of Outpatient Surgery

Surgical
Minimum cost for draping, instruments, electrocautery, pharmaceuticals (e.g., anesthesia, antibotics, and analgesics).
Preoperative blood chemistries, chest x-ray, and electrocardiogram may not be necessary.

Hospital
No operating room, recovery room, or hospital bed charges.

Administrative
Time managment is more efficient.
Patient scheduling is easier because it is directly controlled by one physician rather than a Control Room scheduling many surgeons that perform a variety of operations of varying duration.

Personnel
Does not require specialized operating room nurses (scrub, circulating, other), recovery room personnel, or postoperative surgical floor nurses.

gery often saves time and money and is more convenient for both the patient and physician. Greater efficiency allows more time for the development of a more personal relationship among physician, patient, nurse, and secretary that promotes the continuity and long-term follow-up necessary for patients with skin cancer. Regular quality assurance reviews help identify and resolve problems in a timely manner. Outpatient surgery has several economic advantages over inpatient surgery (Table 2–5).

Operating Facilities

An office-based outpatient surgical facility can be organized into separate groups of rooms. This arrangement should provide specific areas for reception, treatment, and recovery so that all patients can be easily and directly observed from a central nursing station from the beginning to the end of their treatment. No surgery should ever be considered a minor procedure, but a large treatment room where more complicated surgery is performed should be close to the nursing station. Less complicated procedures, such as suture removal, are usually performed in rooms farther away. Over the years, most professional facilities have evolved along this general plan, although the specific amount of space allocated to individual areas often varies. Ideally, the overall layout should convey a comfortable, yet efficient, professional appearance. It should be compact to save steps and have relatively wide hallways for an unimpeded, two-directional flow of traffic. The atmosphere should reflect a clean, meticulous, well-organized, high-quality medical facility.

The three most important things a good treatment room should have are space, lighting, and storage cabinets (Fig. 2–37).

Space. Treatment rooms can be divided into those containing operating chairs and those containing operating tables. Depending on the style of practice, the ratio of chairs to tables may range from 2 to 1 to 4 to 1. Ideally, the rooms should measure about 12 × 14 feet for chairs and 12 × 16 feet for tables; when cabinets and sink are added, the open areas may be reduced to about 12 × 10 feet and 12 × 12 feet. It is useful to divide the room in halves to distinguish the patient changing area from the sterile surgical area where the procedures are performed. The surgical table should be located in the middle of the room, with the patient facing the door so that his or her face can be seen from outside the room. There should be about 3 feet of clearance room at the ends of the table and 4 feet at the sides to allow easy access to the patient by the physician, surgical assistant, and circulating nurse. A circulating nurse is needed for complicated cases to provide additional surgical assistance, to monitor the patient, and to replenish supplies during the operation. The open area allows for the movement of wheelchairs and gurneys, the free rotation of surgical tables, gurneys, and stools, and convenient access to countertop materials and instruments.

Lighting. There should be two sources of light: room light and surgical light. Room light should be from fluorescent bulbs that are located in the ceiling and that light the central working area. Ceiling modules that each contain four 4-foot bulbs (40 watts per bulb) are ideal. The ceiling lights should be offset to accommodate surgical lights. Surgical lighting can be from either tract or point-source lights. Tract lighting with double-point source is best for tables because the entire area from the patient's head to feet can be lit from several directions. Point-source overhead lights are cumbersome for tables unless they can be rotated 360 degrees. Dual lighting is preferred when two surgeons are operating simultaneously at different sites. Single-point source lights are

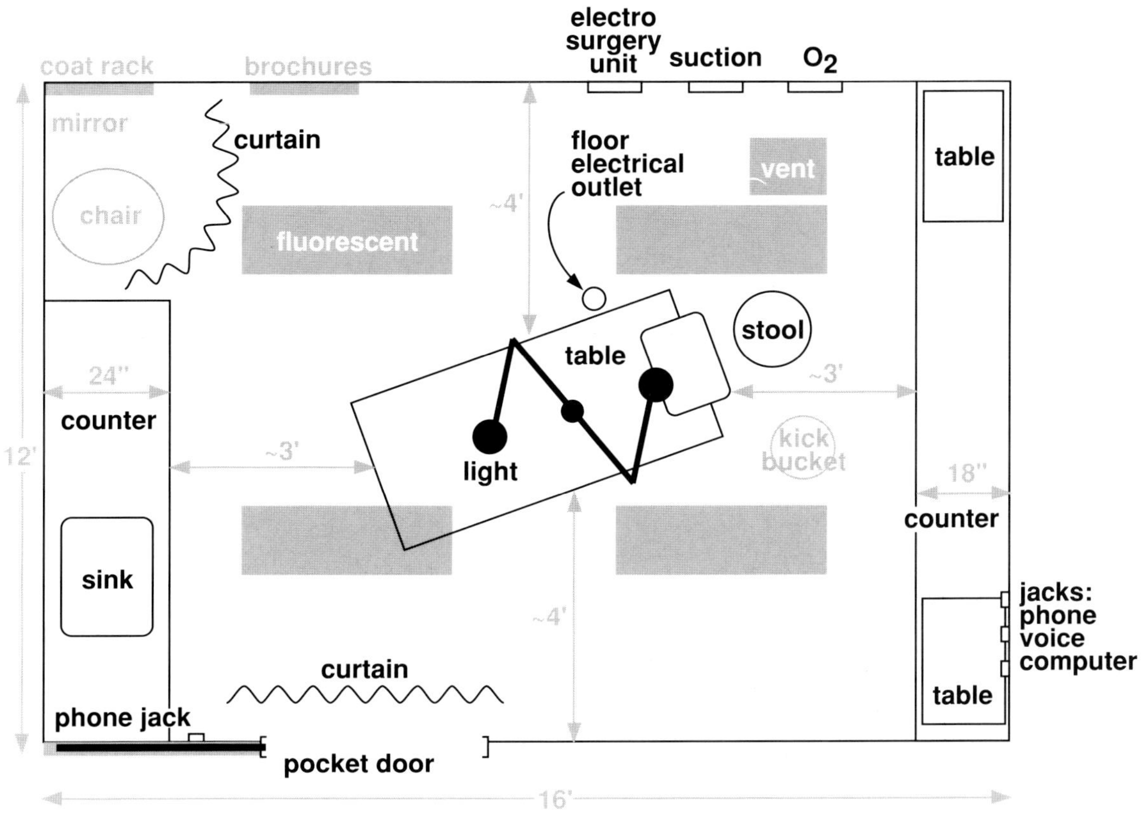

FIGURE 2–37. Layout of surgical room: A pocket door eliminates wasted space behind an opened door. A diagonally placed surgical table increases space to maneuver in the head and neck area. Moveable utility tables are stored under counter top. (Not shown: upper wall cabinets above counter top.)

suitable for chair procedures. Sunlight is best for examining the skin, but it is unpredictable and often fails to light all areas of the body. Floor lamps or additional headlamps are also useful. Halogen lights are the brightest and warmest, and they have a less yellow spectrum than incandescent lights. In addition, we use lightweight battery-powered surgical headlamps that illuminate almost any desired area of the body.

Cabinets. Cabinets are usually placed along one wall in small rooms and along two walls in large rooms. When cabinets are on adjacent walls, the operating chair or table should be oriented diagonally across the room to provide more space around the chair or table. Sinks are usually located close to the door. Each operating room ideally should have the same number of cabinets with identical material and equipment organization. Then, a nurse who learns one room knows them all.

Surgical Table. The operating table should be reserved for complicated procedures on the face, back, genitoanal region, and lower extremities. A wide table (29 inches) provides the advantage of being more comfortable for the patient, who is usually awake during surgery. Patients feel less anxious and more secure if they can easily rest their arms and shoulders without fear of rolling off the table. The use of a wide table often means that the patient must to be positioned off-center, so sometimes the patient must be asked to scoot over. The disadvantage of this off-center position is that the assisting nurse must lean over twice as far as when a narrower chair or table (22 to 24 inches) is used. The nurse and doctor should therefore stand on the same side. Narrow tables should have table belts. During long procedures, patients may prefer a pillow behind their knees to reduce pressure on their back. Pneumatic stools on wide casters that can be adjusted with hand levers or foot pedals (for the gloved surgeon) are the most versatile. Movable tables are versatile and allow the floor to be easily cleaned. Floors should be linoleum or vinyl tile for easy cleaning and to allow free movement of the table, surgical stool, and kick-bucket waste container.

Surgical Chair. Operating chairs are more versatile than tables. Elderly patients with arthritis and back problems prefer a chair that has a relatively low foot rest. Both tables and chairs should support a patient in the Trendelenburg position (either manual or automatic) in case of emergency. Most chairs are narrower than tables and come with removable arms that allow easy access for handicapped patients; ideally, chairs should be adjustable to allow for changes in the patient's position. In general, minor procedures on the face, scalp, neck, and chest are most easily done with the patient seated upright so the physician can get sufficiently close to the lesion. Surgical chairs and tables are easiest to clean if the vinyl covering does not contain seams or breaks that can collect fluids or pieces of tissue.

Other Basic Equipment. An oxygen source, suction equipment, electrosurgical unit, and Mayo stand are other basic components of the surgical room. Optional equipment may include crash cart, large equipment table, intravenous stand, cardiac monitor, blood pressure cuff, and separate lines or jacks for office phone, computer network, and emergency facilities.

Recovery Area

Patients who have just undergone surgery can rest in the recovery area, where they can be periodically observed by the nursing staff, until they are stable enough to leave the outpatient facility. Patients who have had facial surgery may have bandages that cause anxiety or embarrassment. The recovery room is a transition area. Here—in the company of friends, relatives, and medical staff—patients can be given comfort, support, and encouragement while being monitored for bleeding, drainage, pain, and other potential problems. Ideally, the recovery room should be segregated from the reception area for new patients. This separation prevents any confusion or misunderstanding that may arise during the normal course of observation and conversation; for example, a new patient may see a recovering patient with a large nasal bandage in the waiting area and assume that his own nasal cancer will be equally destructive, even though it is actually a small primary tumor. Most dermatologic surgery is performed under local anesthesia, and the patient is discharged immediately afterward. A separate recovery room in which vital signs can be routinely monitored is usually needed in hospitals or ambulatory care centers where general anesthesia or intravenous sedation is administered.

Personnel

A Mohs surgical team ideally includes the physician, one or more nurses and histotechnicians, a receptionist, a typist, and an office manager. In small office practices, the last three roles may be combined. In larger offices, the core staff typically consists of a physician, a lead nurse, and a back-up nurse. The lead nurse prepares the patient and sets up the room before surgery, and the back-up nurse discharges the patient, cleans up the treatment room, and transfers the specimens to the laboratory for processing after the procedure. This organization permits the efficient treatment of patients, one after the other. It is highly desirable that all support personnel have overlapping responsibilities so that during emergencies or absences continuous care can be provided without compromising quality and efficiency.

Follow-up

Long-term follow-up is necessary to recognize new cancerous growths and recurrent lesions. Patients with basal cell or squamous cell carcinoma are routinely followed for 5 years. Approximately one in four patints with basal cell carcinoma will develop another skin cancer during the follow-up period, although this rate varies according to the geographic areas in which these patients live. Patients with melanoma or very large or complicated basal cell or squamous cell cancers are followed for life because they are subject to late recurrence and metastasis. Because of the seriousness of melanoma, some patients may benefit from a support group. More information may be obtained from regional comprehensive clinical cancer centers and from the Skin Cancer Foundation, 245 Fifth Avenue, Suite 4202, New York, NY 10016.

REFERENCES

1. Mohs FE: Chemosurgery in Cancer: Gangrene and Infections. Springfield, IL: Charles C Thomas, 1956, pp 9–23.
2. Mohs, FE: Chemosurgery. Microscopically Controlled Surgery for Skin Cancer. Springfield, IL: Charles C Thomas, 1978, pp 1–29.
3. Tromovitch TA, Stegman SJ: Microscopically controlled excision of skin tumors: Chemosurgery (Mohs): Fresh tissue technique. Arch Dermatol 110:231, 1974.
4. Mikhail GR: Chemosurgery in the treatment of skin cancer. Int J Dermatol 14:33, 1975.
5. Tromovitch TA, Stegman SJ: Microscopic-controlled excision of cutaneous tumors: Chemosurgery, fresh tissue technique. Cancer 41:653, 1978.
6. Robins P: Chemosurgery: My 15 years of experience. J Dermatol Surg Oncol 7:779–789, 1981.
7. Swanson NA: Mohs surgery: Technique, indications, applications, and the future. Arch Dermatol 119:761–773, 1983.
8. Cottel WI, Bailin PL, Albom MJ, et al.: Essentials of Mohs micrographic surgery. J Dermatol Surg Oncol 14:11–13, 1988.
9. Bailin PL, Ratz JL, Wheeland RG: Mohs micrographic surgery technique. In Roenigk RK, Roenigk HH (eds): Dermatologic Surgery: Principles and Practice. New York: Marcel Dekker, 1988.
10. Roenigk RK: Mohs micrographic surgery. Mayo Clin Proc 63:175, 1988.
11. Lang PG Jr, Osguthorpe JD: Indications and Limitations of Mohs Micrographic Surgery. In Lang PG Jr, Osguthorpe JD (eds): Mohs Micrographic Surgery of the Head and Neck: A Multidisciplinary Approach. Philadelphia: W. B. Saunders, 1989, pp 613–644.
12. Burg G, Hirsch RD, Konz B, Braun-Falco O: Histographic surgery: Accuracy of visual assessment of the margins of basal-cell epithelioma. J Dermatol Surg Oncol 1:21–24, 1975.
13. Freeman RG: The handling of pathologic specimens for gross and microscopic examination in dermatologic surgery. J Dermatol Surg Oncol 8:673, 1982.
14. Breuninger H: Histologic control of excised tissue edges in the operative treatment of basal cell carcinomas. J Dermatol Surg Oncol 10:724, 1984.
15. Breuninger H, Schaumburg-Lever G: Control of excisional margins by conventional histopathological techniques in the treatment of skin tumors. An alternative to Mohs technique. J Pathol 154:167, 1988.
16. Abide JM, Nahai F, Bennett RG: The meaning of surgical margins. Plast Reconstr Surg 73:492–496, 1984.
17. Rowe DE, Carroll RJ, Day CL Jr: Long-term recurrence rates in previously untreated primary basal cell carcinoma: Implications for patient follow-up. J Dermatol Surg Oncol 15:315–328, 1989.
18. Rowe DE, Carroll RJ, Day CL Jr: Mohs surgery is the treatment of choice for recurrent (previously treated) basal cell carcinoma. J Dermatol Surg Oncol 15:424–431, 1989.
19. Koranda FC, Heffron ET, Modert CW, Perkins LL: Photo-mapping for microscopically controlled surgery. J Dermatol Surg Oncol 8:463, 1982.
20. Picoto AM, Picoto A: Technical procedures for Mohs fresh-tissue surgery. J Dermatol Surg Oncol 12:134–138, 1986.
21. Bentley TJ, Koranda FC, Miller LM: Histologic evaluation of horizontal frozen sections. Improved staining and special staining techniques. J Dermatol Surg Oncol 8:466, 1982.
22. Cottel WI: Perineural invasion by squamous-cell carcinoma. J Dermatol Surg Oncol 8:589–600, 1982.
23. Hanke CW, Wolfe RL, Hochman SA, O'Brian JJ: Perineural spread of basal cell carcinoma. J Dermatol Surg Oncol 9:742–747, 1983.
24. Lang PG, Maize JC: Histologic evolution of recurrent basal cell carcinoma and treatment implications. J Am Acad Dermatol 14:186, 1986.
25. Mikhail GR, Kelly AP, Elmquist JG: Metastatic basal cell epithelioma discovered by chemosurgery. Arch Dermatol 105:103, 1972.
26. Penneys NS: Immunoperoxidase methods and advances in skin biology. J Am Acad Dermatol 11:284, 1984.
27. Menn H, Robins P, Kopf AW, Bart RS: The recurrent basal cell epithelioma: A study of 100 cases of recurrent, re-treated basal cell epitheliomas. Arch Dermatol 103:628, 1971.
28. Grabaski WJ, Salasche SJ, McCollough ML, Berkland ME, Gutierrez JA, Finstuen K: Interpretation of Mohs micrographic frozen sections: A peer review comparison study. J Am Acad Dermatol 20:670–674, 1989.
29. Zitelli J: Secondary intention healing: An alternative to surgical repair. Clin Dermatol 2:92–106, 1984.
30. Lang P: The partial closure. J Dermatol Surg Oncol 11:966–969, 1985.
31. Robins P, Pollack SV, Robinson JK: Immediate repair of wounds following operations by Mohs fresh-tissue technique. J Dermatol Surg Oncol 5:329–336, 1979.
32. Ceilley RI, Anderson RI: Microscopically controlled excision of malignant neoplasms around eyelids followed by immediate surgical reconstruction. J Dermatol Surg Oncol 4:55, 1978.
33. Albom MJ: The management of recurrent basal-cell carcinomas—Please no grafts or flaps at once. J Dermatol Surg Oncol 3:382–384, 1977.
34. Robins P, Albom MJ: Recurrent basal-cell carcinomas in young women. J Dermatol Surg Oncol 1:49–51, 1975.
35. Mohs FE, Snow SN: Microscopically controlled surgical treatment for squamous cell carcinoma of the lower lip. Surg Gynecol Obstet 160:37–41, 1985.
36. Mohs FE, Larson PO, Iriondo M: Micrographic surgery for the microscopically controlled excision of carcinoma of the external ear. J Am Acad Dermatol 19:729–737, 1988.
37. Mohs FE, Zitelli JA: Microscopically controlled surgery in the treatment of carcinoma of the scalp. Arch Dermatol 117:764–769, 1981.
38. Mohs FE, Snow SN, Messing EM, Kuglitsch ME: Microscopically controlled surgery in the treatment of carcinoma of the penis. J Urol 133:961–966, 1985.
39. Braun M: The case for Mohs surgery by the fixed-tissue technique. J Dermatol Surg Oncol 7:634, 1981.
40. Mikhail GR, Farah RN: Surgery of the skin of the male genitalia. In Epstein E, Epstein E Jr (eds): Skin Surgery, 5th ed, vol 2. Springfield, IL: Charles C Thomas, 1982.

41. Brown MD, Zachary CB, Grekin RC, Swanson NA: Genital tumors: Their management by micrographic surgery. J Am Acad Dermatol 18(1):115–122, 1988.
42. Bernstein G, Forgaard DM, Miller JE: Carcinoma in situ of the glans penis and distal urethra. J Dermatol Surg Oncol 12:450–455, 1986.
43. Mohs FE: Chemosurgery. Microscopically Controlled Surgery for Skin Cancer. Springfield, IL: Charles C Thomas, 1978, pp 215–218.
44. Mohs FE: Fixed-tissue micrographic surgery for melanoma of the ear. Arch Otolaryngol Head Neck Surg 114:625–631, 1988.
45. Mohs FE: Chemosurgical treatment of melanoma: A microscopically controlled method of excision. Arch Dermatol 62:269–279, 1950.
46. Mohs FE: Chemosurgery for melanoma. Arch Dermatol 113:285–291, 1977.
47. Mohs FE, Bloom RF, Sahl WL: Chemosurgery for familial malignant melanomas. J Dermatol Surg Oncol 5:127–131, 1979.
48. Mohs FE: Micrographic surgery for satellites and intransit metastases of malignant melanoma. J Dermatol Surg Oncol 12:471, 1986.
49. Mohs FE, Snow SN, Larson PO: Mohs micrographic surgery fixed-tissue technique for melanoma of the nose. J Dermatol Surg Oncol (December, 1990).
50. Zitelli J, Mohs FE, Larson PO, Snow SN: Mohs micrographic surgery for melanoma. Dermatol Clin North Am 7:833–843, 1989.
51. Johnson OK Jr, Emrich LJ, Karakousis CP, et al.: Comparison of prognostic factors for survival and recurrence in malignant melanoma of the skin, clinical stage 1. Cancer 55:1,107–1,117, 1985.
52. Day CL Jr, Harrist TJ, Gorstein F, et al.: Malignant melanoma. Prognostic significance of microscopic satellites in the reticular dermis and subcutaneous fat. Ann Surg 194:108, 1981.
53. Hruza GJ, Snow SN: Basal cell carcinoma in a patient with acquired immunodeficiency syndrome: Treatment with Mohs micrographic surgery fixed-tissue technique. J Dermatol Surg Oncol 15:545–551, 1989.
54. Sitz, KV, Keppen M, Johnson DF: Metastatic basal cell carcinoma in acquired immunodeficiency syndrome–related complex. JAMA 257:340–434, 1987.
55. Vanderveen EE, Stoner JG, Swanson NA: Chiseling of exposed bone to stimulate granulation tissue after Mohs surgery. J Dermatol Surg Oncol 9:925–928, 1983.
56. Latenser J, Snow S, Mohs FE: Power drills to fenestrate bone to stimulate wound healing. J Dermatol Surg Oncol (March, 1991).
57. Mohs FE: Chemosurgical amputation for gangrene. Surgery 57:427, 1965.
58. Bennett RG, Mitchel MP: Chemosurgical debridement of osteomyelitic bone by zinc chloride fixative. J Dermatol Surg Oncol 13:771, 1987.
59. Stoner JG, Swanson NA: Chronic radiodermatitis with dystrophic calcification treated with Mohs surgery. J Dermatol Surg Oncol 11:160, 1985.
60. Davila de Pedro RL, Mohs FE: Extirpation of a nidus of infection with tetanus bacilii by chemosurgery. J Dermatol Surg Oncol 7:8, 1981.
61. Sebben JE: Surgical Preparation. In Roenigk RK, Roenigk HH (eds): Dermatologic Surgery. New York: Marcel Dekker, pp 11–39.
62. Gross DJ, Jamison Y, Martin K, Fields M, Dinehart SM: Surgical glove perforation in dermatologic surgery. J Dermatol Surg Oncol 19:1,226–1,228, 1989.

CHAPTER 3

Instrumentation for Mohs Surgery

Gerald Bernstein, M.D.

Despite the highly technical nature of Mohs micrographic surgery, most Mohs surgeons can effectively operate with standard surgical instruments. Occasionally, however, special instruments will be required to totally ablate a cutaneous malignancy, as when tumor invades periosteum or bone or when eyelid structures are involved.

When performing an operation, the surgeon has the goal of obtaining maximum accuracy and safety. Therefore, the selection of surgical instruments is made with these objectives in mind. Speed and ease of performance are of secondary importance but are developed with experience. Thus, the Mohs surgeon must constantly search for new instruments to enhance surgical efficiency.

The finest surgical instruments are made of stainless steel, although occasionally tungsten-carbide inserts are bonded to the stainless steel to increase durability. Excellent instruments are manufactured in Germany, Sweden, Great Britain, and the United States. Pakistan has a growing surgical instrument industry, but its instruments are not generally considered to be of the highest quality. It is axiomatic that a surgeon use instruments that must be sharp and kept in optimal operating condition.

Carefully selected, well-maintained surgical instruments are necessary for the Mohs surgeon to effectively remove the tumor-bearing tissue with the least involvement of normal surrounding skin.

Scalpels. Although the scalpel is the primary surgical cutting instrument, it is most effective when used on firm resistant tissue. It is more difficult to manipulate when cutting layers of soft, flaccid, or mobile tissue such as fat, mucous membrane, or eyelid skin. Tensing the skin greatly increases the effectiveness of the scalpel.

The scalpel is held in one of three grips: the pencil, the fingertip, or the palm grip. For most Mohs surgical procedures, the pencil grip is most commonly used and provides the greatest accuracy and control because it utilizes the intrinsic muscles of the hand as well as the forearm muscles. To increase security during cutting, the forearm and elbow can be splinted against the body. Greater accuracy and control are obtained when the blade is drawn or pulled toward, rather than pushed away from, the surgeon. The pencil grip also allows the surgeon to easily and quickly change the blade angle as required during the procedure.

The fingertip grip is used for vertical stabbing or puncture cuts, while the palm grip increases accuracy of long straight cuts. These grips are much less useful for the small deliberate cuts generally used by Mohs surgeons.

There are four main cutting actions: slide cutting, press cutting, sawing, and scraping. Slide cutting provides the most direction and depth control and is the most effective for Mohs surgery. Also, slide cutting usually obtains the best specimens for frozen-section pro-

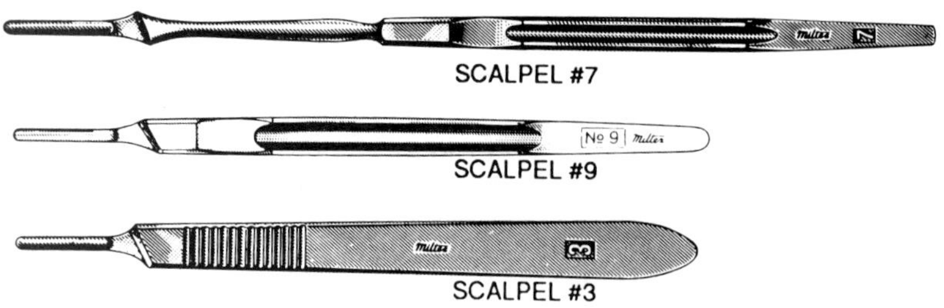

FIGURE 3–1. Three standard scalpel handles from top, are the #7, #9, and #3.

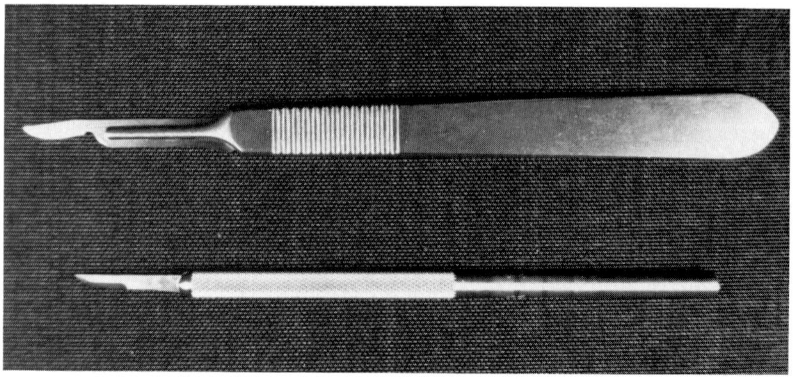

FIGURE 3–2. *Below,* Beaver handle with a #64 blade. *Above,* a # 3 handle with a #15C blade.

cessing. Press cutting is used mostly for entering cavities such as cysts and furuncles. Sawing, although useful for procurement of split-thickness skin grafts, is rarely necessary during Mohs surgery. Scraping is used to remove periosteum or perichondrium.

Modern scalpels consist of a reusable handle with snug-fitting disposable blades. Scalpel handles are available in many shapes and lengths; virtually all use standard disposable blades. The most commonly used is the No. 3 handle. I favor those with a centimeter scale on one side, which cost slightly more than the plain handles. The No. 7 and 9 handles, which are less popular, are thinner and may be difficult to control, especially during lengthy operations (Fig. 3–1).

The Beaver handle is round and thin, much like a pencil (Fig. 3–2). Because of the delicate design, many prefer this scalpel and their specially designed blades. The new Siegel-Quill handle is longer but otherwise similar in design to the Beaver and accepts standard blades.

Scalpel blades are made in several common shapes and sizes. These include the No. 10, 11, 15, and 15C (Fig. 3–3). Blades are made either of stainless steel or carbon steel. The carbon steel blades are sharper but do not keep their sharpness as long as stainless blades do. Stainless steel blades are also somewhat more expensive.

The No. 15 blade is the most versatile and useful for Mohs surgery. The blade is small enough for the most delicate facial surgery, yet sufficiently broad for effective use on virtually all skin surfaces. This is the workhorse blade for Mohs surgeons.

The No. 10 blade is very broad and is thus especially suitable for cutting the thick skin of the nuchal area and the back. Although often neglected in favor of the No. 15 blade, the No. 10 blade should be considered for removal of

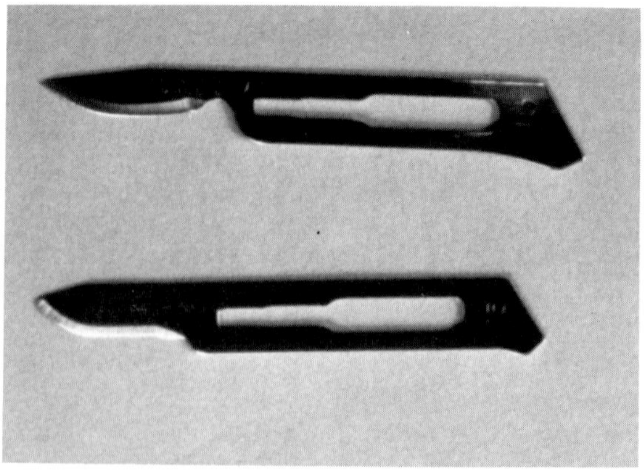

FIGURE 3–3. Scalpel blades for dermatologic surgery: *Below,* a #15 blade—probably the most commonly used blade by Mohs surgeons. *Above,* the #15C blade is finer and more delicate and is appropriate for use on eyelids, nose, and lips.

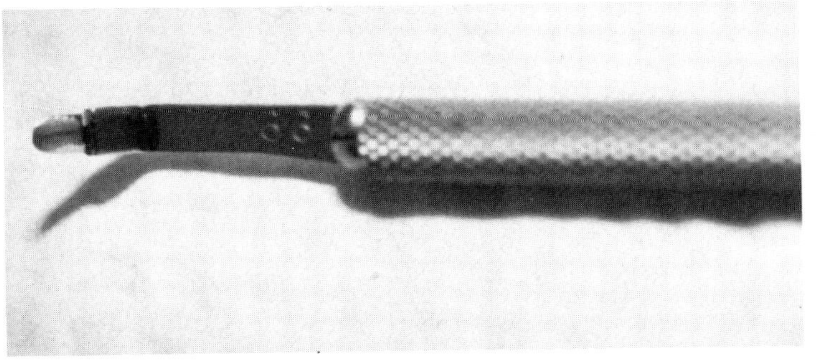

FIGURE 3–4. The angled Beaver blade (#6910): This blade, which fits only the Beaver handle, has a 45-degree angle that makes it very useful in inaccessible areas. Other shapes in the Beaver line are also available.

large tumors on the thick skin of the back and nape.

The No. 11 blade is triangular and used for stab or puncture incisions. Many Mohs surgeons find it ideal for very fine, controlled excisions by only using the tip of the blade.

The No. 15C blade has been used by oral surgeons for many years but has only recently been recognized as a highly effective blade for skin surgery. While resembling a No. 15 blade, it is thinner and has a shallow bevel, thus combining the features of the No. 11 and the No. 15 blades. The No. 15C is ideal for fine, delicate cutting around the eye, ear, nose and lips. It is similar in size and shape to the No. 67 Beaver blade.

Beaver blades are made in a large variety of shapes and sizes. The No. 67 is the usual type for facial surgery. Of greater utility are the curved and bent special application blades made for Beaver handles. Many of these facilitate Mohs surgery in areas not easily accessible, such as the ear canal (Fig. 3–4).

Blade breakers are scalpel handles which are generally round or flat. They are made to grab and break off and securely hold a small fragment of carbon steel razor blade. Developed by ophthalmologists, they are extremely sharp. The broken blade usually has a narrow triangular shape, making it most effective for stab- and saw-type cuts. Blade breakers tend to be expensive. However, they are at times very useful (Fig. 3–5).

Scissors. Scissors are mainly used for cutting and blunt dissection. By stabilizing the tissue

A

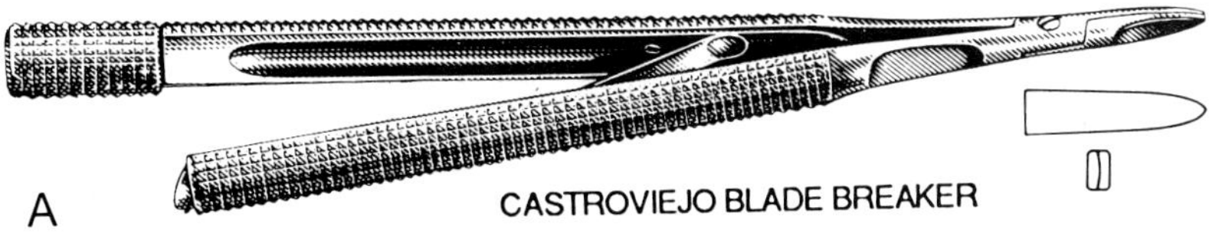

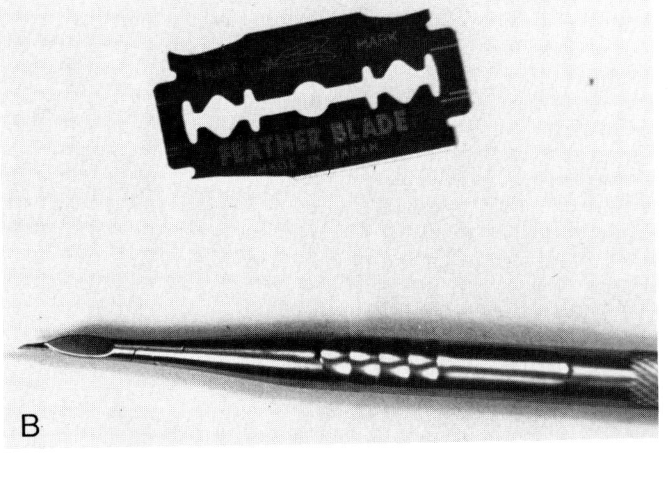

B

FIGURE 3–5. *A*, Castroviejo blade breaker is 5¼″ long. *B*, It holds a small part of a razor blade, which is extremely sharp.

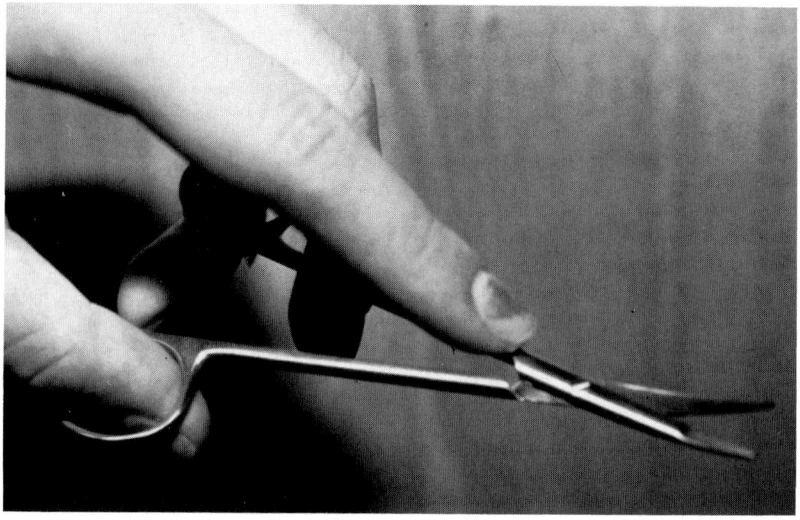

FIGURE 3–6. The proper grasp for the surgical scissors. The thumb and fourth finger go through the loops while the index finger, placed on the hinge, stabilizes the scissors.

between the blades, scissors are able to cut soft, loose, flaccid, or otherwise movable tissues more effectively than scalpels. They also have an advantage over scalpels in that, while blind dissection can be safely performed with blunt scissors, it is rarely possible with a sharp scalpel.

Scissors operate by utilizing three force vectors in cutting: torque, sheering, and closing. These vectors are best utilized by cutting with the distal portion and tips of the scissors. Cutting too close to the fulcrum can cause bunching of the tissue with resultant ragged, irregular cuts and some tissue crushing.

The optimal way to use the scissors, in most cases, is to hold them with the thumb and fourth finger (Fig. 3–6). This provides the greatest stability as the index finger is free to stabilize the blades. Most scissors are made for right-handed surgeons and cannot be easily utilized efficiently with the left hand.

Although scissors are made in a variety of sizes and shapes, there are basically two major categories of scissors. They can be straight or curved and may have blunt or sharp tips.

Curved scissors are more maneuverable and offer approximately a 30% increased visibility and mobility over straight scissors. They are especially useful for horizontal cutting in deep tissue planes. Straight scissors offer more accuracy in making straight cuts than do curved ones. Sharp-tipped scissors are more useful for fine accurate cutting, while blunt-tipped scissors are used more for dissection.

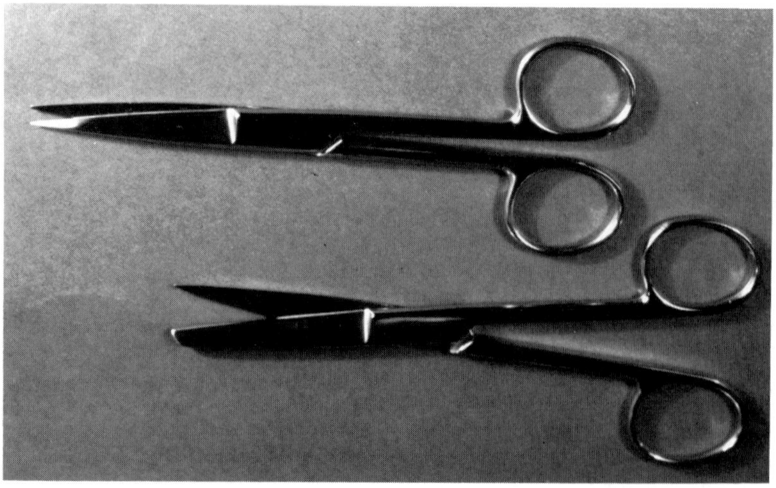

FIGURE 3–7. Utility scissors with sharp/sharp *(top)* and sharp/blunt points.

The great diversity of scissors often makes the selection of the most appropriate instrument difficult. The decision, often influenced by early training and based on teachers' preferences, depends on the application, location, and accessibility of the operative site and the type of tissue being operated on. Those generally most useful for the Mohs surgeon are discussed here.

Utility scissors are useful for cutting paper, gauze, and sutures. They are less expensive than operating scissors. In addition to being available with straight or curved blades and with sharp or blunt tips, they can also be obtained with a composite of both sharp and blunt tips (Fig. 3–7). They are not intended for cutting tissues.

Iris scissors are the workhorse of most Mohs surgeons for tissue-cutting purposes. They are small, ranging in size from 3¼ to 5 inches and can be found with large- or standard-size finger loops. They vary in the ratio of the length of the blades to the handles, with several mechanical advantages. They are appropriate for cutting most tissues, including mucous membranes and eyelids. A common mistake is to cut the thick skin of the back or nape with small delicate iris scissors. This can rapidly blunt the instrument and may permanently damage it. It is important to match the size of the scissors to the thickness of the tissue being cut.

If desired, the lower blade of the iris scissors can be serrated at a small extra cost. This provides increased stability when cutting loose tissue or skin tags. Iris scissors are also used to remove sutures, although some surgeons feel that this causes blunting or damage to the scissors. Common iris scissors and several other specialty types are shown in Figure 3–8. Many

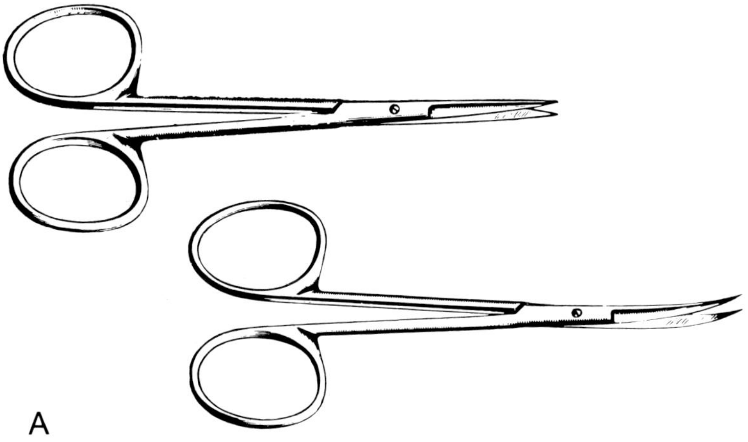

A

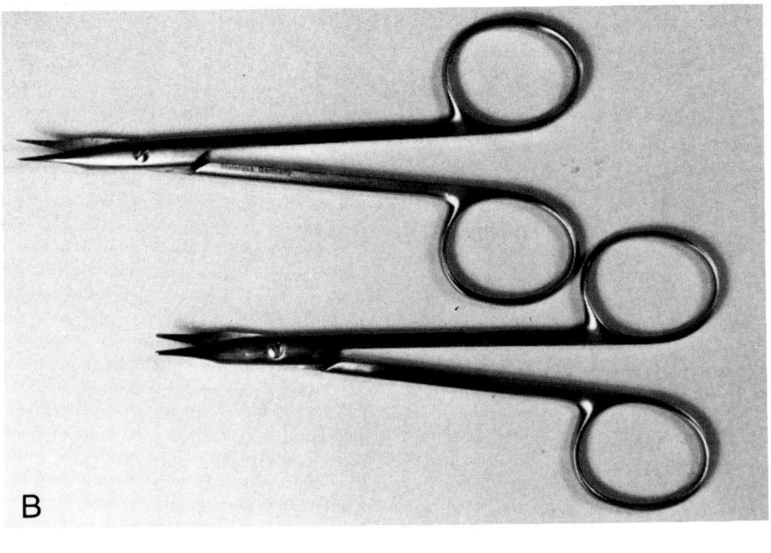

B

FIGURE 3–8. *A*, Standard iris scissors, straight and curved, 3¼″ long—excellent for sharp, delicate work. *B*, Stevens tenotomy scissors are very delicate, ophthalmological scissors for delicate work, such as on eyelids. Sharp, curved tips *(above)*; blunt, curved tips *(below)*.

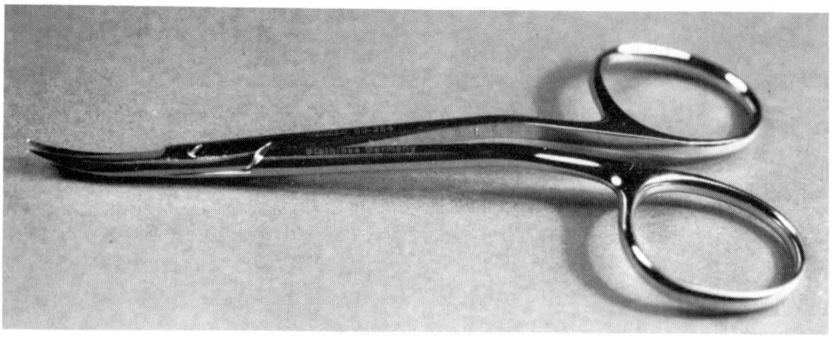

FIGURE 3–9. LaGrange scissors with a double curve.

iris scissors have been developed by ophthalmologists, including the Bonn, which is very delicate.

LaGrange scissors have a double curve which has been borrowed from dentistry. These scissors are commonly used in hair transplants and punch biopsies. The double curve allows the Mohs surgeon to make horizontal cuts in deep spaces (Fig. 3–9).

Gradle scissors are extremely popular

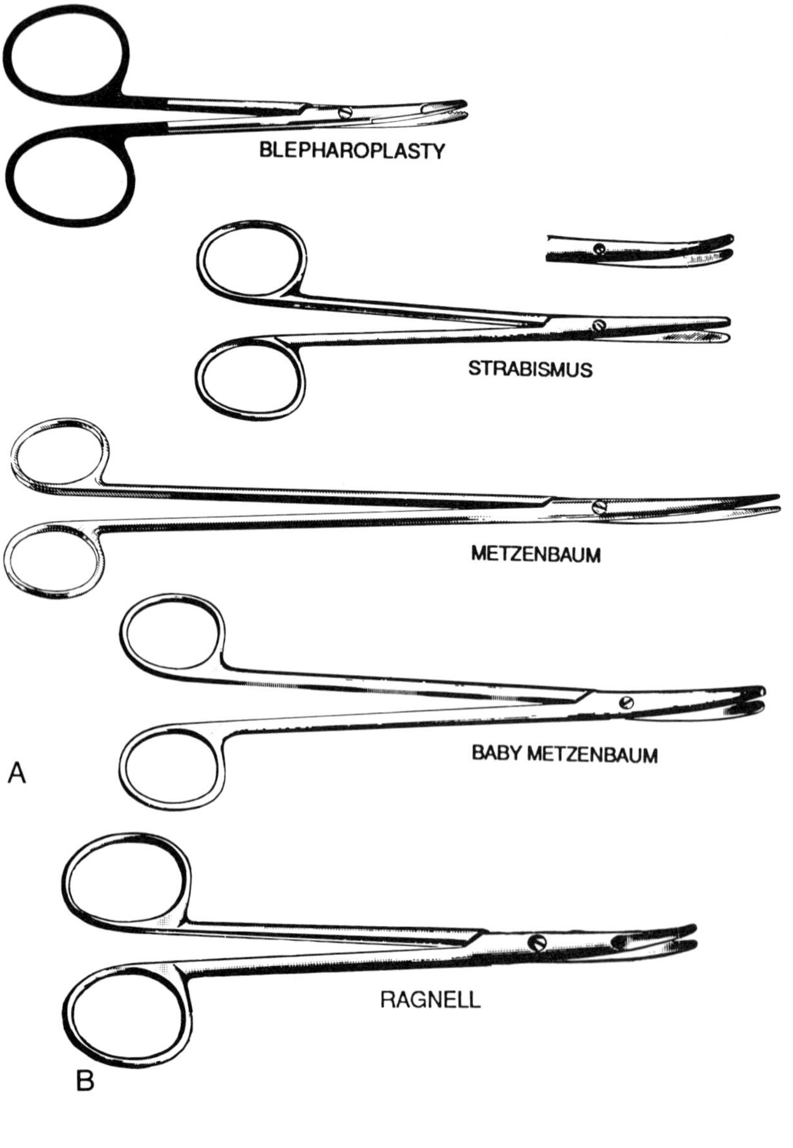

FIGURE 3–10. Blunt-end dissection scissors. *A* (from *top*), Blepharoplasty scissors are 4½″ long and have a serrated lower blade; strabismus scissors are straight and curved; Metzenbaum and baby Metzenbaum are curved. *B*, Ragnell scissors are curved and their distal ½″ is thinned.

among dermatologists and Mohs surgeons. In reality, they are fine-pointed ophthalmologic scissors, originally intended for removal of tiny sutures. They are virtually identical to thc Stevens tenotomy scissors which were also developed for ophthalmologic use.

Stevens tenotomy scissors are available in straight or curved styles with sharp or blunt tips. The curved blunt-tipped Stevens tenotomy scissors are excellent for eyelid surgery and delicate tissue dissections. Similarly, the sharp Stevens tenotomy scissors are suitable for cutting delicate flaccid tissues. They can also be used to remove fine 6-0 or 7-0 sutures.

As mentioned above, blunt scissors are primarily indicated for dissection. A selection of dissecting scissors of varying sizes and shapes is useful for the Mohs surgeon; examples are the Metzenbaum, delicate (or baby) Metzenbaum, Ragnell, blepharoplasty, and Fomon scissors (Fig. 3–10).

Metzenbaum scissors range in size from 5 to 11 or more inches. Delicate, or baby, Metzenbaum's have more delicate blades and are thus more useful for finer dissections. Blepharoplasty scissors are yet smaller and more delicate. One of my favorite blunt scissors are the 5-inch Ragnell scissors which have curved blunt blades. The distal blade halves are thinned, making them unusually delicate. Similar but smaller scissors are the Kaye scissors, which measure 4½ inches and usually have

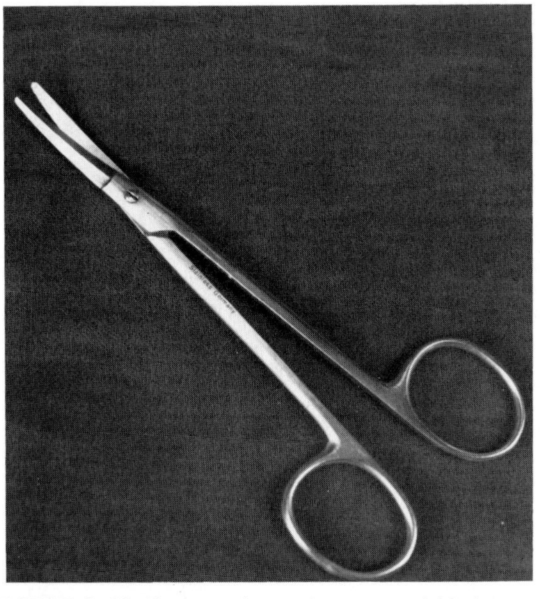

FIGURE 3–11. Fomon scissors have curved blades and semisharp margins.

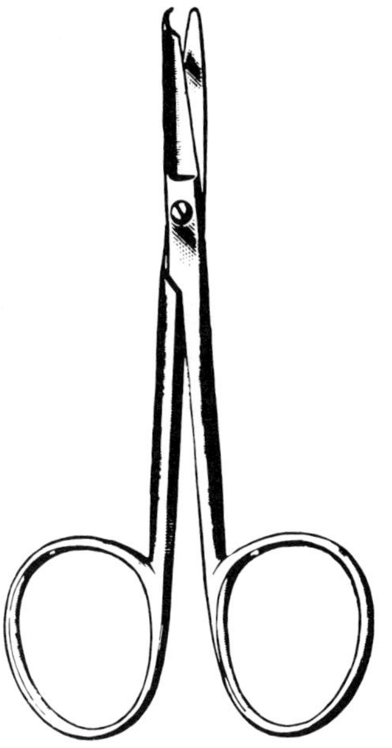

FIGURE 3–12. Spencer stitch scissors: The lower blade has a small hook to facilitate grasping of the suture.

tungsten-carbide blades (the lower blade is serrated). Fomon scissors are curved and have the outside edge of both blades partially sharpened to facilitate blunt dissection (Fig. 3–11).

Tungsten-carbide blade inserts are available for many scissors as well as needle holders. Their extreme hardness insures that the blades maintain their sharpness for long periods. They have a longer, effective life and are ordinarily sold with lifetime guarantees. They traditionally have golden fingerloops.

Additional scissors that may be needed by the Mohs surgeon include bandage scissors, stitch scissors, and other specialty scissors (Fig. 3–12). Bandage scissors are a variation of utility scissors with a guard to prevent accidental skin lacerations beneath dressings. Stitch scissors are preferred by those who feel that the small hook facilitates suture removal.

Forceps. Forceps are intended as grasping tools and are available in an overwhelming array of sizes and shapes. They are ordinarily held in the nondominant hand and are used to hold tissue that is being cut, to retract other tissues, to grasp vessels for hemostasis, and to stablize tissues during suturing. They also have many other uses, such as picking up instruments and supplies.

Forceps are divided into two major categories: the serrated and the toothed. The serrated, also known as dressing forceps, are not in-

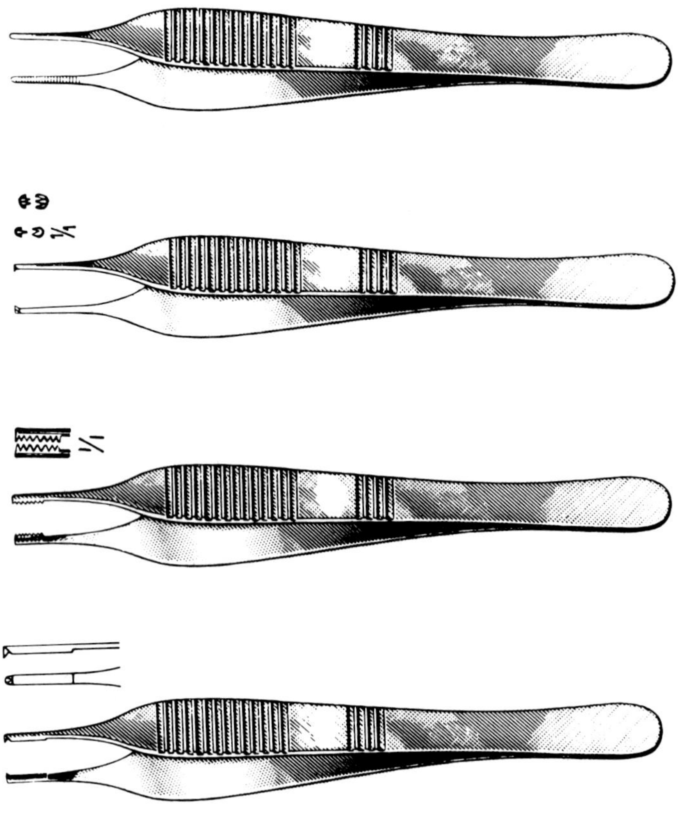

FIGURE 3–13. Adson type forceps (from *top*): Adson dressing forceps; Adson tissue forceps, 1×2 teeth; Adson-Brown forceps, 7×7 teeth; Adson tissue suturing platform forceps.

tended for handling tissue because the force used to hold the tissue can cause crush injury. Tissue forceps have opposing teeth, usually 1× 2, although other forceps such as the Brown-Adson have seven teeth on each side. When gently used, tissue forceps can be used to manipulate tissues without causing significant trauma and can be as trauma-sparing as skin hooks (Fig. 3–13).

The selection of forceps is a matter of personal style and taste. In general, the size and shape of the forceps should be functional for the procedure and the tissue being operated upon. The Adson tissue forceps (1×2 teeth) are probably the type most commonly used. The size of the handle and the teeth make them appropriate for use on most tissues. For a more secure grasp, the Brown-Adson forceps (7×7 teeth) may be more appropriate; the greater number of fine teeth gently fixes the skin and has a more tissue-sparing effect.

Iris forceps, finer and smaller than Adson forceps, are useful for handling delicate tissues such as the eyelids, mucous membranes, lips, and nailbeds. They also allow the Mohs surgeon to excise small tissue fragments.

Examples of iris forceps include the standard iris forceps, the Bishop-Harmon forceps, the Graefe, and the Castroviejo forceps. Most of these were developed for ophthalmologic use and are very delicate; some are available in curved as well as straight types (Fig. 3–14). Also, some can be obtained with suturing platforms which consist of slight thickenings at the distal portion of the forceps to aid in grasping the needle when suturing.

Hemostats. Hemostats are primarily used for achieving hemostasis by grasping bleeding vessels prior to electrocoagulation or ligature. Other uses include retracting tissues, blunt dissection, and probing as well as facilitating the passage of sutures around large vessels. Because clamping of tissue causes crush injury, every effort should be made to clamp only the vessels with as little surrounding tissue as possible. If the vessel is not too large, the hemostats can be touched with the electrocoagulating electrode to seal it.

Hemostats are also manufactured in a variety of sizes, shapes, and degrees of delicacy. They are available with either curved or straight blades, but curved ones are generally more useful. They are made for right-handed

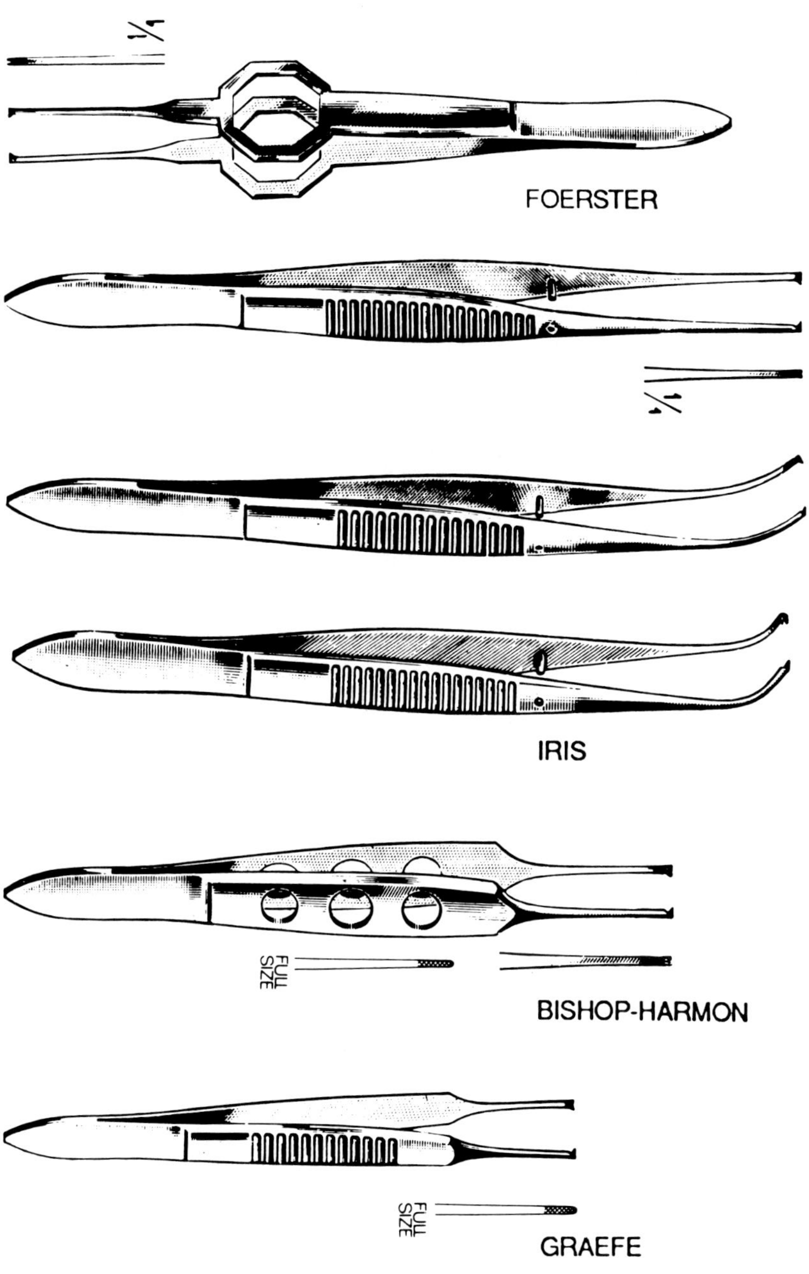

FIGURE 3–14. Iris forceps (from *top*): Foerster; standard iris, straight; standard iris, curved; Bishop-Harmon; Graefe.

use and are most accurately held with the thumb and fourth finger in the loops and the index finger on the fulcrum or along the shaft for stability.

Selection of size and shape of the hemostat is again determined by the preference and style of the Mohs surgeon and the size of the hands and fingers of the operator. Also, the nature and size of the tissue being treated helps to determine the optimal hemostat. Examples of commonly used hemostats include the Kelly, Halsted, and Hartman Mosquito (Fig. 3–15).

Special Clamps. Desmarres chalazion clamps are ophthalmologic clamps that have a flat, stainless steel plate and a ring-shaped opposing jaw. The latter can be tightened against the former with the tissue held in between. The instrument gently, but firmly, immobilizes the treated tissue and also maintains a bloodless field within the ring. It is ideal for eyelid surgery. However, it can also be effectively used for surgery on mucous membranes or other surfaces that are hard to immobilize, such as the lips and tongue (Fig. 3–16).

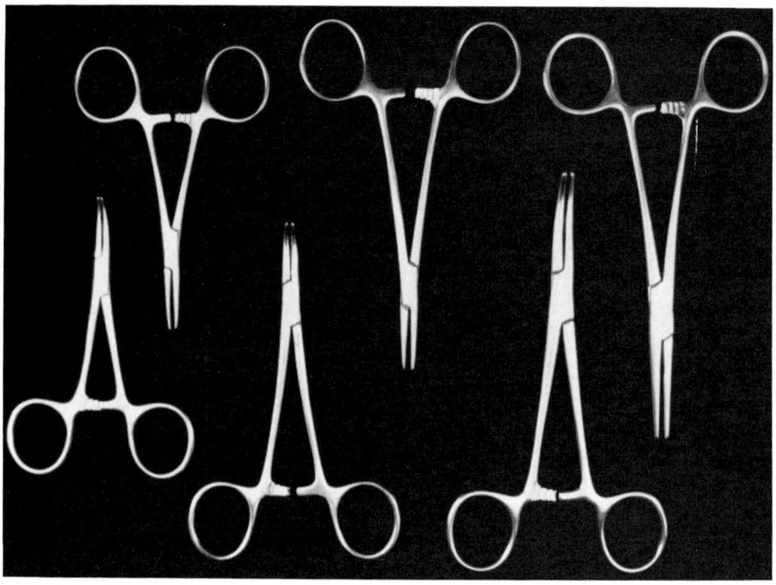

FIGURE 3–15. Hemostats (from *left*): Hartman mosquito hemostat, curved (3½″); Hartman mosquito hemostat, straight; Halstead mosquito hemostat, curved (5″); Halstead mosquito hemostat, straight; Kelly hemostat, curved (5½″); Kelly hemostat, straight.

Self-retractors are not commonly used in Mohs surgery; however, they may occasionally prove handy for the unassisted surgeon operating deeply in tissues. The Alm retractor is illustrated in Figure 3–17.

Allis clamps have opposing jaws which can be fixed with a locking mechanism. They are mainly used as retracting instruments; however, the jaws can severly crush tissue and are therefore not useful for tissue that is to be examined microscopically.

Skin Hooks. Skin hooks are used by Mohs surgeons to hold and retract skin. These instruments are the least damaging to the skin and are preferred by many surgeons over forceps. They do pose some risk to the operator because of the backward projection of the hooks and the possiblity of puncture wounds to the surgeon or the assistants if the hook slips.

Hooks are available with one, two, or more prongs (the latter are referred to as rakes). They are also available with fixed or flexible shafts and vary in size and shape. The prongs can be sharp or blunt. Generally, sharp hooks are preferred because they provide increased stability and security. For those who can comfortably and efficiently suture with hooks, they are the

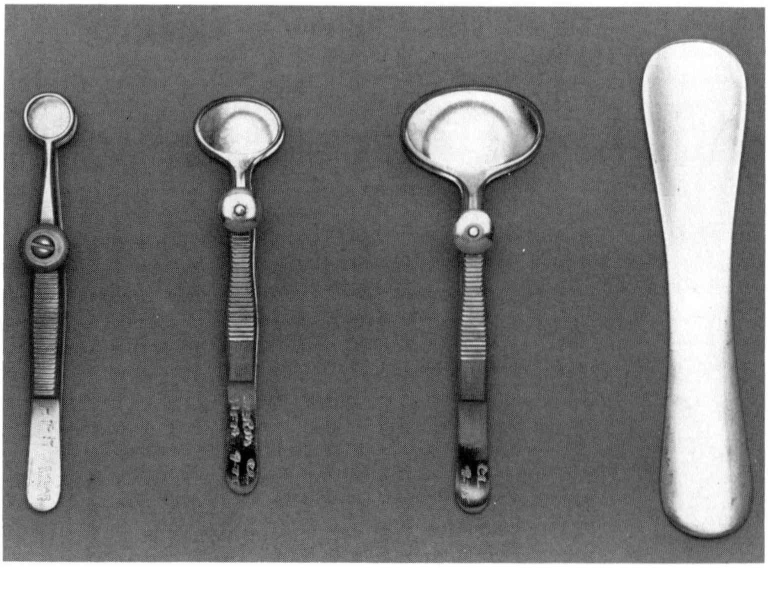

FIGURE 3–16. Desmarres chalazion clamps (from *left*): Lambert chalazion clamps; Desmarres chalazion clamps, medium and large (2½″); Jaeger eyelid retractor.

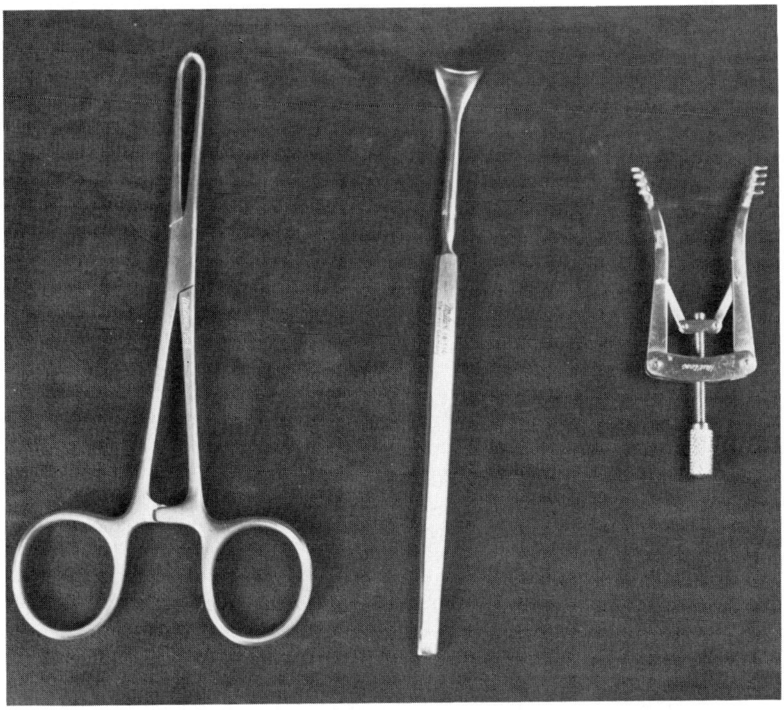

FIGURE 3–17. Examples of retractors (from *left*): Allis clamp, Desmarres lid retractor, and Alm retractor.

instrument of choice. In any event, hooks are ideal for manipulating and retracting tissue.

Skin hooks with single prongs include Frazier, Tyrell, and Guthrie types. The Joseph and several of the rakes are examples of double or multipronged hooks. Many hooks, such as the Senn, have double ends and can be utilized as either a hook or a blunt retractor (Fig. 3–18).

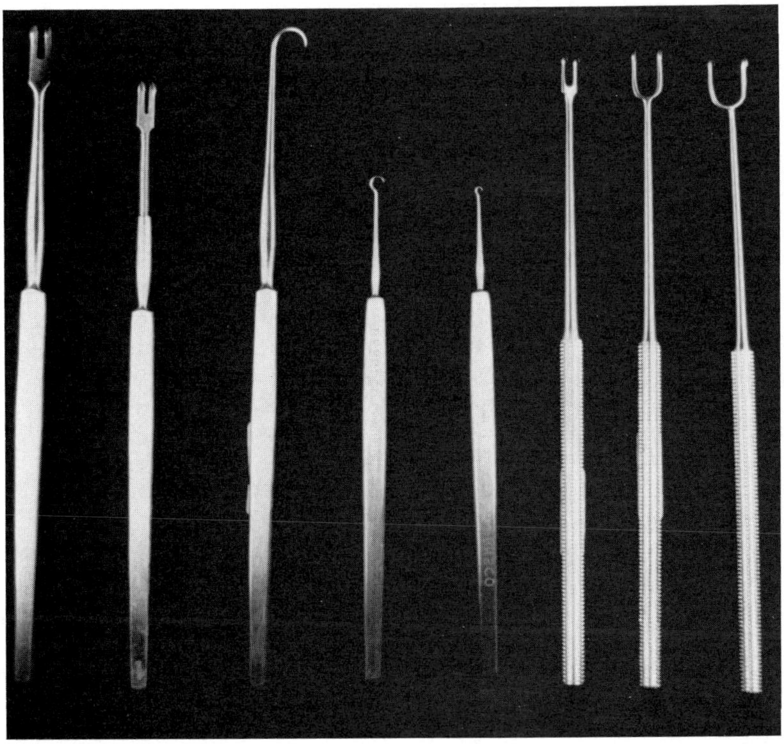

FIGURE 3–18. Skin hooks (from *left*): Double sharp, straight; double sharp, flexible; large single-prong hook; Frazier hook; Tyrell hook; Guthrie delicate hook (3 mm); Joseph hook (5 mm); and double hook (7 mm).

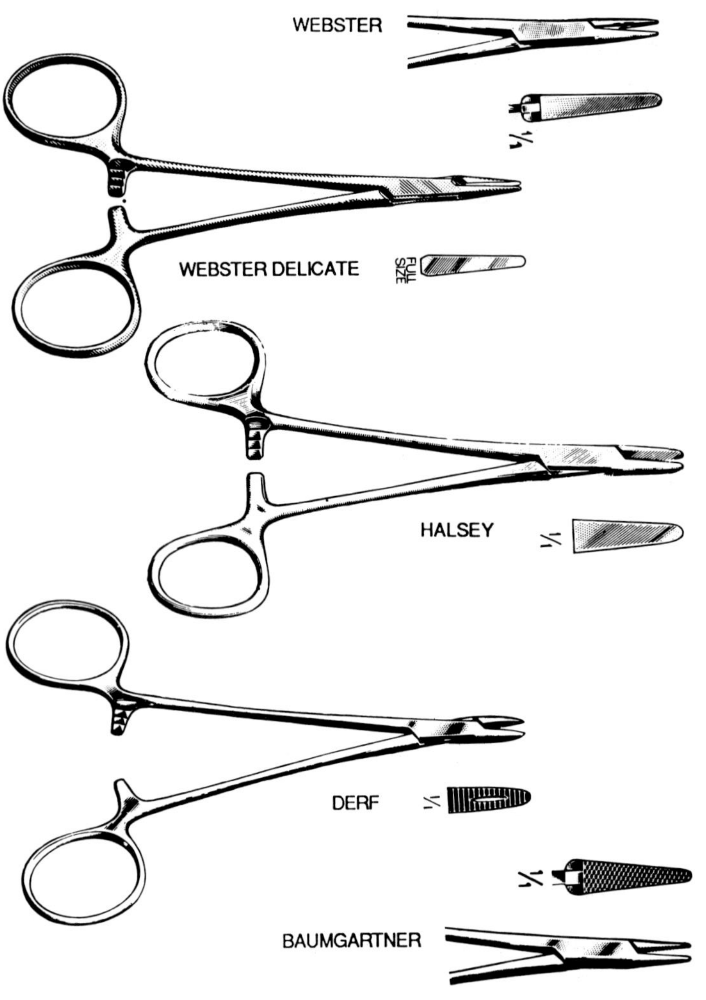

FIGURE 3–19. Some popular needle holders (from *top*): Webster; Halsey; Derf; Baumgartner.

Needle Holders. Mohs surgeons frequently require needle holders capable of securely holding fine curved needles. Needle holders have smooth or very fine serrated jaws and must be constructed of the high-quality stainless steel or have tungsten-carbide inserts to firmly grasp the needle. The larger needle holders have deep transverse ridges and cannot securely hold thin needles. Moreover, fine sutures can be cut inadvertently by the sharp edges of the ridges.

Conventional needle holders are maneuvered by the pronation/supination action of the forearm muscles. The greatest accuracy and precision can be obtained by placing the thumb and fourth finger in the loops with the index finger along the shafts of the needle holder. However, increased power can be obtained by holding the needle holder in the palm. This is less efficient because the fingers have to be replaced back in the loops to release the needle. Most needle holders open and close with a squeeze-lock, release-unlock mechanism. They are made for right-handed surgeons and can only be opened and closed with the fingers in the loops. They are difficult to use with the left hand.

The most popular needle holders for the Mohs surgeons include the Webster (5-inch), Halsey (5-inch), and Derf (4¾-inch) types. The Mayo-Hegar and Crile-Wood are also effective. The Baumgartner (5½-inch) is effective for larger needles (Fig. 3–19).

The Castroviejo needle holder was developed for ophthalmological use. It is pencil-shaped, has a spring-leaf release mechanism which both opens and closes the jaws with the same pushing action. This reduces jarring which might otherwise interfere with suturing delicate tissues. The lock mechanism allows the left-handed surgeon to use this needle

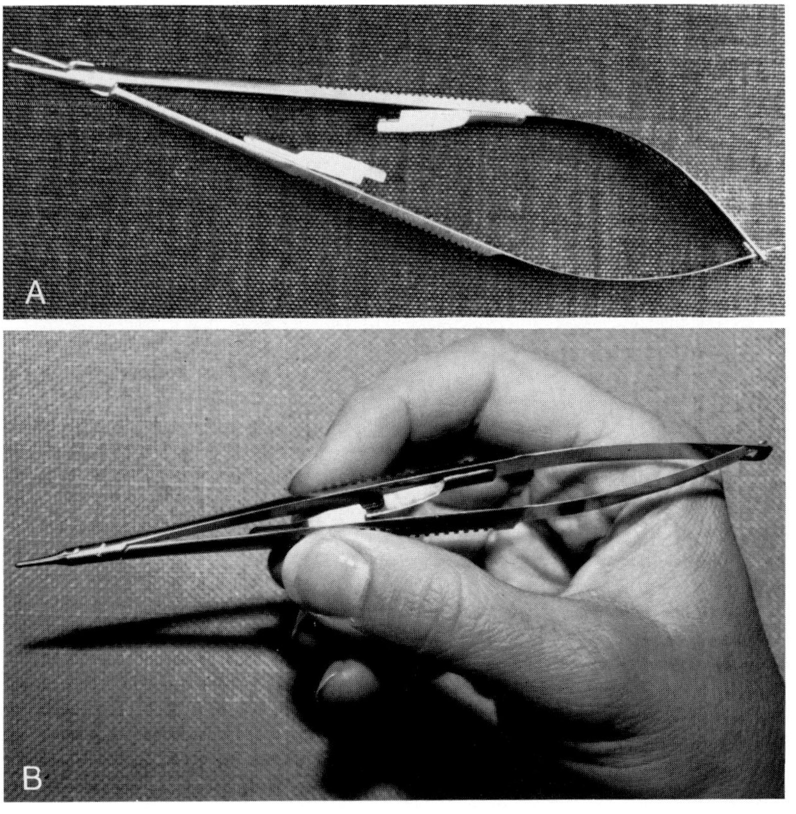

FIGURE 3–20. *A*, Castroviejo needle holders are used to suture very delicate tissues. *B*, Castroviejo needle holder is pencil-shaped, allowing control with the intrinsic muscles of the hand rather than the forearm muscles.

holder as easily as the right-handed surgeon. A further advantage is the tubular shape of the needle holder, which allows the surgeon to grasp it like a pencil. In this fashion, the device can be maneuvered by the fine intrinsic hand muscles, rather than by the forearm muscles, with greater accuracy and precision. This is an expensive needle holder adapted for use with only the finest needles and sutures. Mohs surgeons usually do not require more than one or two of these instruments (Fig. 3–20).

Some variations on the lock mechanisms of more conventional needle holders exist which allow left-handed surgeons equal ease in operation. The jaws can also be both opened and closed by pushing, rather than by locking and unlocking, with greater efficiency and more rapid suturing. These include the Mathieu (5½-inch) and the Boynton (5-inch). Miltex Quick-Release needle holders have conventional shapes but utilize the push-push locking/unlocking mechanism. They are available in Crile-Wood and Mayo-Hegar configurations as well as Webster's.

Finally, the Olson-Hagar needle holder includes scissors in the same mechanism as the needle holder. It can be obtained in small sizes for delicate suturing and allows the surgeon to cut the suture without the need of an assistant. This can be an effective assistant-sparing instrument (Fig. 3–21).

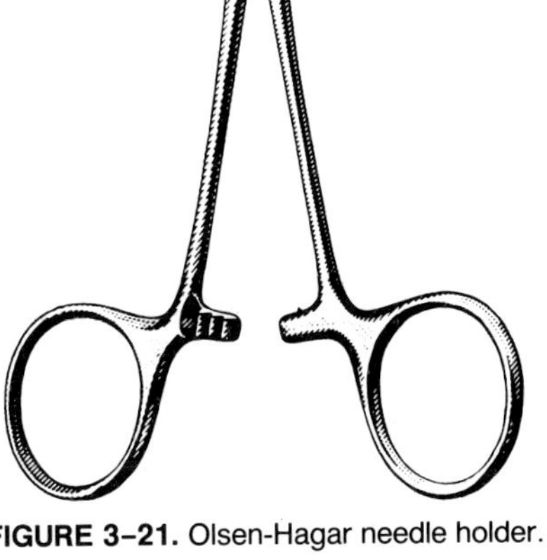

FIGURE 3–21. Olsen-Hagar needle holder.

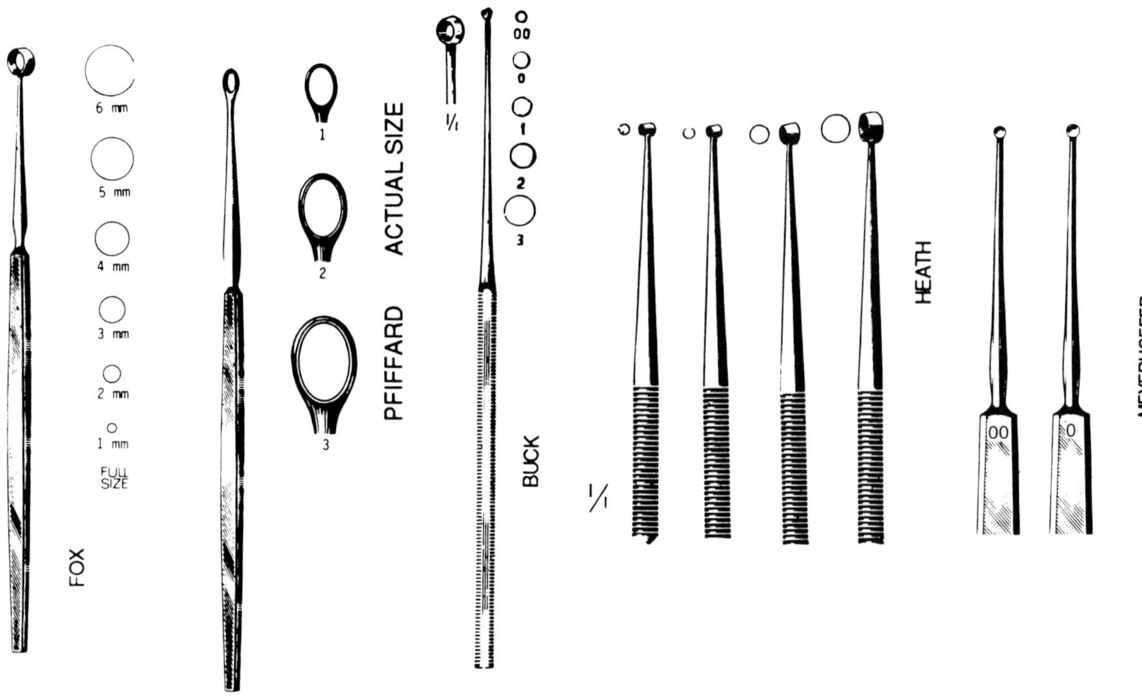

FIGURE 3–22. Dermal curettes (from *left*): Fox, Piffard, Buck, Heath, and Meyerhoeffer (smallest sizes shown)—all come in different sizes.

Curettes. Curettes are tumor debulking instruments and are well known to dermatologic and Mohs surgeons. The selection is based on handling comfort and ease of use. Some prefer the larger Fox-type handles, others the pencil-thin Buck Sharp ear curettes. The Piffard type has an oval, rather than a round, cutting loop which is somewhat easier to keep clean during operation. It may also be easier to sharpen. Small Heath and Meyerhoeffer curettes were developed for ophthalmologic (chalazion) use. Their very fine cutting loops and scoops are preferred by some Mohs surgeons (Fig. 3–22).

Periosteal and Perichondrial Elevators. Periosteal and perichondrial elevators are often essential for the Mohs surgeon to separate the periosteum and perichondrium. The cutting edges vary widely in shape and size. Very often, they are double-ended instruments. The Freer (7-inch) is very effective for periosteal removal and is also an excellent tool for nail avulsion (Fig. 3–23). I have had success with the Cottle for perichondrial separation, although perfect perichondrial removal is rarely obtained with any instrument. The Discoid-Cleoid is a double-ended dental excavator with two small sharp cutting edges. It is operated by pulling the blade toward the surgeon. Early use shows it to be a good instrument for periosteum or perichondrium removal. It is relatively inexpensive.

Osteotomes. Osteotomes (bone chisels) are occasionally utilized by Mohs surgeons to remove bone that has been invaded by tumor or that obstructs access to soft tissues with residual tumor.

There are two major categories of osteotomes: those that separate by pushing the instrument and those in which a mallet is used to pound on the chisel. The latter are the most accurate and provide the greatest control. There is substantial risk of slipping with a push-controlled chisel. By contrast, the mallet-driven chisel can be precisely controlled by varying the strength of the tapping on the chisel.

Bone rongeurs, another type of bone-cutting instrument, chip off bone fragments for histological examination (Fig. 3–24).

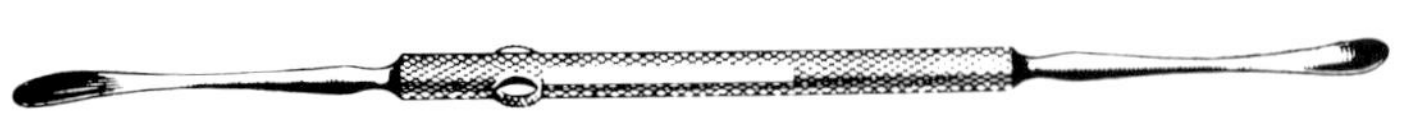

FIGURE 3–23. Freer double-ended periosteal elevator.

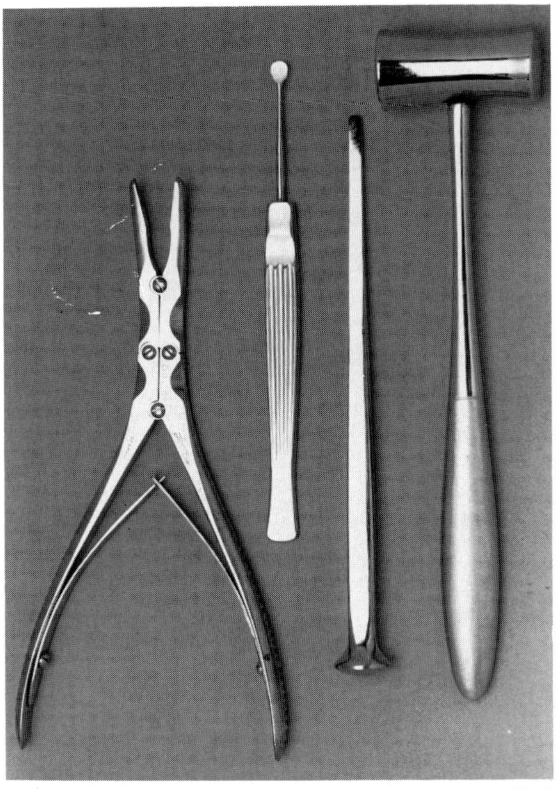

FIGURE 3–24. Bone instruments (from *left*): Rongeur, Wolf periosteal/perichondrial elevator, bone chisel, and Lucae mallet.

Eye Protectors. When operating on eyelids, it is prudent to consider utilizing an eye protector, which has three advantages: (1) the eye is protected from inadvertent trauma, (2) the opaque material protects the eye from the bright operating lights, and (3) the cornea is protected when using the electrocoagulating current on the eyelid. Several types are available. I favor the Kohlberg eye protector, which is very smooth, soft, and easily installed (Fig. 3–25). The Jaeger lid plate is also very popular (Fig. 3–26).

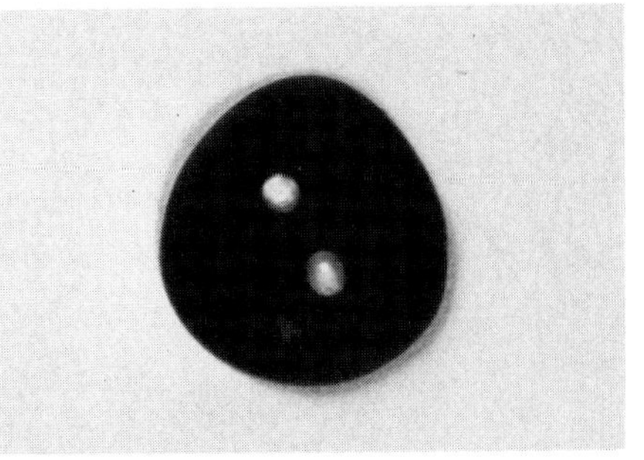

FIGURE 3–25. Kohlberg eye protector made of methylacrylate. Diameter is 2.4 cm..

Standard Mohs Tray. A standard Mohs tray (Fig. 3–27) includes:

- No. 3 scalpel handle, usually with No. 15 or 15C blade
- Sharp curettes—large and small
- Utility scissors
- Curved iris scissors for cutting tissue
- Curved iris scissors for cutting sutures
- Adson-type forceps
- Delicate forceps
- Sterile cotton applicator sticks

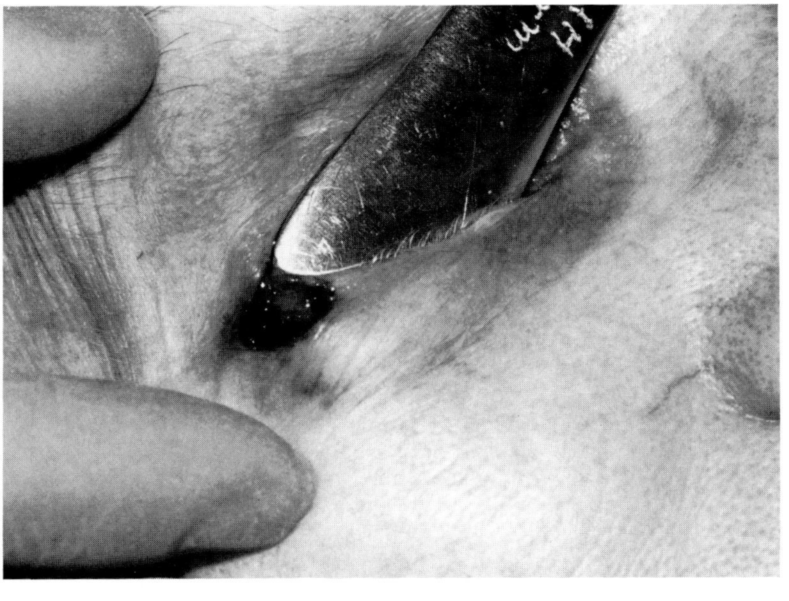

FIGURE 3–26. Jaeger eye protector with lid held in place during surgery.

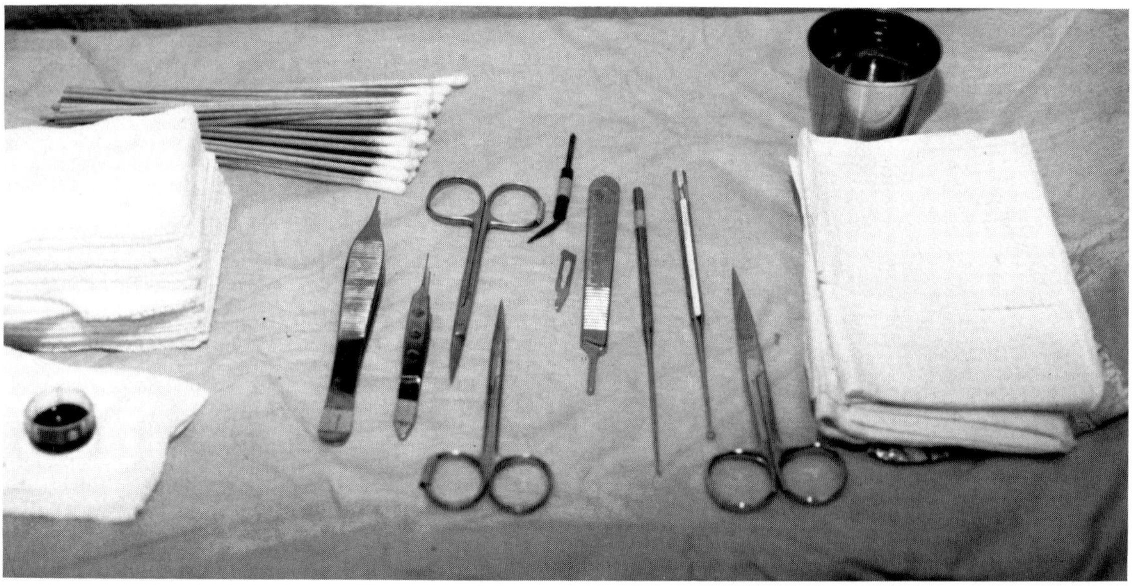

FIGURE 3–27. A standard Mohs tray.

Sterile gauze
Dyes for marking the margins of the tissue sections

Other instruments can be added as necessary for different types of tumor and for repairs.

Conclusion. Above all, instruments must always be kept sharp and in good condition. Ultrasonic cleansers are the most effective way to clean instruments, especially those with hard-to-clean spaces, such as curettes, hemostats, and needle holders with hinges capable of trapping blood and debris. Following washing and ultrasonic cleansing, instruments are most appropriately sterilized in an autoclave or Chemiclave. Glutaraldehyde is an effective form of cold sterilization when properly used according to the manufacturer's instructions. Gas (ethylene oxide) sterilization is also effective, and small office kits are available. All gas-sterilized instruments and supplies must be carefully vented prior to use according to manufacturer's instructions because of the danger of tissue burns to surgeon, staff, and patient.

REFERENCES

1. Anderson RM, Romfh RF: Techniques in the Use of Surgical Tools. New York: Appleton-Century-Crofts, 1980.
2. Bennett RG: Instruments and their care. In Klein E (ed): Fundamentals of Cutaneous Surgery. St. Louis: C. V. Mosby, 1988, pp. 259–270.
3. Bernstein G: The 15C scalpel blade. J Dermatol Surg Oncol 13:969, 1987.
4. Davis RS: New equipment and instruments for excisional surgery. Clinics in Dermatology 5:11–29, 1987.
5. Grande DJ, Neuberg M: Instrumentation for the dermatologic surgeon. J Dermatol Surg Oncol 15:3, 1989.

CHAPTER 4

Neoplasms in Mohs Micrographic Surgery Practice: A Clinicopathologic Correlation

John M. Pelachyk, M.D.
George R. Mikhail, M.D., M.S.

Since the most innocuous-appearing lesion may be a malignancy, early and accurate diagnosis requires critical attention. Adequate biopsy material should be obtained from suspected lesions. Because accurate knowledge of tumor pathology is axiomatic for the practice of Mohs surgery, this chapter is planned as an aid toward learning about and recognizing tumors—benign and malignant, common and rare—that may be encountered in a Mohs surgery practice. It is arranged in an atlas-like format with abundant clinical and histologic illustrations. It is not meant to be an exhaustive account of the lesions described but concentrates on their clinical and histologic features with emphasis on how to make the diagnosis. Larger works on this subject will remain the mainstay for detailed information. It is highly recommended that the surgeon should foster a close relationship with the pathologist. When the diagnosis is in doubt, the slides should be circulated to other pathologists in consultation, and more biopsies may have to be performed before embarking on any form of therapy.

This chapter is arranged in seven sections containing groups of neoplasms that are related by cell origin, anatomic site, or biological behavior. The seven groups of neoplasms that will be reviewed are premalignant epithelial lesions and in situ carcinomas, malignant epithelial neoplasms, epithelial neoplasms of uncertain malignant potential, adnexal neoplasms, melanocytic neoplasms, mesenchymal neoplasms, and malignant neoplasms of uncertain origin and metastatic carcinoma.

PREMALIGNANT EPITHELIAL LESIONS AND IN SITU CARCINOMAS

Actinic Keratoses

Actinic (solar) keratoses are sunlight-induced premalignant lesions that are seen as solitary or multiple lesions on the sun-exposed areas of the skin usually in middle-aged or elderly persons who have fair complexions. They are noted most often on the face and dorsa of the hands in both sexes as well as on the bald portions of the scalp in men and the pretibial area in women. Actinic keratoses typically present as erythematous, oftentimes scaly and occasionally eroded papules or small plaques (Fig. 4–1). Clinical variants of actinic keratoses in-

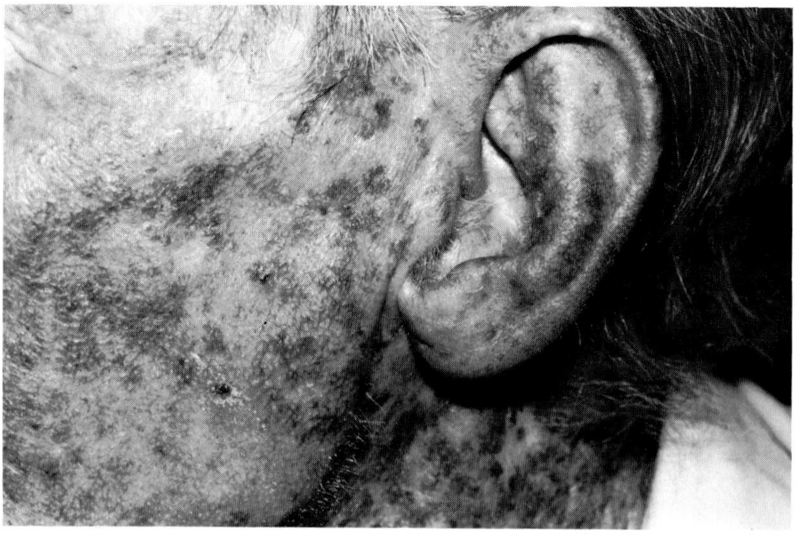

FIGURE 4–1. Actinic keratosis: Note typical clinical presentation of multiple, small scaling papules on actinically damaged skin of face.

clude the hypertrophic (Fig. 4–2) and pigmented types.

All actinic keratoses are characterized histologically by varying degrees of epithelial atypia overlying dermal tissue showing evidence of actinically induced degeneration. Epithelial changes in actinic keratoses include:

Loss of polarity and crowding of nuclei
Cells with an increased nuclear-to-cytoplasmic ratio
Pleomorphic and hyperchromatic nuclei
Increased number of mitotic figures
Dyskeratosis.

Varying degrees of hyperkeratosis and parakeratosis overlie the dysplastic epidermis. Actinically induced dermal changes include fragmentation and degeneration of the dermal collagen fibers, which on hematoxylin and eosin (H&E) stained sections characteristically exhibit a basophilic appearance of grayish hue (Fig. 4–3). Five histologic variants of actinic keratoses are recognized: atrophic, hypertrophic (Fig. 4–4), bowenoid (Fig. 4–5), acantholytic (Fig. 4–6), and pigmented. In advanced lesions, evidence of early invasive squamous cell carcinoma may be noted focally (Fig. 4–7).

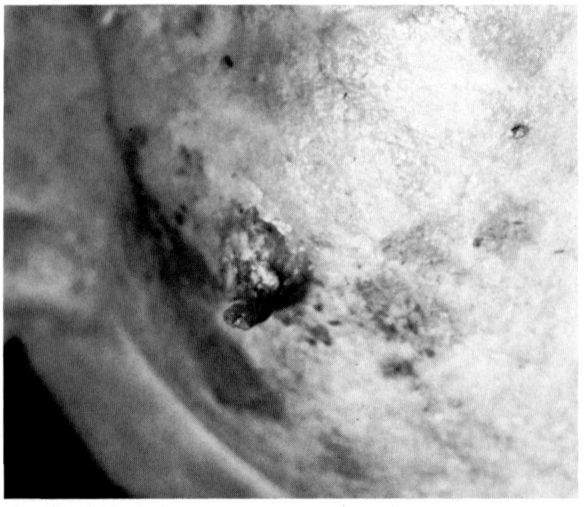

FIGURE 4–2. Actinic keratosis: Hypertrophic variant shows lesion with marked hyperkeratosis forming a cutaneous horn.

Leukoplakia

In the past, leukoplakia was loosely defined as a white patch or plaque on the oral or genital mucosa that histologically showed early, in situ anaplastic epithelial changes. Recently, the term has been redefined by oral pathologists and accepted by the World Health Organization to indicate any persistent white lesion of the oral or genital mucosa that cannot be rubbed off.[1,2] This is a purely clinical description, and does not include or infer any specific histologic or etiologic connotation. Lesions of leukoplakia consist of one or several white, flat patches or slightly raised, ill-defined plaques that can be present on any oral (Fig. 4–8) or genital (Fig. 4–9) mucosal surface. The etiology of leukoplakic lesions can include any number of benign, premalignant, or malignant conditions.

Lesions of precancerous or premalignant leukoplakia histologically show focal, in situ epithelial atypia and, as such, have a similar

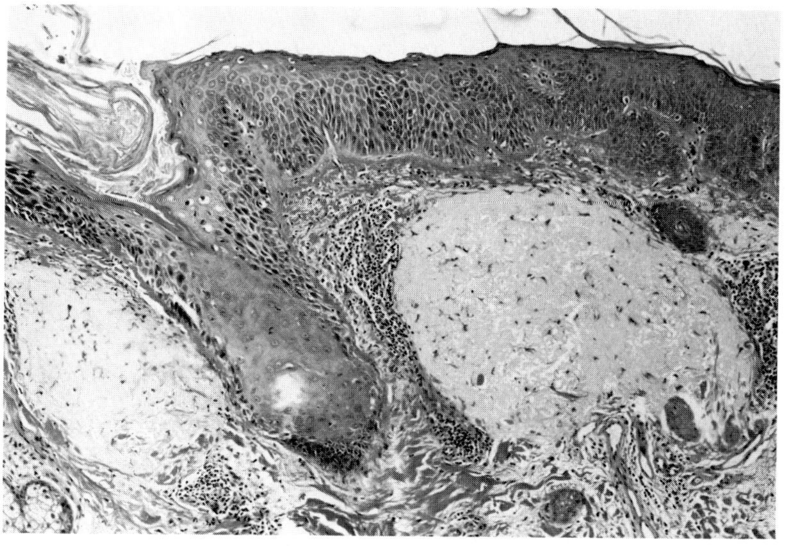

FIGURE 4–3. Actinic keratosis: Atypical squamous epithelium is noted above dermal changes of solar degeneration and chronic inflammation; note relative lack of cellular atypia within follicular epithelium.

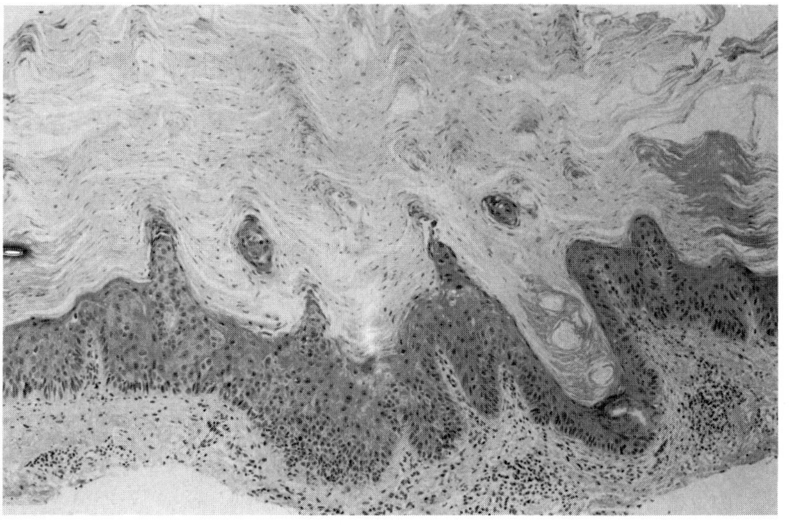

FIGURE 4–4. Actinic keratosis: Hypertrophic variant showing epithelial changes of marked hyperkeratosis, diffuse parakeratosis, mild papillomatosis, irregular hyperplasia, and nuclear atypia.

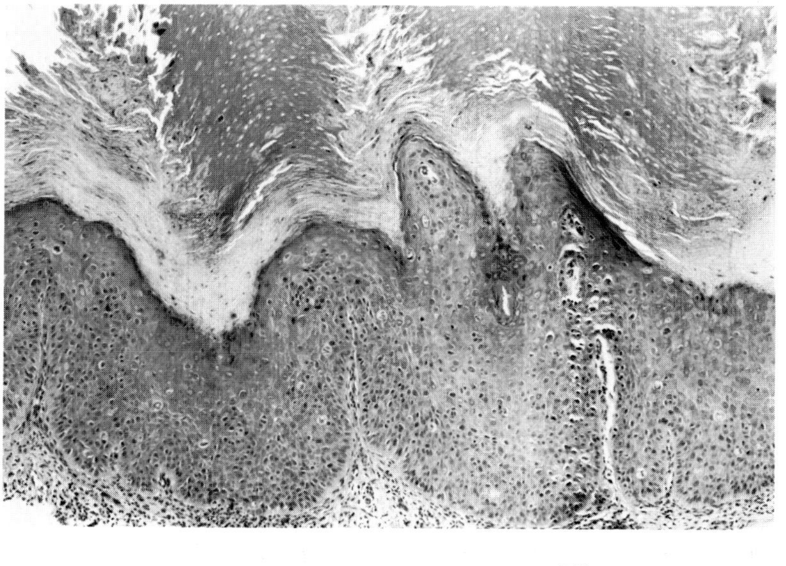

FIGURE 4–5. Actinic keratosis: Bowenoid variant showing focal full-thickness epithelial atypia with overlying hyperkeratosis and parakeratosis.

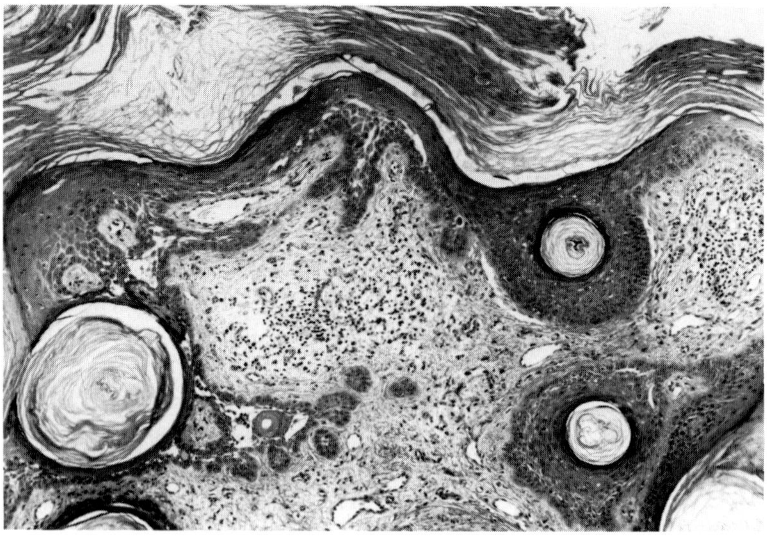

FIGURE 4–6. Actinic keratosis: In acantholytic variant, nuclear atypia is most pronounced in basal layer, which extends into the dermis in short, duct-like structures, showing acantholysis with cleft formation.

histologic appearance to actinic keratoses. These features include varying degrees of hyperkeratosis and parakeratosis, loss of cell polarity, crowding of nuclei, nuclear neopleomorphism and hyperchromatism, and varying numbers of mitotic figures and dyskeratotic cells (Fig. 4–10).

Bowen's Disease and Erythroplasia of Queyrat

Bowen's disease is an epithelial in situ carcinoma, and usually presents as a solitary lesion on either sun-exposed or nonexposed skin. It appears as a slowly enlarging, erythematous, oftentimes scaly or eroded plaque with a sharp but irregular border (Fig. 4–11). Not infrequently, it can involve fingers (Fig. 4–12) and interdigital spaces (Fig. 4–13). It may rarely be pigmented (Fig. 4–14).

The term *erythroplasia of Queyrat* is sometimes applied to lesions of epithelial carcinoma in situ located on mucosal surfaces. It manifests itself clinically as a symptomatic, sharply circumscribed, bright red, slightly infiltrated plaque. The area most often involved is the glans penis (Fig. 4–15), but other mucosal surfaces such as the vulva, and conjunctiva (Fig. 4–16) may also be affected.

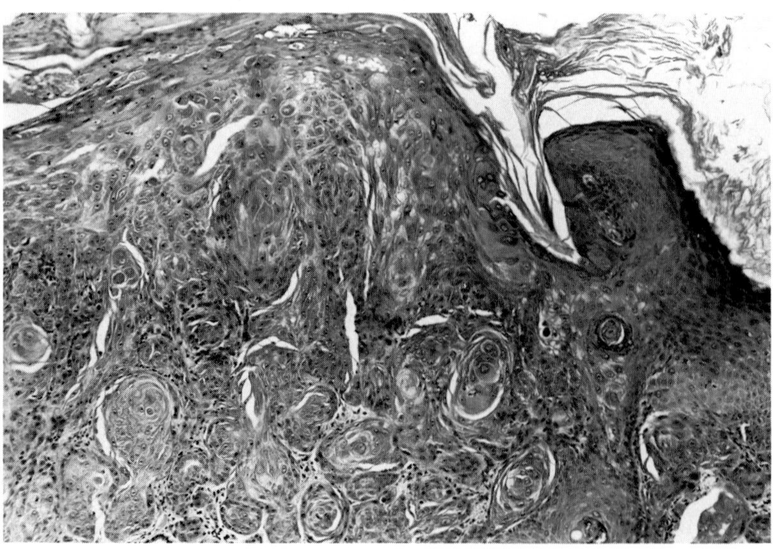

FIGURE 4–7. Actinic keratosis: Note extension of small islands of atypical epithelial cells into the upper dermis, signifying transformation into an early invasive squamous cell carcinoma.

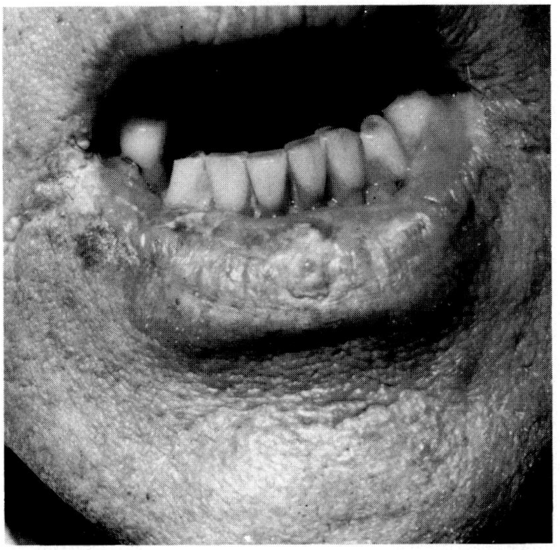

FIGURE 4-8. Leukoplakia: White, raised plaques are present on the lower lip.

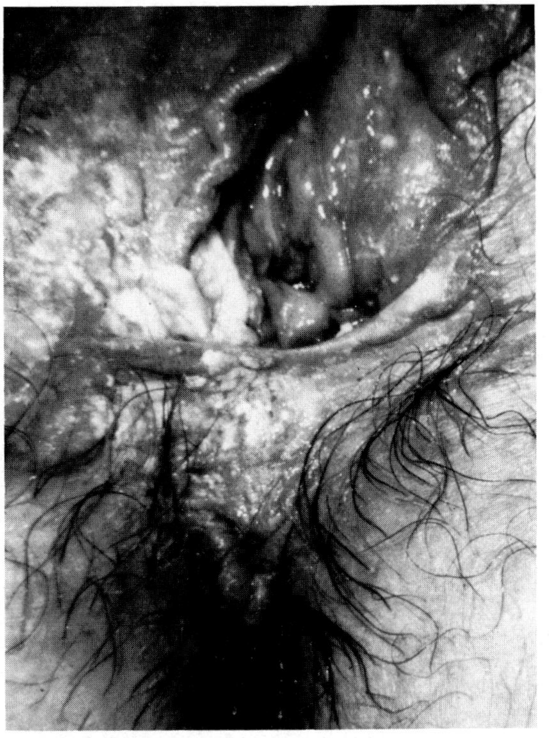

FIGURE 4-9. Leukoplakia: White, ill-defined plaques are noted on vulvar mucosa.

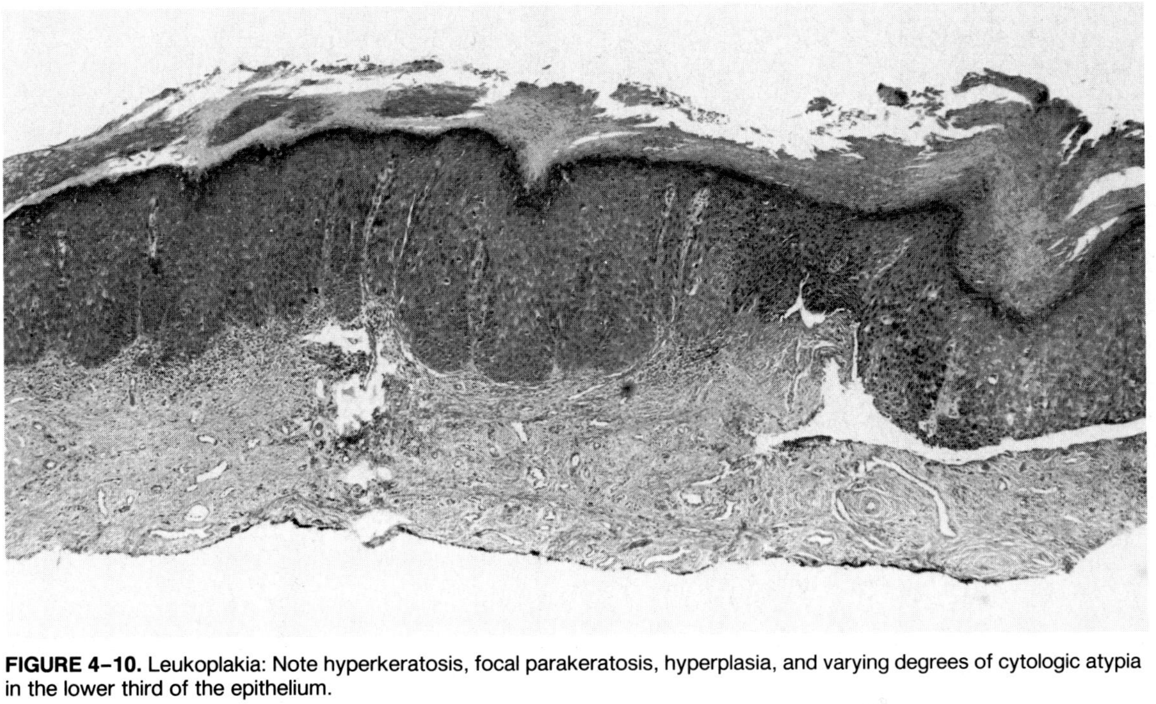

FIGURE 4-10. Leukoplakia: Note hyperkeratosis, focal parakeratosis, hyperplasia, and varying degrees of cytologic atypia in the lower third of the epithelium.

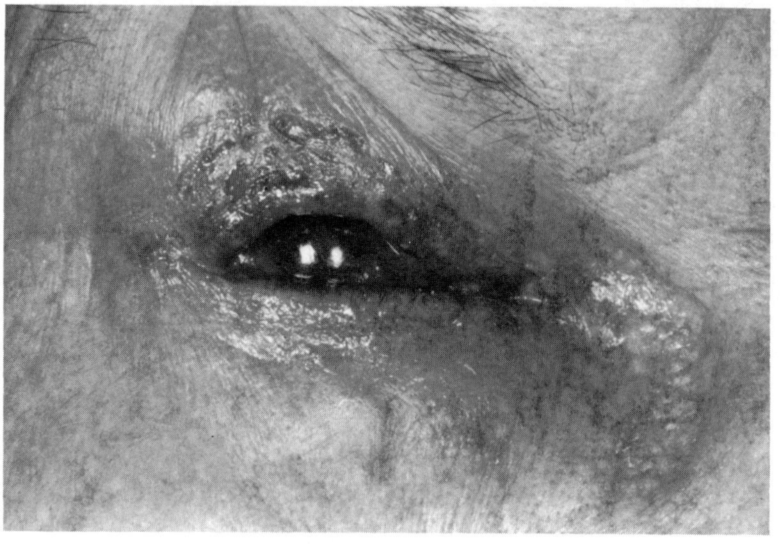

FIGURE 4–11. Bowen's disease: Note scaly, slightly raised, crusted plaque on upper eyelid.

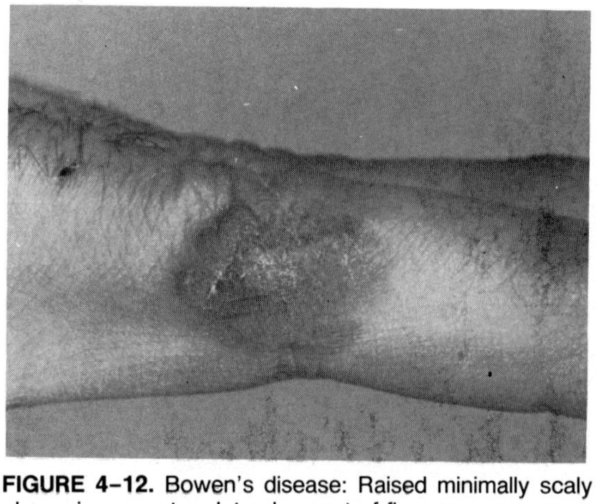

FIGURE 4–12. Bowen's disease: Raised minimally scaly plaque is present on lateral aspect of finger.

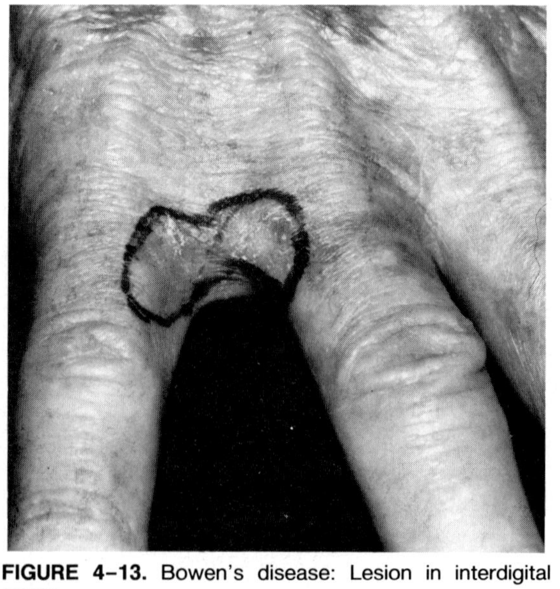

FIGURE 4–13. Bowen's disease: Lesion in interdigital space.

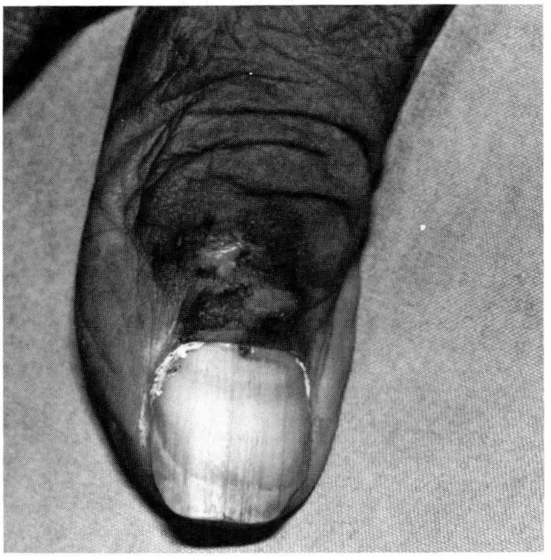

FIGURE 4-14. Bowen's disease: Note pigmentation of lesion on proximal nail fold.

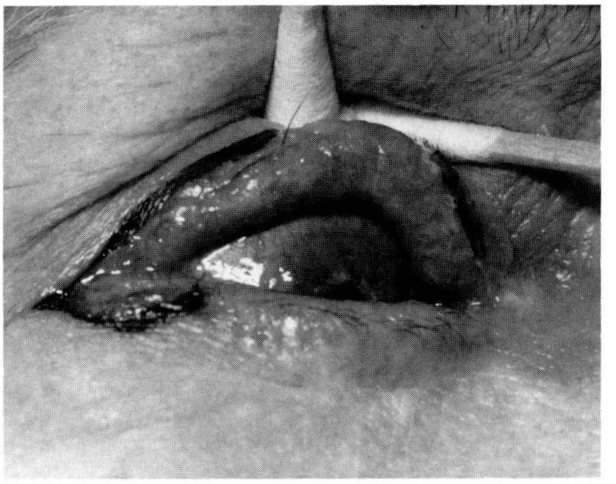

FIGURE 4-16. Erythroplasia of Queyrat: Shiny plaque on conjunctival surface of upper eyelid.

Bowen's disease represents an intraepithelial in situ squamous cell carcinoma and, histologically, is characterized by broad-based hyperplasia and full-thickness epithelial atypia. The dysplastic bowenoid epithelium shows a complete disarray of cellular polarity along with the presence of multiple, large atypical cells with pleomorphic, hyperchromatic nuclei and scattered dyskeratotic cells (Fig. 4-17). Overlying hyperkeratosis and parakeratosis may be present, and mitoses, often atypical, and multinucleated epithelial cells are seen (Fig. 4-18). Occasionally, the atypical epithelial cells are vacuolated and simulate the appearance of Paget's disease (Fig. 4-19). The integrity of the basal membrane is preserved. Erythroplasia of Queyrat has a histologic appearance identical to that of Bowen's disease, except that hyperkeratosis and parakeratosis are often absent (Fig. 4-20).

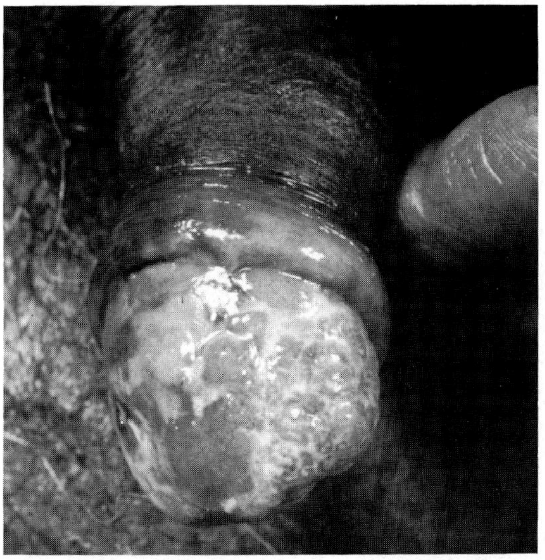

FIGURE 4-15. Erythroplasia of Queyrat: Shiny, indurated, focally macerated plaque involving entire glans penis.

Bowenoid Papulosis

Bowenoid papulosis is a recently recognized but not uncommon entity that involves the genitalia of both men and women. It presents clinically as multiple, small, red-brown, somewhat verrucous, flesh-colored to slightly pigmented papules on the glans and penile shaft in men (Fig. 4-21) and on the perineum and vulva in women (Fig. 4-22). The lesions occur most often in patients under the age of 40 who often have had a history of genital warts. They tend to regress spontaneously or with conservative treatment but can persist and, in rare instances, have been noted to progress to true in situ or invasive carcinoma.[3] Evidence of a viral etiology for bowenoid papulosis has been substantiated, based on the histologic finding of human papilloma virus type 16 antigen in the lesions.[4]

The histologic changes in bowenoid papulosis are often indistinguishable from those of Bowen's disease. However, subtle histologic differences may be noted in some cases. These differences include a more focal or circumscribed

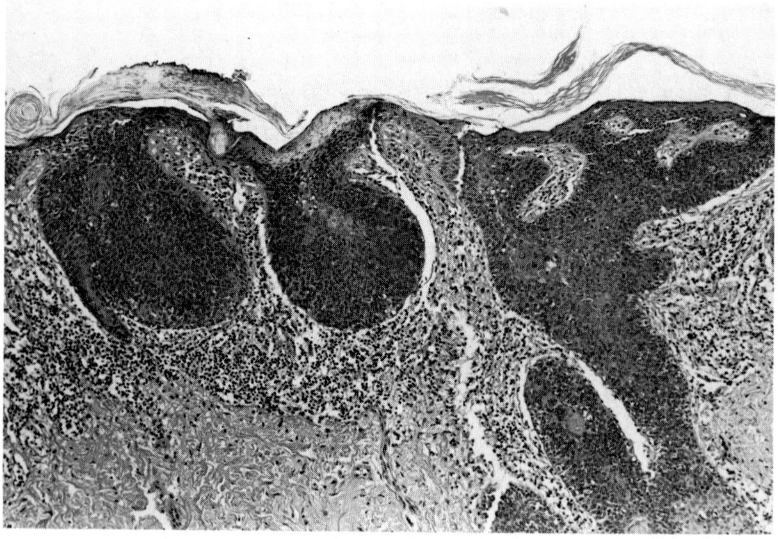

FIGURE 4–17. Bowen's disease: Broad acanthosis and full-thickness epithelial atypia characterize Bowen's disease; note involvement of adnexal (sweat duct) epithelium.

FIGURE 4–18. Bowen's disease: Note numerous mitoses and multinucleated epithelial cells.

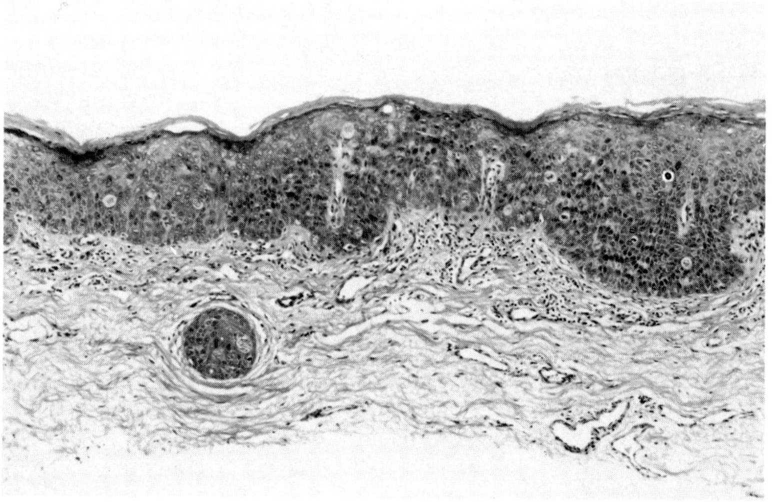

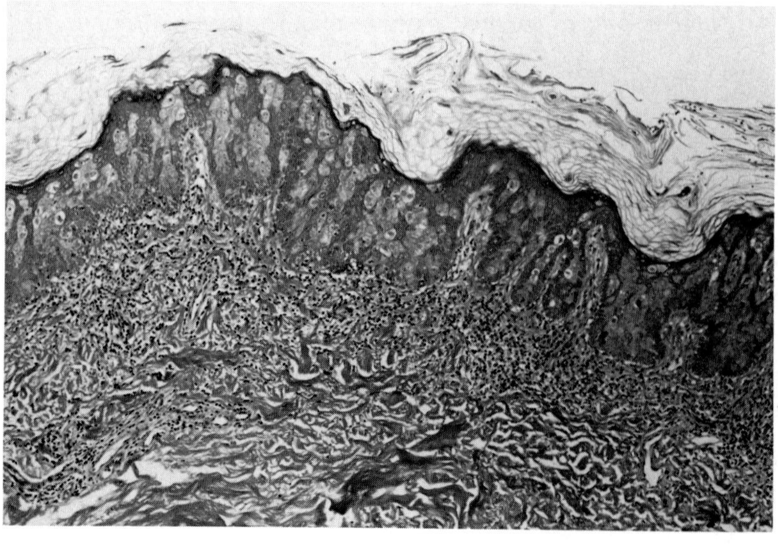

FIGURE 4–19. Bowen's disease: Note similarity of atypical bowenoid epithelium to epithelial changes in Paget's disease in this lesion.

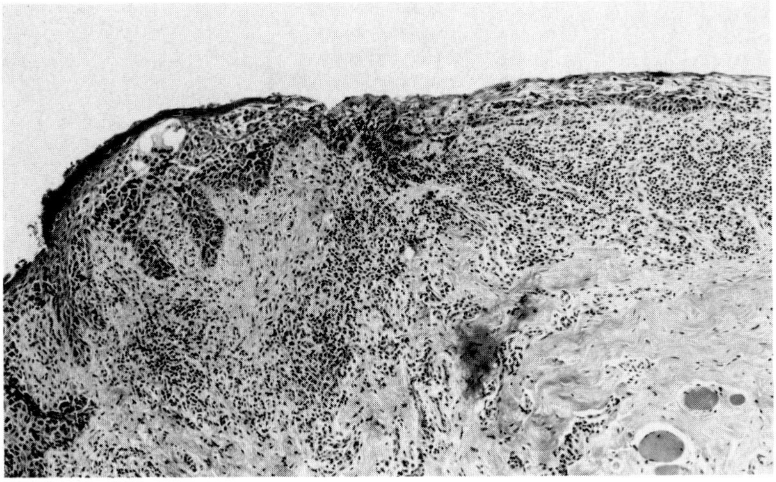

FIGURE 4–20. Erythroplasia of Queyrat: Histology is identical to that of Bowen's disease except for lack of hyperkeratosis and parakeratosis.

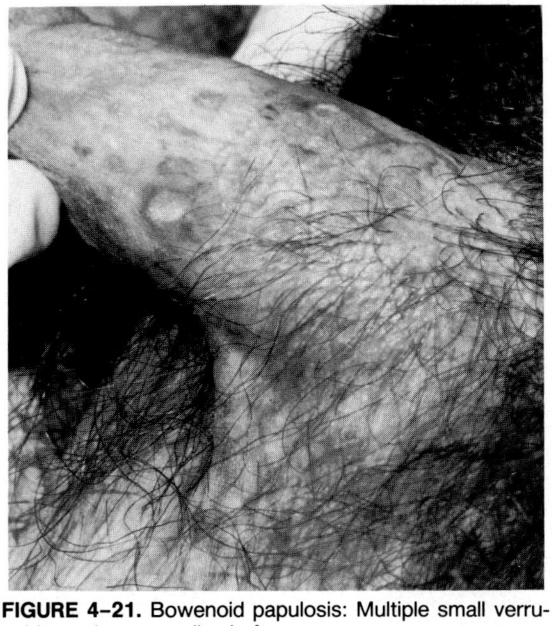

FIGURE 4–21. Bowenoid papulosis: Multiple small verrucoid papules on penile shaft.

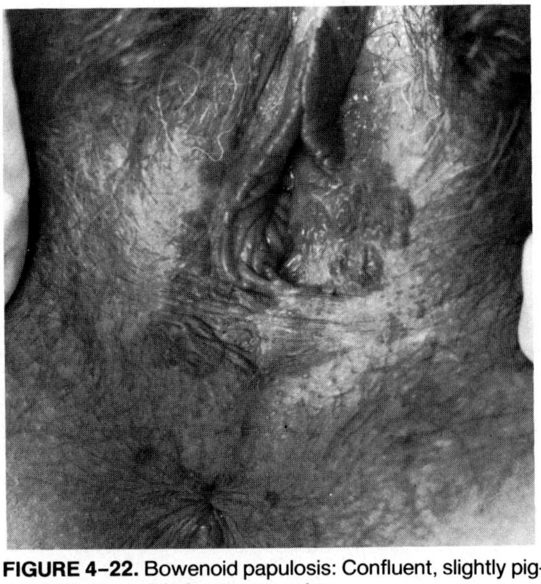

FIGURE 4–22. Bowenoid papulosis: Confluent, slightly pigmented verrucoid plaques on vulva.

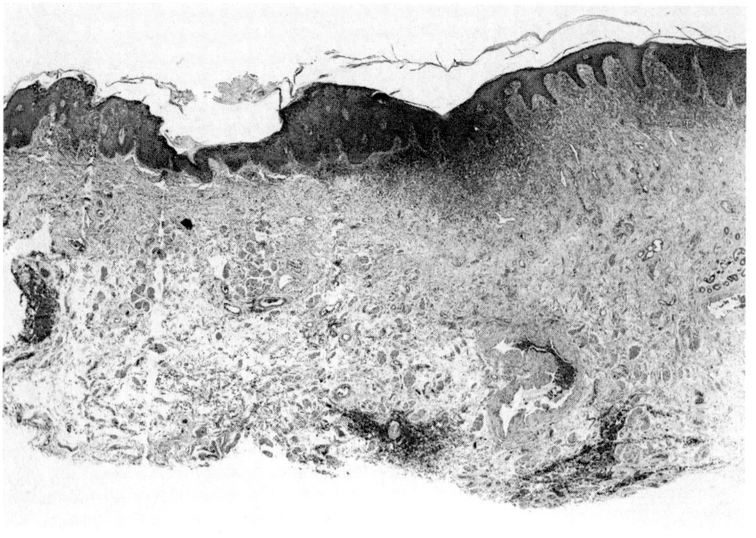

FIGURE 4–23. Bowenoid papulosis: Note focal areas of squamous cell atypia interspersed among normal-appearing epithelium.

area of epithelial atypia (Fig. 4–23), a lesser degree of cytologic atypia, and the fact that the atypical epithelium in bowenoid papulosis shows a more orderly background of keratinocyte maturation than in Bowen's disease (Fig. 4–24). Also, histologic evidence of condylomata acuminata and bowenoid papulosis may coexist in the same lesion.

MALIGNANT EPITHELIAL NEOPLASMS

Basal Cell Carcinoma

Basal cell carcinomas (BCC), or epitheliomas, are neoplasms of epithelial origin seen almost exclusively on hair-bearing skin. They usually occur as solitary lesions in adults, although the occurrence of multiple lesions either simultaneously or subsequently is not uncommon. They are most often encountered on the sun-exposed areas of fair-skinned individuals, and prolonged sun exposure is felt to be the primary predisposing factor in their development. As in squamous cell carcinoma, other less common contributing factors in basal cell carcinoma are large doses of x-rays, burns, scars, and possibly the injection of or exposure to chemical carcinogens.

There are five main clinical types of BCC: noduloulcerative; pigmented; morphea-like, or sclerotic; superficial; and fibroepithelioma. The noduloulcerative BCC is the most common

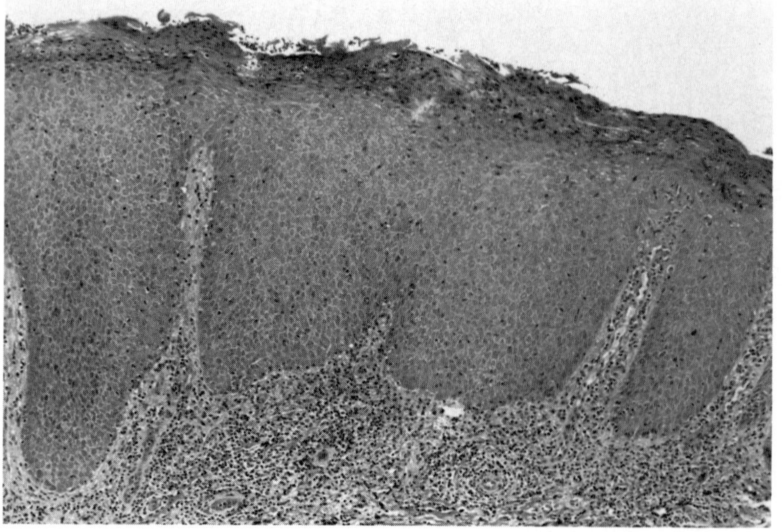

FIGURE 4–24. Bowenoid papulosis: Degree of cytologic atypia is less remarkable, and there is a more orderly maturation of keratinocytes in involved epithelium in Bowenoid papulosis as compared with Bowen's disease.

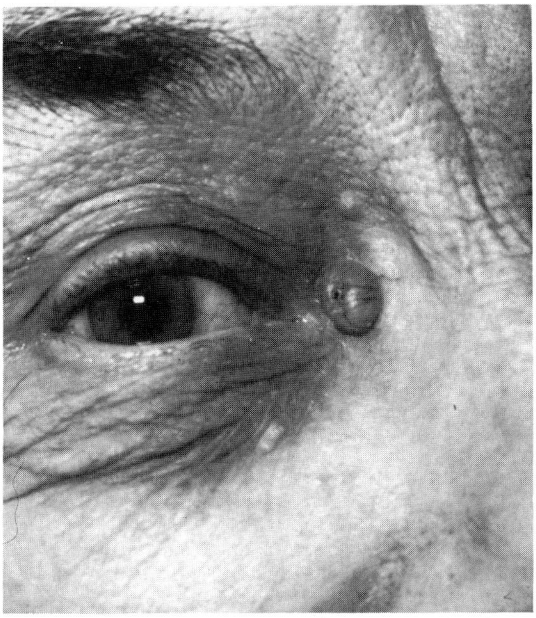

FIGURE 4–25. Basal cell carcinoma: Early nodular basal cell carcinoma consists of a raised telangiectatic nodule with a small central erosion.

clinical variant and usually begins as a small, telangiectatic, waxy nodule with or without a central erosion (Fig. 4–25). It typically gradually increases in size, ulcerates centrally, and is surrounded by a pearly rolled border (Fig. 4–26). If left untreated, it can enlarge in size and

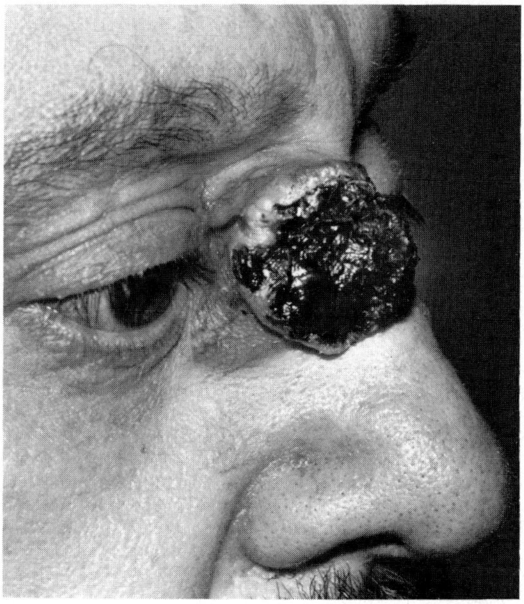

FIGURE 4–26. Basal cell carcinoma: More advanced nodulo-ulcerative basal cell carcinoma shows central ulceration with raised pearly border.

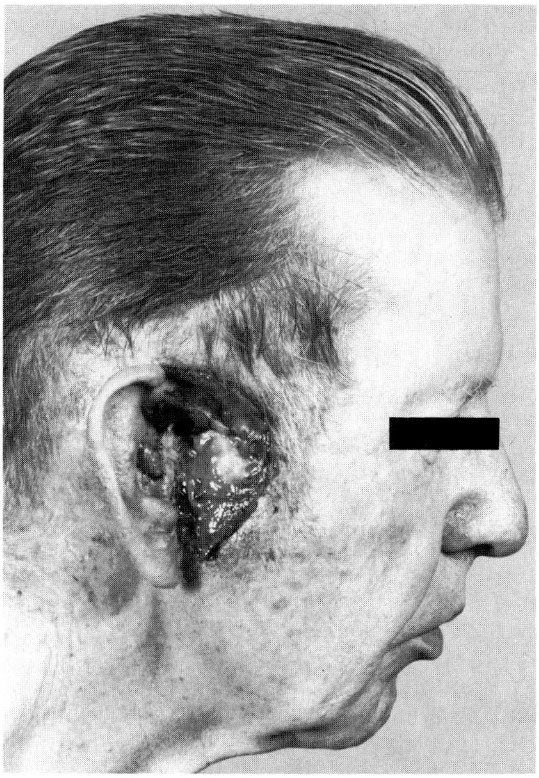

FIGURE 4–27. Basal cell carcinoma: Long-standing nodulo-ulcerative basal cell carcinoma with ulceration and extensive local tissue destruction.

can become more aggressive with direct invasion into the surrounding and underlying tissues (Fig. 4–27). The pigmented BCC differs from the noduloulcerative type by the presence of varying degrees of melanin in the lesion (Fig. 4–28). The morphea-like or sclerotic BCC manifests itself as a slightly raised, shiny, indurated, occasionally telangiectatic plaque with ill-defined borders (Fig. 4–29). The superficial BCC presents as one or several erythematous, scaling, slighty raised plaques that are surrounded by a fine, thread-like raised border. They may show foci of erosion or crusting, and occur predominantly on the trunk (Fig. 4–30). Fibroepithelioma was first described by Pinkus[5] and presents usually as a solitary, raised, firm, sessile to slightly pedunculated nodule with overlying red, smooth skin (Fig. 4–31). It is most commonly seen on the back.

As a rule, BCC does not metastasize, but incidences of metastasis ranging from 0.01% to 0.1% have been reported.[6,7] Typically, metastasis results from a large, long-standing, ulcerated, locally invasive primary lesion or from one that has recurred despite repeated surgical

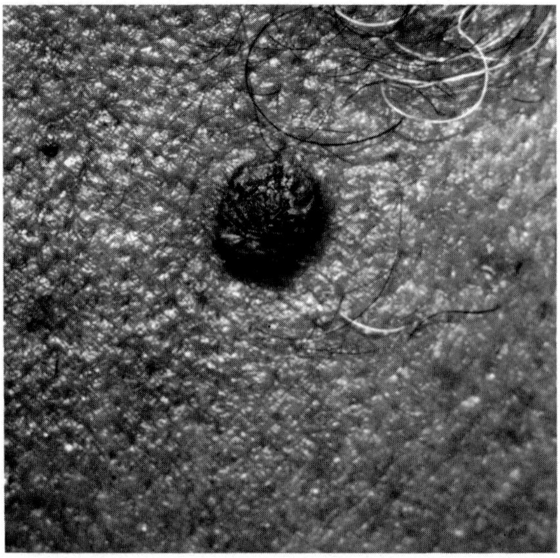

FIGURE 4–28. Basal cell carcinoma: Note raised, slightly shiny pigmented nodule on cheek.

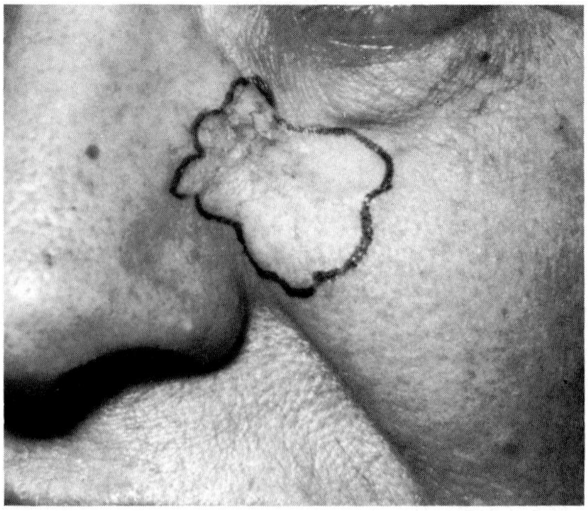

FIGURE 4–29. Basal cell carcinoma: Sclerotic (morphea-like) basal cell carcinomas present as a firm, slightly raised, indurated, ill-defined plaque on the malar region.

excisions or radiotherapy. Also, the morphea-like, or sclerotic type, of BCC seems to have a greater propensity for metastasis than the other types. The most common sites of metastatic spread are lymph nodes, bone, and lungs.

There are three clinical syndromes in which BCC plays an important role: linear unilateral basal cell nevus, the nevoid BCC syndrome, and the Bazex syndrome. The linear unilateral basal cell nevus syndrome is rare, and consists of a unilateral linear or zosteriform eruption consisting of multiple, closely set, nodules of BCC with or without superimposed comedones and striae-like atrophy. The nevoid BCC syndrome is inherited as an autosomal dominant condition with low penetrance. Hundreds of small nodules appear on the face and body between puberty and early adulthood during the "nevoid" stage. During later adulthood, the lesions may become more aggressive, invasive, destructive, and mutilating in the "neoplastic" stage (Fig. 4–32). Death may ensue as a result of invasion of the brain and orbit. Over half of the adult patients with the nevoid BCC syndrome show numerous, small, plantar and palmar pits (Fig. 4–33), which are felt to represent

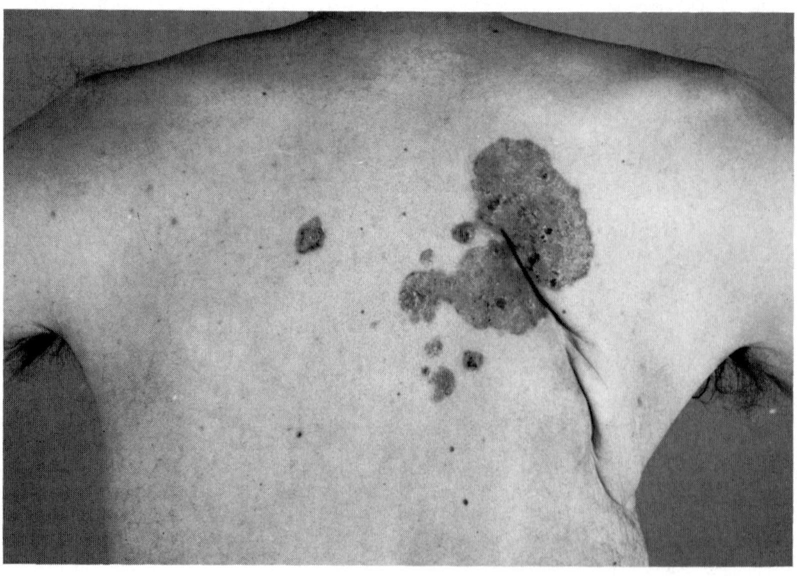

FIGURE 4–30. Basal cell carcinoma: Superficial variant shows multiple solitary and confluent, scaly, focally eroded plaques with a thin raised border.

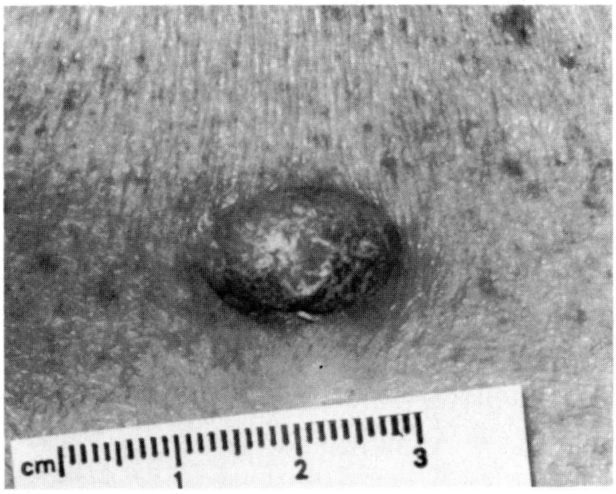

FIGURE 4–31. Basal cell carcinoma: Fibroepithelioma (fibroepithelial tumor of Pinkus) is seen as a firm, dome-shaped, slightly pedunculated nodule with relatively smooth surface.

formes frustes of BCC in those locations. Patients may also show several skeletal and central nervous system anomalies, including odontogenic keratocysts of the jaw, rib anomalies, scoliosis, mental retardation, and intracranial calcification. The Bazex syndrome (dominantly inherited) consists of follicular atrophoderma and multiple small, usually facial basal cell carcinomas. Occasionally localized or generalized hypohidrosis or anhidrosis and congenital hypotrichosis are seen.

The characteristic cell of BCC, the so-called

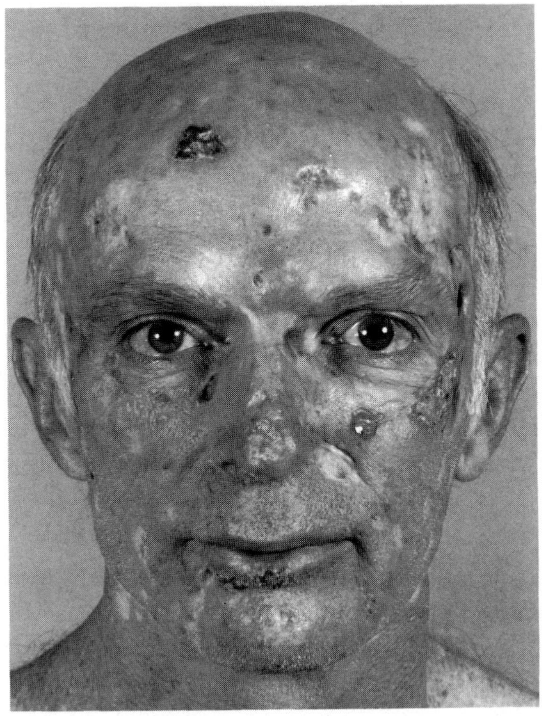

FIGURE 4–32. Basal cell carcinoma: Multiple superficial nodular to focally invasive lesions on the face of a patient with nevoid basal cell carcinoma syndrome.

basalioma cell, has a large, ovoid nucleus and relatively little cytoplasm. The nuclei resemble those of the basal cell layer of the epidermis, except that they have a higher nuclear-

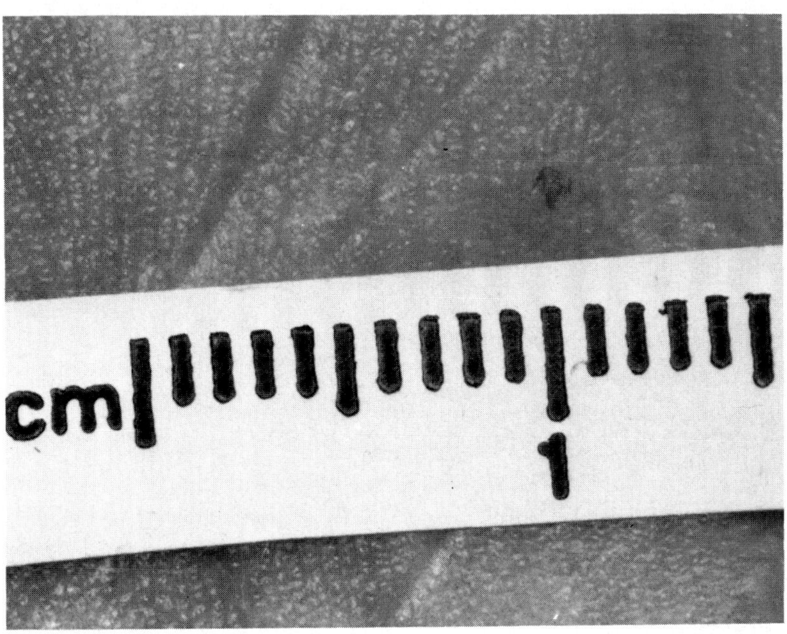

FIGURE 4–33. Basal cell carcinoma: Small palmar pits characteristic of patients with nevoid basal cell carcinoma syndrome.

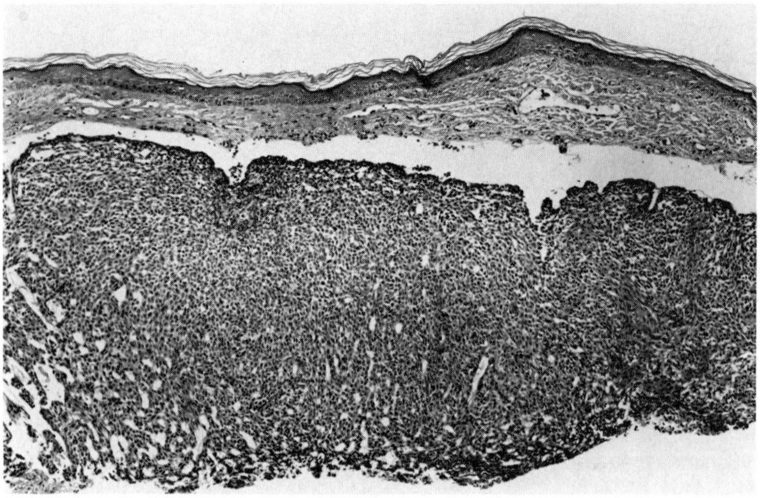

FIGURE 4–34. Basal cell carcinoma: Note mass of characteristic basalioma cells exhibiting peripheral palisading and retraction from dermal stroma.

to-cytoplasmic ratio, and they stain more basophilic on H&E sections than normal epidermal cells. They do not have a particularly anaplastic appearance, although occasionally large multinucleated cells or atypical mitoses may be seen. The cells may contain varying amounts of melanin pigment. They tend to be fairly cohesive, usually forming closely packed islands and nests of cells. Characteristically, the cells at the periphery of the tumor islands show a palisade type of arrangement. The surrounding dermal stroma often appears rarefied and mucinous and may contain numerous spindle-shaped fibroblastic cells in addition to patchy areas of inflammation. Frequently, there are areas of retraction of the stroma from the tumor islands resulting in peritumoral clefts (Fig. 4–34).

From a histologic standpoint, basal cell carcinomas can roughly be divided into seven major types. However, significant overlap between the various types is common. The types are: superficial, solid, cystic, keratotic, adenoid, morphea-like (sclerotic), and fibroepithelioma (fibroepithelial tumor of Pinkus).

Superficial BCC shows multiple buds and irregular proliferations of basalioma cells attached to the undersurface of the epidermis and embedded in a fibrous stroma. The tumor islands usually show peripheral palisading of basalioma cells and retraction from the surrounding dermal stroma (Fig. 4–35).

Solid BCC shows multiple, varying sized masses of basalioma cells with peripheral palisading of nuclei and retraction clefts from the surrounding dermis (Fig. 4–36). Foci of tumor cell necrosis, epidermal ulceration, solar elastosis, and a patchy chronic dermal infiltrate are often seen.

In the cystic variant, one or several large,

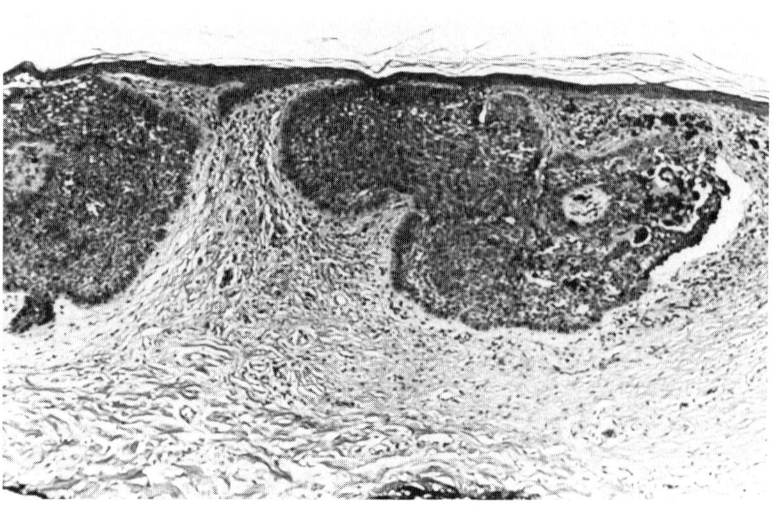

FIGURE 4–35. Basal cell carcinoma: Superficial type of basal cell carcinoma shows multiple small islands of basalioma cells attached to the undersurface of the epidermis.

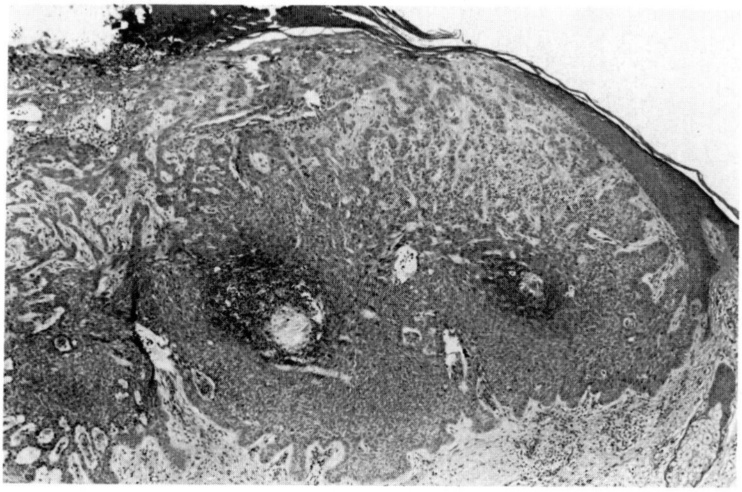

FIGURE 4–36. Basal cell carcinoma: Solid type of basal cell carcinoma shows large aggregates of basalioma cells with peripheral palisading and focal retraction from surrounding dermis. Note associated ulceration and chronic inflammation.

cystic cavities are present within solid aggregates of basalioma cells (Fig. 4–37). The cystic space is most likely formed as a result of extensive necrosis of tumor cells.

The keratotic BCC shows foci of keratotic cells and horn cysts within the islands of basalioma cells (Fig. 4–38). The horn cysts appear to represent abortive attempts at hair shaft formation. Keratotic basal cell carcinomas share this feature in common with trichoepitheliomas, sometimes causing great difficulty in histologic differentation between the two (Fig. 4–39).

The adenoid BCC shows formations resembling tubules or gland-like structures within the tumor islands, which are often surrounded by a mucoid stroma (Fig. 4–40). The morphea-like, or sclerotic, BCC shows multiple, small, narrow strands of basalioma cells, embedded in a dense, fibrous dermal stroma (Fig. 4–41). The tumor cells often extend deep into the dermis and may occasionally be associated with a few, slightly larger and more closely recognizable aggregates of basalioma cells.

The fibroepithelioma type of BCC (also termed fibroepithelial tumor of Pinkus) consists of long, thin, branching, and anastomosing strands of basalioma cells that extend from the overlying epidermis into a fibromucinous dermal stroma (Fig. 4–42). The tumor is usually well demarcated at its lower border. In more advanced lesions, foci of superficial, solid, or cystic types of BCC may be present (Fig. 4–43). Ulceration and deeper dermal extension can also occur.

Other uncommon histologic variants of BCC include the adamantinoid, granular, clear-cell, and matrical types, but discussion of

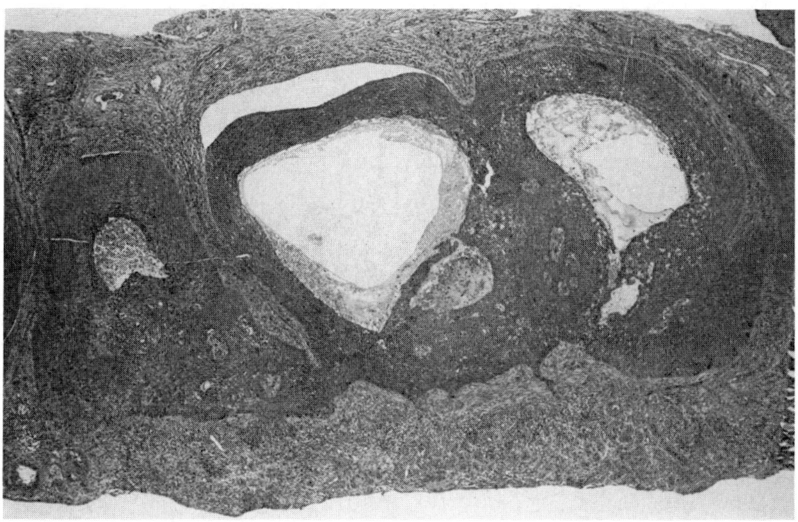

FIGURE 4–37. Basal cell carcinoma: Several large cystic cavities within larger solid islands of basalioma cells define cystic variant of basal cell carcinoma.

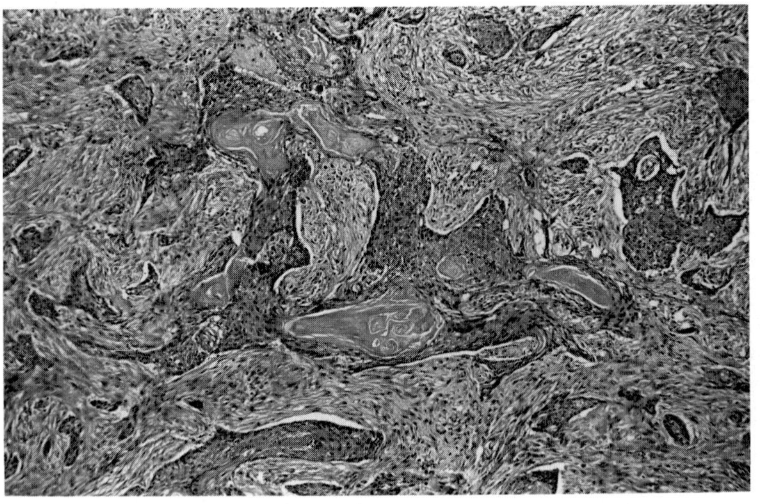

FIGURE 4–38. Basal cell carcinoma: Keratotic basal cell carcinoma shows several foci of keratinization within islands of basalioma cells.

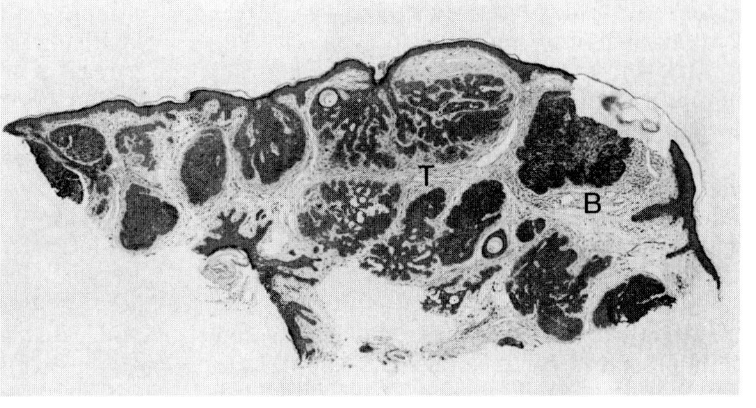

FIGURE 4–39. Basal cell carcinoma: Photomicrograph of lesion showing features of both trichoepithelioma (*T*) and solid variant of basal cell carcinoma (*B*). Features favoring diagnosis of basal cell carcinoma include presence of larger, undifferentiated masses of basalioma cells, focal dermal inflammation, and retraction of tumor islands from surrounding dermal stroma.

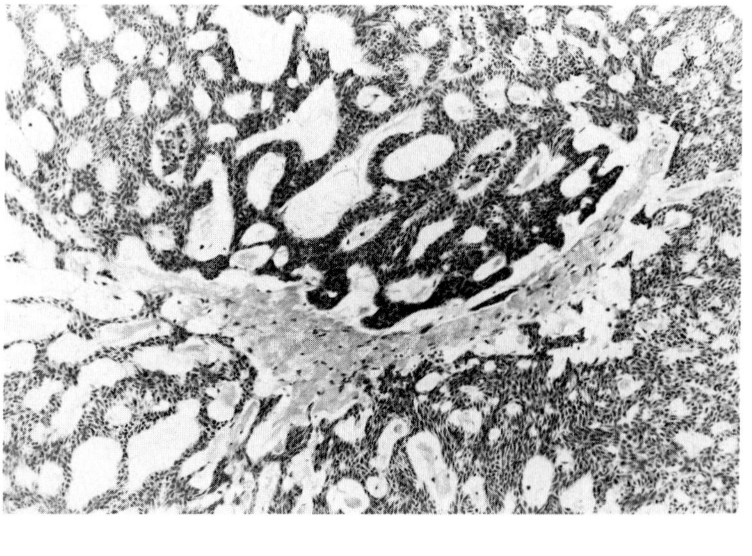

FIGURE 4–40. Basal cell carcinoma: Adenoid basal cell carcinoma shows formations resembling glandular or tubular structures.

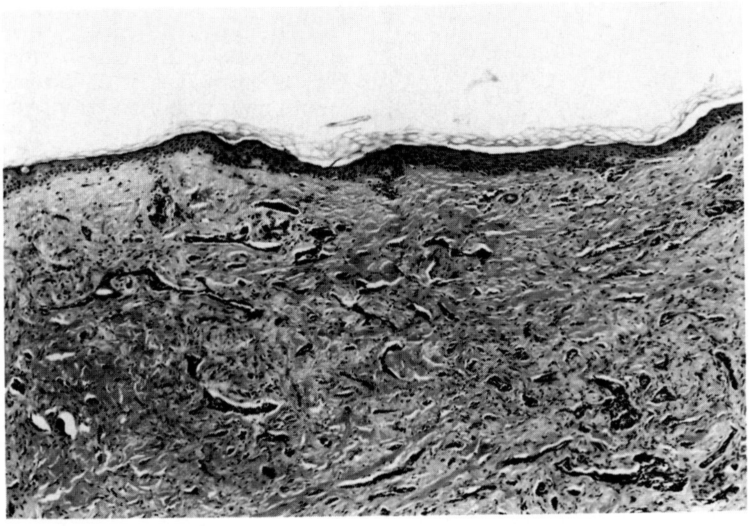

FIGURE 4–41. Basal cell carcinoma: Sclerotic (morphea-like) basal cell carcinoma shows multiple, small, narrow strands of basalioma cells embedded within a dense fibrous stroma.

FIGURE 4–42. Basal cell carcinoma: Fibroepithelioma (fibroepithelial tumor of Pinkus) consists of long, thin, branching, and anastomosing strands of basalioma cells extending from the epidermis into underlying fibrotic dermal stroma.

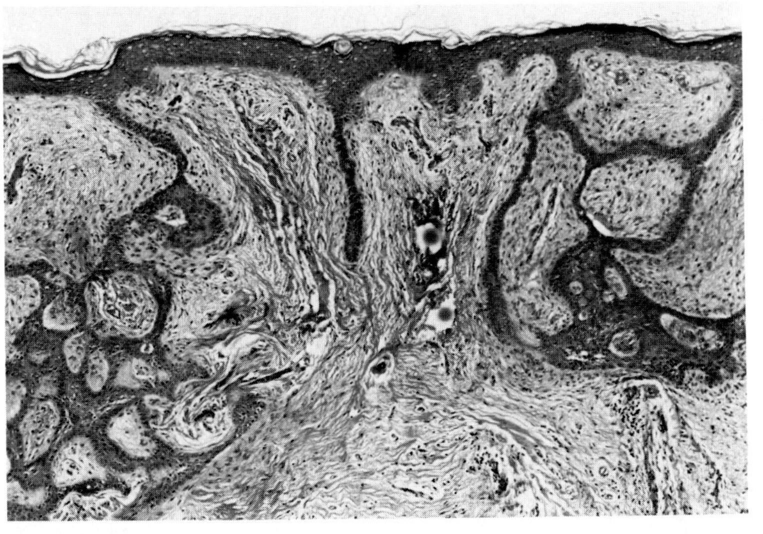

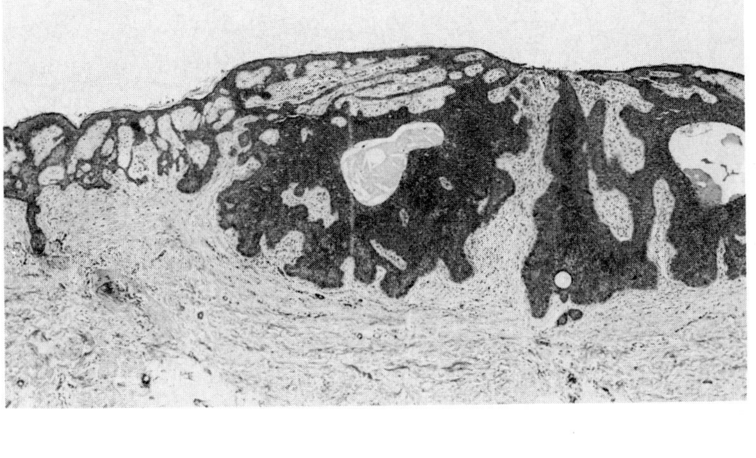

FIGURE 4–43. Basal cell carcinoma: Note islands of solid and cystic basal cell carcinoma *(left)* within lesion of fibroepithelioma *(right).*

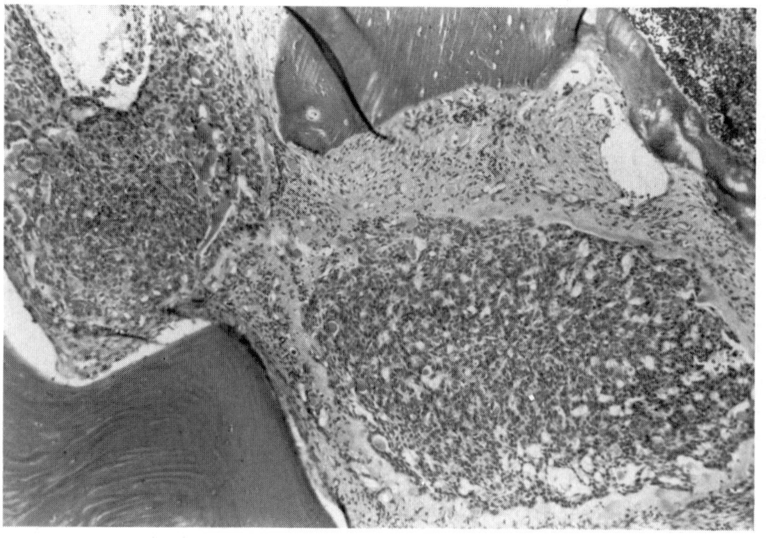

FIGURE 4–44. Basal cell carcinoma: Lesion of metastatic basal cell carcinoma in bone shows features characteristic of primary solid type of basal cell carcinoma.

these variants is beyond the scope of this text. The histologic features of metastatic basal cell carcinoma closely resemble those of the primary cutaneous lesion (Fig. 4–44).

Squamous Cell Carcinoma

Squamous cell carcinoma (SCC) may occur anywhere on the skin and mucous membranes. Clinically, SCC of the skin most commonly presents as either a shallow ulcer surrounded by an irregular raised border (Fig. 4–45) or as a raised, fungating, irregularly shaped nodule with or without ulceration (Fig. 4–46). SCC is usually seen in sun-damaged skin, either de novo or from a preexisting actinic keratosis. The latter apparently has a relatively low propensity for metastasis. Other premalignant epithelial lesions that may give rise to invasive SCC include Bowen's disease (Fig. 4–47) and erythroplasia of Queyrat (Fig. 4–48 and 4–49). SCC may also arise from preexisting burn scars, from foci of chronic irritation, and from long-standing cutaneous ulcerations. SCC aris-

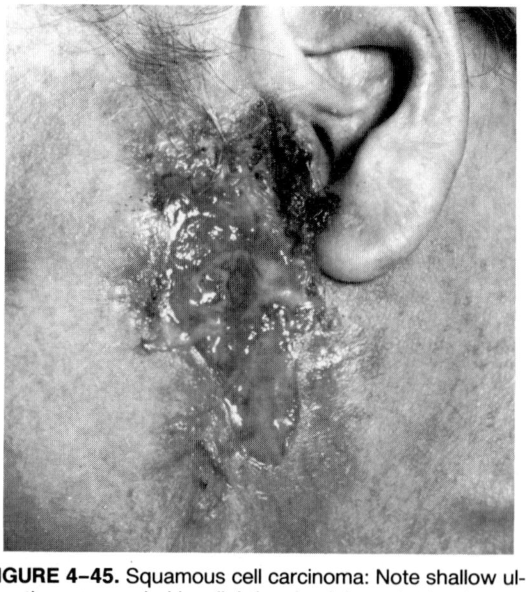

FIGURE 4–45. Squamous cell carcinoma: Note shallow ulceration surrounded by slightly raised, irregular border.

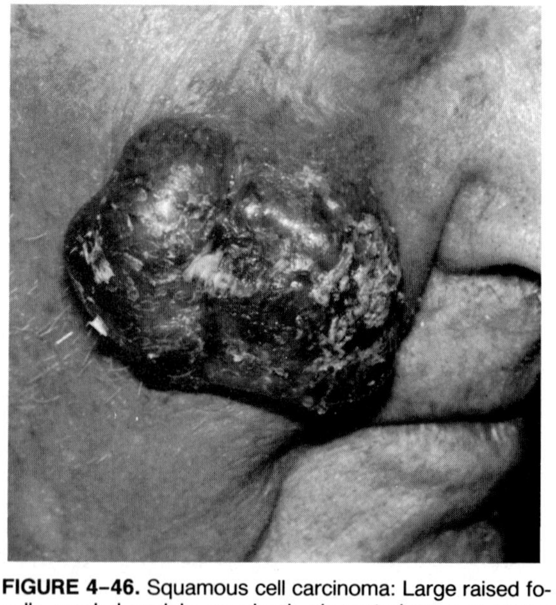

FIGURE 4–46. Squamous cell carcinoma: Large raised focally eroded nodule on cheek characterizes a common presentation of this lesion.

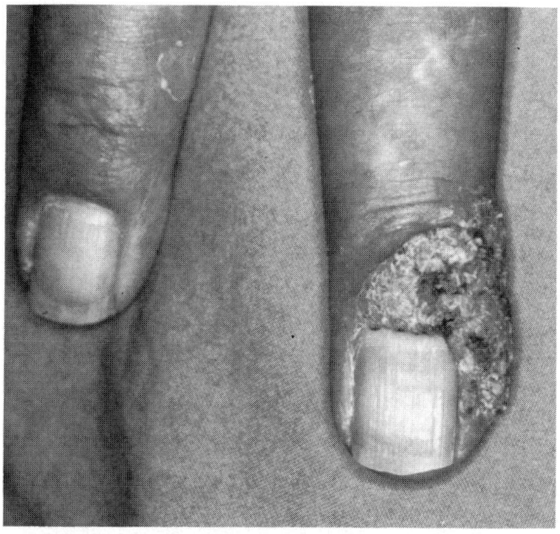

FIGURE 4–47. Squamous cell carcinoma: Invasive squamous cell carcinoma arising from a lesion of periungual Bowen's disease.

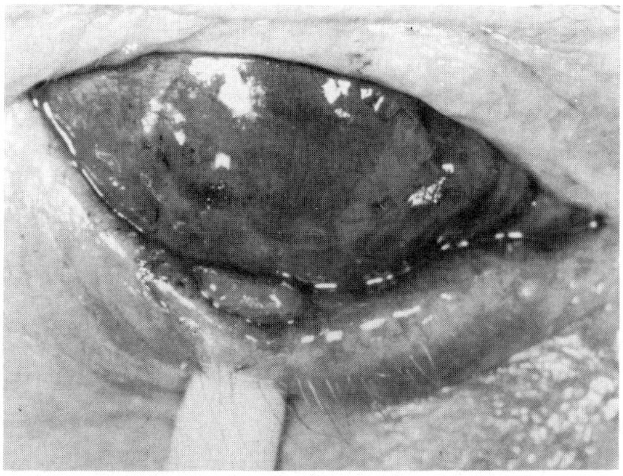

FIGURE 4–49. Squamous cell carcinoma: Small elevated nodular squamous cell carcinoma developing within conjunctival erythroplasia of Queyrat. (From Dixon R, Mikhail GR: Erythroplasia of conjunctiva. *Journal of the American Academy of Dermatology* 4:160–165, 1981. Copyright 1981, The C. V. Mosby Company.)

ing secondary to inflammatory and degenerative processes have a much higher rate of metastasis than those developing within sun-damaged skin or premalignant epithelial lesions. Uncommonly, SCC may arise from preexisting benign lesions, such as porokeratosis (Fig. 4–50) or psoriasis vulgaris (Fig. 4–51).

Histologically, SCC consists of irregular masses of squamous cells that proliferate downward from the surface epithelium into the underlying dermis. The infiltrating tumor masses are composed in varying proportions of

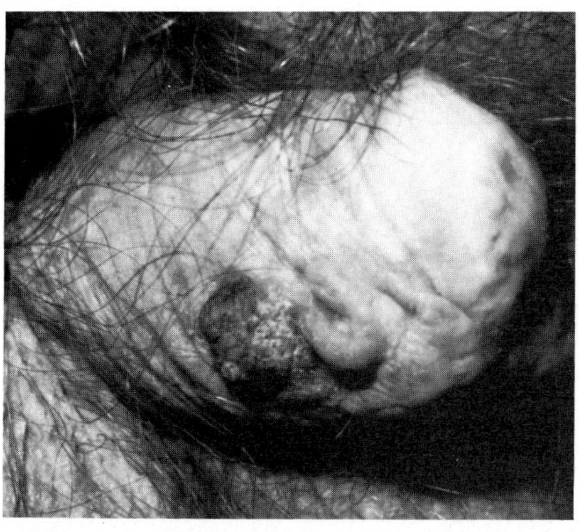

FIGURE 4–48. Squamous cell carcinoma: Raised verrucoid nodular squamous cell carcinoma arising from erythroplasia of Queyrat of the penis.

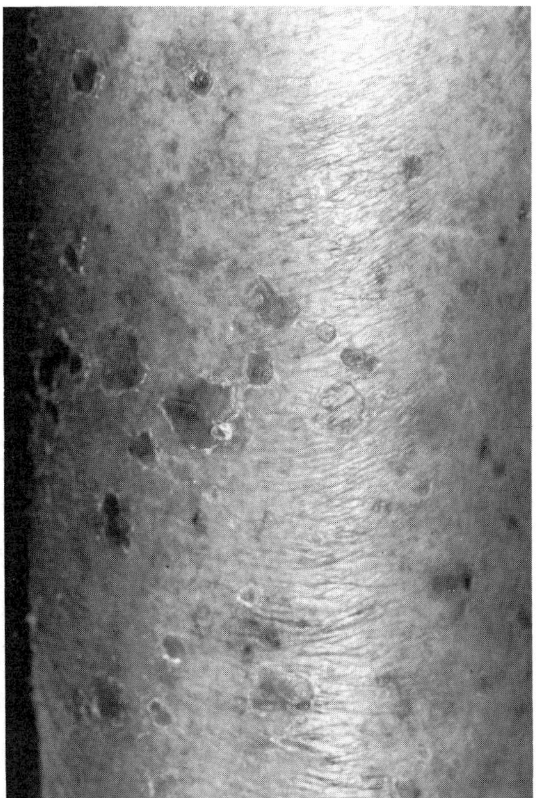

FIGURE 4–50. Squamous cell carcinoma: Multiple circinate lesions of porokeratosis on leg, some of which histologically showed early invasive squamous cell carcinoma (see Fig. 4–61).

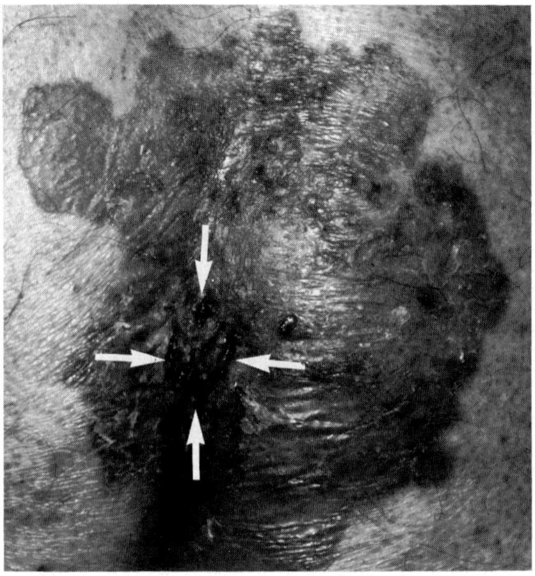

FIGURE 4–51. Squamous cell carcinoma: Note focus of eroded squamous cell carcinoma *(arrows)* developing within a plaque of psoriasis vulgaris in intergluteal region.

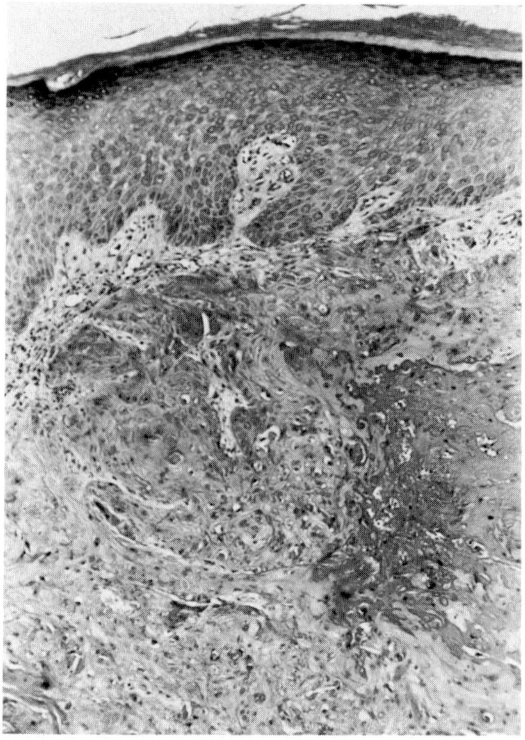

FIGURE 4–52. Squamous cell carcinoma: Representative grade I lesion shows presence of squamous cell tumor masses in upper dermis composed of predominantly mature squamous cells with slight nuclear atypicality and a high degree of keratinization.

normal-appearing and atypical or anaplastic squamous cells. The anaplastic cells are characterized by pleomorphic and hyperchromatic nuclei, the absence of intercellular bridges, individual cell keratinization, and typical and atypical mitotic figures. Differentiation in SCC is toward keratinization, indicated by the formation of horn pearls, structures composed of concentric layers of squamous cells showing gradual progression to keratinization toward the center.

A system for grading cutaneous SCC was developed by Broders in 1921[8] that recognizes four grades of severity (I to IV) according to the proportion of differentiated and undifferenti-

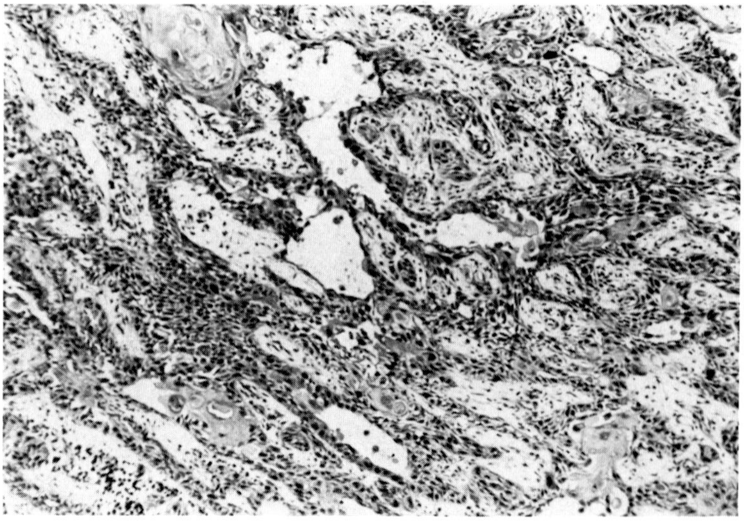

FIGURE 4–53. Squamous cell carcinoma: In grade II lesion, squamous cell masses show much less keratinization than in grade I, and cells exhibit a higher degree of nuclear atypicality.

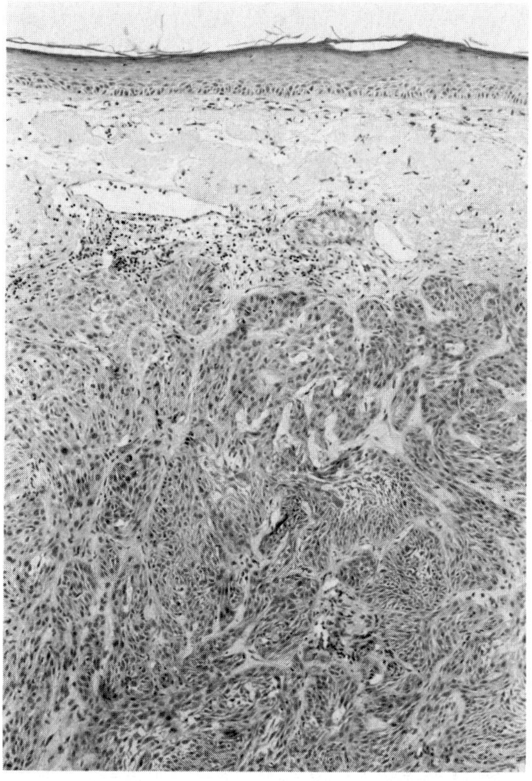

FIGURE 4–54. Squamous cell carcinoma: In grade III lesion keratinization is absent in most areas, many tumor cells are atypical and lack intercellular bridges.

ated cells in the tumor. Broders' grade I is also termed well-differentiated SCC and indicates a lesion with a high proportion of differentiated cells showing relatively slight atypicality and a high degree of keratinization (Fig. 4–52). Broders' grade II, termed moderately well-differentiated SCC, shows much less keratinization than grade I and a higher degree of cytologic atypicality (Fig. 4–53). In Broders' grade III, termed poorly differentiated SCC, keratinization is absent in many areas, intercellular bridges are commonly lacking, and the majority of tumor cells show significant nulcear anaplasia with atypical mitoses (Fig. 4–54). In Broders' grade IV, termed undifferentiated SCC, evidence of keratinization and intercellular bridge formation is absent. The tumor cells are highly anaplastic, containing pleomorphic, often spindle-shaped, nuclei and numerous atypical mitoses (Fig. 4–55). Because of this, grade IV SCC is often classified as spindle cell squamous carcinoma, and differentiation from atypical fibroxanthoma, amelanotic malignant melanoma, and fibrosarcoma becomes difficult without the aid of immunohistochemical examination of the tissue (Fig. 4–56).

Histologic variants of SCC include adenoid (acantholytic), desmoplastic, mucinous, "basosquamous" cell, and mixed carcinomas. Adenoid SCC is characterized by tumor islands with tubular and alveolar structures developing as a result of focal dyskeratosis and acantholysis of the neoplastic cells (Fig. 4–57). Desmoplastic SCC shows small nests and strands of atypical squanous cells surrounded by a densely fibrotic dermal stroma (Fig. 4–58). Basosquamous cell carcinomas are considered by some[9] to represent epithelial neoplasms with clearly definable features of both basal cell and squamous cell carcinoma within the same le-

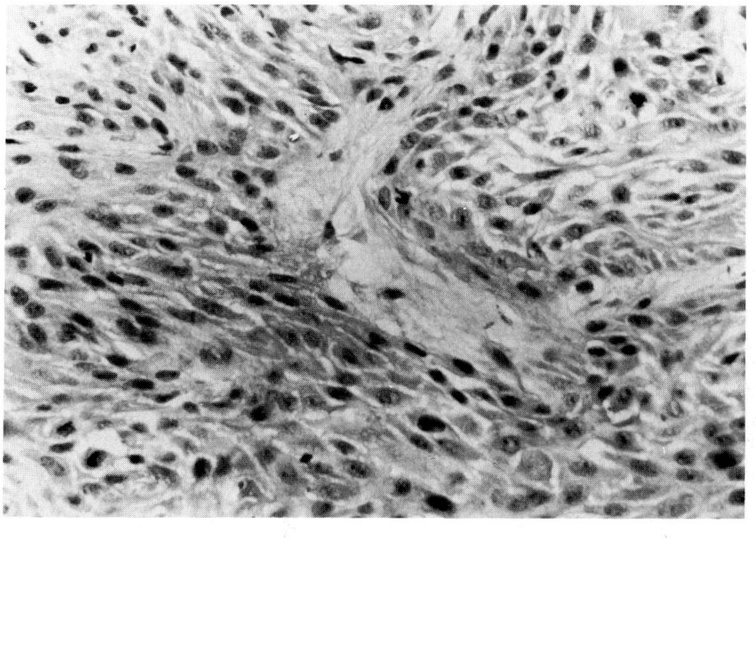

FIGURE 4–55. Squamous cell carcinoma: Grade IV lesion shows complete lack of keratinization and spindle-shaped anaplastic nuclei with numerous mitoses.

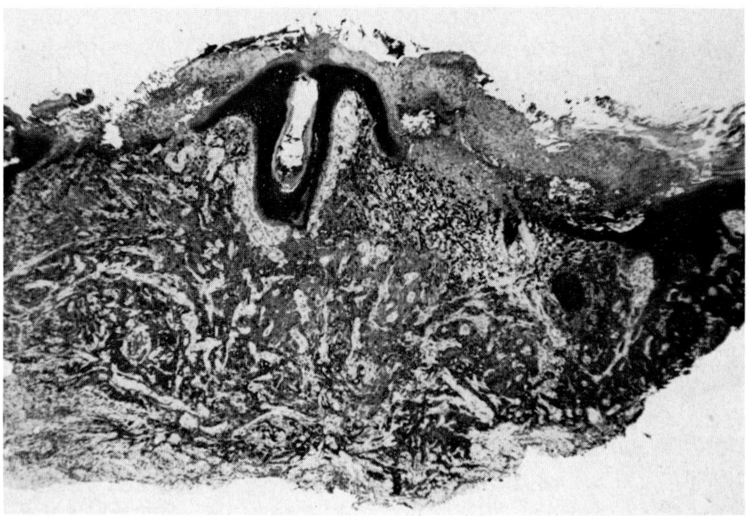

FIGURE 4–56. Squamous cell carcinoma: Immunohistochemical staining of undifferentiated, spindle cell squamous carcinoma with antikeratin antibodies shows positive staining of tumor islands and overlying epidermis.

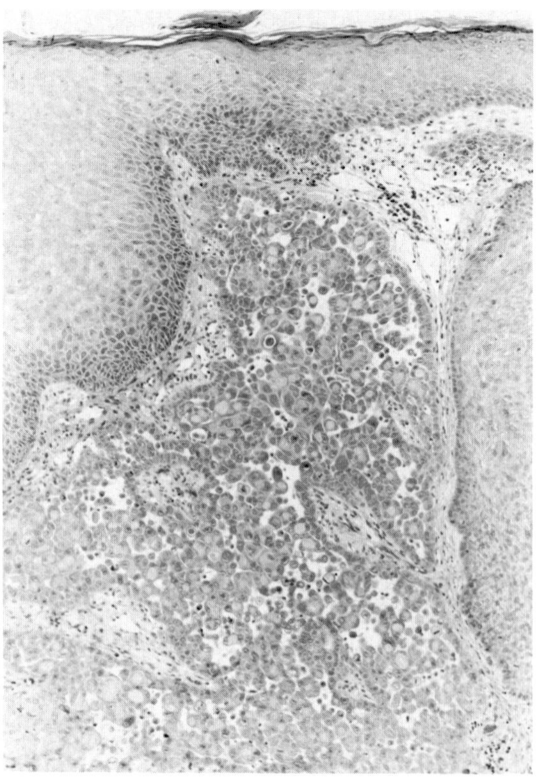

FIGURE 4–57. Squamous cell carcinoma: Adenoid (acantholytic) variant with alveolar morphology of tumor islands which contain acantholytic, dyskeratotic, and anaplastic squamous cells.

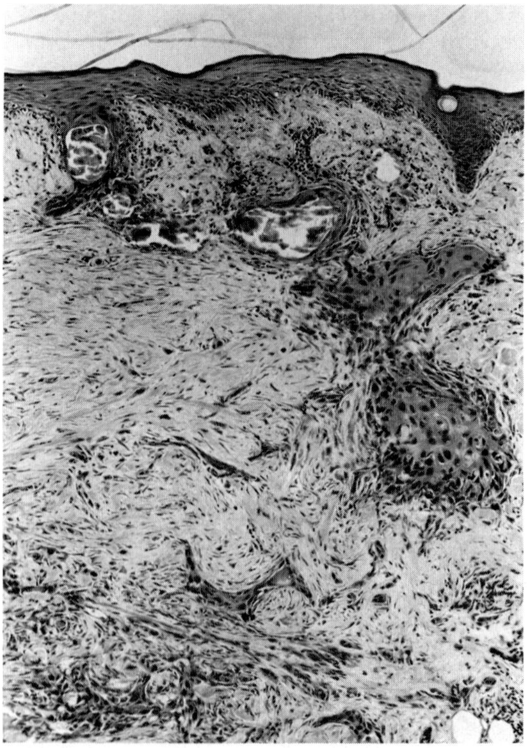

FIGURE 4–58. Squamous cell carcinoma: Desmoplastic variant shows small nests of atypical squamous cells embedded within a dense fibrous stroma.

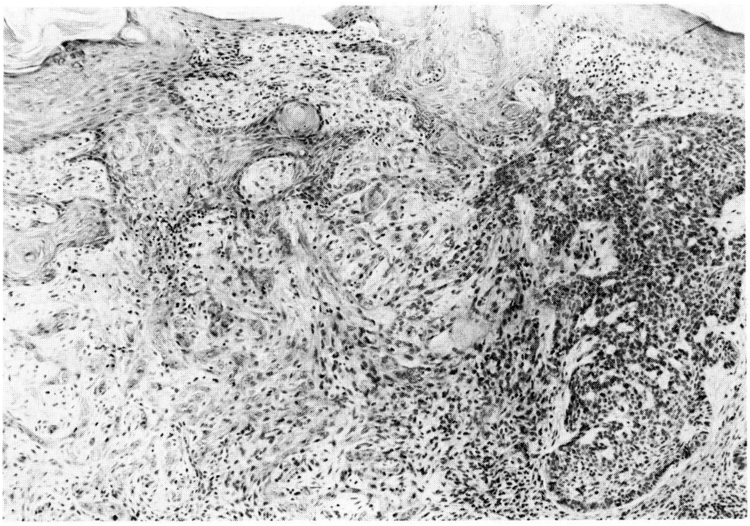

FIGURE 4-59. Squamous cell carcinoma: So-called basosquamous cell carcinoma shows tumor to exhibit features of both squamous cell carcinoma *(left)* and basal cell carcinoma *(right).*

sion (Fig. 4–59). Some authors question the existence of basosquamous cell carcinoma and feel that such lesions are probably basal cell carcinomas with focal squamoid differentiation of the tumor cells (also termed metatypical or metaplastic basal cell carcinoma).[10,11] Mixed carcinoma shows a SCC contiguous to a BCC or so-called collision tumor (Fig. 4–60). Lesions of SCC developing within benign lesions or premalignant lesions show combined features of both the primary lesion and the carcinoma (Fig. 4–61 and 4–62).

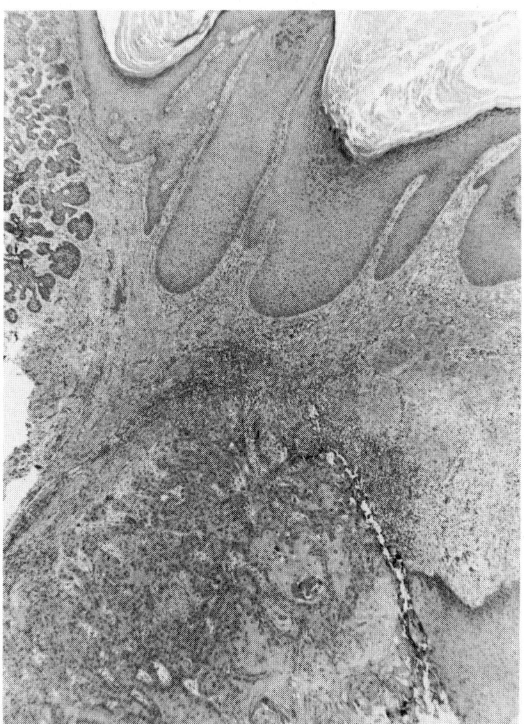

FIGURE 4-60. Squamous cell carcinoma: Mixed carcinoma shows foci of squamous cell carcinoma *(bottom)* and basal cell carcinoma *(upper left)* contiguous to each other in the same lesion.

Verrucous Carcinoma

Verrucous carcinoma is a low-grade squamous cell carcinoma that presents clinically as a slowly growing, initially exophytic, verrucous plaque or nodule that may ultimately penetrate deep into the underlying tissues. It causes local destruction of tissue and metastasizes only very late, if at all. The three regions in which verrucous carcinoma most commonly occurs are the oral cavity, the anogenital region, and the plantar surface of the foot. Verrucous carcinoma of the oral cavity (also called oral florid papillomatosis) presents as large, white, cauliflower lesions on the oral mucosa. Verrucous carcinoma of the anogenital area (also called Buschke-Löwenstein tumor) presents as a large, exophytic papillomatous plaque, most commonly on the glans penis and the foreskin in uncircumcised men or on the vulva in women. Studies have shown evidence of human papilloma virus infection in some cases of anogenital verrucous carcinoma.[12] Plantar verrucous carcinoma (also known as epithelioma cuniculatum) presents as an exophytic, verrucoid mass resembling a wart (Fig. 4–63).

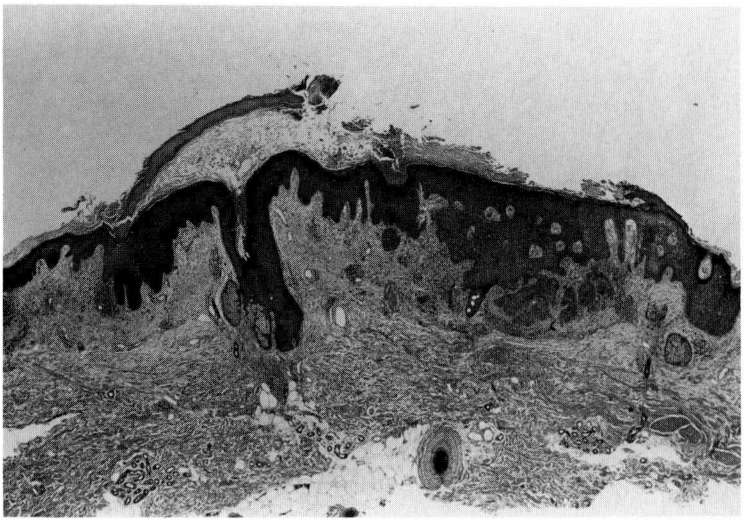

FIGURE 4–61. Squamous cell carcinoma: Early invasive squamous cell carcinoma *(right)* developing within a lesion of porokeratosis; note elongated cornoid lamella near left lateral margin of lesion.

As the lesion grows, it develops crypts, abscesses, and erosions and may eventually penetrate deeply into the underlying bony structures of the foot. Other less common areas of involvement by verrucous carcinoma include the palm (Fig. 4–64), back, and face (Fig. 4–65).

Histologically, the superficial portion of the tumor generally resembles a verruca, and shows hyperkeratosis, parakeratosis, papillomatosis, and irregular acanthosis. However, large bulbous masses of relatively well-differentiated squamous cells extend deeply into the underlying dermis and even into the subcutaneous tissue (Fig. 4–66). There may be mild nuclear atypia of the keratinocytes in the lower layers of the acanthotic epithelium, but significant nuclear anaplasia, horn pearl formation, and individual cell keratinization are usually absent. Optimal evaluation of a lesion suspected of being a verrucous carcinoma requires a large, deep biopsy and correlation of the clinical and microscopic features with the biologic behavior of the neoplasm.

Pseudocarcinomatous Hyperplasia

Pseudocarcinomatous, or pseudoepithelimatous, hyperplasia represents considerable

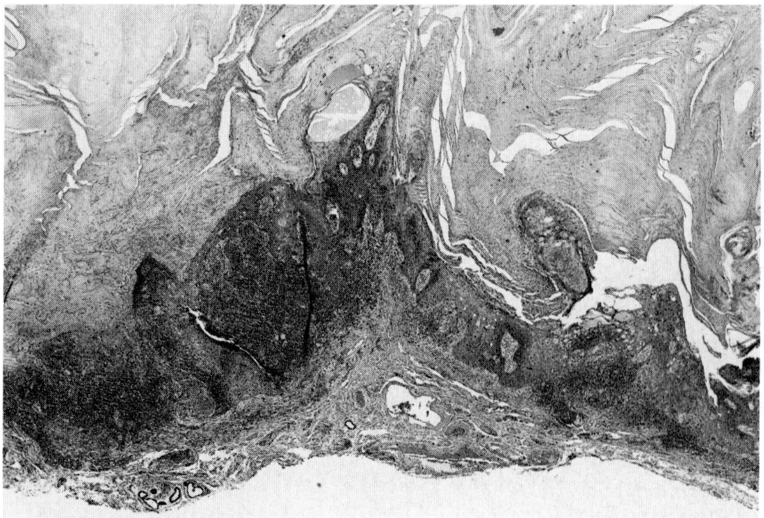

FIGURE 4–62. Squamous cell carcinoma: Invasive squamous cell carcinoma *(left)* arising in a lesion of Bowen's disease.

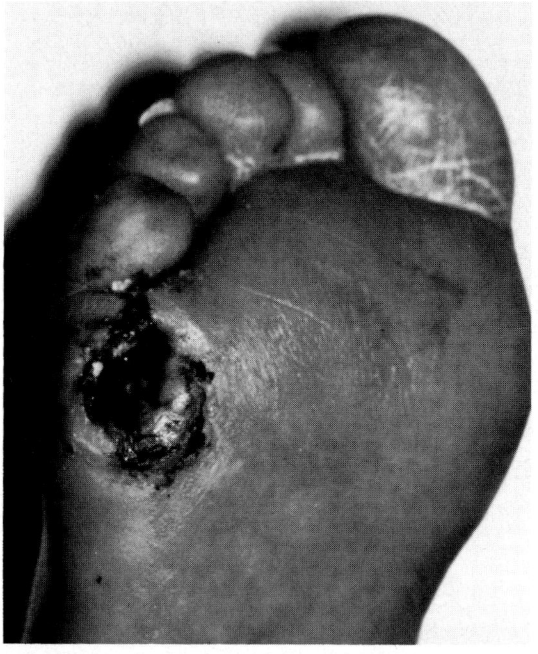

FIGURE 4-63. Verrucous carcinoma: Note verrucoid fungating mass on anterolateral sole.

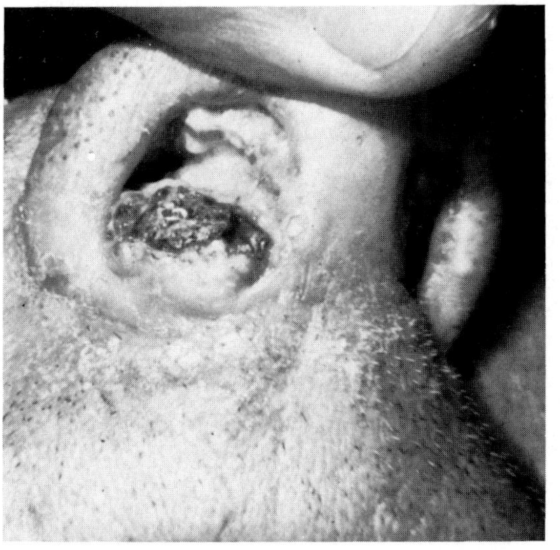

FIGURE 4-65. Verrucous carcinoma: Exophytic verrucoid mass in nasal vestibule.

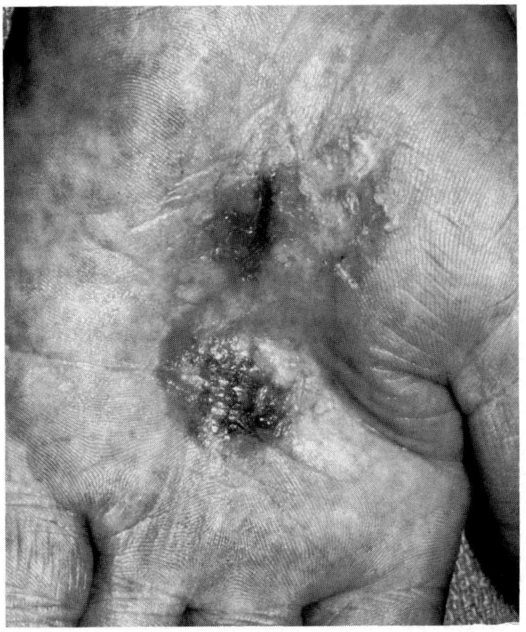

FIGURE 4-64. Verrucous carcinoma: Verrucoid focally-eroded plaque on the palm.

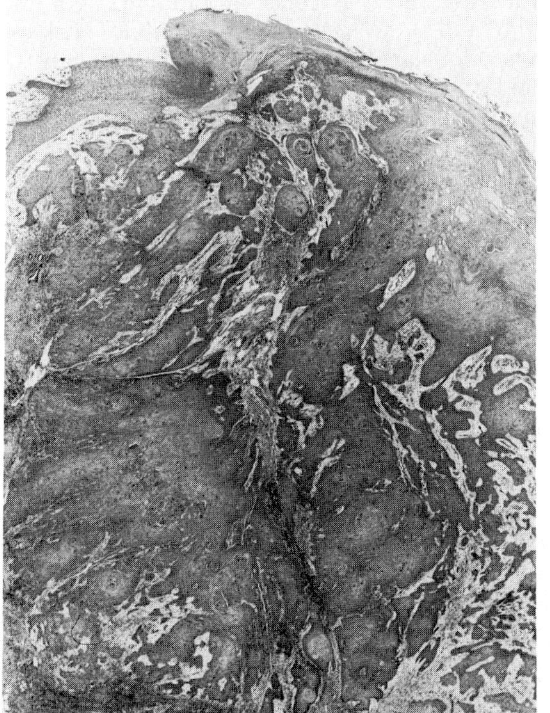

FIGURE 4-66. Verrucous carcinoma: Note multiple large bulbous masses of well-differentiated squamous cells extending deep into the dermis; degree of nuclear atypia is mild.

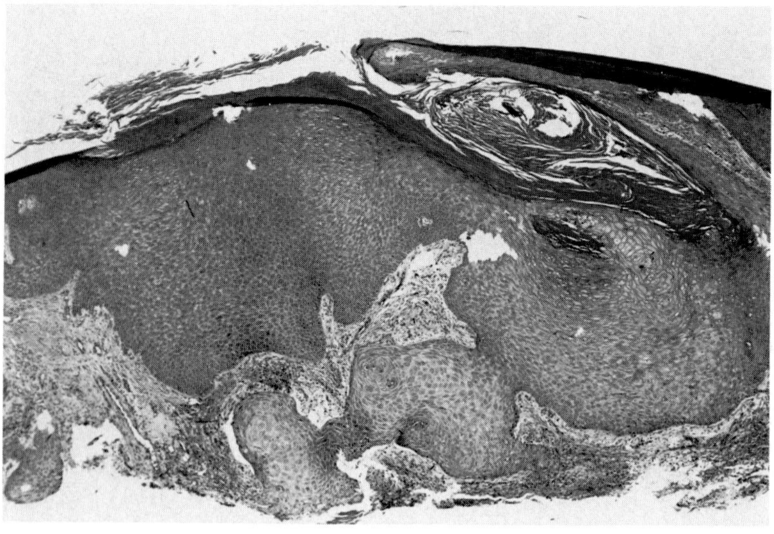

FIGURE 4–67. Pseudocarcinomatous hyperplasia: Note irregularly acanthotic epithelial masses extending into the upper dermis.

downward proliferation of the epidermis into the underlying dermis. Clinically and histologically, it closely simulates squamous cell carcinoma. It occurs most often in chronic proliferative inflammatory processes (e.g., bromoderma, blastomycosis, hidradenitis suppurativa) and at the edges of chronic ulcers such as those associated with burns, stasis dermatitis, pyoderma gangrenosum, lupus vulgaris, osteomyelitis, or syphilitic gumma. It occasionally occurs in association with a granular cell tumor.

The histologic picture of pseudocarcinomatous hyperplasia shows irregular extension into the dermis of uneven, jagged, irregularly acanthotic epidermal masses and strands (Fig. 4–67). There is often an associated inflammatory infiltrate, which frequently surrounds and extends into the acanthotic epithelial masses (Fig. 4–68). The squamous cells comprising the dermal epithelial nests are usually very well differentiated, and anaplastic features such as individual cell keratinization, nuclear hyperchromatism, and pleomorphism are absent (Fig. 4–69). Nevertheless, even when all the above criteria are taken into consideration, it may still be difficult or impossible to differentiate pseudocarcinomatous hyperplasia from a well-differentiated (Broders' grade I) squamous cell carcinoma, and multiple biopsies and detailed clinical information may be necessary to arrive at a final diagnosis.

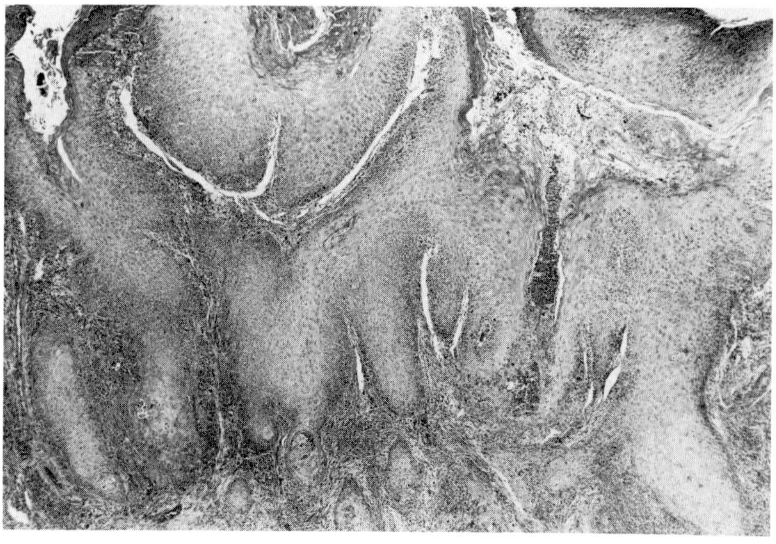

FIGURE 4–68. Pseudocarcinomatous hyperplasia: Dense inflammatory infiltrate surrounds and focally extends into the peripherating epithelial masses.

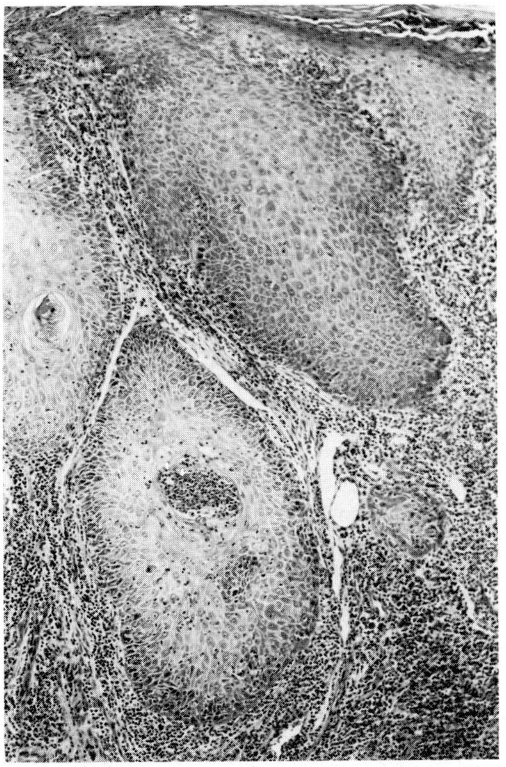

FIGURE 4–69. Pseudocarcinomatous hyperplasia: High-power examination shows lack of significant nuclear atypia and the presence of intraepithelial neutrophilic abscesses—features favoring a diagnosis of pseudocarcinomatous hyperplasia over well-differentiated squamous cell carcinoma.

EPITHELIAL NEOPLASMS OF UNCERTAIN MALIGNANT POTENTIAL

Keratoacanthoma

Keratoacanthoma (KA) is a common, heavily keratinized tumor that is regarded by many as a benign lesion.[13] Characteristically, its onset appears as a rapidly growing nodule that enlarges in 2 to 8 weeks to up to 2.0 cm, remains stationary for 2 to 8 weeks, and then slowly involutes within a similar period. This evolution is much faster than that of a squamous cell carcinoma; however, lesions that are larger and more persistent (up to one year) are known to occur.

Several variants of KA have been recognized. The solitary type is the most common. Multiple, eruptive, giant, and subungual types also exist. In essence, the course and the history are almost identical in all of them. KA has also been reported to occur on the conjunctiva; the nasal, oral, and anal mucosa; and on the tongue, palate, and gingiva.

Keratoacanthoma: Benign or Malignant?

The question of whether solitary KA is benign or malignant deserves special consideration. Baer and Kopf[14] cautioned against making the diagnosis of KA on history and clinical features. They reported a case that was considered a good example of KA but proved to be a squamous cell carcinoma after biopsy. This has been also reported by Rook and Whimster in 1950 and in 1979.[15,16] It is significant that Rook could report spontaneous cure in only two cases out of more than 40 at a scientific meeting in 1950.[17] At the same meeting, Smith made the statement, "He would be a bold man who would say on looking at one of those sections that there was no malignancy."[18] Several observers have reported malignant transformation of KA, including Belisario,[19,20] Smith,[21] Zimmerman,[22] and Beerman.[23] Mikhail[24] reported three cases of squamous cell carcinoma diagnosed histologically as KA by two eminent dermatopathologists. The outcome was disastrous in all three who succumbed due to metastases.

According to Rook and Whimster,[16] certain histologic features help in differentiating KA from squamous cell carcinoma: (1) KA arises in normal skin (GRM: this is not always true), (2) epithelial hyperplasia is mainly in appendages (GRM: this is rarely seen), (3) there is no ulceration, (4) minimal cellular atypia in the fully developed lesion occurs, and (5) absence of truly invasive growth is absent. Pinkus and Mehregan[25] state that none of these criteria is without exception, and that buttress formation may be also seen in squamous cell carcinoma. They recommend that the diagnosis should be based on clinicopathological correlation—rapid growth and histologic pattern—and that it is important the biopsy should include the entire lesion, if feasible, or normal skin in it. In our experience, the main pitfall in differentiating KA from squamous cell carcinoma is relying on a short history because many patients seem unwilling to admit a long history when a cutaneous cancer is in question. In reporting on 30 years of experience, Rook and Whimster have come to believe that KA is "a reactive hyperplasia capable of spontaneous involution but is also capable of summating as a co-carcinogen in the presence of actinic damage to produce a rapid growing squamous cell carcinoma."[16] They also state that KA is the most common precursor of squamous cell carcinoma in the elderly.

Spontaneous involution of KA does not absolve it of malignancy. Cancers, including malignant melanomas, can spontaneously regress.[26–29]

Unfortunately, the diagnosis of KA is often made by clinicians and pathologists. Even those who maintain that KA is a benign self-healing process advise treatment because of the lack of absolutely reliable clinical or histologic criteria to differentiate it from squamous cell carcinoma.[14]

Rook and Whimster[16] have made the observation that there are squamous cell carcinomas that in their early phases may emulate KA both clinically and histologically. Since KA can be very destructive, especially when situated on the nose, the eyelid, and the lip, these lesions should not be relegated to the class of benign lesions.

The modalities that have been recommended for the treatment of KA include electrosurgery, cryosurgery, and excision. Parker and Hanke[30] have treated five large KAs with intralesional 5-fluorouracil with apparently good results. However, this treatment failed in a sixth case. We have found this modality useful in small lesions of eruptive KA; otherwise, we strongly advocate excision. If the KA is small, an excisional biopsy will serve in making the diagnosis and will effect a cure. In case of large lesions, the central portion and part of the marginal skin on two sides should be obtained if a biopsy is needed. The remainder should be excised later and the margins carefully checked. There is no modality in existence that surpasses the Mohs micrographic surgery in this respect. We believe that the welfare of the patient should be the foremost priority. Finally, we strongly agree with other workers that KA may be classified a subtype of squamous cell carcinoma[31] and should be treated as such. This is the course recommended by Lever and Schaumburg-Lever.[32] They state that as squamous cell carcinomas can masquerade as keratoacanthomas, both clinically and histologically, it is best to err on the safe side in case of doubt and assume that the lesion is a squamous cell carcinoma. Illustrative examples are depicted in Figures 4–70 and 4–81.

Multiple Keratoacanthomas

There are two variants of this subtype of KA: the multiple self-healing KAs of the Ferguson-Smith type, which may be familial,[33,34] and the eruptive Grzybowski type.[35] The latter leave scarring after involution. We have reported on a case of eruptive keratoacanthoma that occured in a plaque form in an immunosuppressed patient.[36] We have also observed the eruptive form in another who was receiving chemotherapy. Both cases had renal transplants. Examples are portrayed in Figures 4–70 to 4–85.

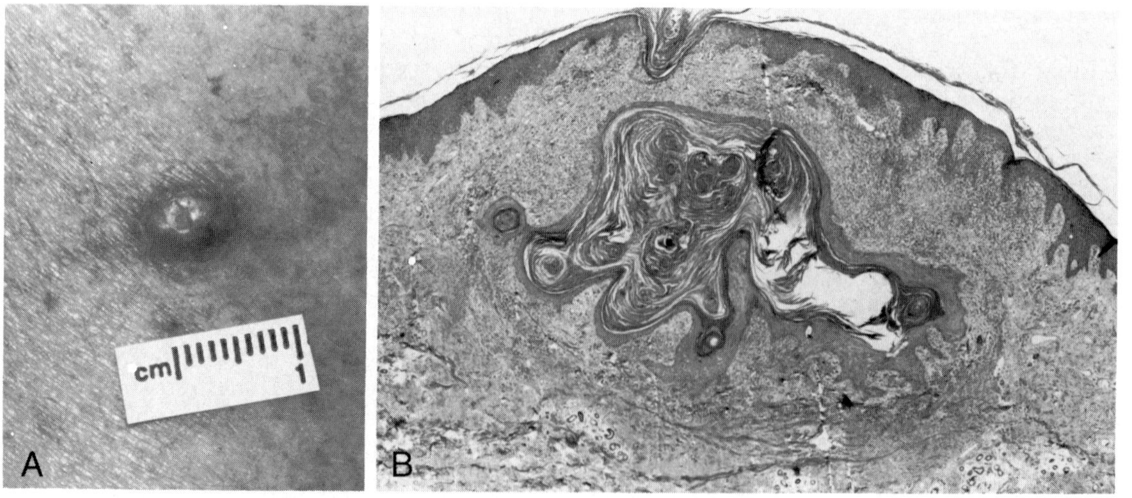

FIGURE 4–70. *A*, Early keratoacanthoma (KA) on arm; note the keratinized center. *B*, Section shows a heavily keratinized epithelial growth invading the dermis. Note relationship to overlying hair follicle.

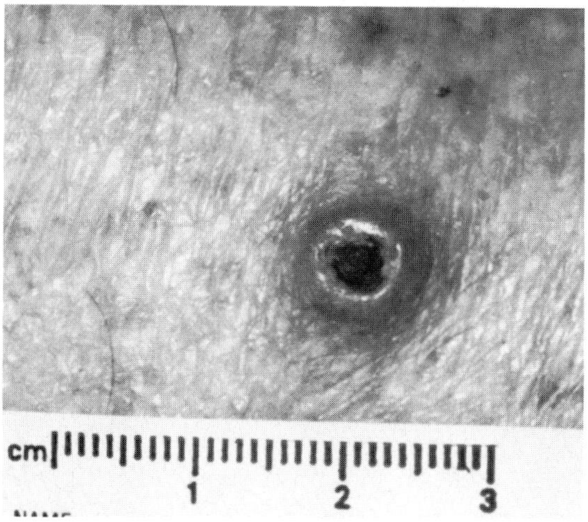

FIGURE 4–71. Early squamous cell carcinoma: Ulceration is the clue to the diagnosis.

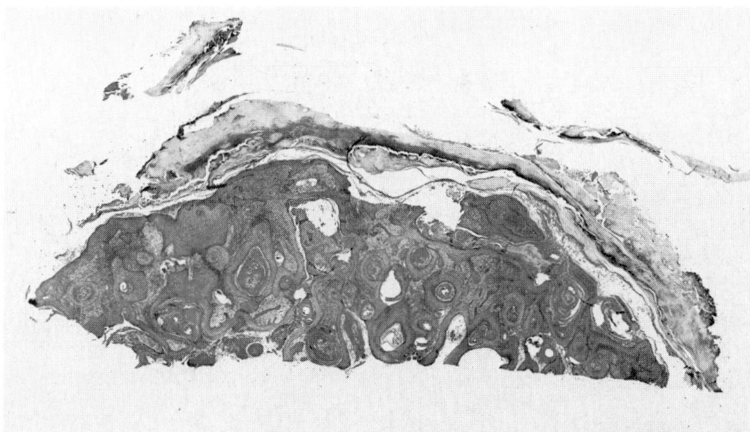

FIGURE 4–72. Section of inadequate biopsy: The margins and the dermis were not included.

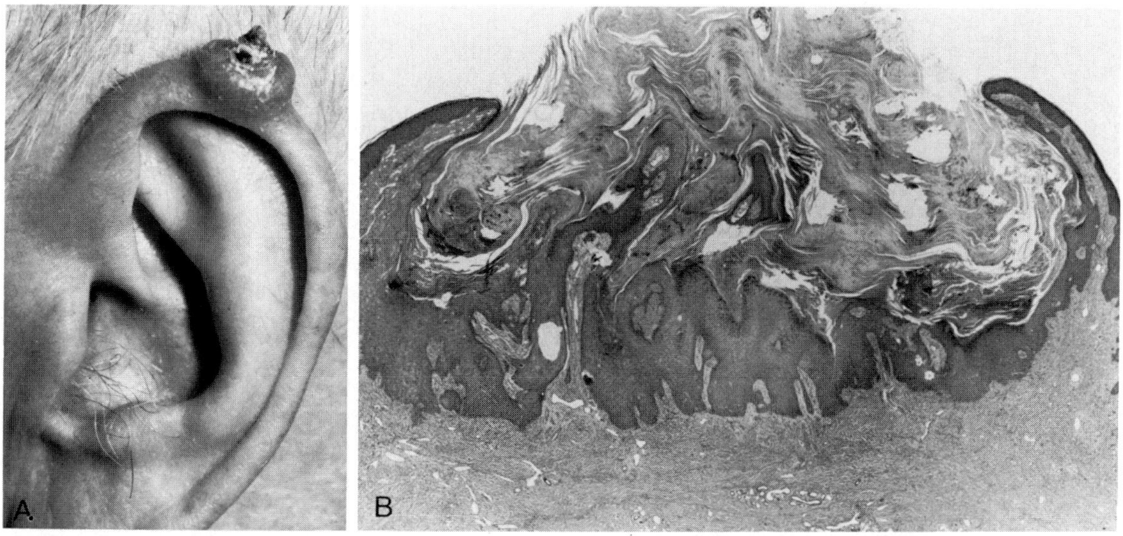

FIGURE 4–73. *A,* Fully developed keratoacanthoma (KA). *B,* Typical histology of a fully developed KA.

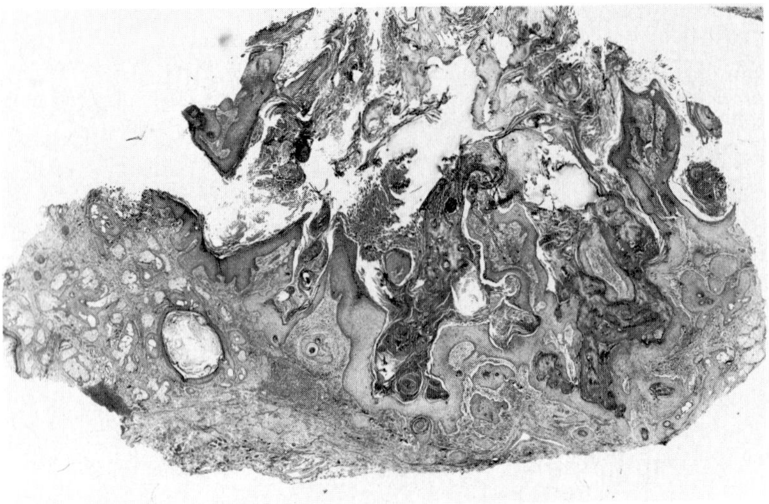

FIGURE 4–74. Early regressive stage of keratoacanthoma: Note increased keratinization and thinning out of the epithelial component.

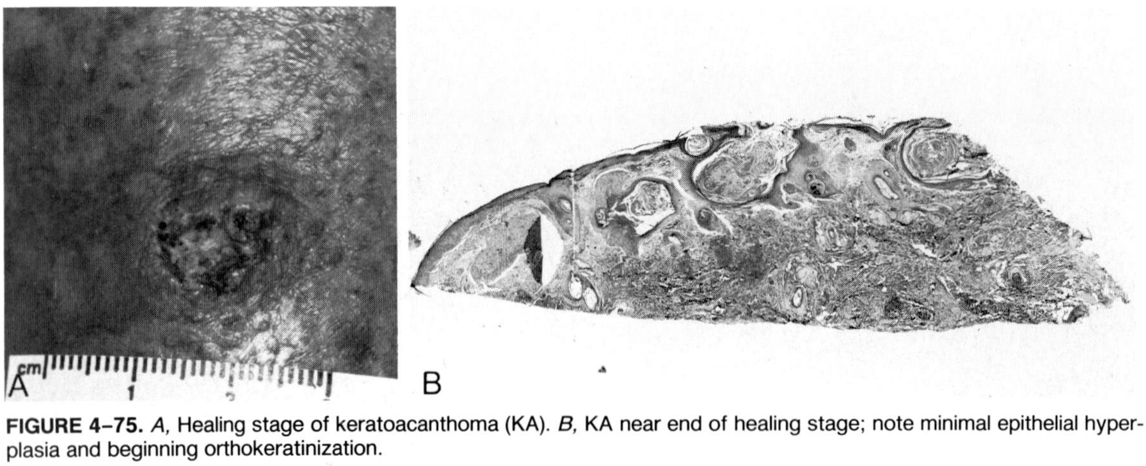

FIGURE 4–75. *A*, Healing stage of keratoacanthoma (KA). *B*, KA near end of healing stage; note minimal epithelial hyperplasia and beginning orthokeratinization.

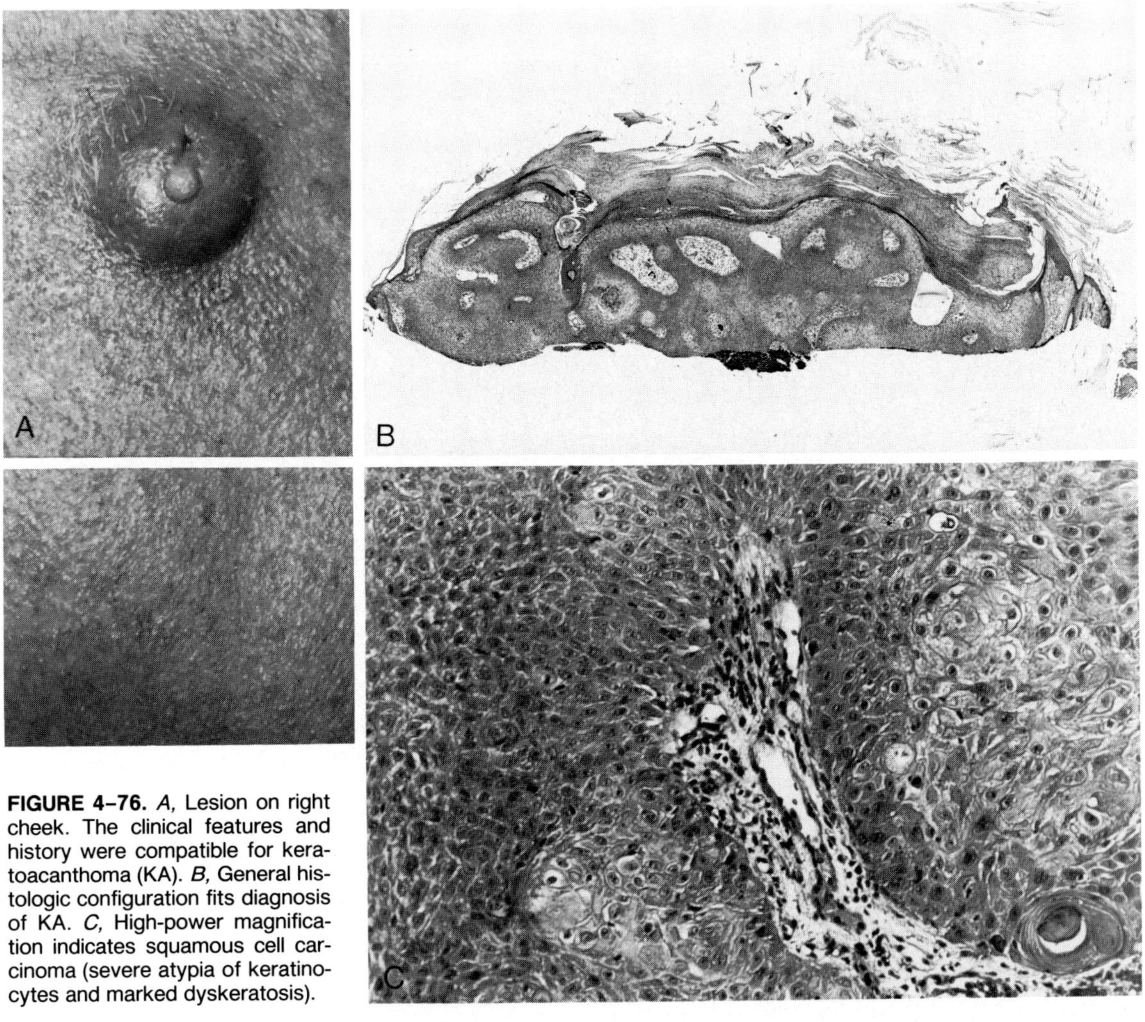

FIGURE 4–76. *A*, Lesion on right cheek. The clinical features and history were compatible for keratoacanthoma (KA). *B*, General histologic configuration fits diagnosis of KA. *C*, High-power magnification indicates squamous cell carcinoma (severe atypia of keratinocytes and marked dyskeratosis).

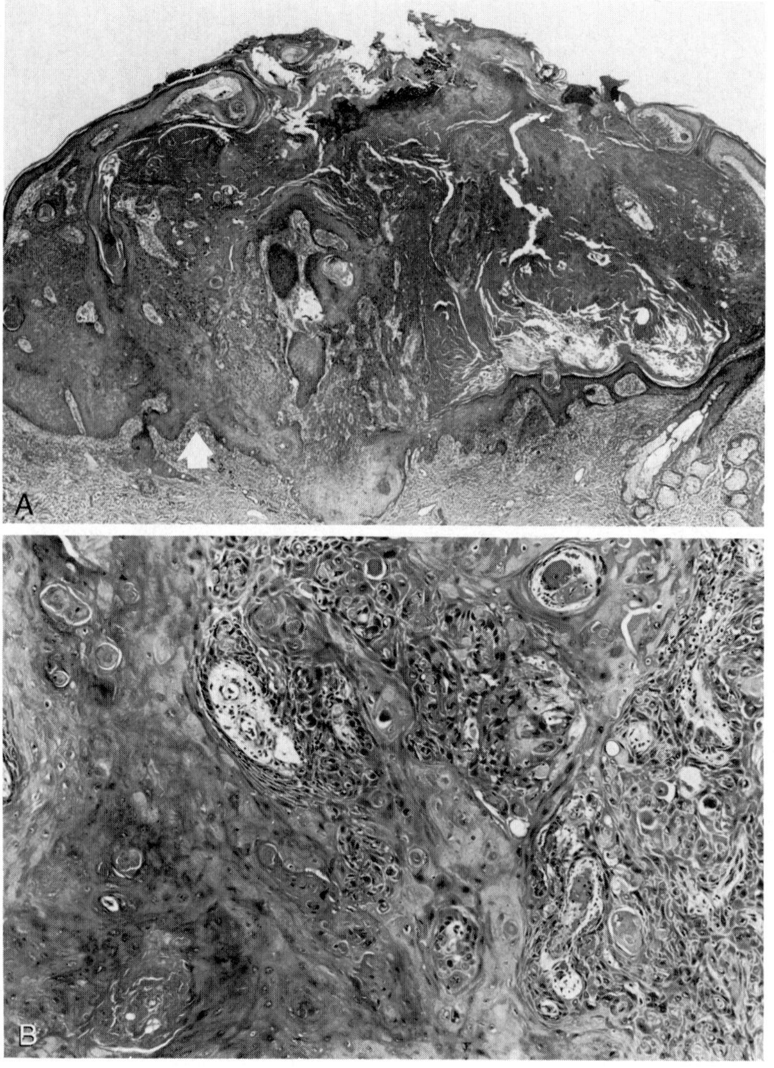

FIGURE 4–77. *A*, Diagnosis of keratoacanthoma by history and scanning power. *B*, Higher magnification of area above arrow in A shows frank squamous cell carcinoma. Whether this was a malignant transformation or the lesion was a carcinoma from the beginning could not be decided.

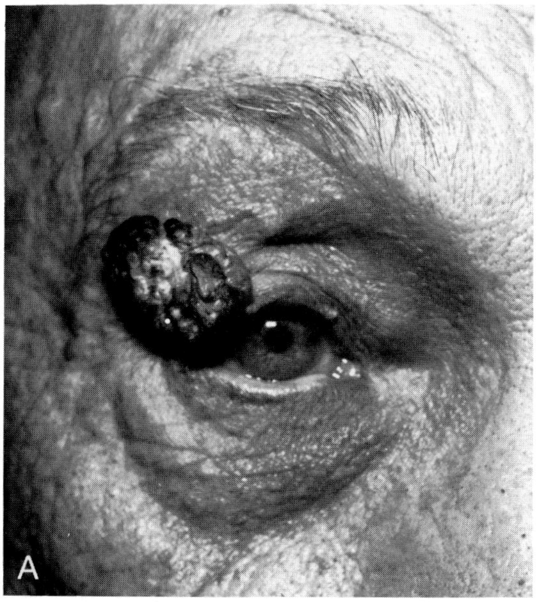

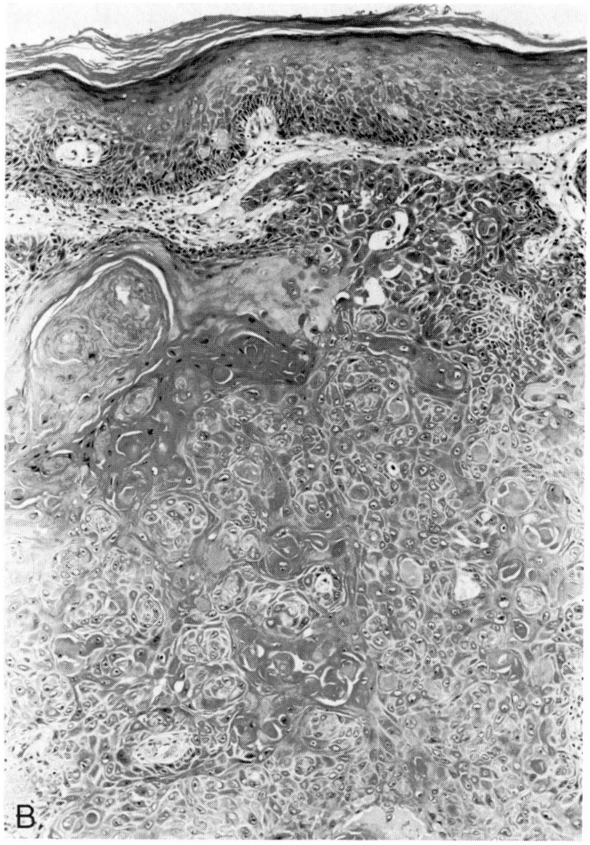

FIGURE 4–78. *A*, By history, the lesion was considered a keratoacanthoma. *B*, By microscopy, the lesion was a squamous cell carcinoma.

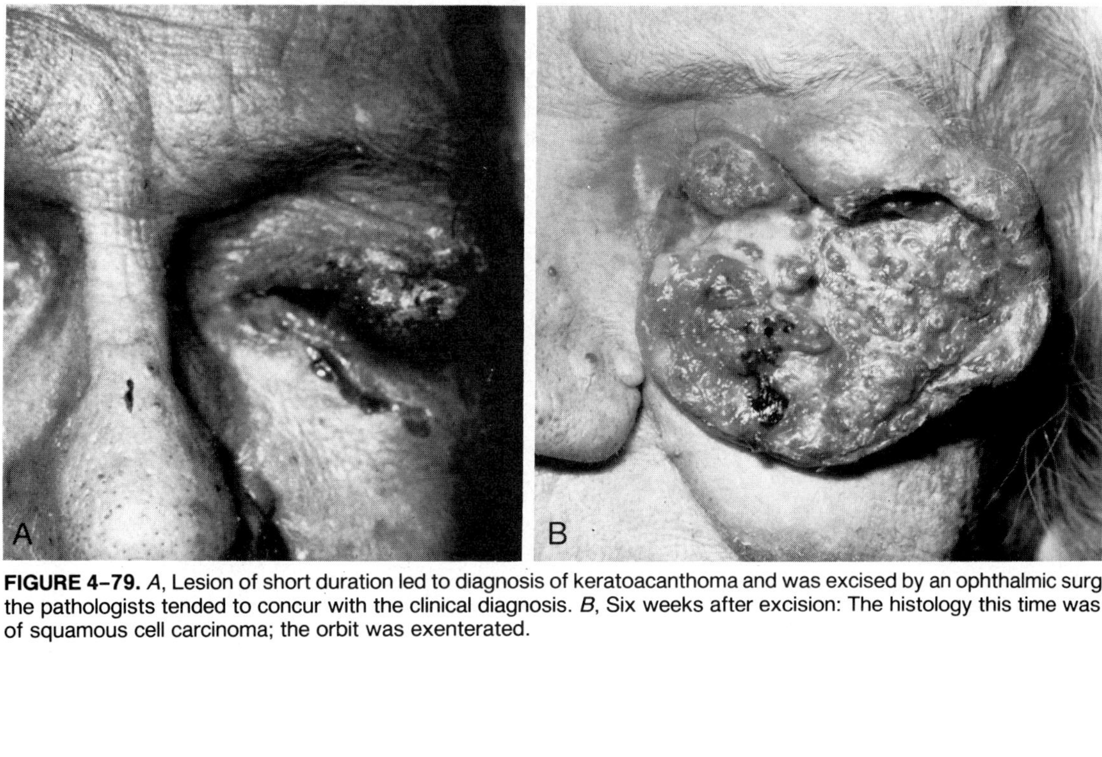

FIGURE 4–79. *A*, Lesion of short duration led to diagnosis of keratoacanthoma and was excised by an ophthalmic surgeon; the pathologists tended to concur with the clinical diagnosis. *B*, Six weeks after excision: The histology this time was that of squamous cell carcinoma; the orbit was exenterated.

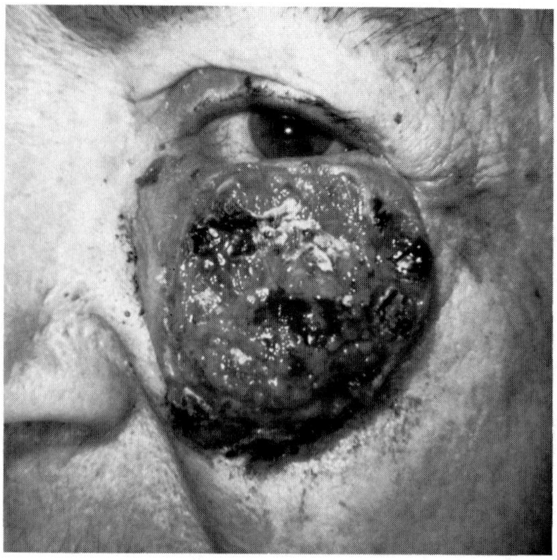

FIGURE 4–80. Original clinical diagnosis was keratoacanthoma; tremendous, life-threatening extension of lesion after intralesional 5-fluorouracil 5%.

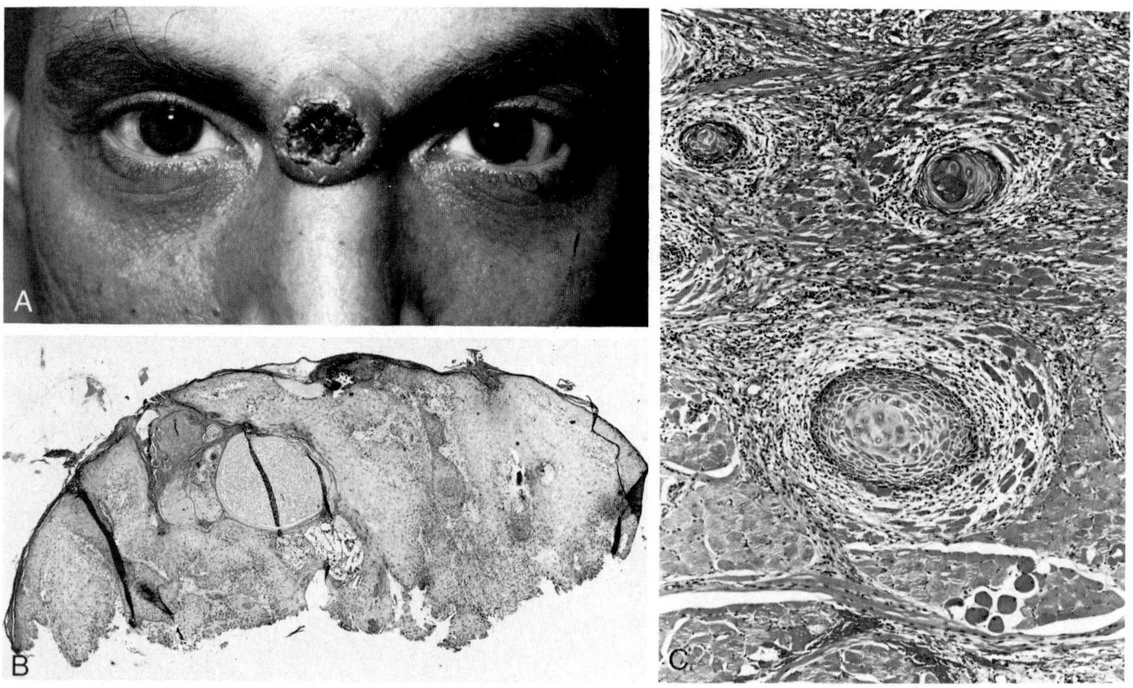

FIGURE 4–81. *A*, Recurrent keratoacanthoma (KA); the original lesion was of a few weeks' duration. *B*, The pathology report read "compatible with KA," despite an inadequate specimen. *C*, Muscle invasion by the tumor was seen after re-excision.

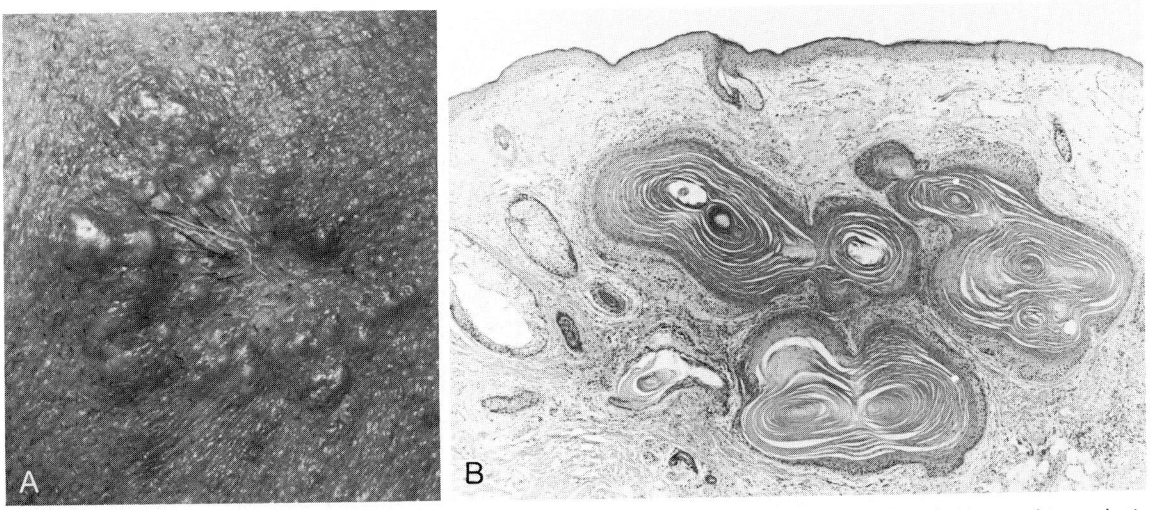

FIGURE 4–82. *A*, Keratoacanthoma (KA) en plaque: Free central area was site of biopsy. Patient had a renal transplant, was receiving chemotherapy, and developed numerous eruptive KAs. *B*, Note relation of KA to overlying follicle. (From Washington C, Mikhail GR: Eruptive keratoacanthoma en plaque in an immunosuppressed patient. *Journal of Dermatologic Surgery and Oncology* 113:1357, 1987. Copyright 1987, the Journal of Dermatologic Surgery and Oncology, Inc.)

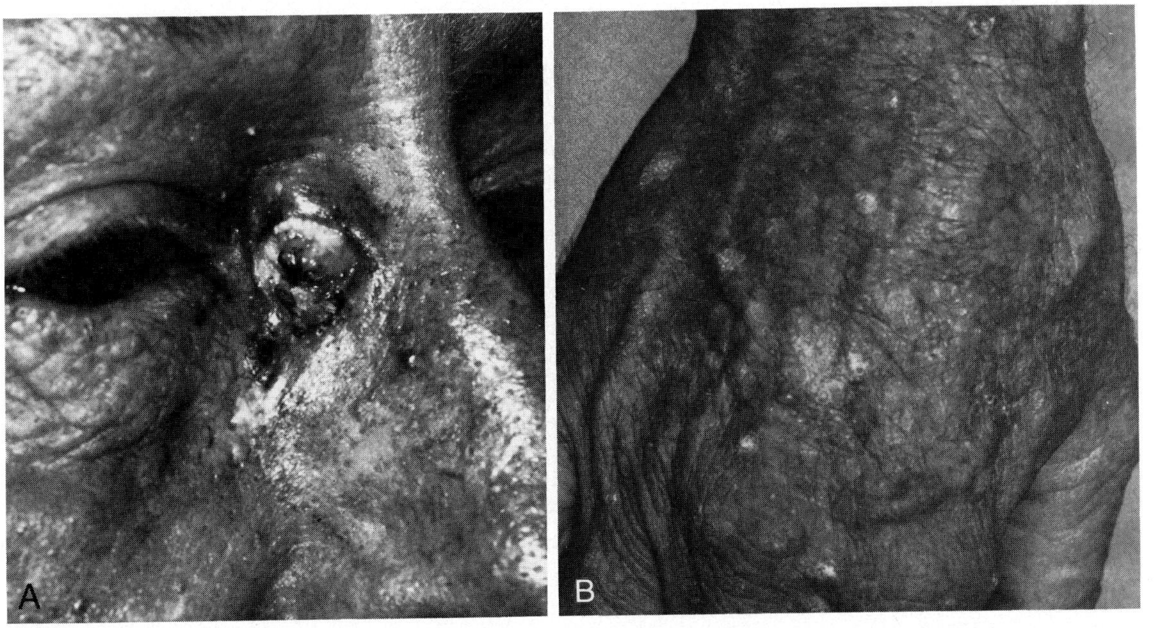

FIGURE 4–83. *A*, Another renal transplant patient with a keratoacanthoma-like squamous cell carcinoma at right medial canthus. *B*, Some of the eruptive keratoacanthomas on dorsa of hands (Grzybowski type).

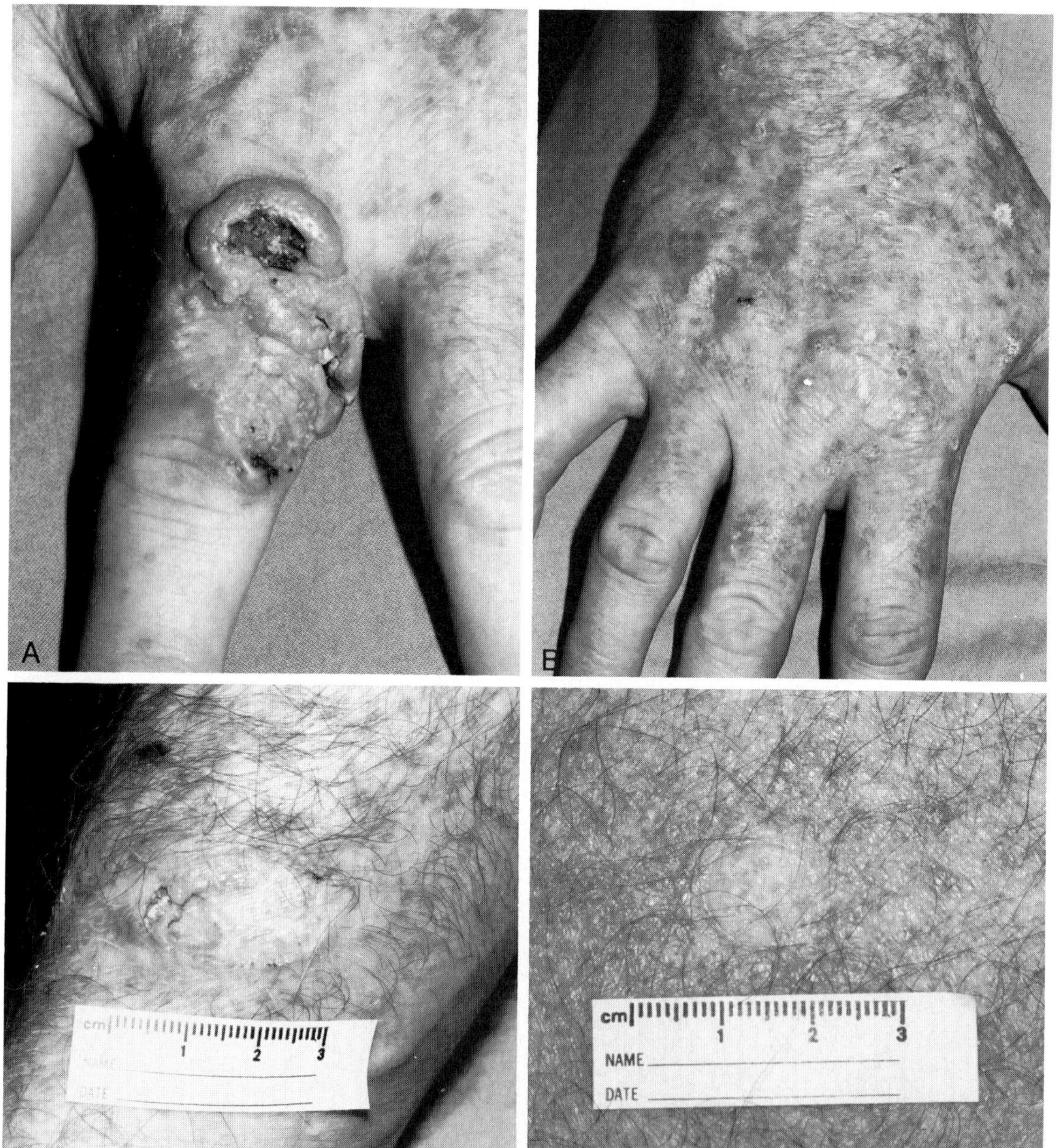

FIGURE 4–84. *A*, Giant keratoacanthoma (KA) on the hand of a man age 40 who had eruptive KAs of the Ferguson-Smith (familial) type for many years. *B*, Eruptive KA. *C* and *D*, Healed and scarred sites of spontaneously involuted KAs.

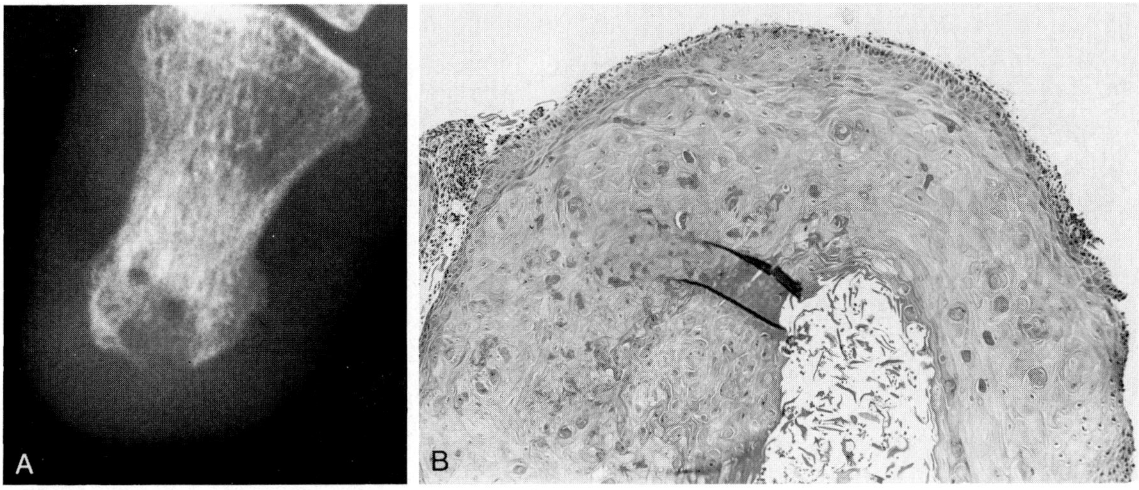

FIGURE 4–85. *A*, The diagnosis of subungual keratoacanthoma is seldom made solely on clinical grounds. The clues are pain, tenderness, and radiologic evidence of destruction of the terminal phalanx. *B*, Distinctive histology: a well-keratinizing circumscribed lesion.

ADNEXAL NEOPLASMS

Neoplasms differentiating in the direction of cutaneous adnexa are divided into four groups: pilar, sebaceous, apocrine, and eccrine. The degree of differentiation of the neoplasms within each group ranges from well-differentiated hyperplasias and adenomas to the less well-differentiated epitheliomas and undifferentiated carcinomas. Although a complete discussion of adnexal neoplasms is beyond the scope of this chapter, representative entities from each of the four groups will be presented.

Adnexal Neoplasms of Pilar Origin

Representative adnexal neoplasms of pilar origin include trichoepithelioma, desmoplastic trichoepithelioma, trichoblastic fibroma, and proliferating trichoilemmal cyst.

Trichoepithelioma (also termed epithelioma adenoides cysticum) occurs as either solitary or multiple lesions, most often on the face. Multiple trichoepithelioma, transmitted as an autosomal dominant trait, may occur simultaneously with multiple cylindromas. The lesions are raised, firm, flesh-colored papules or nodules ranging in size from 2 mm to 2 cm (Fig. 4–86). Clinical differentiation from nodular basal cell carcinoma may be difficult.

Histologically, the lesions consist of multiple islands of basaloid epithelial cells that vary in size and are arranged in a retiform, or lace-like, pattern (Fig. 4–87). Some of the islands show horn cysts, while others show evidence of abortive hair papilla formation. The islands are surrounded by a moderately fibrotic dermal stroma. There is usually no retraction of the tumor islands from the surrounding dermis, and tumor cell necrosis and dermal inflammation are uncommon. These features are helpful in differentiating trichoepithelioma from basal cell carcinoma.

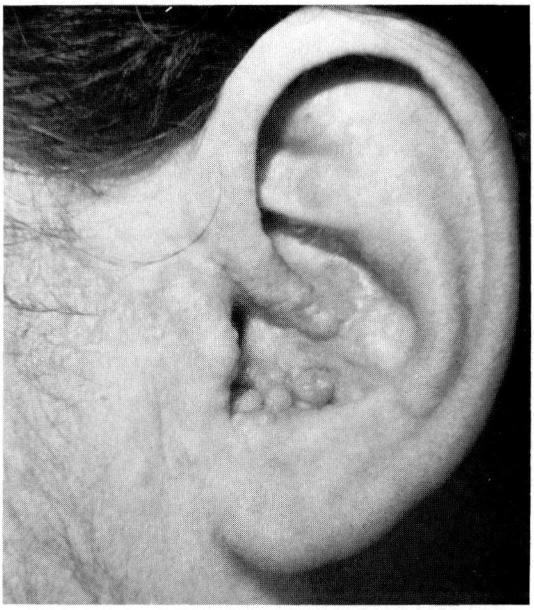

FIGURE 4–86. Trichoepithelioma: Multiple raised papules and small nodules on ear.

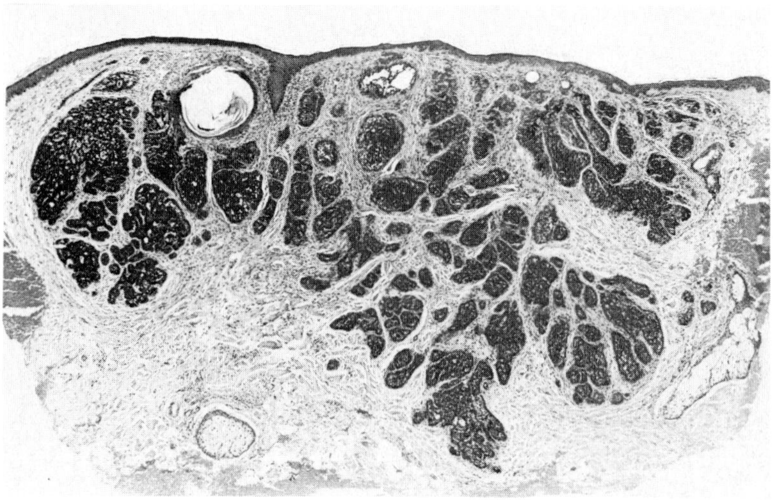

FIGURE 4–87. Trichoepithelioma: Characteristic histology shows multiple islands of basaloid cells arranged in a lace-like pattern surrounded by a moderately fibrotic dermal stroma.

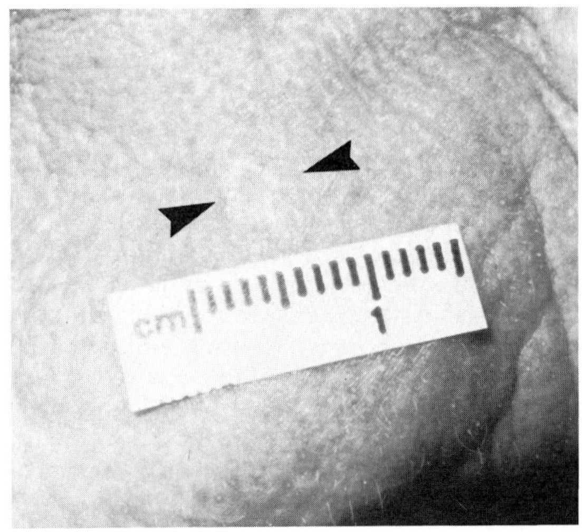

FIGURE 4–88. Desmoplastic trichoepithelioma: Note solitary raised papule with slight central depression on chin *(arrowheads).*

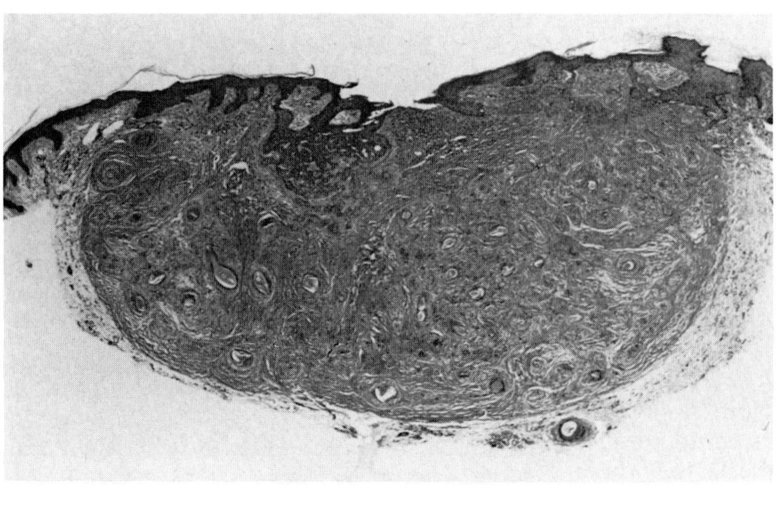

FIGURE 4–89. Desmoplastic trichoepithelioma: Numerous strands of basaloid epithelium, horn cysts, and fibrotic dermal stroma characterize the lesion histologically.

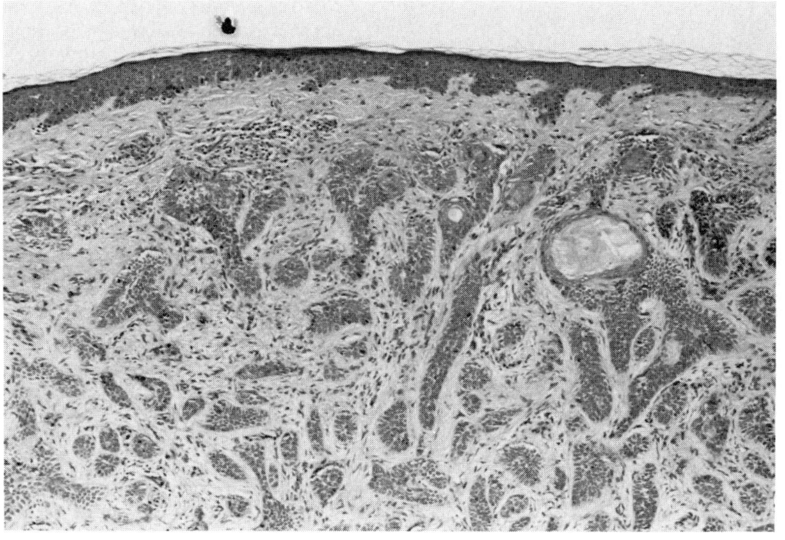

FIGURE 4–90. Desmoplastic trichoepithelioma. High-power view shows histologic details of desmoplastic trichoepithelioma. Presence of horn cysts and lack of stromal retraction help differentiate lesion from sclerotic basal cell carcinoma.

Desmoplastic trichoepithelioma is regarded as a distinct variant of trichoepithelioma, clinically appearing as an oval-shaped, firm, flesh-colored, 3 to 8 mm papule with a shallow central depression (Fig. 4–88). It occurs almost exclusively on the face and is most often seen in women ages 20 to 40.

The three characteristic histologic features of desmoplastic trichoepithelioma include narrow strands of basaloid tumor cells, horn cysts, and a desmoplastic dermal stroma (Fig. 4–89). The tumor islands range from one to five cells in thickness, and do not show significant nuclear atypia (Fig. 4–90). Desmoplastic trichoepithelioma is differentiated from a sclerotic basal cell carcinoma by the lack of horn cysts in the latter.

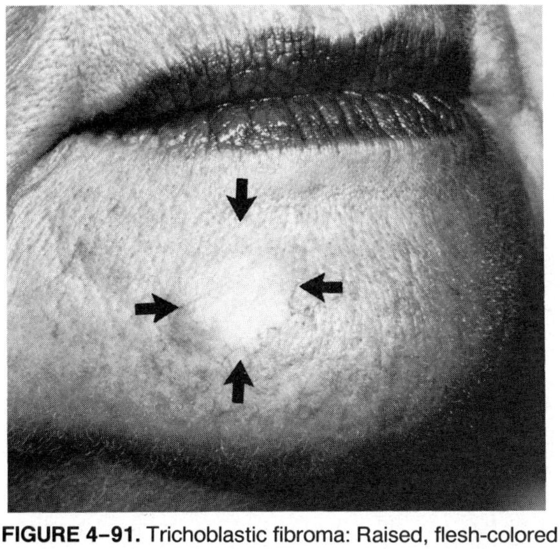

FIGURE 4–91. Trichoblastic fibroma: Raised, flesh-colored nodule with fine superficial telangiectasia on the chin *(arrows).*

Trichoblastic fibroma is a rare epithelial trichogenic neoplasm[37] that presents as a relatively large (greater than 1 cm), flesh-colored, dermal nodule, most often found on the face or extremities (Fig. 4–91). Some lesions may have superficial telangiectasia, rendering the clinical differentiation from basal cell carcinoma difficult. The lesions are usually slow-growing and asymptomatic.

Histologically, trichoblastic fibroma consists of multiple, lobular islands of cuboidal-shaped, basaloid cells that are embedded in a moderately dense fibrotic stroma (Fig. 4–92). Distinctive features include the presence of long, thin strands of epithelium one to three cells thick, and the differentiation of some of the larger islands into primitive hair bulb-like structures (Fig. 4–93). Some of the epithelial islands form small horn cysts, while others may show sebaceous differentiation. Lack of distinct peripheral palisading of the epithelial cells, the absence of inflammation, and the formation of primitive hair structures aid in differentiating this lesion from basal cell carcinoma.

Proliferating trichilemmal cyst or pilar tumor is nearly always a solitary lesion, which most commonly occurs on the scalp of elderly women. The lesion begins as a subcutaneous cystic nodule that grows into a large elevated

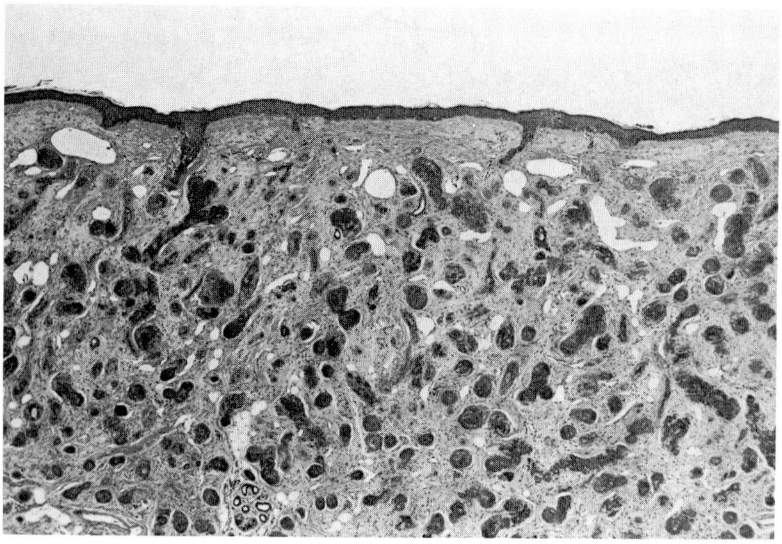

FIGURE 4–92. Trichoblastic fibroma: Multiple varying-sized epithelial islands fill the dermis and are surrounded by a moderately fibrotic stroma.

lobular mass which can ulcerate and then clinically resembles a squamous cell carcinoma (Fig. 4–94). It may be associated with other nonproliferating trichilemmal cysts. Rarely, extremely rapid enlargement of the nodule may indicate malignant transformation.

Histologically, a proliferating trichilemmal cyst is composed of varying-sized lobules of squamous epithelium showing evidence of dyskeratosis (Fig. 4–95). Characteristically, the epithelium in the center of the lobule changes rather abruptly into eosinophilic amorphous keratin (Fig. 4–96). The tumor cells may show a slight degree of nuclear atypia, but their sharp demarcation from the surrounding stroma as well as their abrupt mode of keratinization help in differentiating this lesion from squamous cell carcinoma.

Adnexal Neoplasms of Sebaceous Origin

Adnexal neoplasms of sebaceous origin considered here include sebaceous adenoma, sebaceous epithelioma, and sebaceous carcinoma.

Sebaceous adenoma most commonly presents as a yellowish, circumscribed nodule on

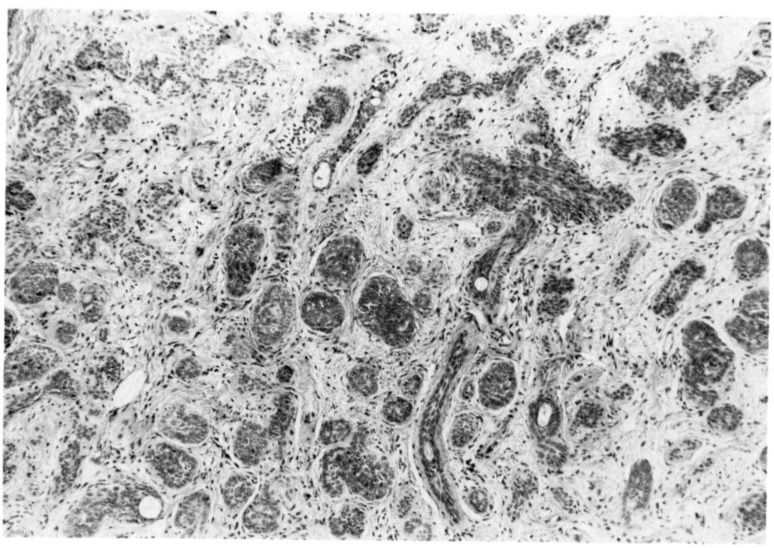

FIGURE 4–93. Trichoblastic fibroma: Note narrow epithelial strands and formation of primitive hair bulb-like structures, occasional small horn cysts, and sebaceous differentiation within the tumor islands.

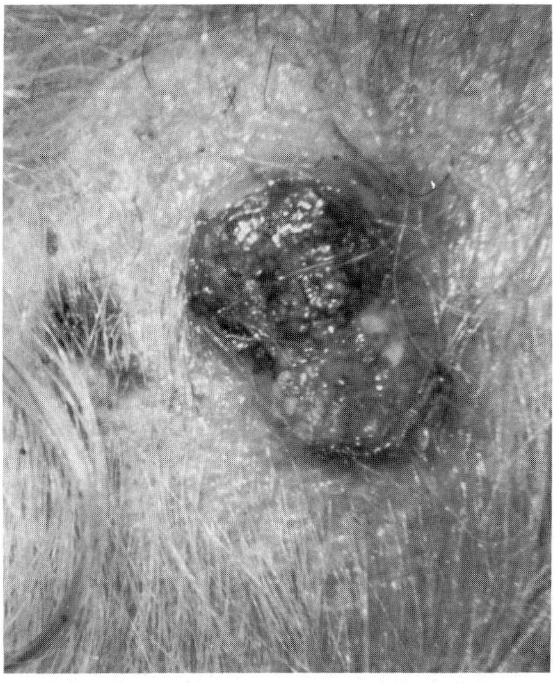

FIGURE 4–94. Proliferating trichilemmal cyst: Lesion most often presents as a large ulcerated nodule on the scalp.

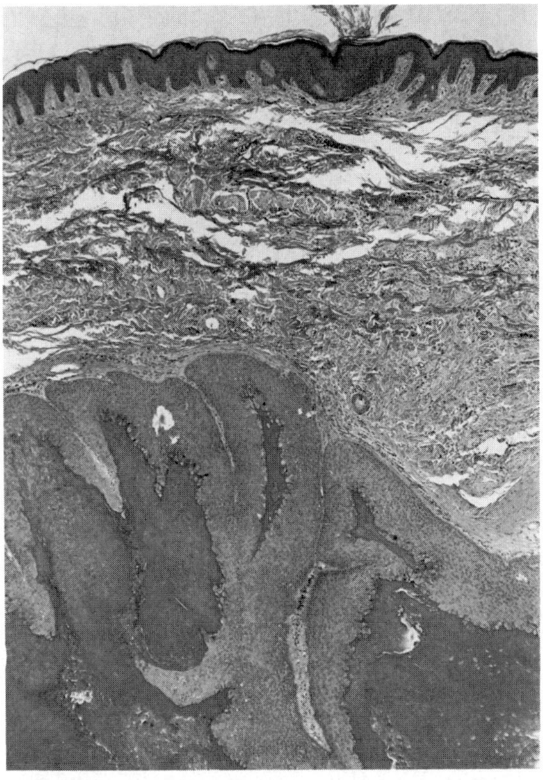

FIGURE 4–95. Proliferating trichilemmal cyst: Note relatively well-demarcated proliferation of squamous epithelium in dermis.

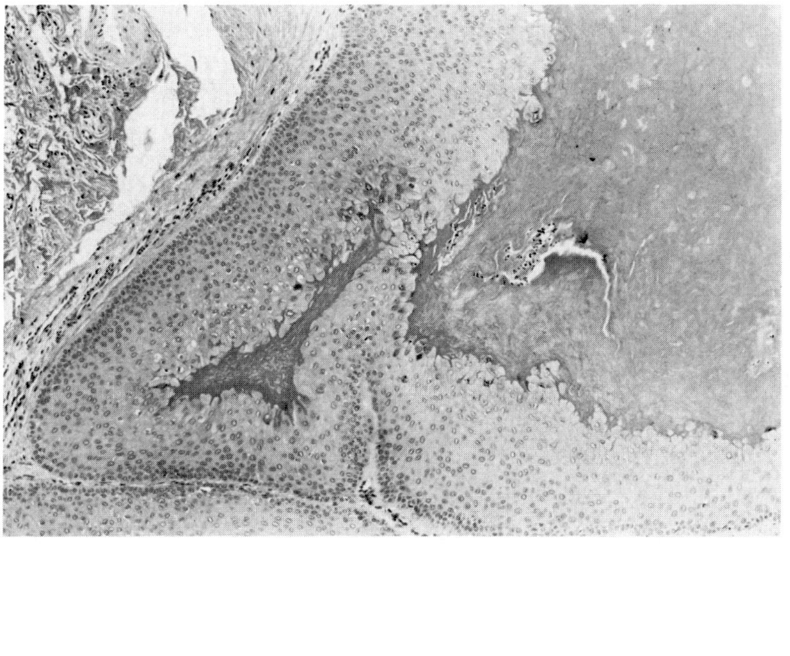

FIGURE 4–96. Proliferating trichilemmal cyst: The epithelium in the center of lobules shows abrupt formation of amorphous keratin.

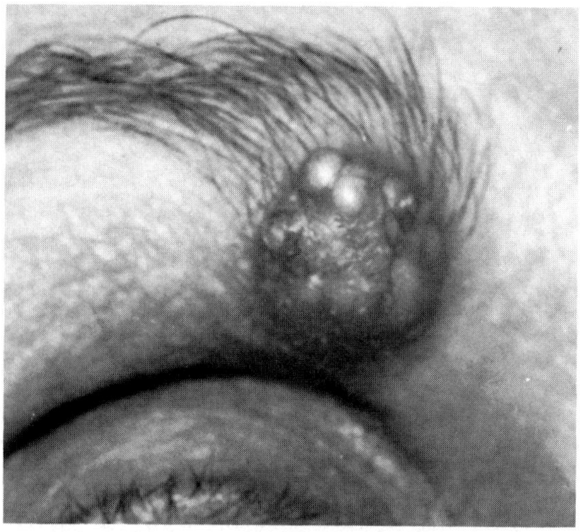

FIGURE 4–97. Sebaceous adenoma: Raised lobulated nodule is present on right medial eyebrow.

the face or scalp (Fig. 4–97). It is not eroded or ulcerated and usually asymptomatic.

Histologically, sebaceous adenoma is composed of well-demarcated, incompletely differentiated sebaceous lobules that are somewhat irregular in size and shape (Fig. 4–98). The lobules are composed of a mixture of basaloid, undifferentiated germinative cells and vacuolated, more mature-appearing sebaceous cells (Fig. 4–99). The two cell types are present in approximately equal proportions in most tumor lobules.

Sebaceous epithelioma clinically presents as a yellow or flesh-colored, varying-sized, well-circumscribed nodule or as an ill-defined plaque (Fig. 4–100). Most sebaceous epitheliomas occur as primary lesions on the face or scalp but may be found in association with a nevus sebaceus (organoid nevus) or the Muir-Torre syndrome.

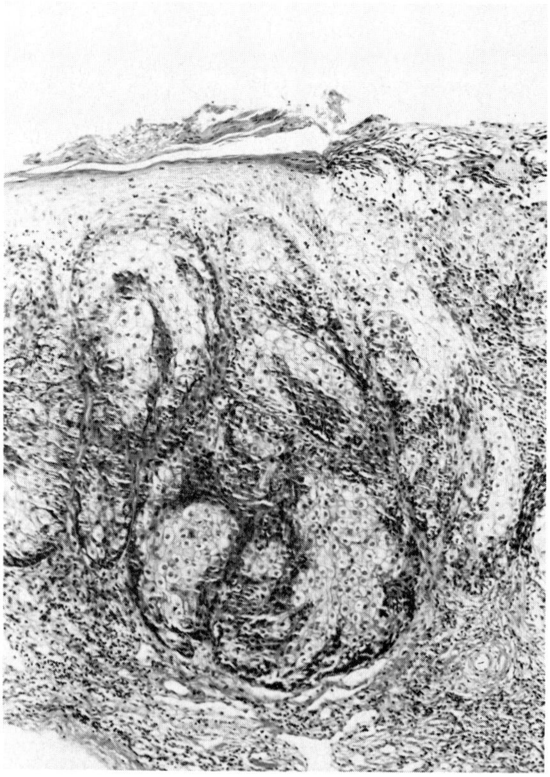

FIGURE 4–99. Sebaceous adenoma: High-power view shows the two cell types comprising the neoplasm; there are approximately equal proportions of germinative and mature sebaceous cells in tumor lobule.

Histologically, sebaceous epithelioma shows irregularly shaped masses and lobules in which significantly more than 50% of the cells are un-

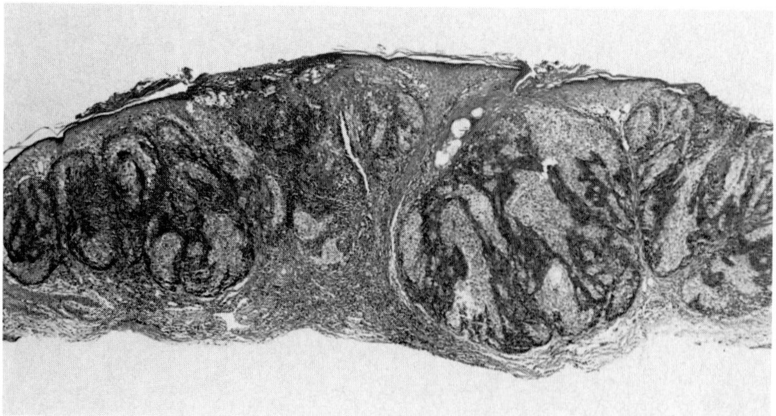

FIGURE 4–98. Sebaceous adenoma: Multiple well-demarcated lobules of incompletely differentiated sebaceous cells.

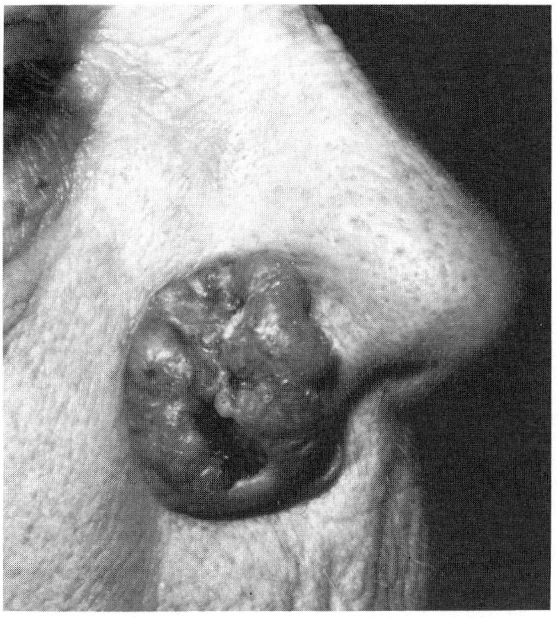

FIGURE 4–100. Sebaceous epithelioma: Large irregularly lobulated nodule on the nasolabial fold area; note clinical resemblance to nodular basal cell carcinoma.

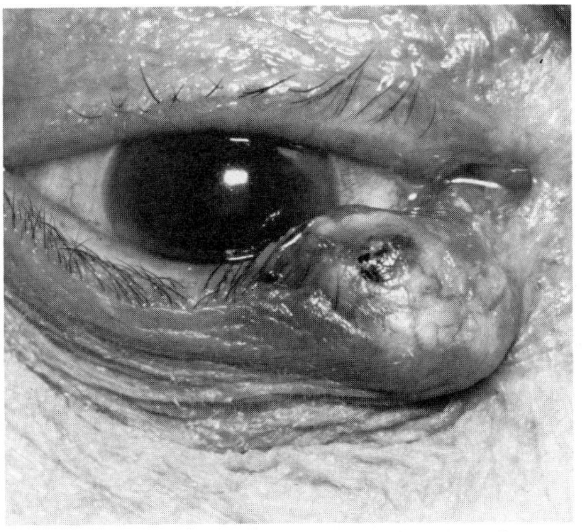

FIGURE 4–102. Sebaceous carcinoma: Large focally eroded nodule on lower eyelid; note clinical resemblance to basal cell carcinoma. (From Dixon R, Mikhail GR, Slater HC: Sebaceous carcinoma of the eyelid. *Journal of the American Academy of Dermatology* 3:241-243, 1980. Copyright 1980, The C. V. Mosby Company.)

differentiated basaloid cells with a much lower percentage of mature sebaceous cells (Fig. 4–101). Necrosis of the sebaceous cells may be seen in some of the tumor lobules. Differentiation of sebaceous epithelioma from a basal cell carcinoma with sebaceous differentiation is difficult, if not impossible, in some cases.

Carcinoma of the sebaceous glands occurs most commonly on the eyelids, where it originates either from the meibomian or zeisian glands. Sebaceous carcinoma of the eyelids clinically may simulate chronic blepharoconjunctivitis or chalazion or may present as a nodular growth (Fig. 4–102). Extraocular lesions almost always present as nodules, with or without ulceration, and may resemble basal cell carcinomas. Sebaceous carcinoma of the eyelid has a relatively high propensity for metastasis, except for those lesions associated with the Muir-Torre syndrome.

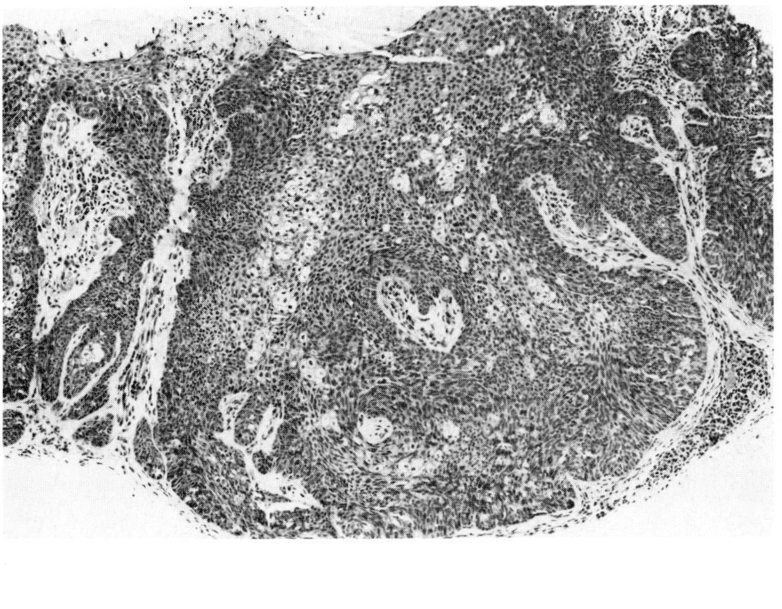

FIGURE 4–101. Sebaceous epithelioma: Note significantly greater proportion of undifferentiated basaloid cells compared to mature sebaceous cells.

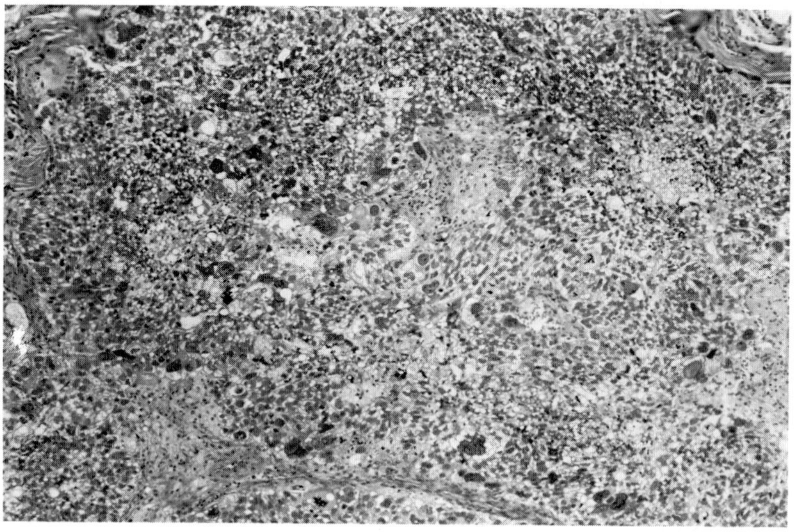

FIGURE 4–103. Sebaceous carcinoma: Irregular lobules composed of an admixture of undifferentiated and partially differentiated sebaceous cells.

Histologically, sebaceous carcinoma presents as irregular lobular formations composed of an admixture of undifferentiated and partially differentiated sebaceous cells (Fig. 4–103). Many of the cells are highly atypical and show significant pleomorphism of their nuclei (Fig. 4–104). Many of the neoplastic cells have a vacuolated or eosinophilic cytoplasm, which upon staining of frozen sections with fat stains, are shown to contain fine lipid granules (Fig. 4–105).

Adnexal Neoplasms of Apocrine Origin

Two adnexal neoplasms of apocrine origin that can cause difficulties in both clinical and histologic differential diagnosis will be considered here: erosive adenomatosis of the nipple and extramammary Paget's disease.

Erosive adenomatosis of the nipple represents an adenoma of the major lactiferous ducts. In early lesions, the nipple appears

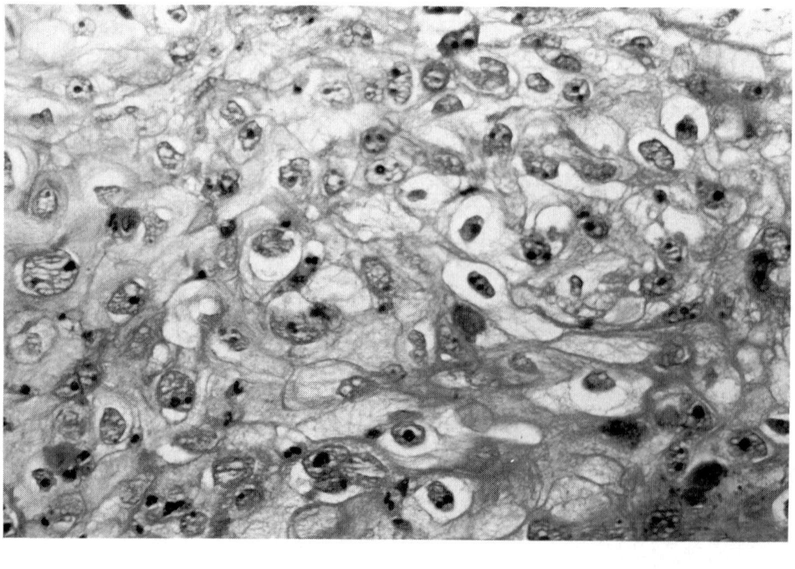

FIGURE 4–104. Sebaceous carcinoma: Note vacuolated cells with pleomorphic nuclei.

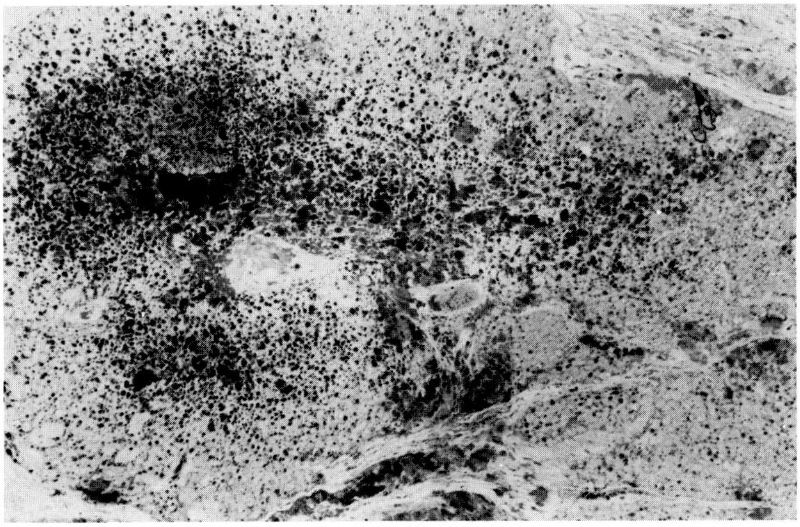

FIGURE 4–105. Sebaceous carcinoma: Note presence of lipid within tumor cells (Sudan black B stain).

eroded and inflamed, and clinical differentiation from mammary Paget's disease may be impossible (Fig. 4–106). In later stages, the nipple shows diffuse nodular thickening that is suspect of breast carcinoma.

Histologically, erosive adenomatosis of the nipple is characterized by multiple, irregular, dilated tubular structures extending from the epidermis into the dermis (Fig. 4–107). The lobules are lined by a peripheral layer of cuboidal cells and a luminal layer of columnar cells, some of which may protrude into the lumen. There is no significant nuclear atypicality. In some lesions, considerable acanthosis of the overlying epidermis may be present. Differentiation of erosive adenomatosis of the nipple from intraductal breast carcinoma rests upon identifying the larger cuboidal cells and greater nuclear atypia of intraductal carcinoma.

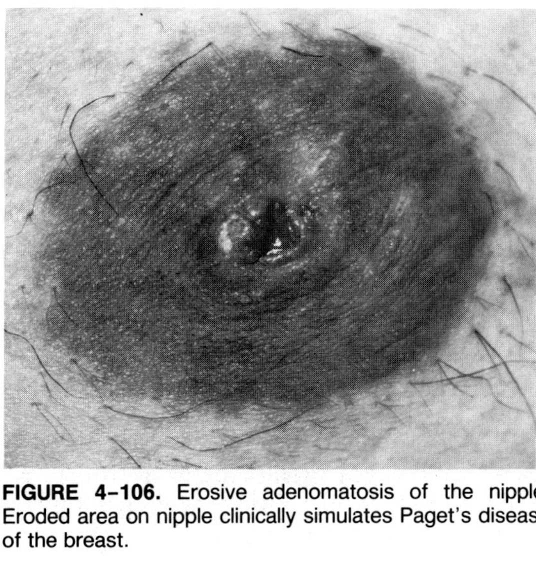

FIGURE 4–106. Erosive adenomatosis of the nipple: Eroded area on nipple clinically simulates Paget's disease of the breast.

Extramammary Paget's disease clinically presents as a slowly enlarging, reddish, eroded, or crusted plaque with a sharp but irregular border. It often clinically simulates Bowen's disease (Fig. 4–108) and most commonly occurs on the vulva, less commonly on the male genitalia or the perianal area, and rarely, in the axilla or ear canal. Since extramammary Paget's disease involves areas in which apocrine glands are commonly present, an apocrine derivation of the neoplasm has been proposed,[38,39] although this opinion is not universally accepted.[40,41] However, more recent immunohistochemical studies support the apocrine origin of most cases of extramammary Paget's disease.[42,43] Rarely, extramammary Paget's disease is a secondary event caused by extension of a primary adenocarcinoma, e.g., rectal or urogenital, to the skin. Long-standing cases of primary extramammary Paget's disease can extend into the dermis along cutaneous glandular structures.

Histologically, extramammary Paget's disease shows permeation of the epidermis by single and small nests of large, round cells that lack intercellular bridges and contain large, somewhat atypical nuclei and ample cytoplasm

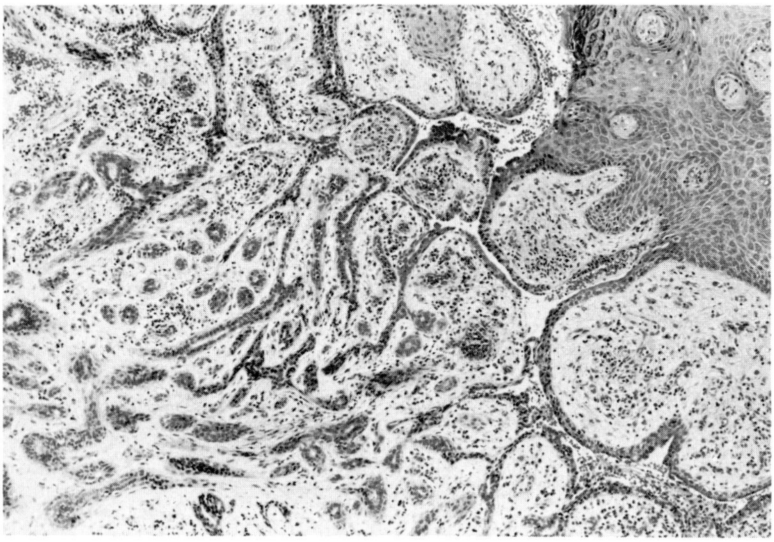

FIGURE 4–107. Erosive adenomatosis of the nipple: Multiple irregular dilated tubular structures extend into the dermis from the overlying acanthotic epidermis.

(Fig. 4–109). Flattened basal cells lie between the tumor cells and the dermis in many areas. This feature is useful in the differentiation of extramammary Paget's disease from in situ superficial spreading malignant melanoma. Also, the tumor cells show little tendency to clumping of nuclei, lack of multinucleated giant cells, and no evidence of dyskeratosis—features important in differentiating extramammary Paget's disease from pagetoid Bowen's disease (Fig. 4–110). Histochemical and immunohistochemical studies can be useful in differentiating extramammary Paget's disease from either Bowen's disease[43] or superficial spreading malignant melanoma in situ.[44] In advanced cases, nests of neoplastic Paget cells are found in the dermis, sometimes in association with sweat duct structures (Fig. 4–111).

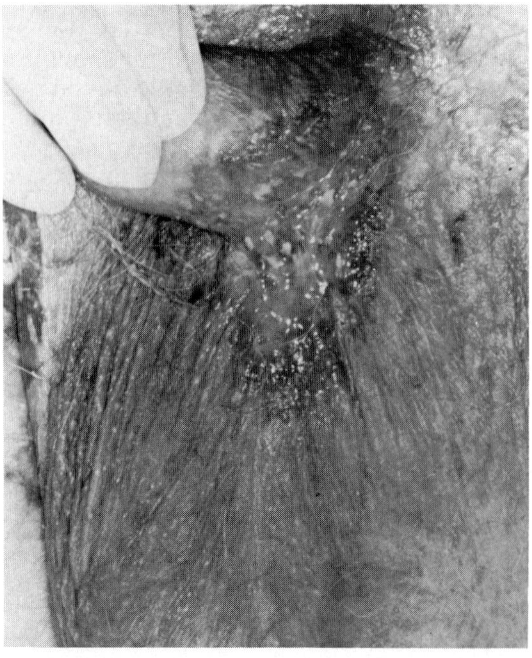

FIGURE 4–108. Extramammary Paget's disease: Note the irregularly bordered, eroded plaque at base of penis.

Adnexal Neoplasms of Eccrine Origin

Some of the adnexal neoplasms of eccrine origin that might be encountered in a Mohs micrographic surgery practice will be reviewed here, including benign and malignant eccrine poroma, malignant chondroid syringoma, and the mucinous and microcystic adnexal variants of primary eccrine carcinoma.

Eccrine poroma is a fairly common tumor, usually occurring on the sole or side of the foot, and less commonly on the hand, finger, arm, or leg. It generally occurs in middle-aged persons and presents as a firm, slightly raised, occasionally eroded nodule usually measuring less than 2 cm in diameter (Fig. 4–112). Malignant eccrine poroma or porocarcinoma may arise de novo but usually develops from a preexisting eccrine poroma.[45] Although initially solitary, it can progress to multiple cutaneous

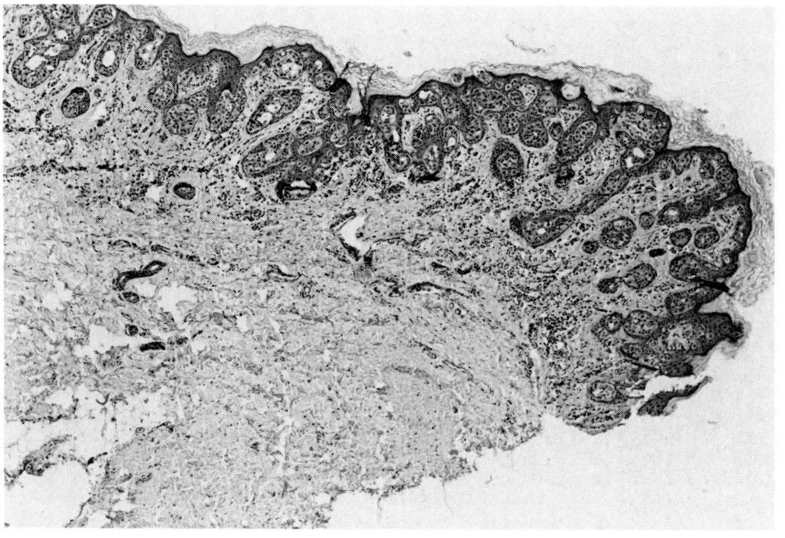

FIGURE 4–109. Extramammary Paget's disease: Multiple nests of atypical Paget cells are scattered throughout the epidermis; note the histologic similarity to in situ superficial spreading malignant melanoma and pagetoid Bowen's disease.

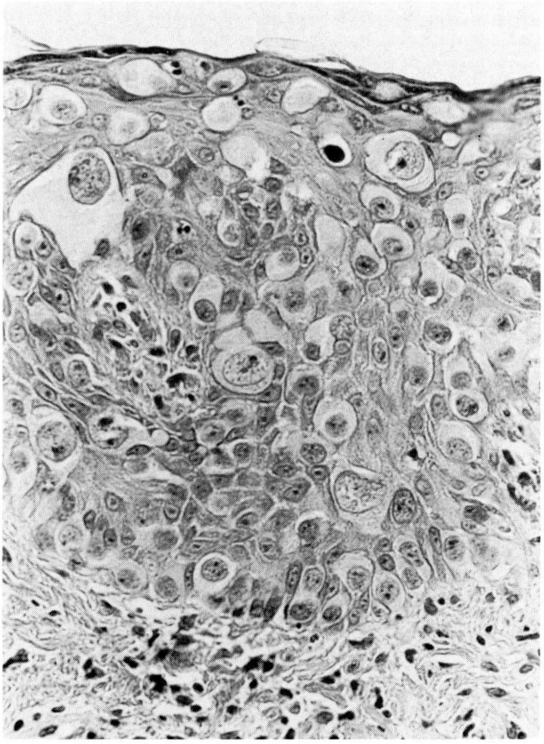

FIGURE 4–110. Extramammary Paget's disease: Note numerous Paget cells with large round atypical nuclei and ample cytoplasm. The presence of flattened basal cells and lack of dyskeratotic cells help to differentiate this lesion from superficial spreading malignant melanoma in situ and pagetoid Bowen's disease, respectively.

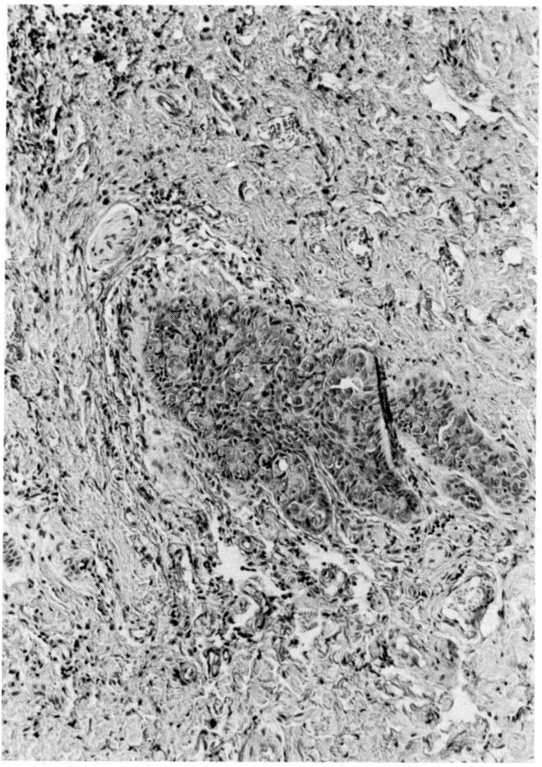

FIGURE 4–111. Extramammary Paget's disease: Nest of atypical Paget cells within the dermis indicates a more advanced or aggressive lesion.

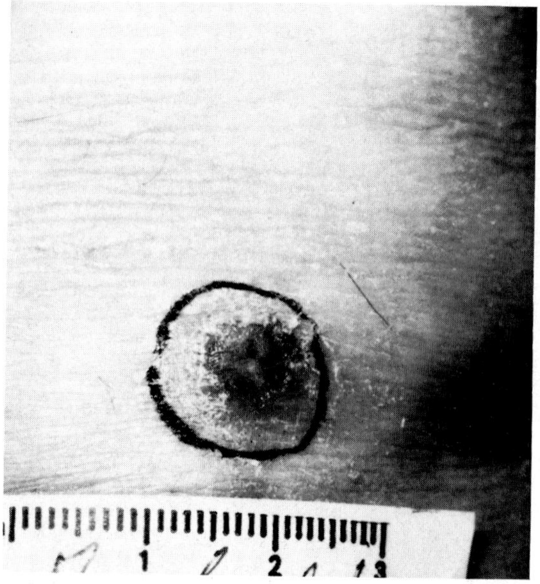

FIGURE 4–112. Eccrine poroma: Raised slightly eroded nodule on knee; the lesion may clinically represent either a benign or malignant eccrine poroma.

and visceral metastases, occasionally resulting in death.

Benign eccrine poroma histologically consists of broad and anastomosing bands of tumor islands that extend from the epidermis into the underlying dermis. The cells comprising the tumor islands have a uniform, cuboidal appearance, contain significant amounts of glycogen, are connected by intercellular bridges, and may show evidence of duct formation (Fig. 4–113). Malignant eccrine poromas that arise from preexisting benign eccrine poromas show histologic features of both lesions with areas of poroma cells with a benign appearance adjoining areas of anaplastic cells (Fig. 4–114). The malignant cells have large, hyperchromatic, pleomorphic nuclei and may be multinucleated (Fig. 4–115). As in the benign lesion, focal glycogen accumulation and cystic, ductal lumina may be present.

Malignant chondroid syringomas, like their benign counterparts, also occur on the head and neck and consist of firm, intradermal, or subcutaneous nodules with or without ulceration (Fig. 4–116). Most lesions of malignant chondroid syringoma arise de novo rather than from preexisting benign chondroid syringomas, and the degree of malignant potential varies from local recurrence to widespread metastases.

Malignant chondroid syringoma is recognizable through its chondroid stroma and tubular structures (Fig. 4–117). Most of the epithelial cells show varying degrees of nuclear atypia and are arranged in irregular cords and islands (Fig. 4–118). Infiltration into blood vessels and surrounding tissue and necrosis can also be seen.

Lesions such as malignant eccrine poroma and malignant chondroid syringoma represent secondary eccrine carcinomas, since they either arise from or have benign counterparts. Primary eccrine carcinomas do not have benign counterparts and arise as independent neoplasms. They clinically present as raised,

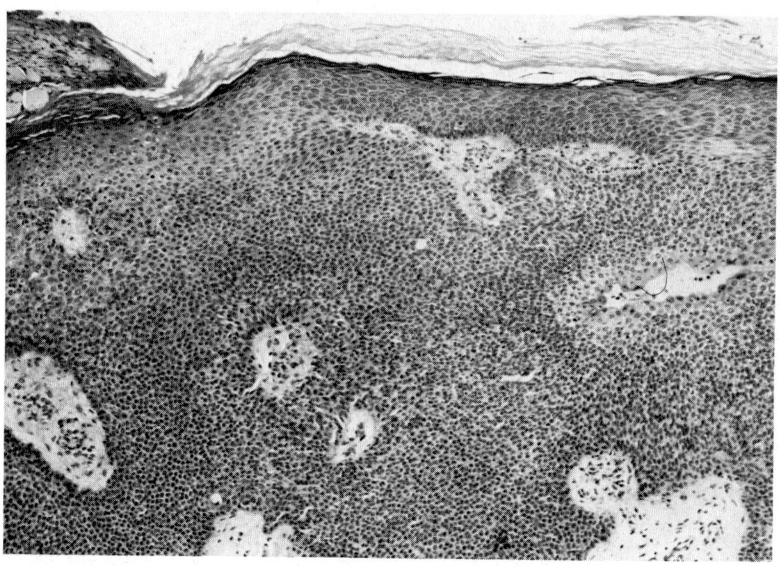

FIGURE 4–113. Eccrine poroma: Benign lesion shows broad anastomosing bands of uniform, small cuboidal epithelial cells extending from the epidermis into the dermis.

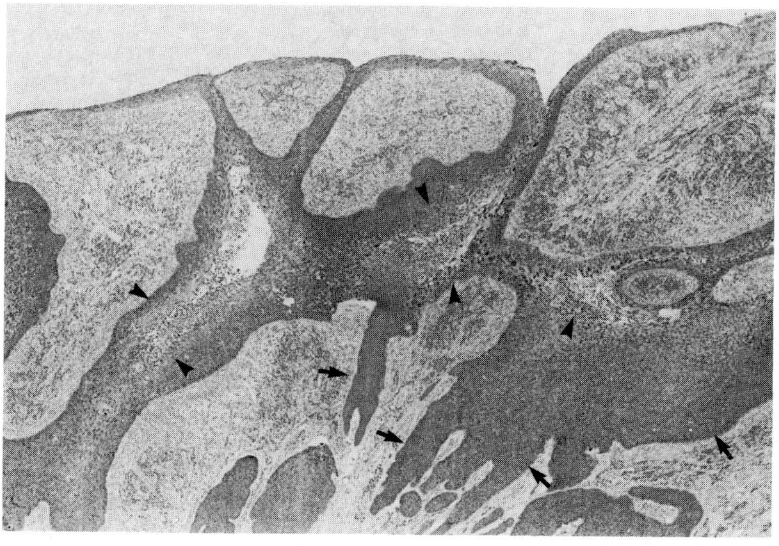

FIGURE 4–114. Malignant eccrine poroma: In this lesion, foci of benign appearing eccrine poroma *(arrow)* are seen adjacent to foci of anaplastic poroma cells *(arrowheads).*

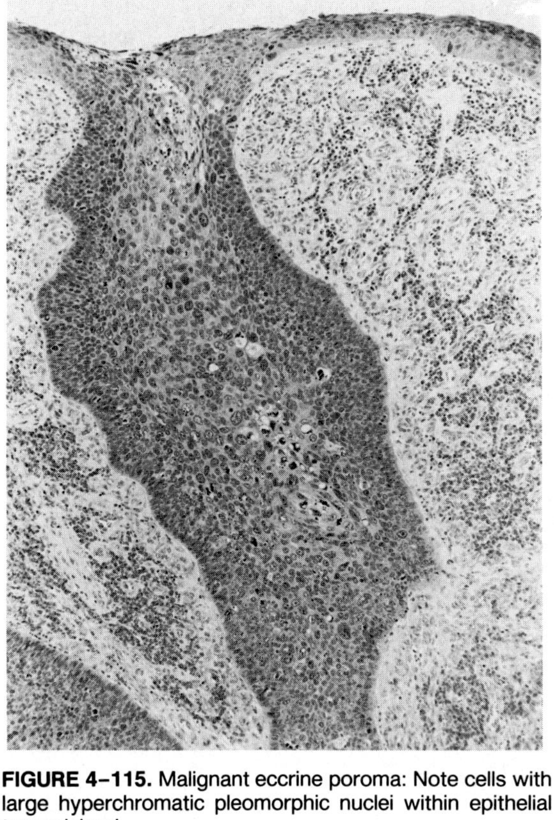

FIGURE 4–115. Malignant eccrine poroma: Note cells with large hyperchromatic pleomorphic nuclei within epithelial tumor island.

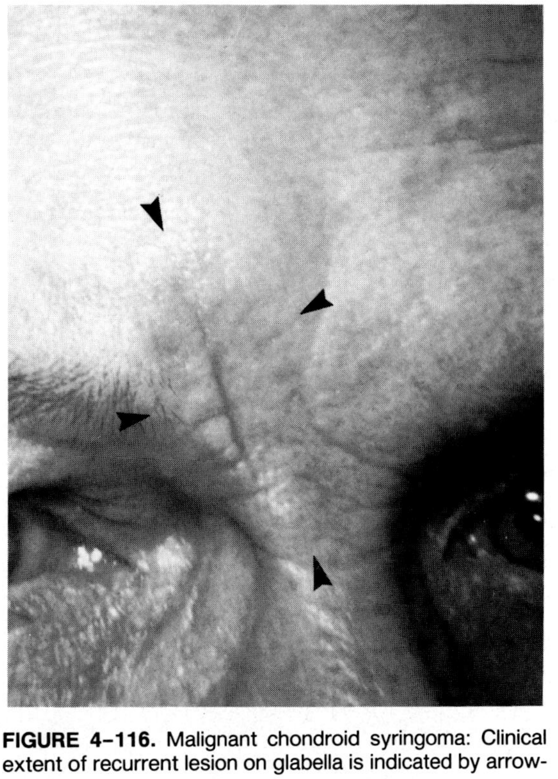

FIGURE 4–116. Malignant chondroid syringoma: Clinical extent of recurrent lesion on glabella is indicated by arrowheads.

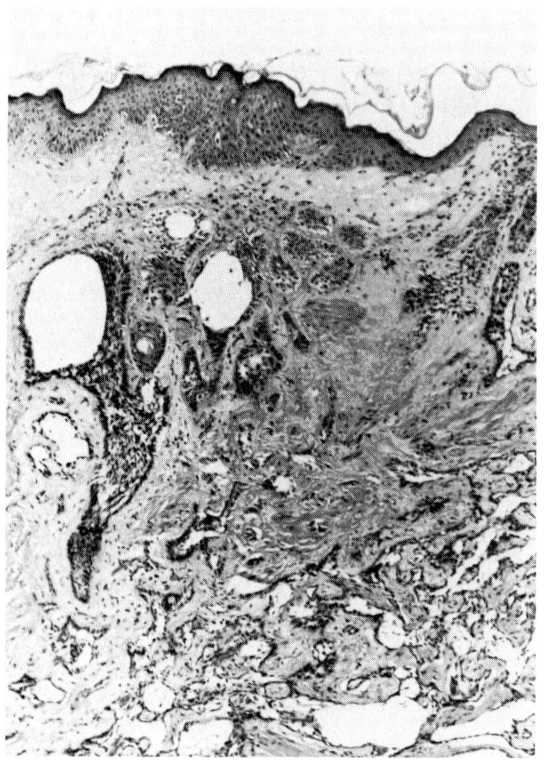

FIGURE 4–117. Malignant chondroid syringoma: Note multiple varying-sized tubular structures embedded in chondroid stroma.

occasionally ulcerated dermal nodules or plaques. Although they can occur on the palm and sole, they appear more commonly elsewhere, particularly on the head and neck.[46] The group of primary eccrine carcinomas includes the classic syringoid, microcystic adnexal, adenoid cystic, mucinous (adenocystic), and the aggressive digital papillary adenocarcinoma variants.

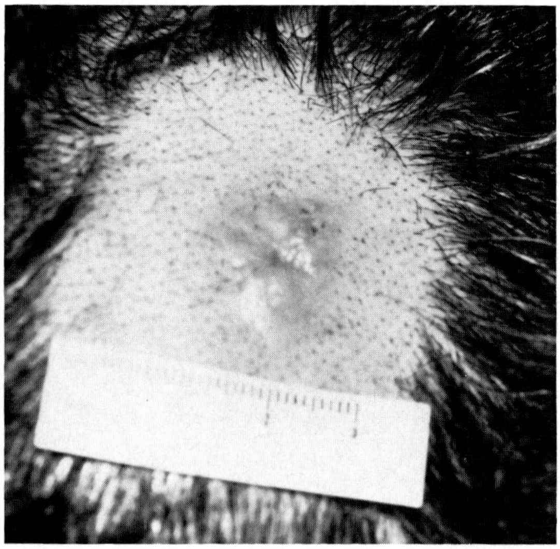

FIGURE 4–119. Mucinous (adenocystic) eccrine carcinoma: Note raised nodule on scalp with irregular surface.

Primary mucinous (adenocystic) eccrine carcinoma[47,48] most commonly occurs on the head and neck, and often presents as a raised cutaneous nodule measuring 1 to 4 cm in diameter (Fig. 4–119).

The histologic appearance of this lesion characteristically shows the tumor to be divided into numerous compartments by thin

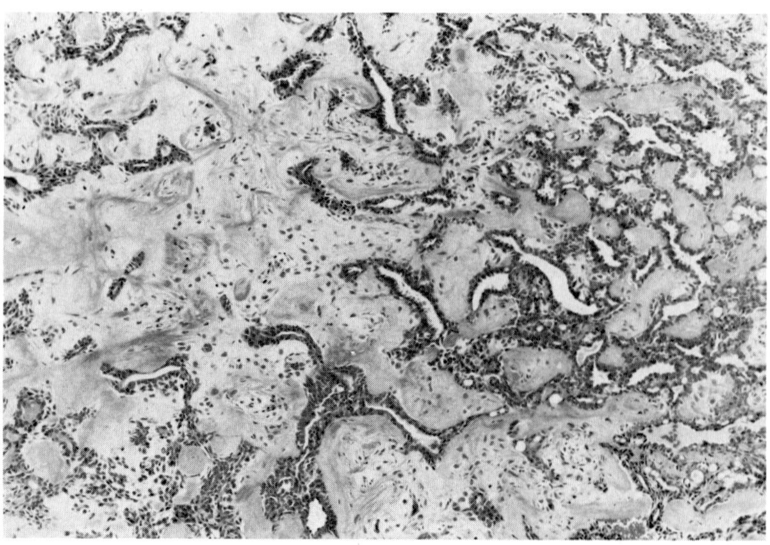

FIGURE 4–118. Malignant chondroid syringoma: Tubular epithelial islands contain cells with a mild to moderate degree of nuclear atypia.

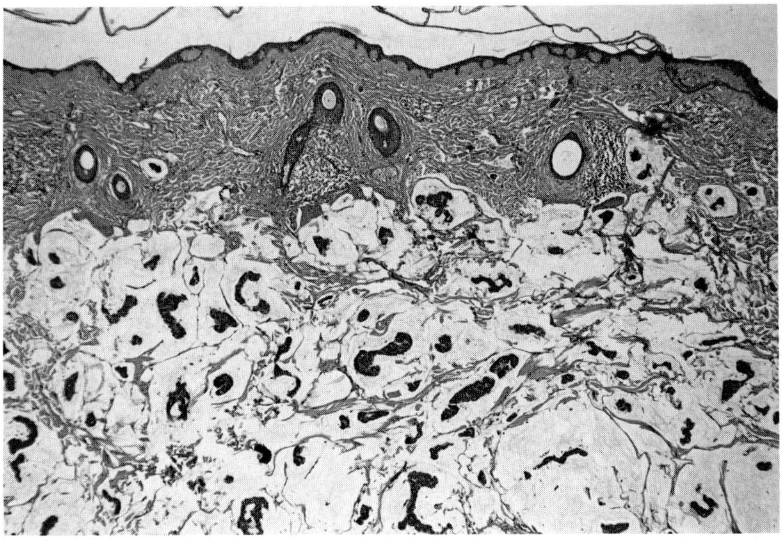

FIGURE 4–120. Mucinous (adenocystic) eccrine carcinoma: Dermal tumor is divided into numerous mucin-containing compartments by thin strands of fibrous tissue.

strands of fibrous tissue (Fig. 4–120). In each compartment, abundant amounts of pale-staining mucin surround nests and cords of moderately anaplastic epithelial cells, some of which may show a tubular lumen (Fig. 4–121). Histochemical reactions show the mucin to be composed of nonsulfated sialomucin.[48]

Microcystic adnexal carcinoma, although most commonly seen on the upper lip, may occasionally occur on the nasolabial fold, the cheek, or the chin.[49,50] The lesions clinically appear as raised, flesh-colored to yellow, solitary plaques (Fig. 4–122), and are most commonly seen in white middle-aged women.

Histologically, the tumor islands show both pilar and glandular components embedded within a desmoplastic stroma. Islands of basaloid cells showing abortive hair follicles and containing horn cysts are intermingled with narrow epithelial islands containing ducts and forming gland-like structures (Fig. 4–123). The tumor often extends deep into the dermis or subcutis, and perineural and muscular invasion is common (Fig. 4–124). The presence of both pilar and eccrine structures aids in the differentiation of this lesion from desmoplastic trichoepithelioma, syringoid eccrine carcinoma, and sclerotic basal cell carcinoma.

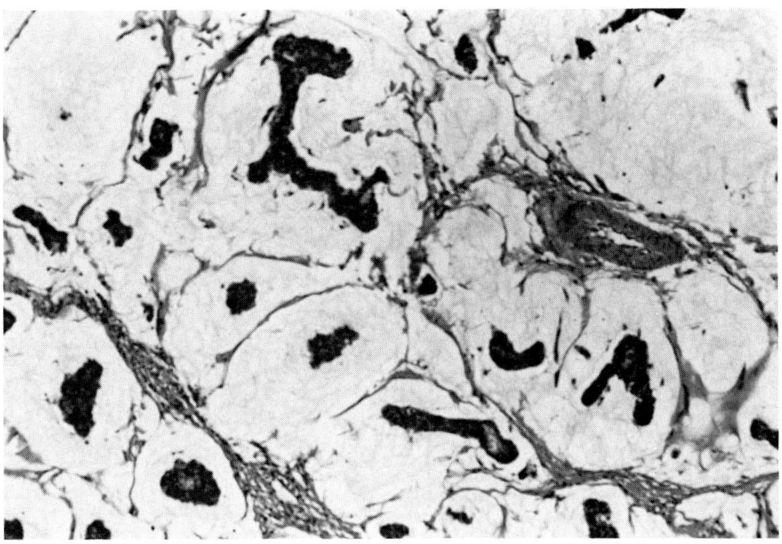

FIGURE 4–121. Mucinous (adenocystic) eccrine carcinoma: Abundant amounts of mucin surround islands of moderately anaplastic epithelial cells.

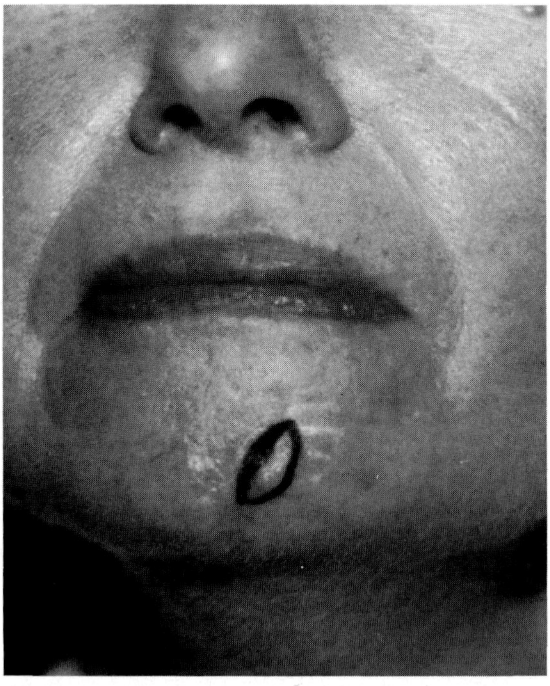

FIGURE 4-122. Microcystic adnexal eccrine carcinoma: Note raised nodule protruding from plaque of recurrent tumor on chin.

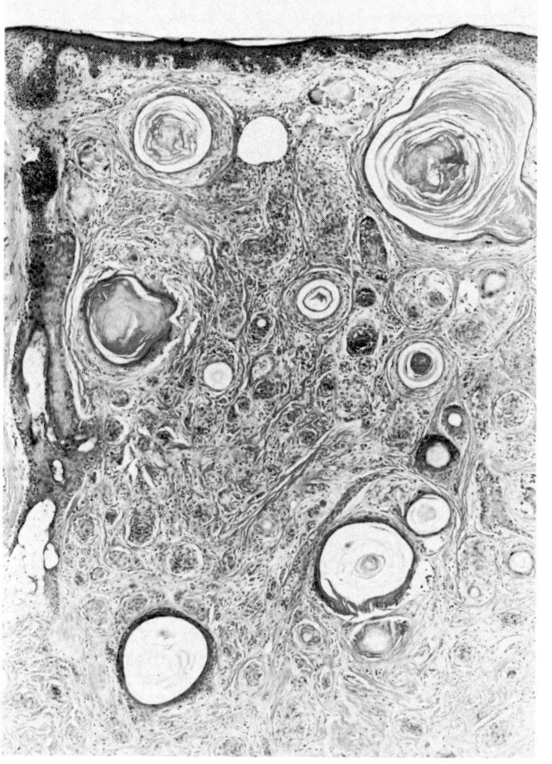

FIGURE 4-123. Microcystic adnexal eccrine carcinoma: Nests of tumor cells showing pilar differentiation and horn cyst formation are intermingled with narrow basaloid strands containing ductal elements.

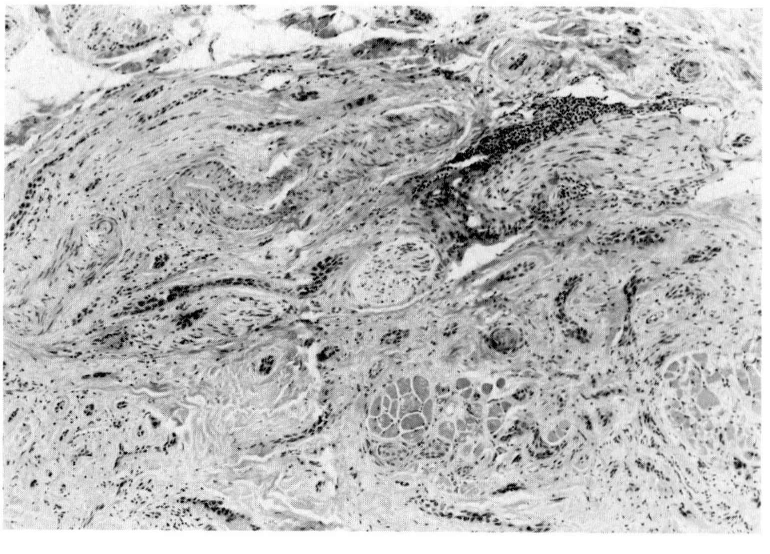

FIGURE 4-124. Microcystic adnexal eccrine carcinoma: Small tumor islands present in deep dermis show both perineural and muscular invasion.

MELANOCYTIC NEOPLASMS

The Mohs surgeon may be called upon to treat certain melanocytic lesions including lentigo maligna, lentigo maligna melanoma, superficial spreading malignant melanoma, nodular malignant melanoma, and acral lentiginous malignant melanoma. Representative cases of these lesions will be presented in this section.

It is generally agreed that there are four types of malignant melanoma. Three types have an early radial or horizontal (in situ) growth phase within the epidermis, followed by a vertical or invasive growth phase that involves the dermis. These three types are: lentigo maligna melanoma, superficial spreading malignant melanoma, and acral lentiginous malignant melanoma. The fourth type, referred to as nodular malignant melanoma, is felt to exhibit a vertical growth phase only.[51,52] The incidence of the four types of malignant melanoma in whites is approximately 70% for superficial spreading malignant melanoma; 15% for nodular melanoma; 8% for acral lentiginous malignant melanoma; and 5% for lentigo maligna melanoma, with 2% of cases unclassifiable.[52] Clinical staging of malignant melanoma includes three levels:

Stage I: No clinical evidence of metastases.
Stage II: Only regional lymph node metastases.
Stage III: Disseminated metastases.

The prognosis involves many factors, including clinical and histologic parameters. Favorable clinical prognostic parameters include location of the tumor on hair-bearing skin of the extremities, small lesion diameter, lack of ulceration, female gender, and lack of lymph node involvement or metastasis. Favorable histologic prognostic factors include the type of melanoma (lentigo maligna and superficial spreading), a low mitotic index of tumor cells, the presence of a host response, the lack of vascular invasion, and the lack of significant depth (tumor thickness). Tumor thickness is the single most important factor in predicting survival in Stage I patients. Originally, the depth of invasion was determined by assessing the extent of dermal involvement, and five levels were defined by Clark, as follows:[51]

Level I: Confinement of the malignant melanoma cells to the epidermis and its appendages.
Level II: Extention into the papillary dermis with at most only a few melanoma cells extending to the interface between the papillary and reticular dermis.
Level III: Extension of the tumor cells throughout the papillary dermis, filling it and impinging upon the reticular dermis without, however, extending into it.
Level IV: Involvement of the recticular dermis.
Level V: Involvement of the subcutaneous fat.

In 1970, Breslow[53] recommended measuring the depth of invasion with an ocular micrometer. In his method, tumor depth in millimeters is measured from the top of the granular cell layer (or ulceration) to the deepest extension of the tumor in the dermis. Using a combination of these two methods of thickness measurements, Bagley and coworkers[54] divided Stage I melanomas into three prognostic groups:

1. Low risk:
   - Melanomas less than 0.76 mm thick and Level II or III.
2. Moderate risk:
   - Melanomas less than 0.76 mm thick and Level IV.
   - Melanomas between 0.76 mm and 1.5 mm thick.
   - Melanomas more than 1.5 mm thick and Level III.
3. High risk:
   - Melanomas more than 1.5 mm thick and Level IV or V.

Bagley found that the five-year survival rates for the three risk groups were 100%, 77%, and 63%, respectively.

The tumor cells in all forms of in situ and invasive malignant melanoma show marked variation in size and shape with two major cell types, spindle and epithelioid, predominating in most lesions. Mitotic figures are generally present in malignant melanoma but are oftentimes few in number. The amount of melanin pigment varies greatly in malignant melanoma. Some lesions may show large amounts of melanin in both tumor cells and dermal melanophages, while other lesions contain no discernible melanin on H&E staining, the so-called amelanotic malignant melanoma. Positive staining of amelanotic lesions with Fontana-Masson or S-100 protein is often extemely helpful in confirming the melanocytic nature of the tumor cells. The amount of inflammatory infiltrate in malignant melanomas also varies greatly.

Lentigo Maligna and Lentigo Maligna Melanoma

Lentigo maligna, also referred to as melanotic freckle of Hutchinson and melanosis circumscripta preblastomatosa of Dubreuilh, occurs on the sun-exposed cutaneous surfaces of older people, especially the face. It most commonly presents as an irregularly circumscribed, unevenly pigmented, nonindurated patch that may show foci of depigmentation or regression (Fig. 4–125). It is very slow-growing, and progression into an invasive lentigo maligna melanoma usually does not occur until the in situ lesion has been present for many years. Progression into an invasive melanoma is clinically indicated by the presence of a papule or nodule within the primary lesion (Fig. 4–126). Lentigo maligna melanoma may rarely present as a nonpigmented, indurated plaque known as a desmoplastic malignant melanoma (Fig. 4–127).

Histologically, early lesions of lentigo maligna show irregular epidermal atrophy, hyperpigmentation, and a significant increase in the

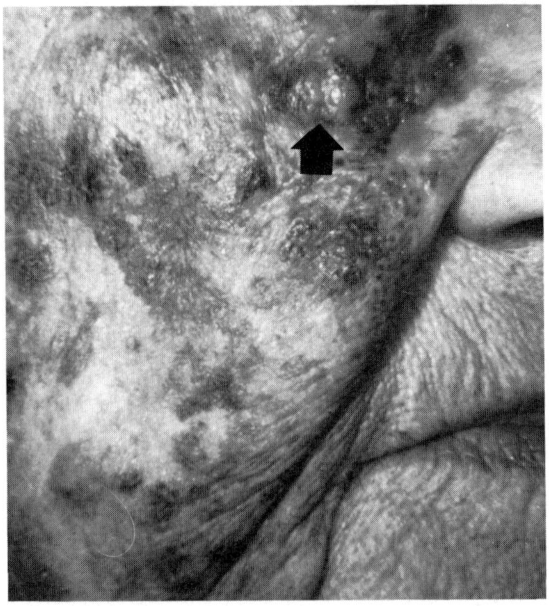

FIGURE 4–126. Lentigo maligna melanoma: Note raised nodule *(arrow)* developing over a background of an irregularly pigmented patch of lentigo maligna, indicating transformation into lentigo maligna melanoma.

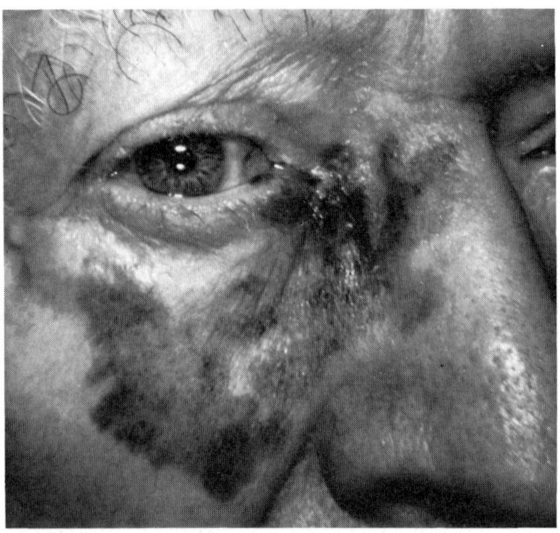

FIGURE 4–125. Lentigo maligna presenting as a large irregularly circumscribed and unevenly pigmented patch on the cheek.

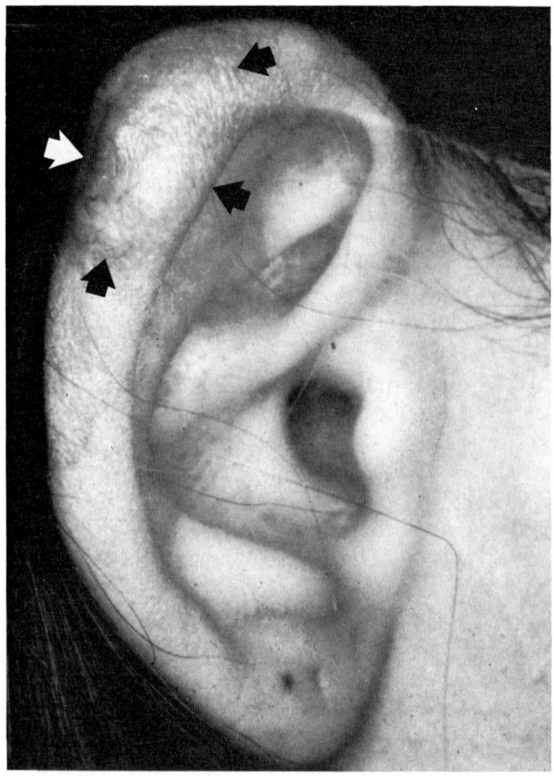

FIGURE 4–127. Lentigo maligna melanoma: Desmoplastic variant of malignant melanoma occurring at the site of previously excised lentigo maligna on the ear.

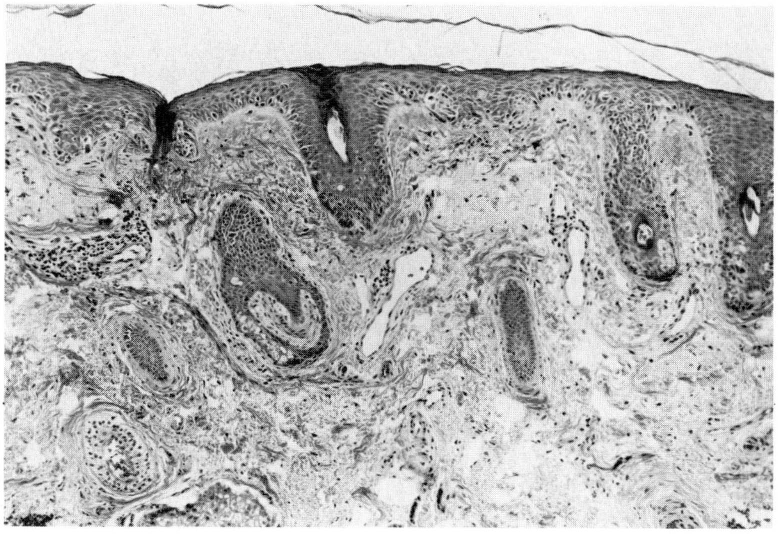

FIGURE 4–128. Lentigo maligna: Atypical melanocytes are present singly and in small nests along the dermal-epithelial junction of the epidermis and hair follicle. Telangiectasia, solar elastosis, and a sparse inflammatory infiltrate characterize dermal changes.

number of basal melanocytes, some of which show mild nuclear atypia and irregularity in their arrangement. More advanced lesions show a marked increase in the concentration of basal melanocytes, which are haphazardly arranged along the dermal-epithelial junction of the epidermis and its appendages. The atypical melanocytes are often spindle-shaped, contain elongated, hyperchromatic nuclei, and may show some tendency to nest formation (Fig. 4–128). However, extension of the atypical melanocytes into upper layers of the epidermis, which is characteristic of the acral lentiginous and superficial spreading variants, is minimal or absent in lentigo maligna. The upper dermis shows solar elastosis, melanophages, and varying degrees of inflammation.

Transformation of lentigo maligna into a lentigo maligna melanoma is indicated by dermal involvement with the atypical melanocytes (Fig. 4–129). Rarely, a desmoplastic histologic variant of malignant melanoma can occur in association with a primary or, more commonly, in a recurrent lentigo maligna melanoma. This variant is characterized by the presence of elongated, amelanotic, atypical melanocytes that are scattered diffusely, although sometimes sparsely, throughout a fibrotic dermal stroma (Fig. 4–130). Absence of melanin makes differentiation of the abnormal melanocytes from dermal fibroblasts difficult, but immunohistochemical staining with S-100 protein identifies the nature of the tumor cells (Fig. 4–131).

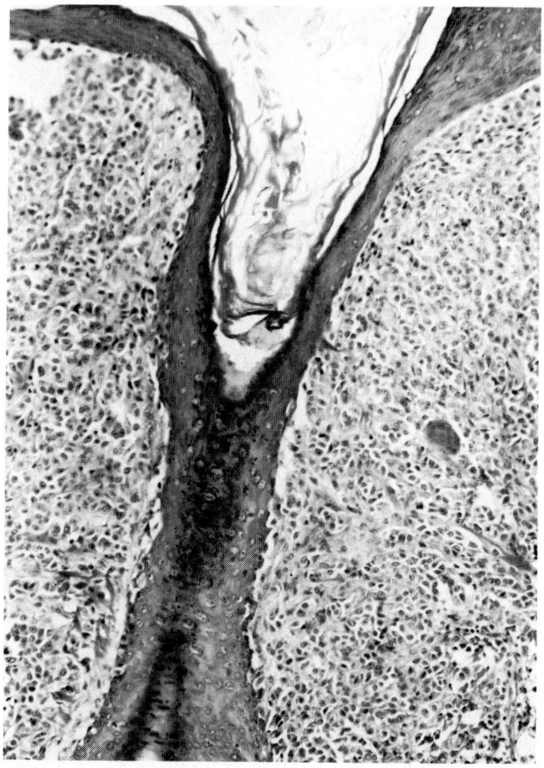

FIGURE 4–129. Lentigo maligna melanoma: High-power view of nodular portion of lesion showing numerous atypical melanocytes in dermis; note presence of a few atypical melanocytes along basal layer of follicular epithelium.

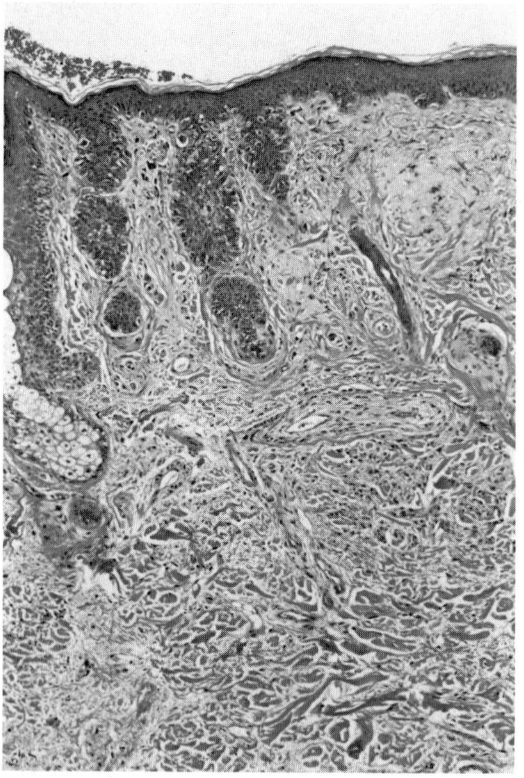

FIGURE 4–130. Desomoplastic malignant melanoma: Spindle-shaped atypical melanocytes are scattered throughout a fibroblastic dermis but are difficult to identify on sections stained with hematoxylin and eosin; note the presence of atypical melanocytes at dermal epidermal junction.

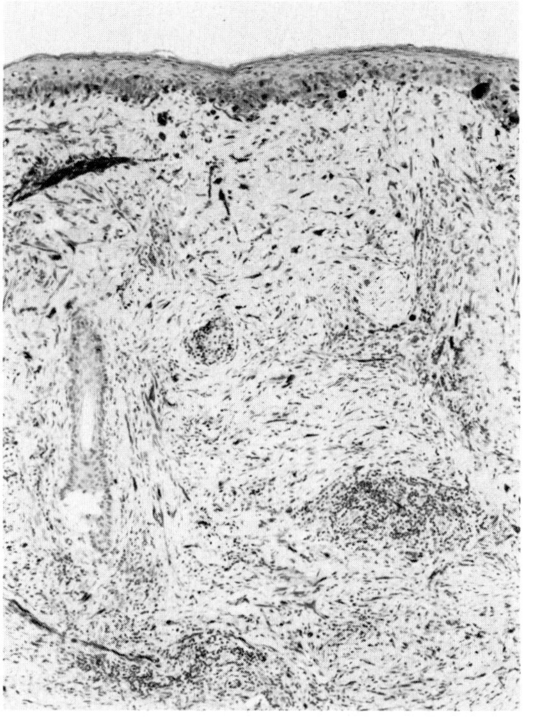

FIGURE 4–131. Desmoplastic malignant melanoma: S-100 staining of sections from lesion in Figure 4–130 confirms the presence of atypical melanocytes at the dermal-epidermal junction and throughout the fibrotic dermal stroma.

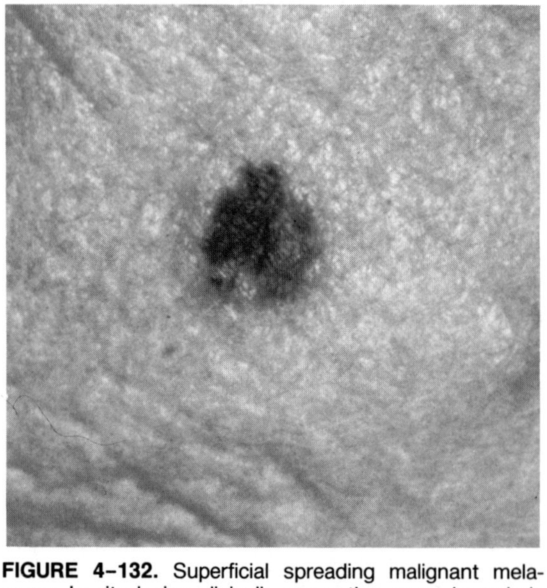

FIGURE 4–132. Superficial spreading malignant melanoma: In situ lesion clinically presenting as an irregularly pigmented, eroded plaque on the temple.

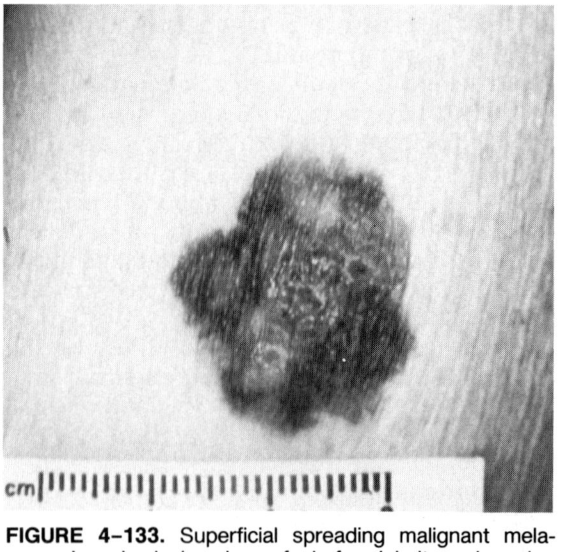

FIGURE 4–133. Superficial spreading malignant melanoma: Invasive lesion shows foci of nodularity and erosion over a background of irregularly pigmented plaque.

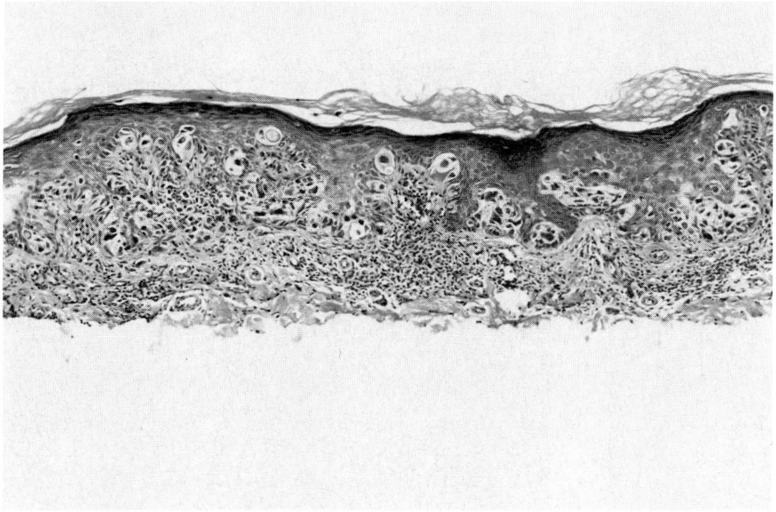

FIGURE 4–134. Superficial spreading malignant melanoma: In situ lesion shows numerous rounded atypical melanocytes present throughout the epidermis.

Superficial Spreading Malignant Melanoma

Superficial spreading malignant melanoma, also called pagetoid malignant melanoma, can occur on both sun-exposed and nonexposed skin. It most frequently involves the upper back in men and the lower legs in women. Early lesions often present as an irregularly outlined, unevenly pigmented patch or a slightly elevated papule or plaque (Fig. 4–132). Variation in color is often great and includes shades of black, brown, tan, red, blue, pink, gray, and white. Dermal involvement occurs much sooner than in lentigo maligna, and is often indicated by the development of nodularity or ulceration (Fig. 4–133). Superficial spreading malignant melanoma usually develops de novo, but can evolve from a preexisting nevus.

Histologically, in situ superficial spreading malignant melanoma is characterized by the presence of rounded, somewhat uniform appearing, atypical melanocytes scattered singly and in small nests throughout an often acanthotic epidermis (Fig. 4–134). The tumor cells have atypical, hyperchromatic nuclei with abundant cytoplasm, often containing fine "dust-like" melanin granules. Extension of the atypical melanocytes into the dermis indicates transformation into an invasive superficial spreading malignant melanoma (Fig. 4–135).

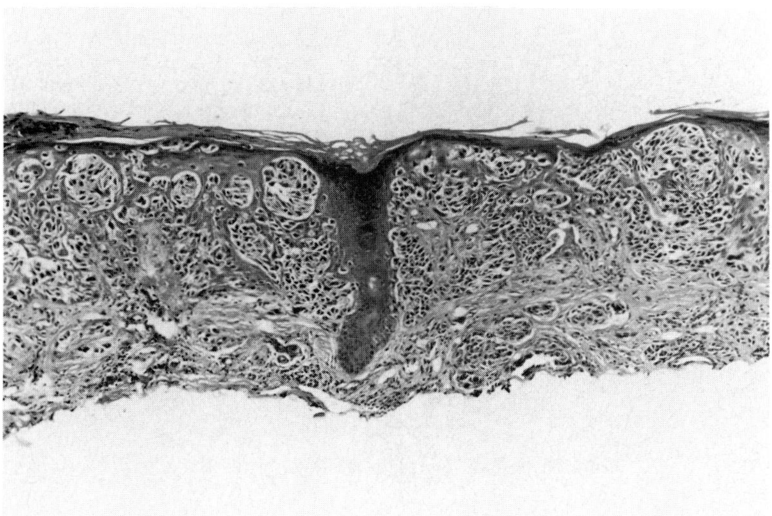

FIGURE 4–135. Superficial spreading malignant melanoma: Nests of atypical melanocytes permeate epidermis and extend into upper dermis in invasive superficial spreading malignant melanoma.

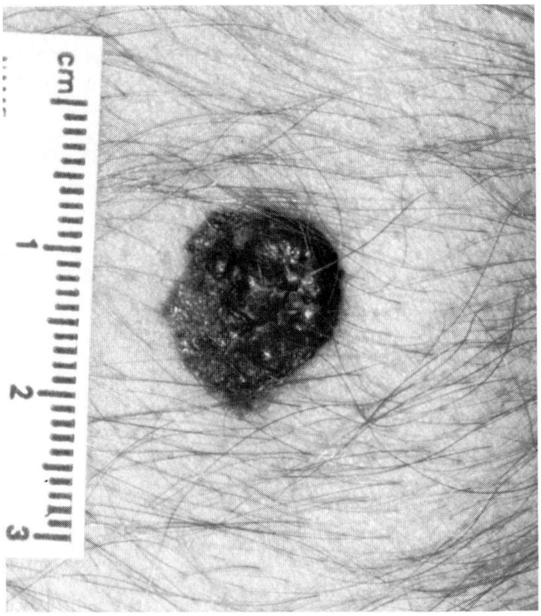

FIGURE 4–136. Nodular malignant melanoma: Elevated deeply pigmented nodular melanoma on thigh.

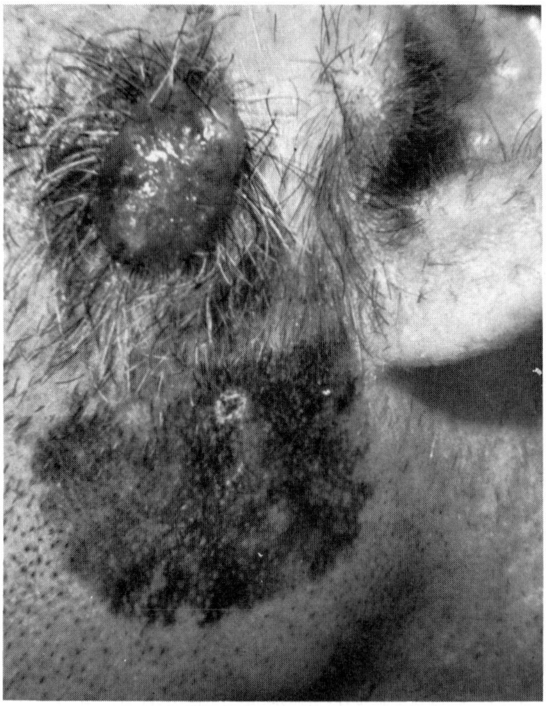

FIGURE 4–137. Nodular malignant melanoma: Large hypomelanotic nodule in preauricular area; note diffusion of pigment into surrounding skin.

Nodular Malignant Melanoma

Nodular malignant melanoma can occur on any cutaneous site and, because of its rapid vertical growth phase, often has a poor prognosis by the time diagnosis is made. It begins as an elevated, usually deeply pigmented, nodule that grows rapidly in size and often undergoes erosion or ulceration (Fig. 4–136 and 4–137).

Histologically, nodular malignant melanoma consists of large dermal aggregates of atypical melanocytes with little, if any, evidence of epidermal involvement (Fig. 4–138). The amount of surrounding dermal inflammation and tumor pigmentation is quite variable.

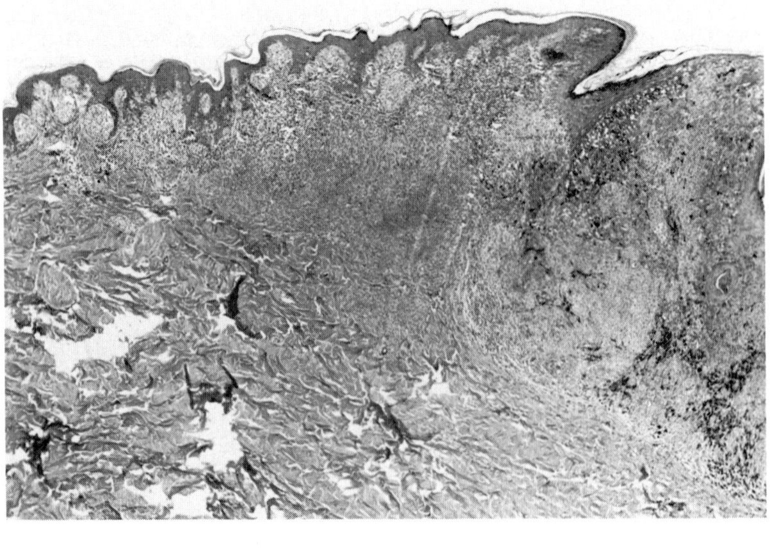

FIGURE 4–138. Nodular malignant melanoma: Large dermal aggregates of atypical melanocytes without significant epidermal or junctional involvement characterize nodular malignant melanoma histologically.

Acral Lentiginous Malignant Melanoma

Acral lentiginous malignant melanoma occurs on the hairless skin of the palms and soles and in the ungual and periungual regions. It is more common in races with dark skin. Clinically, in situ lesions present as an uneven pigmentation with an irregular, ill-defined border (Fig. 4–139). Invasive acral lentiginous malignant melanoma is most often indicated by the presence of a nodular growth over a background of irregular patchy pigmentation (Fig. 4–140). Lesions involving mucocutaneous junctions are variants of acral lentiginous malignant melanoma and are termed juxtacutaneous melanoma. They often have a striking clinical presentation (Fig. 4–141).

Early in situ lesions of acral lentiginous melanoma may present a deceptively benign histologic picture, consisting of an increase in basal melanocytes and hyperpigmentation but with only mild focal atypia of the melanocytic cells (Fig. 4–142). Atypical melanocytes in early lesions are often spindle or stellate in shape. In more advanced lesions, both spindle and epithelioid or rounded cells are seen, with dermal involvement indicating invasive tumors (Fig. 4–143). The juxtacutaneous variant of acral lentiginous malignant melanoma shows involvement of continguous cutaneous and mucosal surfaces with tumor cells (Fig. 4–144).

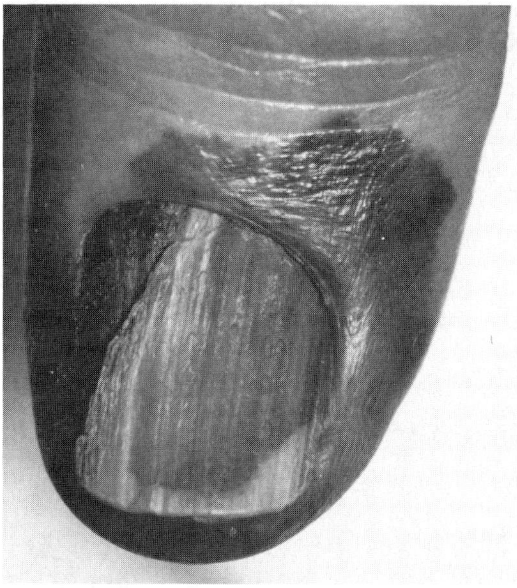

FIGURE 4–139. Acral lentiginous malignant melanoma: Lesion shows irregular patchy pigmentation of nailbed and periungual region (melanotic freckle of Hutchinson).

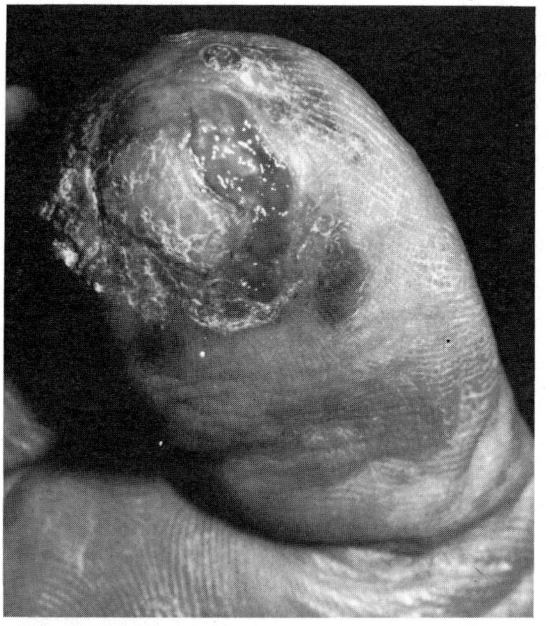

FIGURE 4–140. Acral lentiginous malignant melanoma: Invasive lesion presented as ulcerated nodule on plantar aspect of great toe.

MESENCHYMAL NEOPLASMS

Mesenchymal neoplasms arise from tissue structures derived from embryonic mesen-

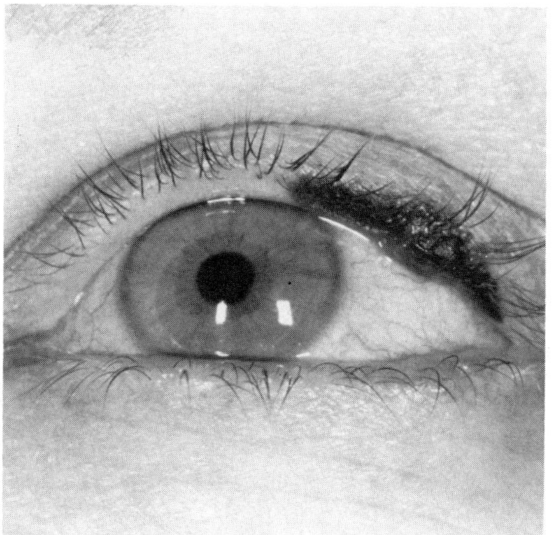

FIGURE 4–41. Acral lentiginous malignant melanoma: Juxtacutaneous variant involving eyelid margin at mucocutaneous junction.

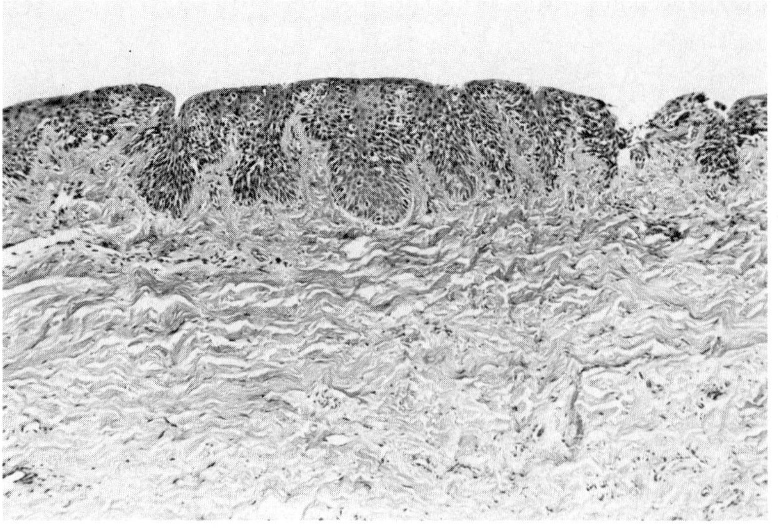

FIGURE 4–142. Acral lentiginous malignant melanoma: Histologic features of early in situ nailbed lesion show increase in number of slightly atypical melanocytes in nailbed epithelium.

FIGURE 4–143. Acral lentiginous malignant melanoma: Invasive lesion shows atypical melanocytes in both epidermis and dermis.

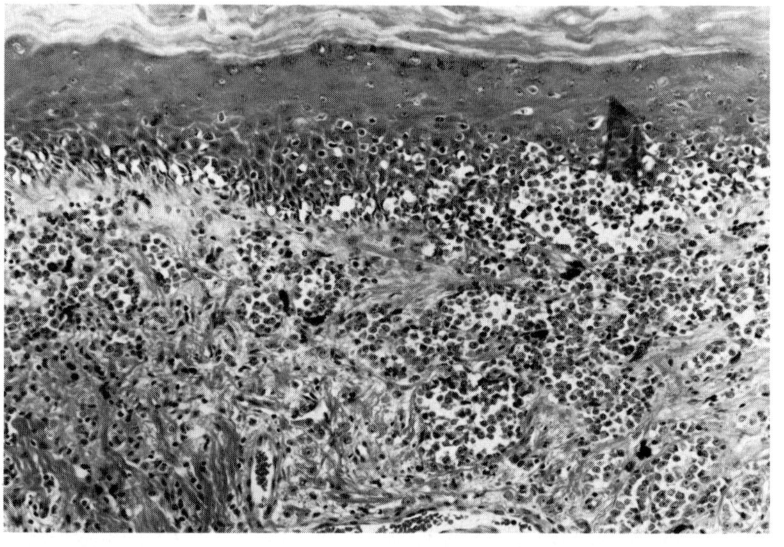

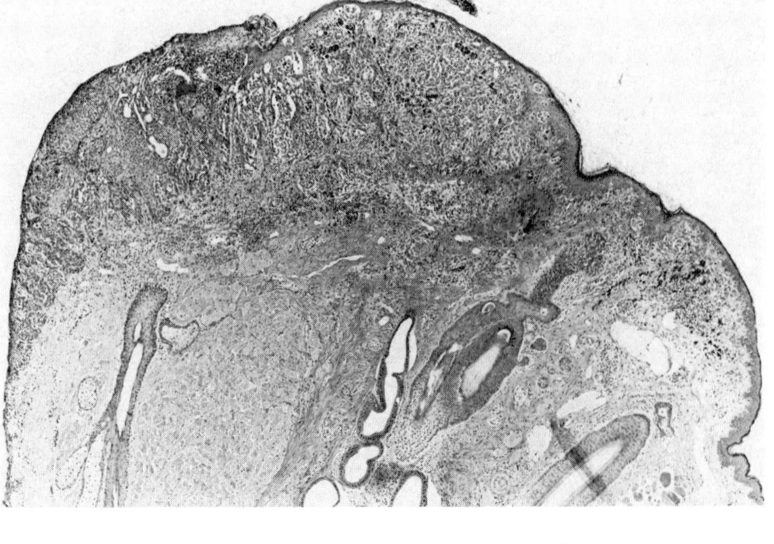

FIGURE 4–144. Acral lentiginous malignant melanoma: Juxtacutaneous variant shows atypical melanocytes involving both cutaneous surface *(right)* and conjunctival epithelium *(left)* as well as underlying dermis.

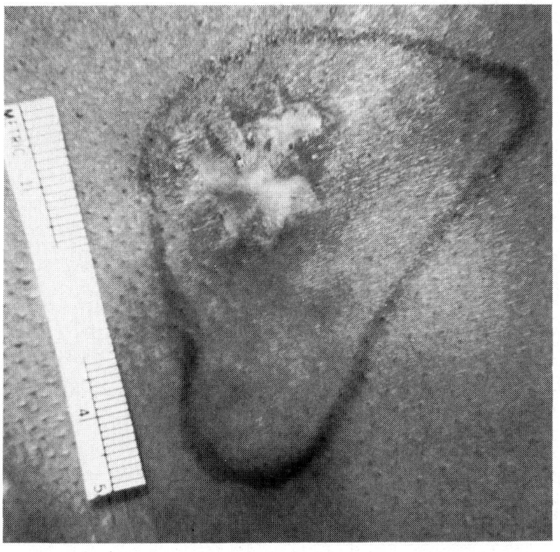

FIGURE 4–145. Dermatofibrosarcoma protuberans: Note large plaque with superimposed nodularity in the intermammary region.

chyme and include tumors of fibrous, vascular, fatty, osseous, and muscular tissues. Although the number of neoplasms included in this category is large, we will limit consideration here to examples of lesions that might be encountered by the Mohs micrographic surgeon: dermatofibrosarcoma protuberans, malignant fibrous histiocytoma, atypical fibroxanthoma, angiosarcoma, and rhabdomyosarcoma.

Dermatofibrosarcoma Protuberans

Dermatofibrosarcoma protuberans represents a slowly growing dermal neoplasm that, although locally invasive, rarely gives rise to metastases. It usually begins as an indurated plaque upon which multiple, firm nodules may develop (Fig. 4–145). The lesions are often dusky red or violaceous in color and may ulcerate as they increase in size. The actual extent of tissue involvement may not be clinically discernable, making it a lesion amenable to histographic excision (Fig. 4–146). It occurs most frequently on the trunk and proximal extremities, with rare involvement of the face, scalp, or neck.

The histologic appearance of the tumor is that of a well-differentiated fibrosarcoma. The tumor is composed predominantly of cells with large, spindle-shaped nuclei and little cytoplasm. The cells are often arranged in intertwining fascicles, forming a so-called storiform pattern, or the cells may radiate outward from a central hub of fibrous tissue resulting in a cartwheel appearance (Fig. 4–147). Mitoses can be seen, but are often rare. Differentiation from a benign dermatofibroma can be difficult, but the greater degree of cellularity, greater nuclear atypicality, larger number of mitoses, and infiltration into the subcutaneous tissue favor a diagnosis of dermatofibrosarcoma protuberans.

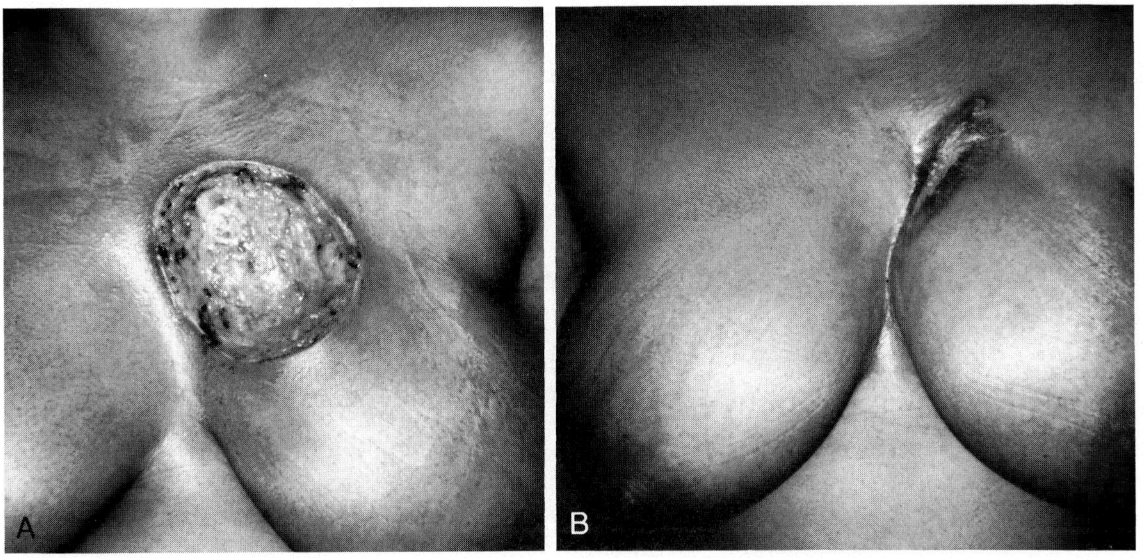

FIGURE 4–146. Dermatofibrosarcoma protuberans: *A*, Actual extent of cutaneous involvement is indicated by final wound size following Mohs micrographic surgery. *B*, Result after healing by second intention.

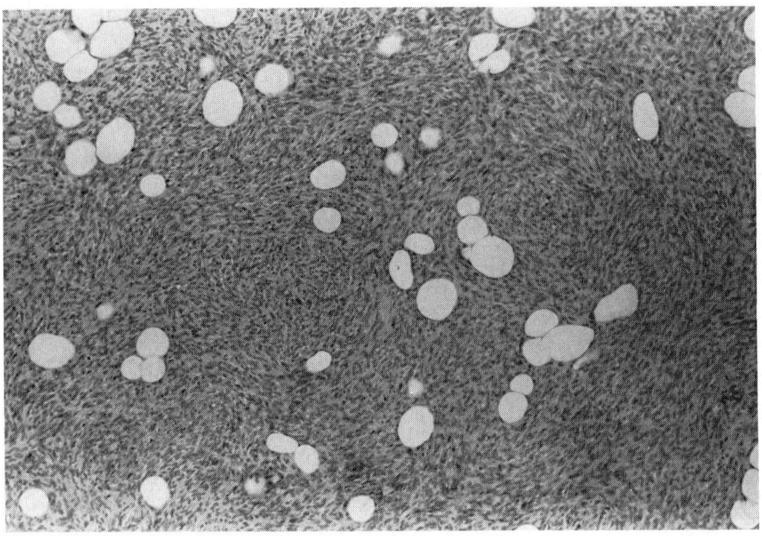

FIGURE 4–147. Dermatofibrosarcoma protuberans: Note atypical fibroblastic nuclei, arranged in intersecting bundles forming the so-called storiform and cartwheel patterns and extending into subcutaneous tissue.

Malignant Fibrous Histiocytoma

Malignant fibrous histiocytoma is a pleomorphic sarcoma that probably represents the most common soft tissue sarcoma of middle and late adulthood.[55] The most common site of involvement is the thigh, including the buttock. Malignant fibrous histiocytomas are subdivided into superficial and deep types, depending upon the site of origin in the tissue. The superficial variant arises in the subcutaneous tissue and rarely involves the skin, where it usually presents as an ulcerated nodule (Fig. 4–148). Deep tumors are more common. They arise from the deep muscle fascia and are associated with a much poorer prognosis. Because of poor demarcation, local recurrences following presumed "adequate" excision are approximately 50%.[55]

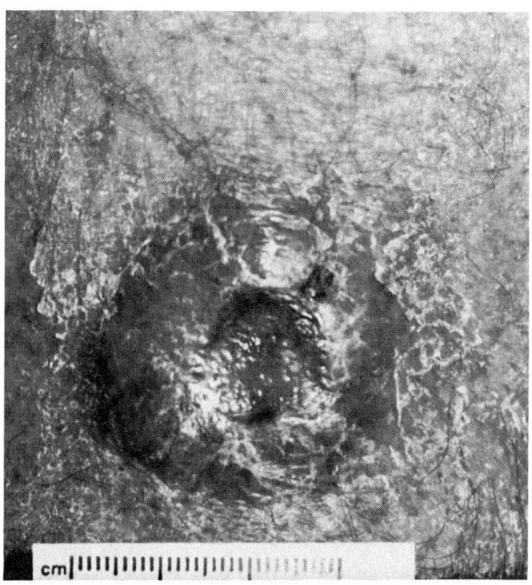

FIGURE 4–148. Malignant fibrous histiocytoma: Large ulcerated nodule characterizes this cutaneous presentation.

Histologically, malignant fibrous histiocytoma is a highly cellular tumor with pleomorphic components. Some of the tumor cells are spindle-shaped and fibroblastic, while others possess irregularly shaped nuclei and ample cytoplasm and resemble histiocytes (Fig. 4–149). Multinucleated giant cells with bizarre, hyperchromatic nuclei are common, as are atypical mitotic figures (Fig. 4–150). Several histologic variants of malignant fibrous histiocytoma have been described and include the xanthomatous, inflammatory, myxoid, angiomatoid, and giant cell types.

Atypical Fibroxanthoma

Atypical fibroxanthoma is a relatively common lesion which occurs most often on sun-exposed or irradiated areas of the head and neck in elderly persons. It often presents as a raised, firm nodule of relatively recent origin and usually measures less than 2 cm in diameter. Some lesions are covered by normal skin (Fig. 4–151), while others are eroded (Fig. 4–152). The lesion was originally felt to be a benign reactive neoplasm,[56] but has been regarded more re-

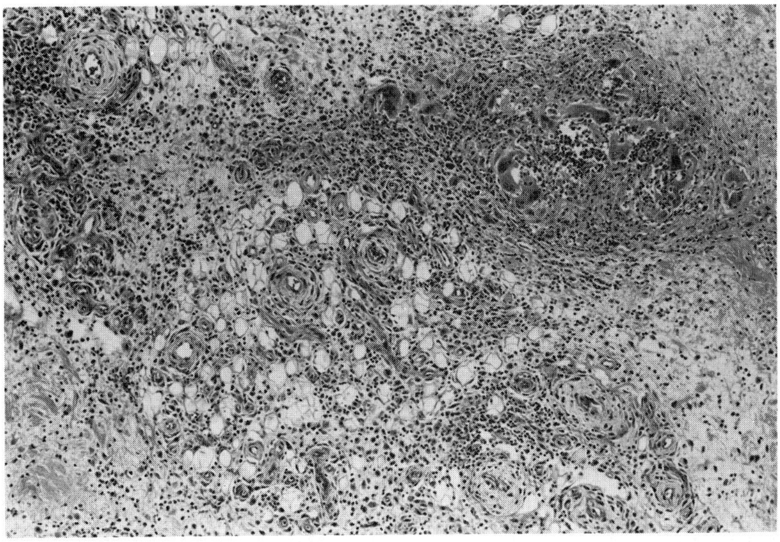

FIGURE 4–149. Malignant fibrous histiocytoma: Spindle-shaped, fibroblast-like cells are intermingled with atypical histiocytoid cells and bizarre giant cells.

cently as a variant of malignant fibrous histiocytoma with low-grade malignant potential and a more favorable prognosis.[57]

Histologically, atypical fibroxanthoma is characterized by a highly cellular dermal infiltrate composed of cells with pleomorphic, hyperchromatic nuclei (Fig. 4–153). Some cells are spindle-shaped while others are polygonal with a foamy, vacuolated cytoplasm, resembling histiocytes (Fig. 4–154). A striking feature is the presence of large, bizarre, multinucleated giant cells and numerous atypical mitoses. A histologic differential diagnosis of atypical fibroxanthoma includes malignant melanoma and spindle cell squamous carcinoma. Immunohistochemical staining for keratin, vimentin, and S-100 protein greatly aids in the differentiation of these lesions (Fig. 4–155).

Angiosarcoma

Angiosarcomas of the skin, also called malignant angioendotheliomas, are rare except for angiosarcomas occurring on the scalp and face of the elderly and those that develop secondary to chronic lymphedema (Stuart-Treves angiosarcoma). Angiosarcomas of the face and scalp may present as rather innocuous erythematous or purple patches or slightly raised plaques (Fig. 4–156). Lesions spread by gradual centrif-

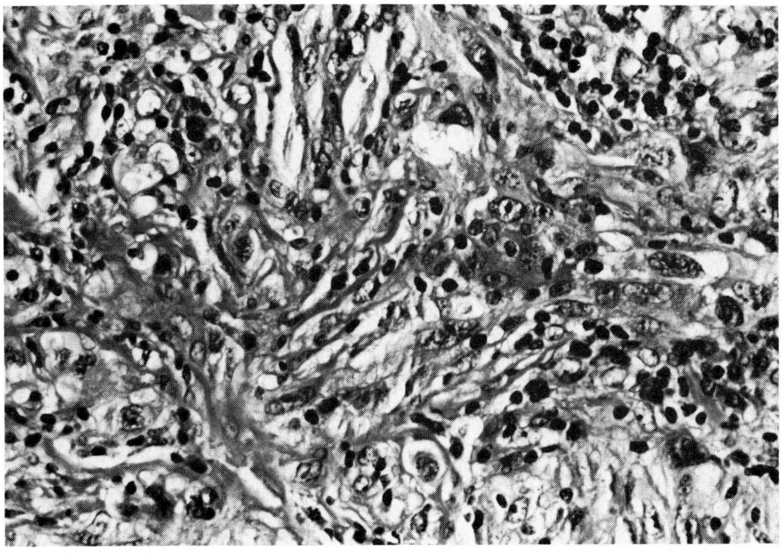

FIGURE 4–150. Malignant fibrous histiocytoma: High-power detail of atypical histiocytoid giant cells.

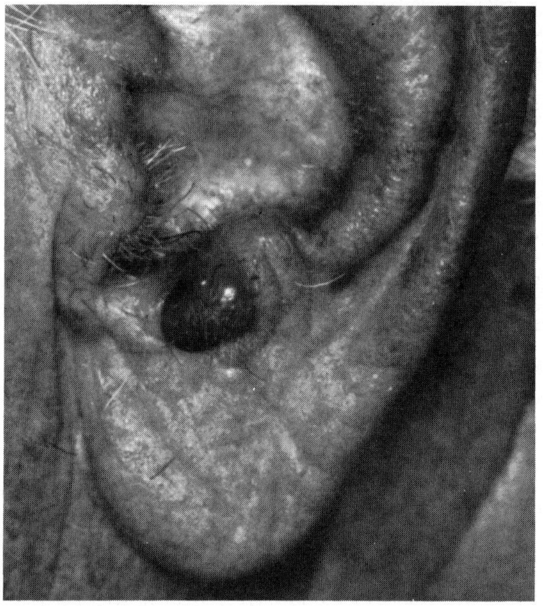

FIGURE 4–151. Atypical fibroxanthoma: Note smooth-surfaced dermal nodule on the ear.

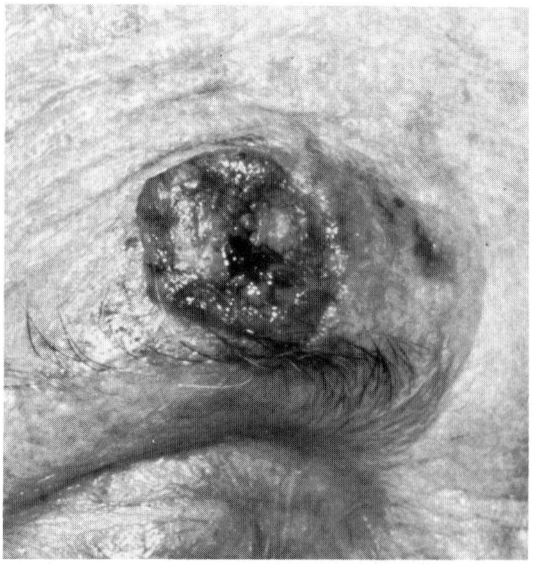

FIGURE 4–152. Atypical fibroxanthoma: Eroded plaque represents another clinical presentation of atypical fibroxanthoma.

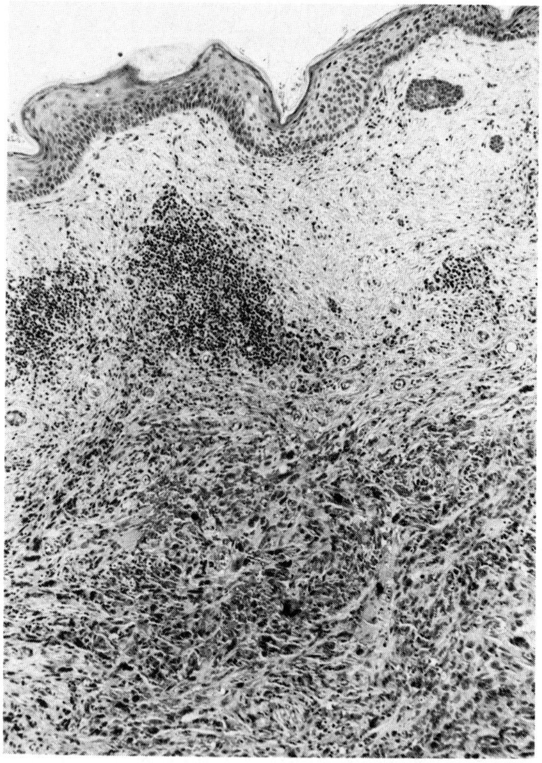

FIGURE 4–153. Atypical fibroxanthoma: Note dense dermal infiltrate of cells with pleomorphic, hyperchromatic nuclei.

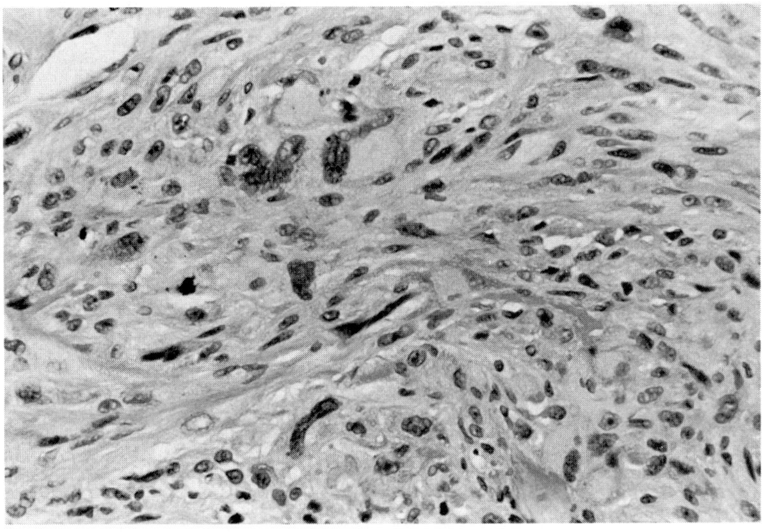

FIGURE 4–154. Atypical fibroxanthoma: Bizarre multinucleated cells and histiocytoid cells with foamy cytoplasm are often present.

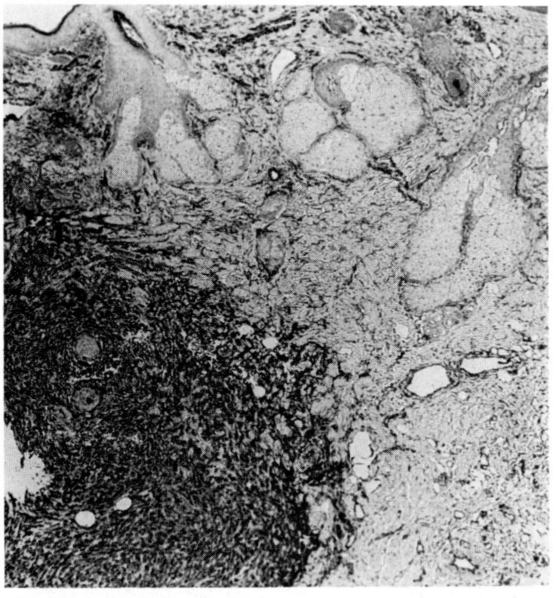

FIGURE 4–155. Atypical fibroxanthoma: Positive staining of tumor cells with vimentin aids in differentiation of atypical fibroxanthoma from malignant melanoma and spindle cell squamous carcinoma.

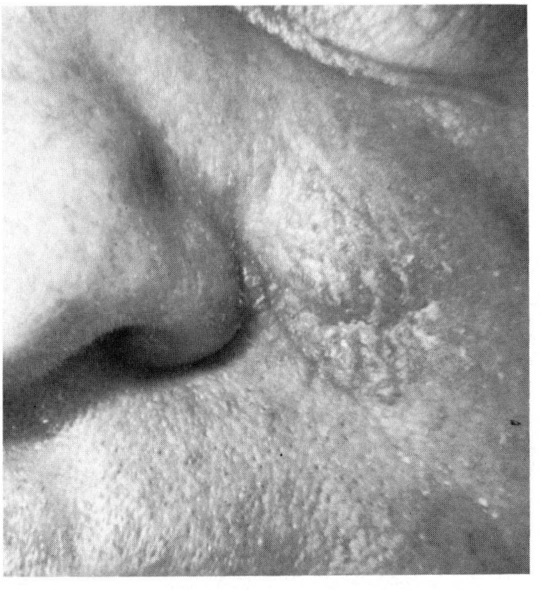

FIGURE 4–156. Angiosarcoma: Ill-defined, slightly raised, irregularly surfaced plaque belies vascular nature of lesion on cheek.

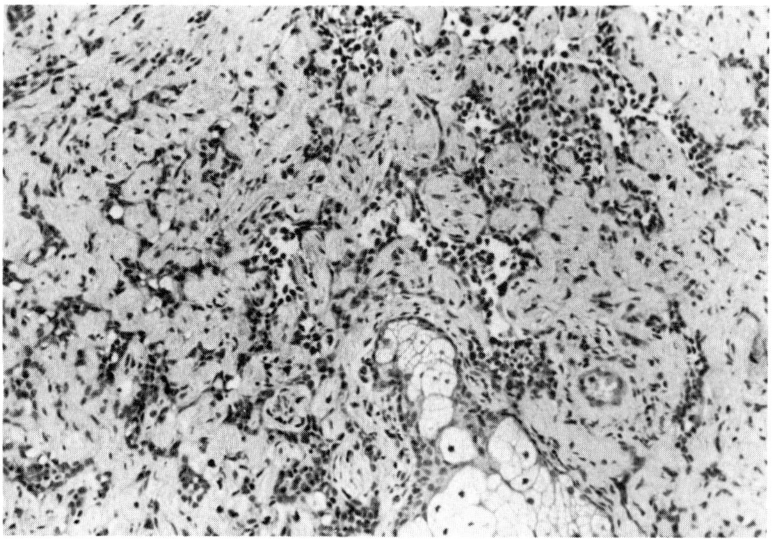

FIGURE 4–157. Angiosarcoma: Relatively well-differentiated tumor shows numerous and anastomosing vascular spaces lined by endothelial cells with mild degree of atypia.

ugal infiltration, and eventually nodules, ulcerations, and severe facial edema develop. Lesions associated with chronic lymphedema often begin as purplish or blue nodules that undergo rapid increase in size and eventually ulcerate. They occur most commonly on the ipsilateral upper extremity of women following mastectomy. Death may occur from extensive local destruction or distant metastases.

The histology of both types of angiosarcoma is similar. The well-differentiated lesions feature multiple, irregular, often anastomosing vascular channels lined by endothelial cells with varying degrees of atypia (Fig. 4–157). In less well-differentiated lesions, the vascular spaces are lined with frankly atypical, cuboidal endothelial cells that protrude into the lumen (Fig. 4–158). In poorly differentiated lesions, solid cords of anaplastic endothelial cells displace the dermal connective tissue, and a syncytium of cells forms in some areas. Positive immunohistochemical staining with Factor VIII–related antigen or *Ulex europaeus* antigen aids in confirming the vascular nature of the tumor.

Rhabdomyosarcoma

Although rare in adults, rhabdomyosarcomas are one of the most common soft tissue sarcomas in children. Most tumors are extramus-

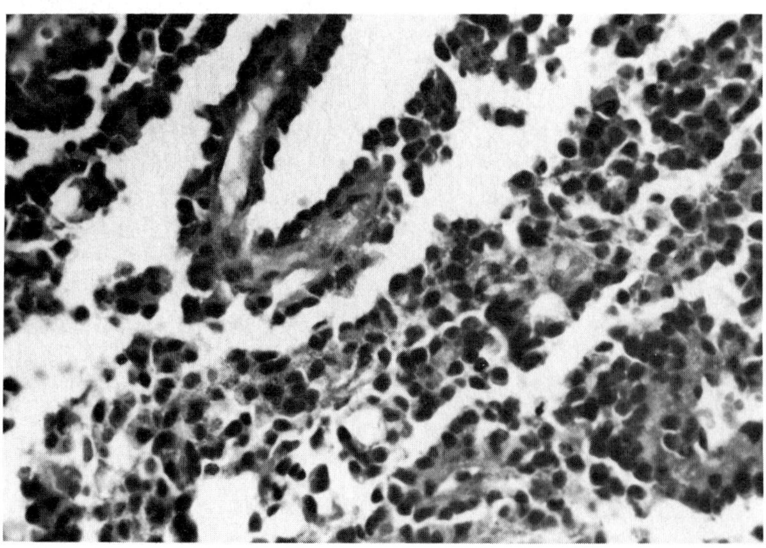

FIGURE 4–158. Angiosarcoma: Less well-differentiated lesion shows vascular channels lined by frankly atypical, cuboidal endothelial cells.

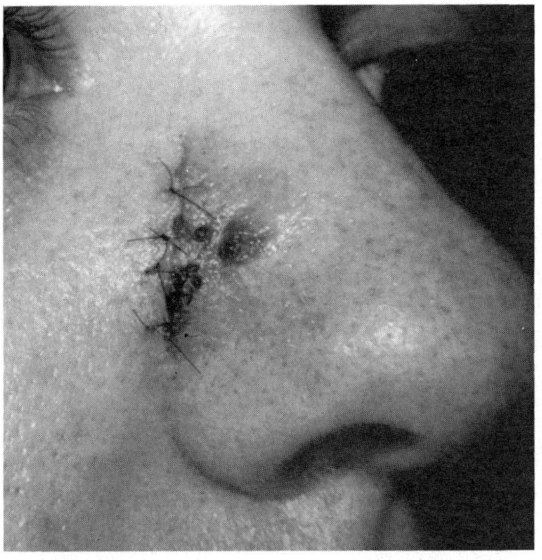

FIGURE 4–159. Rhabdomyosarcoma: Ill-defined subcutaneous plaque on side of nose in a young person.

cular in location, and primary involvement of the skin is rare. When found in the skin, they present as dermal nodules or ill-defined subcutaneous plaques (Fig. 4–159).

Histologically, rhabdomyosarcomas often show only proliferation of undifferentiated spindle-shaped, sarcoma-like cells, although some tumors possess cells with cross-striations recognizable as rhabdomyoblasts. Cells with elongated eosinophilic cytoplasm, so-called strap cells are suggestive but not diagnostic of rhabdomyosarcoma (Fig. 4–160). Application of immunohistochemical stains including desmin, myoglobin, and vimentin to tissue sections is often valuable in the identification of lesions suspected of being rhabdomyosarcomas (Fig. 4–161).

MALIGNANT NEOPLASMS OF UNCERTAIN ORIGIN AND METASTATIC CARCINOMA

In this chapter, we briefly consider two other types of lesions that the Mohs micrographic surgeon may be called upon to treat. These are the Merkel cell carcinoma, a malignant neoplasm of uncertain origin, and examples of carcinoma metastatic to the skin.

Merkel Cell Carcinoma

Merkel cell carcinoma, also referred to as neuroendocrine or trabecular carcinoma, is a not uncommon skin tumor. It most often occurs as a solitary nodule, usually located on the head and extremities. The tumors present as firm red or pink, usually nonulcerated nodules varying in size from 0.8 to 4.0 cm in diameter. Ulceration, though uncommon, may occur (Fig. 4–162). Approximately 50% of patients have regional lymph node involvement at the time of diagnosis, and death from metastatic dissemination occurs in over 25% of the cases.[58] Merkel cell carcinoma was originally felt to be a sweat gland neoplasm,[59] but recent studies have indicated a neuroendocrine derivation of the tumor cells, since they possess histochemi-

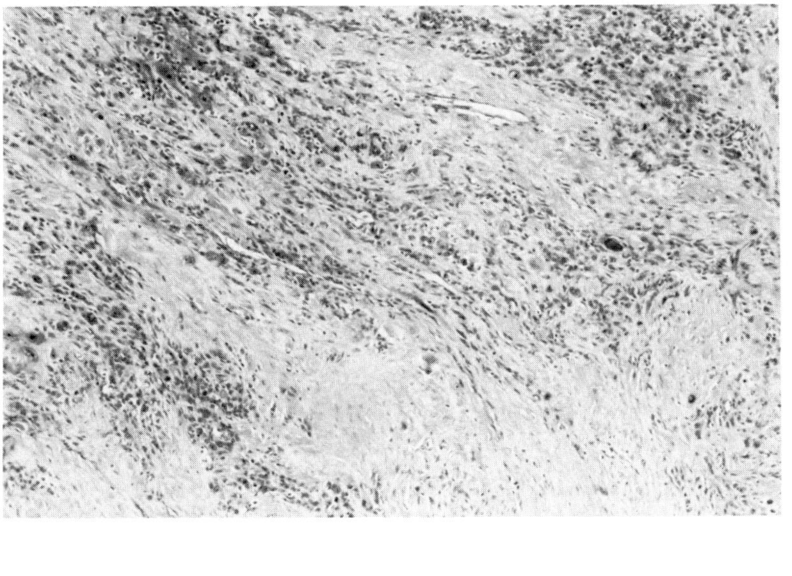

FIGURE 4–160. Rhabdomyosarcoma: Note proliferation of spindle-shaped and elongated cells with pleomorphic nuclei.

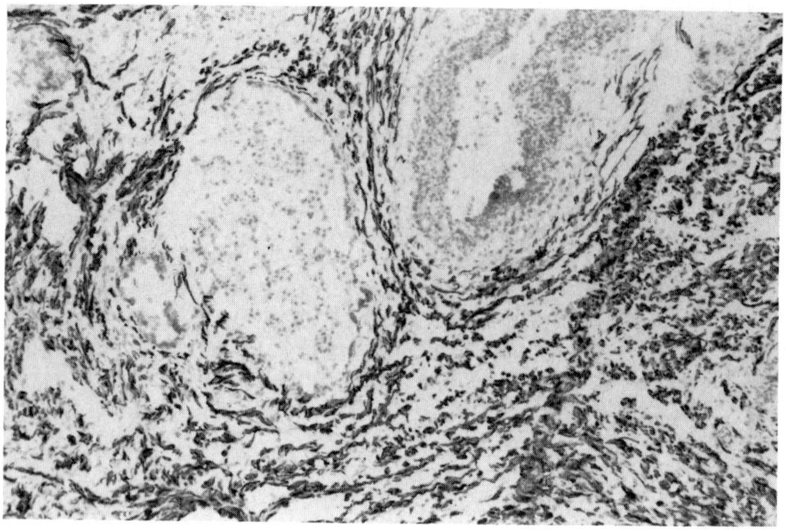

FIGURE 4–161. Rhabdomyosarcoma: Tumor cells stain positive with desmin, confirming their muscular origin.

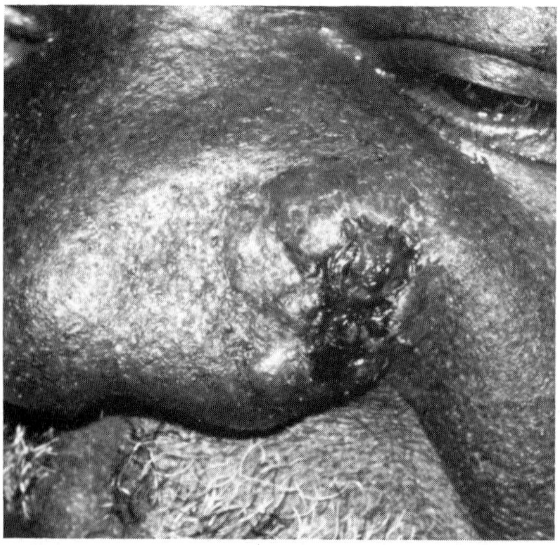

FIGURE 4–162. Merkel cell carcinoma: Note large ulcerated nodule on side of nose.

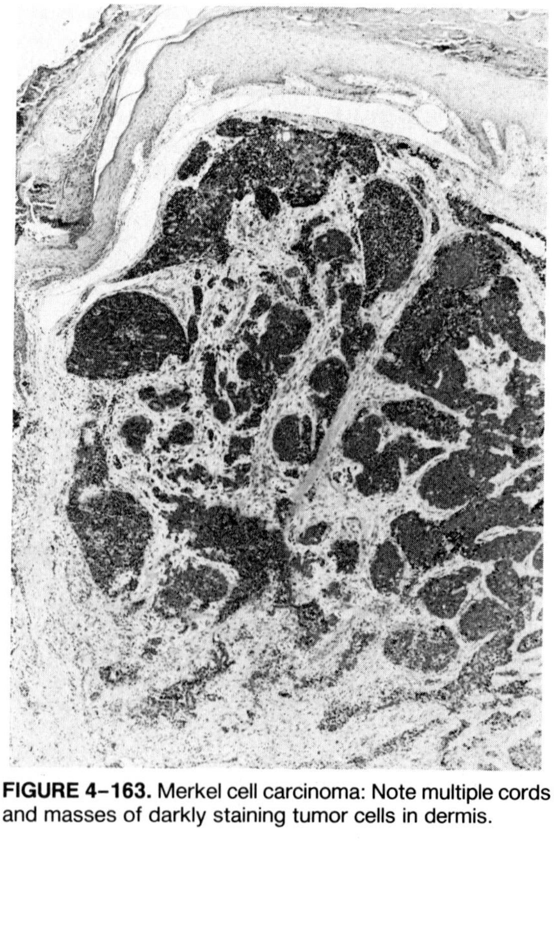

FIGURE 4–163. Merkel cell carcinoma: Note multiple cords and masses of darkly staining tumor cells in dermis.

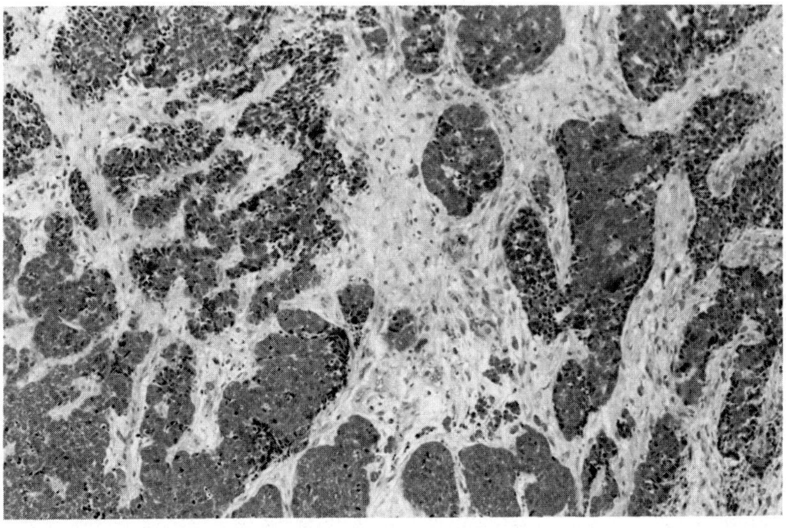

FIGURE 4–164. Merkel cell carcinoma: Characteristic features of tumor cells include closely spaced, round, vesicular nuclei and numerous mitoses.

cal and ultrastructural features similar to cells of the *a*mine *p*recursor *u*ptake and *d*ecarboxylation (APUD) system.[60]

The histologic picture of Merkel cell carcinoma is quite distinct and consists of multiple, varying-sized cords and masses of darkly staining tumor cells in the dermis which extend into the subcutis (Fig. 4–163). The cells have a uniform appearance and contain closely spaced, round vesicular nuclei and scanty, ill-defined cytoplasm. Numerous mitoses are usually present (Fig. 4–164). Differentiation of Merkel cell carcinoma from a small cell malignant lymphoma or metastatic oat carcinoma of the lung may be difficult. However, use of electron microscopy and immunohistochemical stains, including chromograffin, synaptophysin, neuron-specific enolase, and antibodies directed against neurofilaments and neuroproteins, may be particularly rewarding in confirming a diagnosis of Merkel cell carcinoma.

Carcinoma Metastatic to the Skin

Cutaneous metastasis from visceral carcinoma is uncommon and usually occurs late in the course of the primary carcinoma. It results by either direct extension or hematogenous or lymphatic spread. The most common cutaneous metastatic neoplasm in woman originates from carcinoma of the breast and in men from colonic carcinoma. We will consider an example of each.

The four types of cutaneous metastases occurring from lymphatic dissemination of carcinoma of the breast include inflammatory carcinoma, telangiectatic carcinoma, nodular carcinoma and carcinoma en cuirasse. All of these varieties involve either the skin overlying or adjacent to the affected breast and present as indurated erythema, purpuric plaques, multiple nodules, and indurated plaques, respectively. In hematogenous dissemination of breast carcinoma, usually a single distant metastasis is found, most often in the scalp, where it results in an area of hair loss referred to as alopecia neoplastica (Fig. 4–165). The actual extent of the lesion may be difficult to determine clinically.

The histologic picture of hematogenous metastatic breast carcinoma shows an infiltration of the dermis with large and small groups of tumor cells, some of which may show a glandular arrangement (Fig. 4–166). Single files of tumor cells are also seen extending between thickened collagen bundles (Fig. 44–167). The associated dermal fibrosis usually seen in scalp lesions leads to atrophy of the hair follicles and alopecia.

Cutaneous metastases from carcinoma of the colon are caused by hematogenous spread and most often present as solitary nodules or plaques. Lesions of metastatic colonic carcinoma may appear on the scalp, abdominal wall, or umbilicus (Sister Mary Joseph's nodule), but may involve other, less common sites (Fig. 4–168).

Histologically, metastatic colonic carcinoma shows within the dermis varying-sized masses of epithelial cells, some of which show gland-like formations (Fig. 4–169). Many of the cells

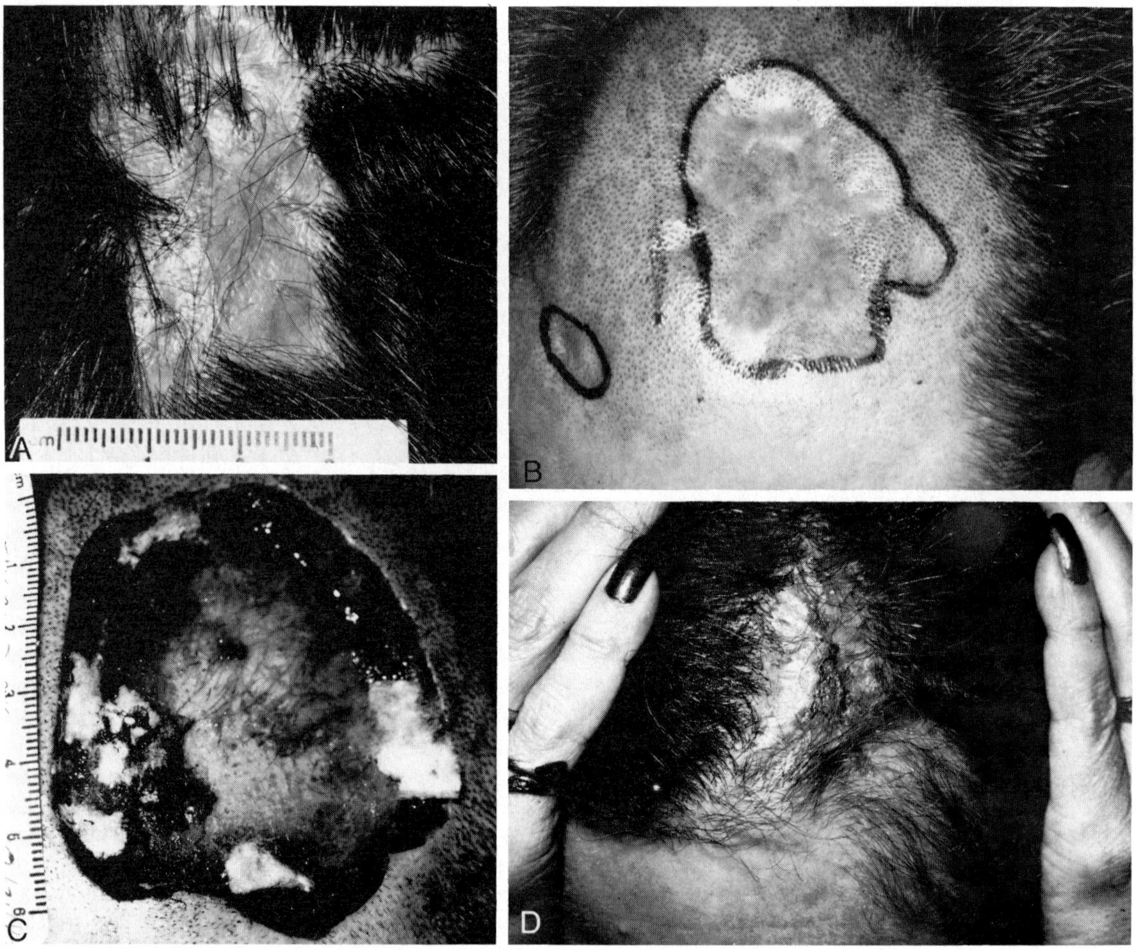

FIGURE 4–165. Metastatic carcinoma of breast: *A,* Irregularly shaped plaque with uneven surface and associated alopecia of scalp. *B,* Extent of primary lesion and smaller secondary lesion after shaving of scalp. *C,* Final wound after Mohs excision of lesion. *D,* Small scar after healing by second intention.

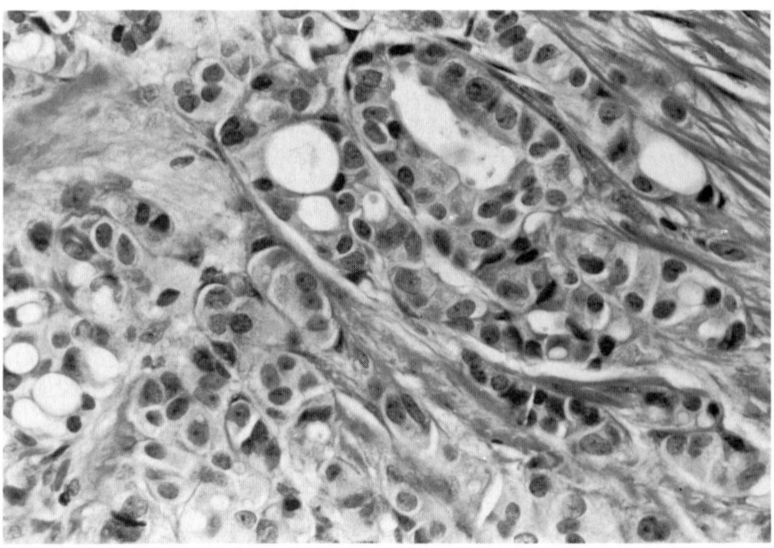

FIGURE 4–166. Metastatic carcinoma of breast: Note varying-sized groups of tumor cells, some of which show glandular formation.

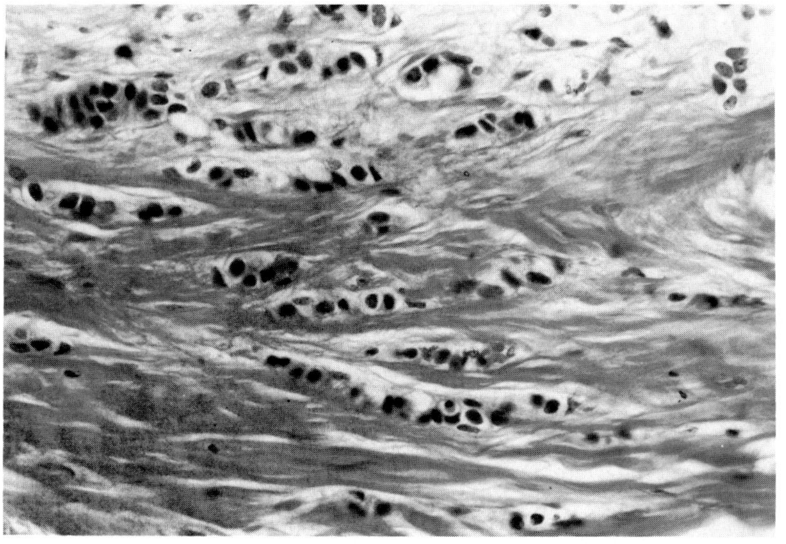

FIGURE 4–167. Metastatic carcinoma of breast: Single rows of tumor cells are present between thickened collagen bundles.

FIGURE 4–168. Metastatic colonic carcinoma: Unusual location for plaque of metastatic colonic carcinoma on the penis.

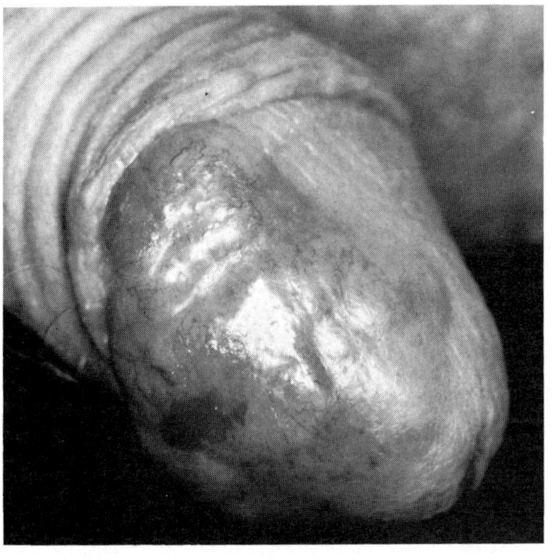

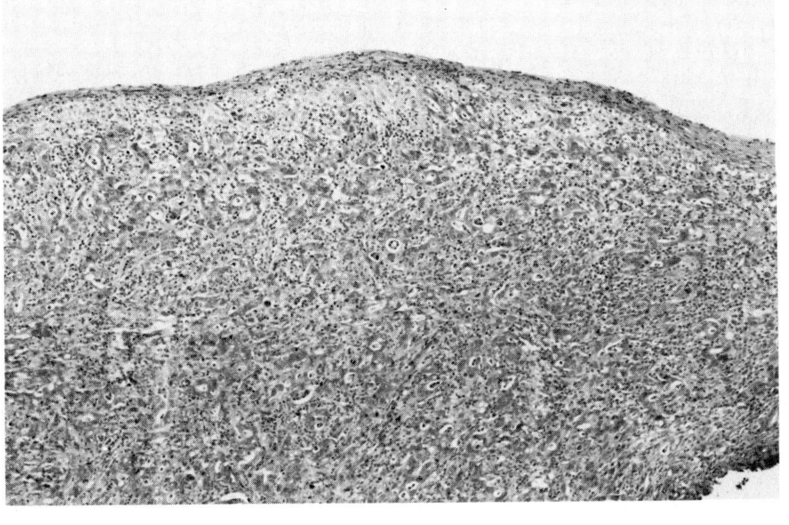

FIGURE 4–169. Metastatic colonic carcinoma: Numerous nests of tumor cells, some of which form gland-like structures fill the dermis.

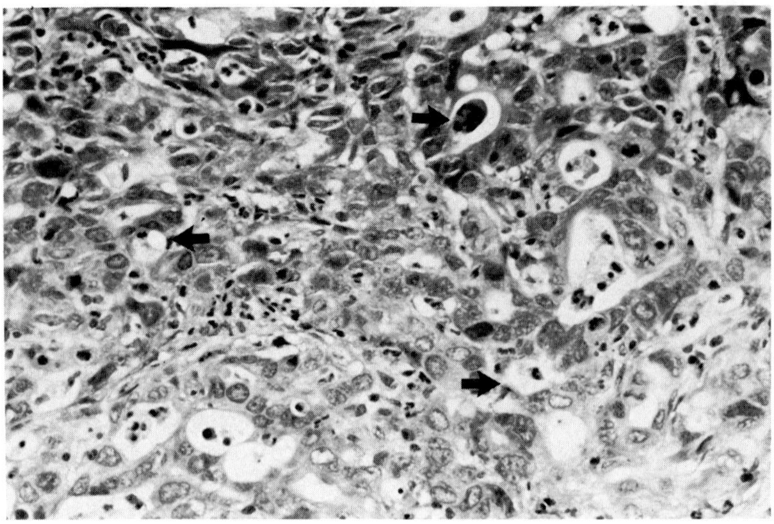

FIGURE 4–170. Metastatic colonic carcinoma: Note abortive glandular lumen formation and presence of signet-ring cells *(arrows).*

contain mucin, and some show a tendency to form signet ring cells characteristic of gastrointestinal adenocarcinoma (Fig. 4–170). The mucin in metastatic colonic carcinoma contains both neutral and acid mucopolysaccharides and therefore stains with both digested periodic acid–Schiff and alcian blue stains. Immunohistochemical staining for carcinoembryonic antigen is also helpful in confirming the gastrointestinal origin of the tumor cells.

REFERENCES

1. Pinboard JJ: Pathology of oral leukoplakia. Am J Dermatopathol 2:277–278, 1980.
2. Shklar G: Modern study and concepts of leukoplakia in the mouth. J Dermatol Surg Oncol 7:996–1,003, 1981.
3. Bonnekok B, Mahrle G, Steigleder GK: Übergang in kutanes Plattenepithelkarzinom bei zwei Patienten mit Bowenoider Papulose (HPV-16). Z Hautkr 62:773–785, 1987.
4. Gross G, Hagedorn M, Ikenberg H, et al.: Bowenoid papulosis: Presence of human papilloma virus structural antigen and HPV-16 related DNA sequences. Arch Dermatol 121:858–863, 1985.
5. Pinkus H: Premalignant fibroepithelial tumor of the skin. Arch Dermatol 67:598–615, 1953.
6. Weedon D, Wall D: Metastatic basal cell carcinoma. Med J Aust 2:177–179, 1975.
7. Costran RS: Metastasizing basal cell carcinoma. Cancer 14:1036–1040, 1961.
8. Broders AC: Squamous cell epithelioma of the skin. Ann Surg 73:141–160, 1921.
9. Borel DM: Cutaneous basosquamous carcinoma. Review of the literature and report of 53 cases. Arch Pathol 95:293–297, 1973.
10. Smith OD, Swerdlow MA: Histogenesis of basal cell carcinoma. Arch Dermatol 74:286–292, 1956.
11. Pinkus H: Epithelial and fibroepithelial tumors. Arch Dermatol 91:24–37, 1965.
12. Okagaki T, Clark BA, Zachov K, et al.: Presence of human papilloma virus in verrucous carcinoma of the vulva. Arch Pathol 108:567–570, 1984.
13. Lever WF, Schaumburg-Lever G: Histopathology of the Skin, 6th ed., Philadelphia: J. B. Lippincott, 1983, pp. 506–509.
14. Baer RL, Kopf AW: Year Book of Dermatology. Chicago: Year-Book Medical Publishers, 1963, pp. 7–41.
15. Rook A, Whimster I: Le Kérato-Acanthome. Arch Belges Dermatol Syphiligraph 6:137–146, 1950.
16. Rook A, Whimster I: Keratoacanthoma a thirty-year retrospect. Brit J Dermatol 100:41–47, 1979.
17. Rook A: Discussion. Proc R Soc Med 43:839, 1950.
18. Smith JF: Discussion. Proc R Soc Med 43:839, 1950.
19. Belisario JC: Brief review of keratoacanthoma and description of keratoacanthoma centrifugum marginatum. Aust J Dermatol 8:65–72, 1965.
20. Belisario JC: Cancer of the Skin. London: Butterworth, 1959, pp. 80–96.
21. Smith JF: Discussion. Proc Roy Soc Med 49:428, 1956.
22. Zimmerman M: Discussion. Arch Dermatol 74:325, 1956.
23. Beerman H: Some aspects of cutaneous malignancies. Am J Med Sci 233:456, 1957.
24. Mikhail GR: Squamous cell carcinoma diagnosed as keratoacanthoma. Cutis 13:378–382, 1984.
25. Pinkus H, Mehregan AH: Keratoacanthoma. A Guide to Dermatohistopathology, 3rd ed. New York: Appelton-Century-Crofts, 1981, pp. 413–414.
26. Everson TC, Cole WH: Spontaneous Regression of Cancer. Philadelphia: W. B. Saunders, 1966, pp. 1–10, 164–220.
27. Spitler LE: Malignant melanoma. J Invest Dermatol 67:437–441, 1976.
28. Smith JL, Stehlin JS, Jr: Spontaneous regression of primary malignant melanomas with regional metastases. Cancer 18:1399–1415, 1965.
29. Mikhail GR: Spontaneous regression of metastatic melanoma. J Dermatol Surg Oncol 12:497–500, 1986.
30. Parker CM, Hanke CW: Large keratoacanthomas in

difficult locations treated with 5-fluorouracil. J Am Acad Dermatol 14:770–777, 1986.
31. Kwitken J: A histologic chronology of the clinical course of the keratocarcinoma (so-called keratoacanthoma). The Mount Sinai Journal of Medicine 52:127–135, 1975.
32. Lever WF, Schaumburg-Lever G: Histopathology of the Skin, 6th ed, Philadelphia: J. B. Lippincott, 1983, p. 508.
33. Smith JF: A case of multiple primary squamous-cell carcinomata of the skin in a young man, with spontaneous healing. Brit J Dermatol 46:267–274.
34. Smith JF: Multiple primary, self-healing squamous epithelioma of the skin. Brit J Dermatol 60:315–318, 1945.
35. Grzybowski M: A case of peculiar generalized epithelial tumors of the skin. Brit J Dermatol 62:310–313, 1950.
36. Washington CV, Mikhail GR: Eruptive keratoacanthoma en plaque in an immunosuppressed patient. J Dermatol Surg Oncol 13:1,357–1,360, 1987.
37. Headington JT: Tumors of the hair follicle: A review. Am J Pathol 85:480–513, 1976.
38. Pinkus H, Mehregan AH: A Guide to Dermatohistopathology, 3rd ed. New York: Appleton-Century-Crofts, 1981, pp. 471–475.
39. James RE, Jr, Austin C, Ackerman AB: Extramammary Paget's disease. Am J Dermatopathol 1:101–132, 1979.
40. Gunn RA, Galagher HS: Vulvar Paget's disease. Cancer 46:590–594, 1980.
41. Caputo R, Califono A: Ultrastructural features of extramammary Paget's disease. Arch Clin Exp Dermatol 236:121–132, 1970.
42. Meiot Y, Mazoujian G, Pinkus G, et al.: Extramammary Paget's disease of perianal and perineal regions. Evidence of apocrine derivation. Arch Dermatol 121:750–752, 1985.
43. Karinemi AL, Forsman L, Wahlstrom T, et al.: Expression of differentiation antigens in mammary and extramammary Paget's disease. Br J Dermatol 110:203–210, 1984.
44. Glasgow BJ, Wen DR, Al-Jitawi S, et al.: Antibody to S-100 protein aids in the separation of pagetoid melanoma from mammary and extramammary Paget's disease. J Cutan Pathol 14:223–226, 1987.
45. Krinz K: Malignes intraepidermales ekkrines Porom. Z Hautkr 47:9–17, 1972.
46. Swanson PE, Cherwitz DL, Neuman P, et al.: Eccrine sweat gland carcinoma. J Cutan Pathol 14:65–86, 1987.
47. Mendoza S, Helwig EB: Mucinous (adenocystic) carcinoma of the skin. Arch Dermatol 103:68–78, 1971.
48. Mehregan AH, Hashimoto K, Rahbari H: Eccrine adenocarcinoma. Arch Dermatol 119:104–114, 1983.
49. Goldstein DJ, Barr RJ, Santa Cruz DJ: Microcystic adnexal carcinoma: A distinct clinicopathological entity. Cancer 50:566–572, 1982.
50. Nicholoff BJ, Fleischman HE, Carmel J: Microcystic adnexal carcinoma. Arch Dermatol 122:290–294, 1986.
51. Clark WH, From L, Bernardino EH, et al.: Histogenesis and biologic behavior of primary human malignant melanoma of the skin. Cancer Res 29:705–727, 1969.
52. Lopransri S, Mihm MC: Clinical and pathologic correlation of malignant melanoma. J Cutan Pathol 6:180–194, 1979.
53. Breslow A: Thickness, cross sectional area and depth of invasion in the prognosis of cutaneous melanoma. Ann Surg 172:902–908, 1970.
54. Bagley FH, Cady B, Lee A, et al.: Changes in clinical presentation and management of malignant melanoma. Cancer 47:2126–2134, 1981.
55. Weiss SW, Enzinger FM: Malignant fibrous histiocytoma. Cancer 41:2250–2266, 1978.
56. Helwig EB: Atypical fibroxanthoma. Tex State J Med 59:644–667, 1963.
57. Enzinger FM: Atypical fibroxanthoma and malignant fibrous histiocytoma. Am J Dermatopathol 1:185, 1979.
58. Tang CK, Toker C: Trabecular carcinoma of the skin. Cancer 42:2311–2321, 1978.
59. Toker C: Trabecular carcinoma of the skin. Arch Dermatol 105:107–110, 1972.
60. Raaf JH, Urmacher C, Knapper WK, et al.: Trabecular (Merkel cell) carcinoma of the skin. Cancer 57:178–182, 1986.

CHAPTER 5

Anatomy of the Head and Neck

Hubert T. Greenway, M.D.
Eric A. Breisch, Ph.D.

Surgical removal of cutaneous and deep neoplasms utilizing Mohs micrographic surgery requires an intimate knowledge of the underlying anatomy. The most critical area and, indeed, the area where the vast majority of Mohs surgical procedures are performed involves the head and neck. The scalp, eyelid, and periorbital area, the nasal area, the ear, the cheek, the lip and perioral area, and the neck each possess specialized structures in addition to the underlying important vasculature, muscles, and nerves. Because one of the goals of Mohs surgery is the preservation of the maximum amounts of normal tissue, knowledge of the anatomy is extremely clinically relevant.

THE SCALP

The scalp consists of the overlying soft tissues as well as the underlying calvarium. The soft tissues composing the scalp are easily remembered via the following mnemonic:

*S*kin
*C*onnective tissue (subcutaneous)
*A*poneurosis (galea aponeurotica)
*L*oose areolar connective tissue
*P*ericranium

The skin of the scalp extends from the supraorbital ridges of the frontal bone to the superior nuchal lines of the occipital bone. Its lateral extent is considered to include the skin and tissues overlying the temporalis muscle. The forehead consists of that region of the scalp extending from the skin overlying the supraorbital ridges of the frontal bones to the highest wrinkle exhibited on the skin covering that frontal bone. Regional descriptions of the scalp are based upon the underlying bones of the cranium, consisting of the frontal, the occipital, and the paired parietal and temporal bones. These bones are divided by the coronal, sagittal, lambdoid, and squamosal sutures. The bones of the calvarium consist of an outer and inner layer of cortical bone separated by a spongy diploë layer. At times, portions of the outer layer may be removed for tissue examination to evaluate the possibility of tumor invasion. Additionally, the Mohs surgeon has traditionally utilized various techniques to provide defects in the outer layer entering the spongy cancellous diploë in order to stimulate the formation of granulation tissue to provide coverage of bony areas where the overlying pericranium had to be removed. The parietal bone consistently provides the greatest thickness. There exists an inherent risk in penetrating the inner table when removing or penetrating the outer table of the calvarium. The blood supply of the bones of the scalp is contributed by both intracranial and extracranial sources.

Pertinent surface anatomy can be easily generated from the bony foundation of the scalp. Localization of cutaneous lesions can be augmented by referring to the underlying calvarial bone. Anteriorly, the supraorbital arches of the frontal bone, elevated ridges just deep to the eyebrows, are readily palpable. The large flattened area of the forehead is formed by the squamous portion of the frontal bone. The crown, or vertex, is a midline point that marks the most superior point of the skull. Posteriorly, the external occipital protuberance, or inion, is palpable at midline. The ridges extending laterally from the inion are the superior nuchal lines.

The connective tissue layer (subcutaneous) contains the vast majority of the vasculature and nerve supply of the scalp. This layer is laced with strong fibrous retinacula that hold the vessels open when the scalp is cut, causing profuse bleeding. The aponeurosis (galea aponeurotica) is a dense fibrous sheet of connective tissue, connecting the anterior and posterior bellies of the occipitofrontalis muscle. Below the galea is the relatively loose areolar connective tissue layer; the loose nature of this layer accounts for the relative mobility of the overlying skin, connective tissue, and aponeurosis. The use of undermining within the loose areolar connective tissue layer allows movement of significant portions of scalp tissue for the reconstruction of large scalp defects. This loose layer is also known as the danger area of the scalp because it provides a site for significant accumulations of blood and other fluids. The possibility of an unintended infection in this area spreading intracranially exists via emissary veins.

The occipitofrontalis muscle is the primary muscle of the scalp consisting of a frontal and occipital belly connected by the galea aponeurotica. The frontal belly originates from the anterior aspect of the galea and inserts into the skin and subcutaneous tissue of the forehead (Fig. 5–1). The occipital belly originates from the posterior aspect of the galea aponeurotica to insert into the supreme nuchal line and mastoid portion of the temporal bone. This region is complicated by the existence of emissary veins of the underlying cortical bone, and bleeding may be more of a problem in this area. The occipitofrontalis muscle pulls the

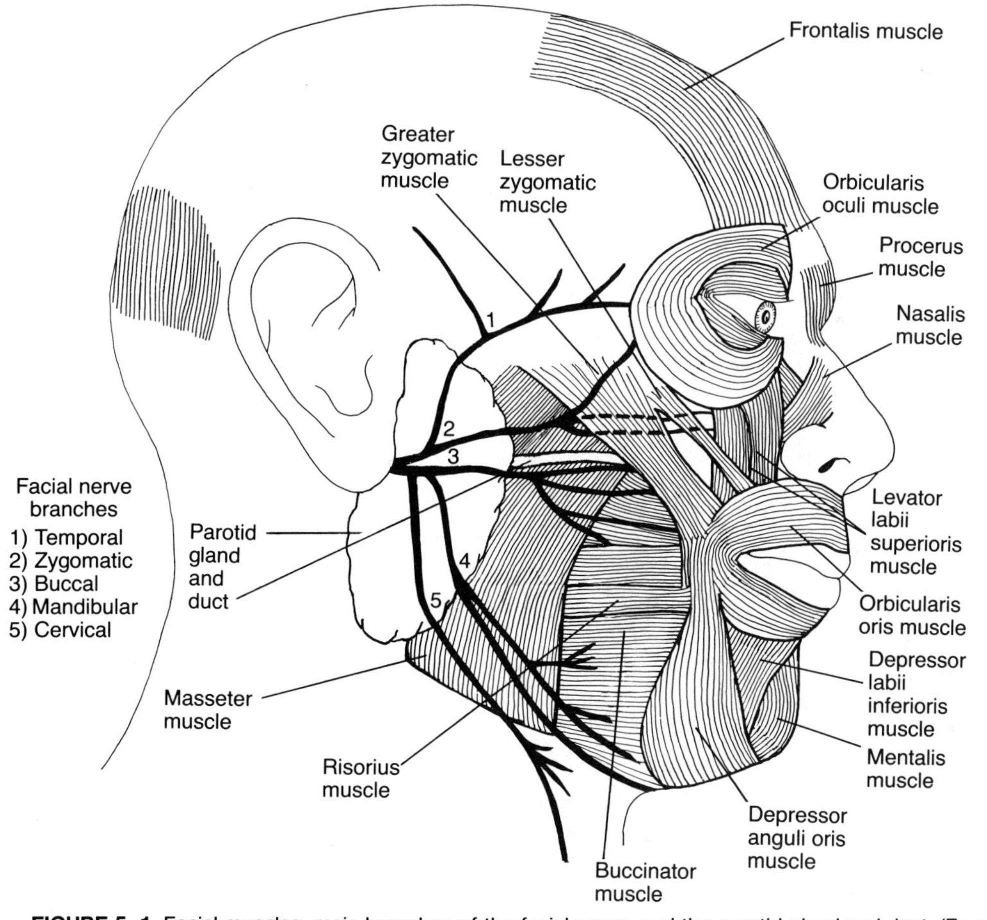

FIGURE 5–1. Facial muscles, main branches of the facial nerve, and the parotid gland and duct. (From Adams J P, Feffer H L, Vailas J C, Wiesel S W: Neck Pain. Charlottesville, Va, The Michie Co, 1988, p. 85.)

skin of the forehead superiorly, elevating the eyebrows and creating horizontal wrinkle lines. Innervation of the frontalis muscle is by the temporal branch of the facial nerve; the occipitalis muscle is innervated by the posterior auricular branch of the facial nerve.

The scalp is an extremely vascular area with the external carotid and internal carotid artery each providing vessels to the scalp with extensive anastomoses. The external carotid artery provides the occipital and postauricular artery before terminating as the superficial temporal artery supplying the scalp (Fig. 5–2). The internal carotid artery, via the ophthalmic artery, provides supraorbital, supratrochlear, and lacrimal branches that supply the anterior portion of the scalp and forehead.

Vascular drainage of the scalp parallels the arterial supply with extensive anastomotic networks connecting different regions. The occipital and parietal regions of the scalp are drained by the occipital vein, which communicates with the superficial temporal veins, the posterior auricular veins, the suboccipital venous plexus, and the vertebral venous plexus. The postauricular veins drain the scalp behind the ear and join the posterior division of the retromandibular vein to form the external jugular vein. The superficial temporal vein drains temporal, parietal, and frontal regions of the scalp, passing just in front of the ear to enter the parotid gland, and there, the superficial temporal vein is joined by the maxillary vein to form the retromandibular vein. Drainage of the frontal (forehead) region of the scalp is via the supratrochlear and supraorbital veins, which anas-

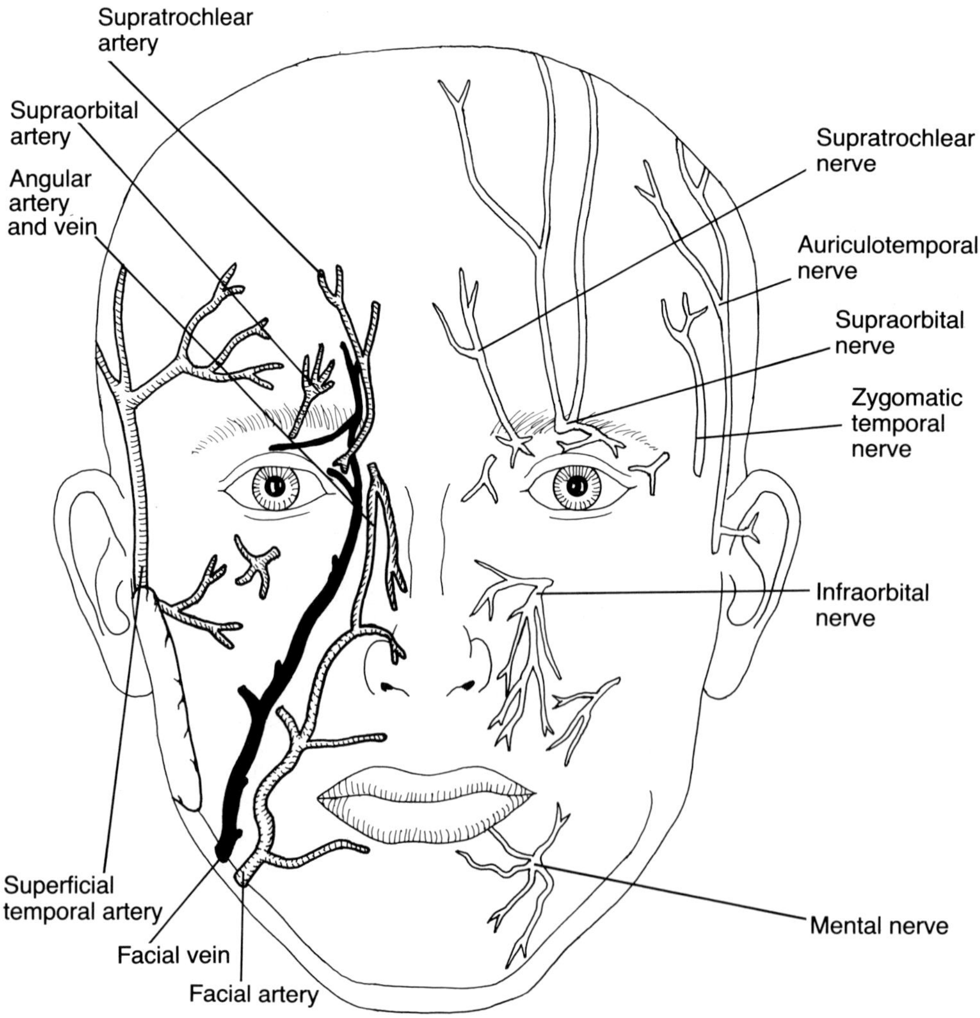

FIGURE 5–2. Vascular and sensory supply to the face.

tomose with the superficial temporal venous system. These supraorbital and supratrochlear veins drain into the ophthalmic venous system with additional connections into the angular vein (facial venous system). There are also extensive venous connections extending between the superficial venous network and emissary veins. Emissary veins pass through the skull to empty directly into dural venous sinuses, thereby allowing venous communication between extracranial and intracranial systems. This network provides a route for the spread of both tumor and infectious processes from the scalp into the intracranial area. The veins of the head and neck are devoid of valves, so blood flow is determined by pressure gradients. In the superficial regions of the head and neck, the normal direction of blood flow is into the superficial venous network.

The lymphatic drainage of the scalp is into regionally located lymph nodes. The occipital nodes, located over the origin of the trapezius muscle, receive lymphatic drainage from the occipital and parietal regions of the scalp; drainage from the occipital nodes is into the superficial and deep cervical nodes. The retroauricular nodes, positioned over the mastoid prominence, drain the occipital, parietal, and temporal regions of the scalp as well as the ear. These retroauricular nodes drain into the superficial and deep cervical nodes. Located in front of the ear and superficial to the parotid gland are the preauricular nodes, which drain the parietal, temporal, and forehead regions of the scalp as well as the ear, eyelids, and cheek. These preauricular nodes drain into the superficial and deep cervical nodes.

The innervation of the scalp consists of a motor and sensory portion. The motor innervation to muscles of the scalp is derived from the postauricular and temporal branches of the facial nerve (see Fig. 5–1). The postauricular branch is the first branch yielded from the facial nerve after its exit from the stylomastoid foramen at the base of the skull. This postauricular branch passes over the mastoid prominence to reach the occipital belly of the occipitofrontalis muscle. In humans, innervation of this muscle is of limited benefit. After the facial nerve enters the parotid gland and divides into its five main branches, the most superior, or temporal, branch leaves the superior pole of the parotid gland, passing above the zygomatic arch to innervate the frontalis muscle (frontal belly of the occipitofrontalis muscle). This temporal branch of the facial nerve is extremely superficial as it passes the zygomatic arch and must be considered during surgical procedures in this area. This branch of the facial nerve runs perpendicular to relaxed skin tension lines in this area, so at times, incisions or excisions may be performed lying parallel to the direction of the nerve, providing a scar line perpendicular to the skin tension lines. In addition, recurrent tumors and occasionally primary tumors may involve this branch, necessitating removal of portions of the nerve. If possible, this should be explained to the patient preoperatively so that he or she may be aware of the possible deficit. If the nerve is sectioned or removed, the normal innervation of the frontalis muscle will not occur, and the patient will have the inability to elevate the eyebrow on that side. This results in the lack of horizontal forehead lines, a sagging eyebrow, and a possible visual field defect.

Correction may involve a coronal lift, a brow lift, a blepharoplasty, or a combination of these. While injury to the nerve may occur and be required in order to eliminate an aggressive tumor, reconstruction of defects in this area should be chosen to avoid damage to the temporal branch of the facial nerve. While nerve involvement by tumor growth may create a deficit after surgery, nerve deficit produced by reconstruction should be avoided. The most common cause of a deficit involving the temporal branch of the facial nerve fortunately is local anesthesia, which is self-limited.

The sensory innervation of the scalp is derived from terminal branches of the fifth cranial nerve as well as from the cervical plexus and dorsal rami. The most important and most frequently encountered nerves are the supraorbital and supratrochlear nerves, which are supplied by the ophthalmic division of the fifth cranial nerve (see Fig 5–2). The supraorbital nerve accesses the face through the supraorbital notch, a landmark located approximately 2.5 cm lateral from the midline along the superior margin of the orbit. The supraorbital nerve supplies most of the forehead and scalp as far posteriorly as the vertex. The smaller supratrochlear nerve emerges onto the face just medial to the supraorbital nerve, providing sensory innervation in the medial region of the forehead. Sectioning of these nerves may provide a feeling of numbness posterior to the surgical site and, if it occurs, is noted by the vast majority of patients. The mandibular division of the fifth cranial nerve provides the auriculotemporal nerve. This nerve emerges onto the face just in front of the ear, passes superficial to the zygomatic arch, and supplies the temporal and parietal regions of the scalp. The lesser occipital nerve is supplied by the cervical plexus, and after arising in the neck this nerve parallels the posterior edge of the sternocleidomastoid muscle to supply the skin over the mastoid region and occipital region of the scalp. The greater occipital nerve is the dorsal ramus of the second cervical spinal nerve, penetrating the trapezius muscle to provide sensation to the occipital and parietal regions of the scalp as far anteriorly as the vertex.

The scalp consists of several layers that provide natural barriers for tumor extension. The galea acts as a barrier, since tumors tend to extend peripherally rather than penetrate this thick, fibrous layer. Once penetration has occurred, the underlying bony foundation also acts as a barrier. Tumor spread may also occur via the lymphatic network as opposed to direct invasion through the galea. Because of the scalp's rich lymphatic supply, significant risk for metastatic disease exists in a number of tumors. In its normal state, the underlying cortical bone is kept moist, and this environment should be duplicated by the use of antibiotic ointments where cortical bone has been exposed.

THE EYELID

The eyelids form a protective screen in front of the eyeball or globe. The eyelid skin is extremely thin and continuous with the conjunctiva at the free margins. The underlying layer of dermis is also very thin and is unique in that, because of its looseness, it allows large accumulations of fluid to occur. The palpebral fissure is the space between the open eyelids. The medial commissure of the lid joins the upper and lower lids medially and is separated from the surface of the eyeball by the lacrimal caruncle. The space filled by the lacrimal caruncle is known as the lacrimal lake. Along the free margin of the upper and lower lids, near the medial commissure, are small elevations (lacrimal papillae) surrounding openings known as the lacrimal puncta, which lead into the lacrimal canaliculi. The lacrimal canaliculi continue medially to empty into the lacrimal sac, which is drained by the nasolacrimal duct into the nasal cavity. Surgical procedures around the medial aspect of the eye may involve the lacrimal drainage system. This is especially important over the lower medial eyelid, as procedures in this area can result in disruption of the lacrimal system. Consideration for probing the lacrimal drainage system should be given in order to aid in its identification during surgery (Fig. 5–3).

Palpation of the bony margins of the orbit can provide the Mohs surgeon with several useful landmarks (Fig. 5–4). The superior margin of the orbit is formed by the frontal bone and the supraorbital notch can be palpated approximately 2.5 cm from the midline. The supraorbital nerve exits the orbital cavity at this point. The lateral margin of the orbit is formed

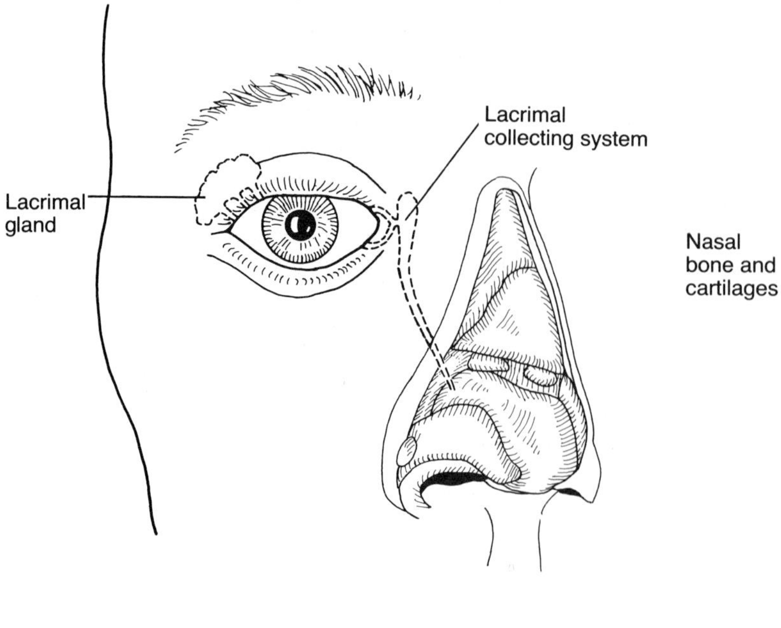

FIGURE 5–3. The lacrimal gland and collecting system; nasal bone and cartilages.

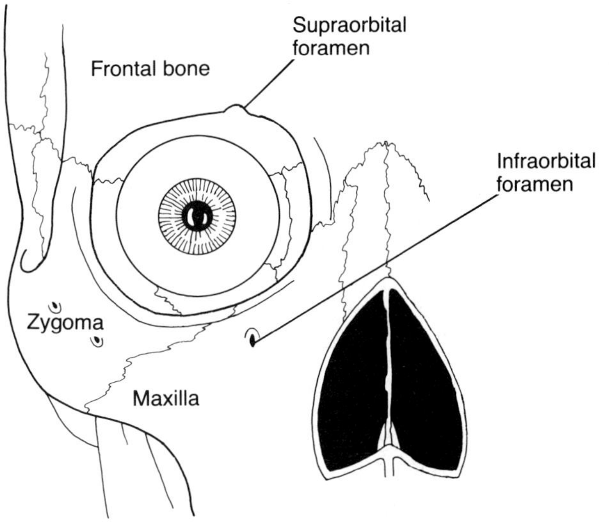

FIGURE 5–4. Bony structure of the periorbital and nasal areas.

by the zygomatic process of the frontal bone and the frontal process of the zygomatic bone. A small bony tubercle, called the tuberculum marginale (Whitenall's tubercle), may be palpated and marks the insertion of the lateral palpebral ligament. The inferior margin of the orbit is formed by the maxillary process of the zygomatic bone and the maxilla. Approximately 5 mm below the inferior margin of the orbit, the infraorbital foramen will be present on a vertical line drawn beginning at the supraorbital foramen. The infraorbital nerve enters the face via the infraorbital foramen and supplies sensory innervation to the lower eyelid. The medial margin of the orbit is formed by the frontal bone and the maxilla, with the maxilla providing a small ridge of bone called the anterior lacrimal crest. The medial palpebral ligament, which can be demonstrated by pulling the eyelid laterally, inserts into this small ridge. Posterior to the medial palpebral ligament is the lacrimal sac.

The tarsal plate provides shape and form for the eyelid and consists of a small semilunar plate of dense connective tissue (Fig. 5–5). Each tarsal plate is anchored medially to the anterior lacrimal crest via the medial palpebral ligament and is also attached to the lateral margin of the orbit via the lateral palpebral ligament. Arising from the bony margins of the orbit is a fibrous sheet of connective tissue called the orbital septum. This septum forms a screen of tissue which seals off the orbital cavity from the superficial aspect of the eyelid and extends from the margins of the orbit to attach to the tarsal plates. The lacrimal gland provides the primary lubrication to the eye and lies behind this orbital septum.

The key muscles associated with the eyelid are the orbicularis oculi muscle and the levator palpebrae superioris muscle, providing closure and opening of the eye, respectively. The orbicularis oculi muscle surrounds the eyelid, acting as a sphincter (see Fig. 5–1). The muscle can be divided into a palpebral and orbital portion. The orbicularis oculi muscle is innervated primarily by the zygomatic branch of the facial nerve with a possible contribution by the temporal branch. Functionally, the orbicularis oculi muscle is responsible for closing the eyelids both gently and tightly, resulting in the spreading of tears across the surface of the eye in addition to its protective mechanism. Paralysis may result in an ectropion of the lower eyelid. The second important muscle of the eyelid is the levator palpebrae superioris. This muscle arises from the apex of the orbit, continuing forward and forming a flattened aponeurosis that blends with the inferior portion of the orbital septum and inserts into the anterior aspect of the superior tarsal plate. The levator palpebrae superioris acts to elevate the upper eyelid and is innervated by the third cranial nerve, the oculomotor nerve.

The vascular supply of the eyelid consists of an arterial supply that is derived from both the internal and external carotid arteries. The ophthalmic artery arising from the internal carotid artery supplies the medial palpebral, supraorbital, supratrochlear, and lacrimal arteries. The medial palpebral arteries consist of a superior and an inferior portion that penetrate through

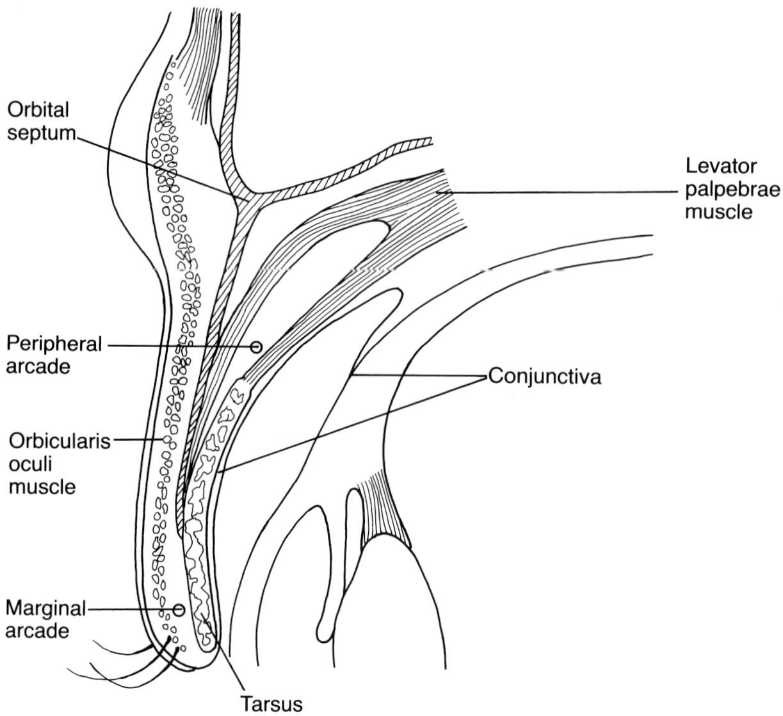

FIGURE 5–5. Sagittal section of the upper eyelid; tarsus provides eyelid form.

the orbital septum medially and then arch laterally over the eyelid. The supraorbital and supratrochlear arteries reinforce the palpebral vessels medially, while the lacrimal artery reinforces the palpebral arteries laterally. Contributions via the external carotid artery include the maxillary artery and the superficial temporal artery. The maxillary artery provides the infraorbital artery, which transverses the infraorbital foramen to supply the lower eyelid. The transverse facial artery arises off the superficial temporal artery, which anastomoses with the lateral distribution of the infraorbital artery to the lower eyelid. A medial anastomosis between the medial palpebral artery (inferior) and the infraorbital artery also exists.

The eyelid veins parallel the arterial system with an extensive surrounding venous network. These veins may drain into the ophthalmic venous system, the superficial temporal vein, or the angular vein (facial venous system). The ophthalmic venous network drains directly into a dural venous sinus.

The lymphatic drainage of the eyelid is divided into two parts. The medial aspect of the eyelids drains into the facial and submandibular nodes, with the lateral aspect of the upper and lower eyelids draining primarily into the preauricular nodal area.

The motor nerve supply to the eyelids is via the zygomatic and temporal branches of the facial nerve supplying the orbicularis oculi muscle (see Fig. 5–1) and the oculomotor nerve supplying innervation for the levator palpebrae superioris muscle. The trigeminal nerve (fifth cranial nerve) provides sensory innervation for the upper and lower eyelids. The ophthalmic division of the trigeminal nerve provides the supraorbital, supratrochlear, and lacrimal nerves for innervation of the upper eyelid. Innervation of the lower eyelid is via the infraorbital nerve arising off the maxillary division of the trigeminal nerve.

Visual acuity should be documented prior to any surgical procedure in the eyelid or periorbital area. This may be done via the use of charts. Additionally, consideration should be given for the measurement of ocular pressure. If it is necessary to patch the eye during Mohs' surgery, it is important to remember that the eye should be patched in a closed position.

THE NOSE

With its location in the central face and its protuberant anatomy, the nose is frequently involved in cutaneous neoplasms of the face. The surface anatomy of the external nose consists of the root, the dorsum, the ala, the columella, the tip, the vestibule, and the nasal labial crease. The root of the nose, located between the two orbits, is marked by a small depression called the nasion. The nasion indicates the midline articulation of the two nasal bones with the frontal bone. The dorsum of the nose extends from the nasion to the tip, with the bridge of the nose identified as that portion of the dorsum that is supported by underlying bone. The ala extends from the tip of the nose, laterally and inferiorly, to attach to the skin of the upper lip. The skin covering the nasal septum in the midline is referred to as the columella. The nares are openings bounded medially by the columella and laterally by the ala with the entrance via the nares into the nasal cavity. The alar crease consists of a small groove in the skin separating the ala from the cheek region of the face. Inferiorly, the alar crease separates the ala from the upper lip and then this area is referred to as the nasolabial crease. This area of the nose and face represents the site of multiple embryonic fusion planes, where the underlying tissues are unusually dense. Partially because of this, neoplasms may be difficult to define clinically in this area.

The skeleton of the nose is provided by both bone and cartilage (Fig. 5–3 and 5–4). The two nasal bones articulate with the maxilla laterally and with the frontal bone superiorly. The remainder of the skeleton is provided by the five major cartilages of the nose: the two lateral cartilages, the two greater alar cartilages, and the single septal cartilage. The superior aspect of the lateral nasal cartilage articulates with the inferior aspect of the respective nasal bone, and the lateral aspect of the lateral cartilage is joined at the frontal process of the maxilla. In the midline, each lateral nasal cartilage is joined to the septal cartilage. The greater alar cartilages are C-shaped, with the lateral crus articulating with the inferior aspect of the lateral nasal cartilage and each medial crus articulating in the midline with the septal cartilage to help form the nasal septum.

There are several muscles in association with the nose: the nasalis (transverse and alar portions) muscle, the levator labii superioris alaeque nasi muscle, the procerus muscle, and the depressor septi muscle. The nasalis muscle arises from the maxilla and its transverse portion extends across the bridge of the nose, joining its associate from the opposite side via an aponeurotic sling; this portion of the muscle helps to compress the nares. The alar part of the nasalis is a small slip of muscle that inserts into the lateral crus of the greater alar cartilage; it acts to dilate the nares. The nasalis is innervated by the buccal branches of the facial nerve. The levator labii superioris alaeque nasi muscle originates from the frontal process of the maxilla and passes inferiorly, with a small slip of muscle inserting into the ala of the nose before the main body of the muscle inserts into the skin of the upper lip. The alar portion of this muscle helps to dilate the nares and is innervated by buccal branches of the facial nerve. The procerus muscle arises from the nasal bones to pass superiorly, inserting into the skin overlying the glabella, acting to pull the skin downward and creating horizontal folds in the skin over the bridge of the nose. The procerus is innervated by temporal branches of the facial nerve. The depressor septi muscle has its origin from the incisive fossa of the maxilla and inserts into the nasal septum. It acts in conjunction with the nasalis to assist in widening the nares and is innervated by the buccal branches of the facial nerve.

The arterial supply to the external nose is primarily from the facial artery via the lateral nasal and the septal branch of the superior labial artery. Secondary branches from the infraorbital artery, nasal branches from the infratrochlear via the ophthalmic and the dorsal nasal branch of the anterior ethmoidal form the ophthalmic artery.

The veins of the external nose, which parallel the arteries, are tributaries of the anterior facial vein. As part of the facial venous system with a central location on the face, the nose lies within the "danger area" of the face. Open communication exists between the anterior facial vein and the ophthalmic veins, which drain into the cavernous sinus; the anterior facial vein communicates with the pterygoid venous plexus through the infraorbital vein, and the pterygoid venous plexus communicates with the cavernous sinus. The lymphatic drainage of the nose is into the buccal nodes of the facial lymphatic chain, with subsequent drainage into the submandibular nodes.

The sensory innervation of the external nose is provided from the trigeminal nerve via its ophthalmic and maxillary divisions. The ophthalmic division of the trigeminal nerve yields the infratrochlear and supratrochlear nerves, which supply the skin over the root and bridge of the nose, while the dorsal external nasal branch of the anterior ethmoidal nerve supplies skin over the dorsum of the nose, extending down to the tip of the nose. The lateral sides of the nose, the ala, and the columella are supplied by the infraorbital nerve via the maxillary division of the trigeminal nerve. The primary motor innervation to the muscles of the nose is derived from the buccal branches of the facial nerve.

The skin overlying the bony bridge of the nose is quite mobile in contrast to the skin over the tip and cartilaginous bridge. This is due to the rather loose subcutaneous tissue in the region of the bony bridge, whereas the subcutaneous tissue in the tip region is very dense and unyielding. Neoplastic lesions in the regions of the root and bridge of the nose tend to spread peripherally, since the bony framework of the nose acts as a barrier, preventing deep penetration. Occasionally a carcinoma may penetrate the underlying bone and spread into the nasal cavity and ethmoid bone. If there is involvement of the cribiform plate of the ethmoid this is particularly dangerous, since the neoplasm may easily invade the cranial cavity. Cancers of the cartilaginous bridge tend to expand peripherally as well as deeply, since the cartilage does little to impede tumor growth. Carcinomas of the nasolabial region of the nose are particularly difficult to delineate, probably because this region is of a complex embryologic nature. Along the embryonic fusion lines the tissues are quite dense and allow numerous avenues for the peripheral expansion of the cancer, which may be extremely difficult for the Mohs surgeon to identify clinically.

THE EAR

The ear is composed of three portions: the external ear, the middle ear, and the inner ear. The external ear is composed of an auricle and an external acoustic meatus, which terminates at the tympanic membrane (Fig. 5–6). The auricle is represented by an irregularly shaped plate of elastic cartilage and a small tag of adipose tissue called the lobule, which is suspended from the inferior aspect of the auricular cartilage. The skin overlying the auricle is relatively loosely attached to its posteromedial aspect compared with the anterolateral surface. Several distinctive surface features mark the auricular cartilage: the helix, the crura, the antihelix, the antitragus, the tragus, the concha, the scaphoid fossa, the triangular fossa, and the concha (Fig. 5–7). The helix forms the outer rim of the auricle, beginning at the crus anteriorly and terminating at the lobule inferiorly. The antihelix is a ridge of cartilage positioned just internal to the helix; two small ridges of cartilage (the superior and inferior crura) sep-

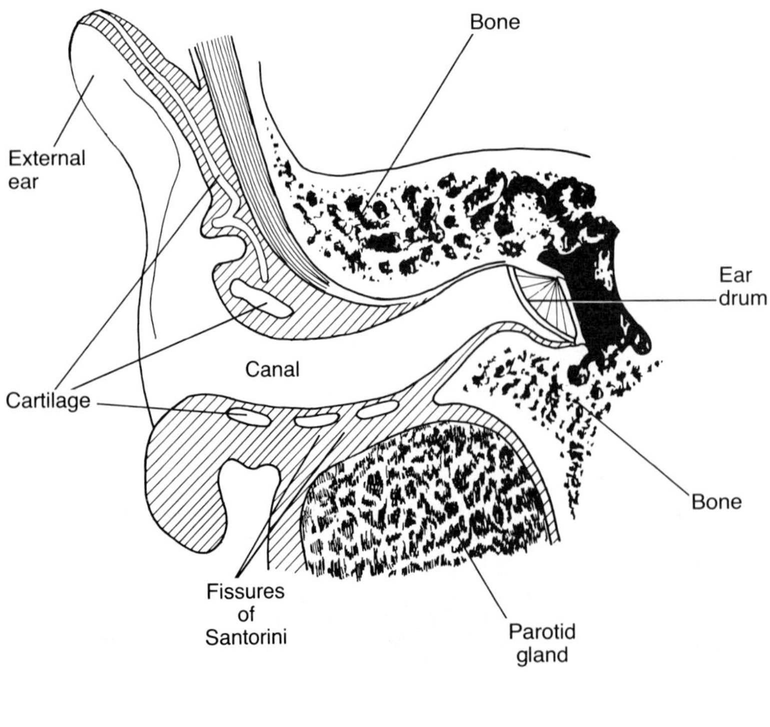

FIGURE 5–6. External ear and canal; note cartilaginous and bony support as well as fissures.

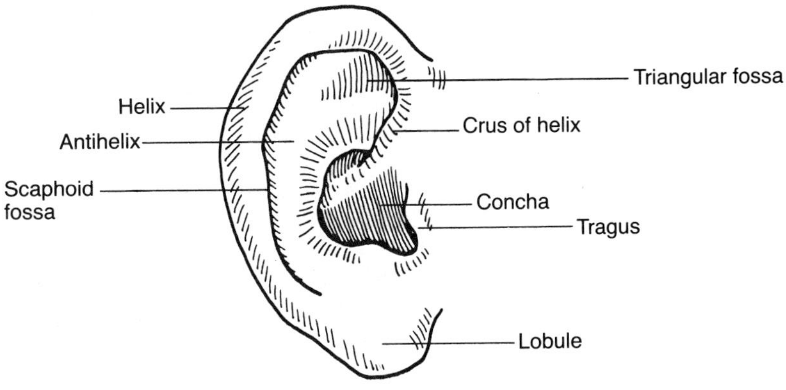

FIGURE 5–7. Components of the external ear.

arated from one another by a small fossa (triangular fossa) join to form a single ridge of cartilage that continues inferiorly to end at the antitragus. The tragus is represented by a triangular projection of cartilage that lies just anterior to the external meatus. The space separating the tragus from the antitragus is called the intertragal notch. The concavity existent beneath the rim of the helix is called the scaphoid fossa, while the space separating the crura of the antihelix is called the triangular fossa. The region of cartilage positioned directly anterior and medial to the antihelix is called the concha. Extending from the medial aspect of the cartilaginous auricle is a trough of cartilage that helps to form the lateral third of the external acoustic meatus. The entire auricle is well attached to the cranium via auricular ligaments.

The external acoustic meatus is a canal lined by skin that terminates medially at the tympanic membrane. The underlying foundation of the meatus is cartilaginous and bony. The lateral third is partly cartilaginous in its anterior and inferior boundaries, but the posterosuperior aspect is bone; the foundation of the entire medial two-thirds of the meatus is formed by the surrounding temporal bone. The isthmus of the external meatus is its most narrow point, a site where foreign objects may become lodged. The trough of cartilage supporting the meatus in its lateral extent is frequently perforated by fissures called the fissures of Santorini. The parotid gland lies directly anterior and inferior to the cartilaginous segment of the meatus. Neoplasms of the external ear reaching the external acoustic meatus may use the fissures of Santorini to reach the parotid gland (see Fig. 5–6).

There are three rudimentary extrinsic muscles of the ear: the anterior, the superior, and the posterior auricular muscles. The anterior auricular muscle originates from the galea aponeurosis to insert into the crus of the helix. The superior auricular muscle arises from the galea aponeurosis to insert into the cranial aspect of the auricle. The posterior auricular muscle arises from the mastoid portion of the temporal bone to insert into the posterior aspect of the concha. The anterior and superior auricular muscles are innervated by the temporal branch of the facial nerve, while the posterior auricular muscle is innervated by the posterior auricular branch of the facial nerve.

The external carotid artery supplies the auricle via the superficial temporal artery, the posterior auricular artery, and the occipital artery. The superficial temporal artery supplies the lateral surface via anterior auricular branches. The posterior auricular and occipital arteries supply the medial surface of the auricle. The veins of the auricle accompany the arteries. The venous drainage of the anterolateral aspect of the ear is into the superficial temporal vein, while the posteromedial region is drained by the posterior auricular vein. The lymphatic drainage of the ear is into the preauricular nodes, the superficial cervical nodes and the postauricular nodes.

The sensory supply to the ear is derived from several different sources with significant overlap. The mandibular division of the trigeminal nerve yields the auriculotemporal nerve, which innervates the anterosuperior quadrant of the anterolateral aspect of the auricle and the entire anterior half of the external acoustic meatus; on the posteromedial surface this nerve innervates a small portion of the auricle superiorly. The seventh, ninth, and tenth cranial nerves supply the skin covering the concha and the posterior half of the external acoustic meatus; these nerves also supply a small patch of skin over the posterior aspect of the auricle. The cervical plexus provides the greater auricular nerve and the lesser occipital nerve, which innervate the remainder of the auricle. The greater auricular nerve ascends across the sternocleidomastoid muscle directly toward the inferior aspect of the auricle to supply its anterolateral surface as well as most of the posteromedial surface. Ascending from the neck, the lesser occipital nerve parallels the posterior edge of the sternocleidomastoid muscle to supply a small portion of the posteromedial surface of the auricle.

THE CHEEK

The cheek is a rather loosely defined area on the face which begins immediately anterior to the tragus of the ear and continues forward to the lateral commissure of the lips. Its supperior boundary begins roughly along a line paralleling the zygomatic arch and the inferior margin of the body orbit, extending inferiorly to the inferior margin of the body of the mandible. A useful landmark is the melolabial crease, which extends from the alar crease inferiorly to help separate the oral region from the cheek.

The cheek can be conveniently subdivided into four regions: the masseteric, malar, infraorbital, and buccal regions. The masseteric region is represented by an area of skin that overlies the masseter muscle. The malar region is an area of the cheek that has the malar prominence of the zygomatic bone as its bony foundation. The infraorbital region is a small semilunar area located just below the bony margin of the orbit. The buccal region represents the largest area of the cheek, extending from the anterior edge of the masseter muscle to the lateral commissure of the lip and from the infraorbital region inferiorly to the mandible.

The surface anatomy of the cheek region includes both bony structures and soft tissues. The bony foundation of the cheek is derived from the maxilla and zygomatic bones. The anterior surface of the maxilla is the predominant bone of the cheek and face. A vertical line drawn on the face beginning at the supraorbital notch intersects the infraorbital foramen approximately 5 mm below the inferior margin of the orbit. This foramen, which perforates the maxilla, transmits the infraorbital nerve onto the face and cheek. The malar portion of the zygomatic bone is responsible for the prominence of the cheek. Extending from the malar prominence posteriorly to the ear is the zygomatic arch. This structure marks the superior extent of the cheek region in the posterolateral aspect of the face. The mandible—its ramus, angle, and body—are easily palpated on the face. The important soft tissue structures that are palpable and useful as landmarks are the masseter muscle and the parotid duct. The masseter muscle, easily identified by asking the patient to clench the teeth, overlies the ramus of the mandible as it extends from the zygomatic arch superiorly to the angle and body of the mandible inferiorly.

The parotid gland, while not palpable, occupies an important position superficial to the masseter muscle. The superior pole of the parotid extends nearly to the zygomatic arch, its posterior boundary on the face parallels the posterior edge of the ramus of the mandible, the inferior pole extends to the angle of the mandible, and its anterior border extends a variable distance out over the masseter muscle. Halfway between the zygomatic arch and the labial commissure the parotid duct is palpable as it crosses the anterior edge of the masseter muscle to penetrate through the muscular wall of the cheek. The buccal fat pad lies in the subcutaneous layer of the cheek positioned between the buccinator muscle and the skin. A well-developed buccal fat pad is responsible for the fullness of the buccal region of the cheek. An important extension of the buccal fat pad that passes between the buccinator muscle and the masseter muscle continues into the deep face, passing superiorly into the temporal fossa and infratemporal fossa. This superior extension of the buccal fat pad provides a route for the transmission of neoplasms from the superficial face into the deep face, with potential invasion into the maxilla and the maxillary sinus.

The muscles of the cheek include a superficial group (the zygomaticus major and minor, the orbicularis oculi, the risorius, the levator labii superioris, and the platysma) and a deep group (the levator anguli oris and the buccinator) (see Fig. 5–1). The zygomaticus major and minor muscles both arise from the zygomatic bone, insert into the skin of the upper lip, and elevate the upper lip. The orbicularis oculi muscle has been previously described in the orbital region, and its primary function is upon the eyelids, but its fibers do extend well into the infraorbital region of the cheek. The risorius muscle arises from the parotid fascia and continues anteriorly across the face to insert into the skin at the corner of the mouth; it acts to pull the corners of the mouth laterally. The levator labii superioris muscle originates from the maxilla just above the infraorbital foramen and inserts into the skin and mucosa of the upper lip; it elevates the upper lip. The platysma muscle originates from the superficial fascia of the upper thoracic region and the neck, and its fibers sweep over the body of the mandible to insert into the skin of the corners of the mouth; it pulls the corners of the mouth inferiorly. The levator anguli oris muscle arises from the maxilla just below the infraorbital foramen, inserts into the corner of the mouth, and acts to elevate the corner of the mouth. The buccinator, the key muscle of the cheek, has an extensive origin from the posterolateral aspect of the maxilla, the pterygomandibular raphe, and the medial aspect of the mandible and inserts into the skin and mucosa of the upper and lower lips. The buccinator forms the muscular wall of the cheek and acts to compress the cheek. All of the muscles associated with the cheek are innervated by branches of the facial nerve (see Fig. 5–1). The zygomaticus major and minor, the levator labii superioris, the levator anguli oris, the risorius, and the buccinator muscles receive their primary innervation from the buccal branches of the facial nerve. The orbicularis oculi muscle receives its primary innervation from the temporal and zygomatic branches of the facial nerve. The platysma muscle is innervated by the cervical branches of the facial nerve.

Vascular supply to the cheek region of the face is derived from branches of the external carotid artery (see Fig. 5–2). The terminal branches of these vessels form an anastomotic network that supplies the face and cheek. The facial artery arises from the external carotid artery within the neck and enters onto the face at the anterior edge of the masseter as it inserts into the mandible. The facial artery continues onto the face, lying directly on top of the buccinator muscle and immediately deep to the platysma, risorius, zygomaticus major and minor, and levator labii superioris muscles. Near the angle of the mouth, the facial artery yields the superior and inferior labial arteries and continues along the lateral aspect of the nose as the angular artery. Numerous muscular branches from the facial artery penetrate the muscular wall of the cheek. The maxillary artery, a branch of the external carotid, yields the buccal and infraorbital arteries. The buccal arises from the maxillary artery just medial to the mandible, descending inferiorly on the superficial aspect of the buccinator muscle; it supplies the skin and mucosa of the buccal cheek region. The infraorbital artery emerges onto the cheek through the infraorbital foramen and supplies the infraorbital cheek area. The superficial temporal artery, a terminal branch of the external carotid, yields the transverse facial artery, which passes through the superior pole of the parotid gland and parallels the parotid duct; this vessel supplies the malar region of the cheek.

Venous drainage of the cheek is via the buccal, infraorbital, superficial, temporal, and anterior facial veins. The most important collecting vein of the cheek is the anterior facial vein, which parallels the facial artery. There are extensive venous communications between the anterior facial vein and the buccal and infraorbital veins, both of which present possible pathways to the cavernous sinus. The lymphatic drainage of the cheek flows into either the preauricular nodes or the facial nodes. The preauricular or parotid nodes drain the masseteric, posterior half of the buccal, and lateral half of the infraorbital regions of the cheek. The facial nodes, which parallel the anterior facial vein, drain the remainder of the cheek regions.

The muscles of the cheek are all innervated by branches of the facial nerve. The facial nerve enters the posterior border of the parotid gland as a single trunk, and as the nerve continues through the gland, it begins to subdivide into five branches which emerge from the protection of the gland, fanning out over the face. The branches that course through the area of the face defined as the cheek are the temporal, zygomatic, buccal, and marginal mandibular. Only the zygomatic and buccal branches of the facial nerve supply muscles associated with the cheek. The zygomaticus major and minor, levator labii superioris, risorius, levator anguli oris, and buccinator muscles receive their primary innervation from the buccal branches, with the zygomaticus muscles receiving secondary innervation from the zygomatic branches. The temporal branch of the facial nerve, although it does not innervate any muscles of the cheek, leaves the superior pole of the parotid gland and travels a very short distance through the masseteric region of the cheek before it enters the temporal region of the scalp. The zygomatic branches of the facial nerve leave the protection of the parotid near its upper pole and run obliquely across the cheek toward the lateral margins of the orbit. After leaving the parotid gland, both the temporal and zygomatic branches may be damaged during superficial surgical procedures, since they are covered only by skin and a variable amount of subcutaneous tissue. Consequently, deep incisions placed parallel to the zygomatic arch may sever multiple branches of these nerves before they have had a chance to arborize extensively, with a resultant muscle paralysis. The buccal branches leave the anterior border of the parotid to run parallel with the parotid duct. Vertically placed incisions over the top of the masseter increase the possibility of cutting these buccal branches. The marginal mandibular branch of the facial nerve has a course through the masseteric region of the cheek, which is roughly parallel to the inferior margin of the mandible. This nerve is covered only by skin, a variable amount of subcutaneous tissue, and the platysma muscle. Since the nerve does not arborize extensively until it reaches the lower lip musculature, any vertically placed incisions over the mandible increase the risk of damage to this branch of the facial nerve. The sensory supply to the cheek is derived from the trigeminal nerve and the greater auricular nerve (see Fig. 5–2). The trigeminal nerve provides terminal branches to the cheek from the maxillary division (infraorbital and zygomaticofacial nerves) and the mandibular division (auriculotemporal and buccal nerves). The infraorbital nerve exits through the infraorbital foramen to supply the skin of the infraorbital cheek, portions of the malar and buccal cheek, lower eyelid, lateral nose, and upper lip. The zygomaticofacial nerve penetrates through small foramina in the malar bone to supply the skin of the malar cheek. The auriculotemporal nerve runs through the parotid gland and emerges just in front of the ear and supplies skin innervation over the masseteric cheek, a portion of the ear, and the temporal region of the scalp. The buccal nerve leaves the infratemporal fossa and descends into the cheek along the superficial surface of the buccinator muscle to supply the skin and mucosa of the buccal cheek. The greater auricular nerve, a branch of the cervical plexus, ascends from the neck to supply the skin in the lower portion of the masseteric cheek region.

LIPS AND PERIORAL REGION

Encircling the mouth or buccal orifice, the lips are represented by a core of musculature covered externally by skin and lined internally by a mucosal membrane. The upper and lower lips are united laterally at the labial commissures. The perioral region is bounded superiorly by the nose, laterally by the cheek and inferiorly by the chin. The melolabial crease, which extends from the ala of the nose inferiorly and obliquely, passes approximately 1 cm lateral to the labial commissure and helps to separate the cheek from the lips. The labiomental crease, a horizontal crease approximately 1 cm below the lower lip, helps separate the chin from the lower lip. The modiolus, a small elevation of skin just lateral to the labial commissure, is created by the muscles of the perioral region as they insert into the skin of this area.

Each lip has a vermilion border, a region of abrupt transition from normal skin to a modified epithelium devoid of hair, sweat glands, and sebaceous glands. The free margin of each lip is referred to as the vermilion zone. The upper lip is marked by the philtrum, a midline depression which extends from the columella of the nose to the vermilion border. The junctional zone of the vermilion border with the philtrum is called Cupid's bow.

The primary lip muscle is the orbicularis oris, a concentrically arranged muscle that inserts into the skin and mucosa of the lips, performing a key sphincteric function (see Fig. 5–1). This muscle is innervated by the buccal branches of the facial nerve. The buccinator muscle, which forms the muscular wall of the cheek, contributes a large number of muscle fibers that help to form the orbicularis oris muscle. The buccinator helps to flatten and retract the lips; it is innervated by the buccal branches of the facial nerve.

The elevators of the upper lip are the zygomaticus major and minor, levator labii superioris, the levator labii superioris alaeque nasi, and the levator anguli oris muscles. The zygomaticus major arises from the malar portion of the zygomatic bone to insert into the skin at the angle of the mouth; it raises the corners of the mouth. The zygomaticus minor muscle arises just medial to the major muscle and inserts into the skin of the upper lip. The levator labii superioris originates from the maxilla just above the infraorbital foramen and inserts into the skin of the upper lip. The levator labii superioris alaeque nasi muscle arises from the maxilla near the medial margin of the orbit and descends along the lateral aspect of the nose to insert into the ala of the nose and the skin of the upper lip. The levator anguli oris muscle originates from the maxilla just below the infraorbital foramen and inserts into skin and mucosa at the angle of the mouth; it is an elevator of the angle of the mouth. All of these muscles are primarily innervated by the buccal branches of the facial nerve with secondary input from the zygomatic branches of the facial nerve. The risorius muscle widens the mouth as in smiling; it arises from the parotid fascia and passes horizontally across the cheek to insert into the skin at the corner of the mouth.

The muscles that act to depress the lips are the platysma, the depressor anguli oris, and the depressor labii inferioris. The platysma muscle arises from the neck region and passes over the mandible to insert into the skin at the corner of the mouth. The depressor anguli oris muscle originates from the body of the mandible to insert into the skin and mucosa at the corner of the mouth. The depressor labii inferioris muscle arises from the mandible just anterior to the depressor anguli oris and inserts into the skin of the lower lip. The mentalis muscle originating from the front of the mandible and inserts into the skin overlying the lip; it acts to protrude the lower lip and provide a horizontal shelf. The motor innervation of the muscles of the lip are derived from the zygomatic, buccal, marginal mandibular, and cervical branches of the facial nerve.

The vascular supply to the lips is derived from the facial artery via its first branches on the face, the inferior and superior labial arteries (see Fig. 5–2). These vessels have a tortuous course through the muscle fibers of the orbicularis oris as they anastomose across the midline with their companion vessels from the opposite side. An important aspect of this anastomotic communication is that a facial artery may be tied off at its point of entry onto the face without fear of ischemic insult to the ipsilateral face. In the elderly patient, the course of the labial arteries through the lips becomes more tortuous and the vessels pass quite superficially to the mucosal surface of the lips, rendering them at some risk of laceration during lip shave procedures.

The venous drainage is via the superior and inferior labial veins, which join the anterior facial vein. The lymphatic drainage of the lips follows several areas. The central and lateral regions of the upper lip flow into the ipsilateral submandibular nodes; the lateral regions of the lower lip flow into the ipsilateral submandibular nodes, and the central regions of the lower lip flow into both ipsilateral and contralateral submandibular and submental nodes. Since the central region of the lower lip drains to either side, the clinician should carefully examine the submandibular and submental nodes for possible metastasis of carcinomas from the lip.

The sensory supply to the lips is derived from branches of the trigeminal nerve. The maxillary division of the trigeminal nerve provides the infraorbital nerve, which innervates the entire upper lip, the lower eyelid, the infraorbital cheek, portions of the buccal cheek, the malar cheek, and the lateral aspect of the nose. The mandibular division of the trigeminal nerve provides the mental nerve that is sensory to the entire lower lip. By dropping a vertical line on the face beginning at the supraorbital notch, the infraorbital foramen and nerve are intersected approximately 5 mm below the inferior margin of the orbit; the mental foramen and nerve are intersected by this line approximately midway in the height of the body of the mandible.

THE NECK

The neck can be divided into an anterior and posterior triangle with the anterior triangle of the neck defined by the anterior border of the sternocleidomastoid muscle, the inferior margin of the mandible, and the midline border from the tip of the chin to the jugular notch. The posterior triangle of the neck is delineated by the sternocleidomastoid muscle, the clavicle inferiorly, and the anterior edge of the trapezius muscle (Fig. 5–8). These triangles are useful both in terms of localization of lesions and in terms of the underlying superficial anatomy. The anterior triangle can be further divided into four smaller triangles: the submental, the submandibular, the carotid, and the muscular. The submental is bordered by the anterior belly of the digastric muscle, the body of the hyoid bone and the midline of the neck. The submandibular triangle is bordered by the two muscular bellies of the digastric and the mandible. The carotid triangle is bordered by the sternocleidomastoid muscle, the posterior border of the digastric muscle, and the superior belly of the omohyoid muscle. The muscular triangle is bordered by the sternocleidomastoid muscle, the superior belly of the omohyoid muscle, and the midline of the neck. Similarly, the posterior triangle of the neck can be di-

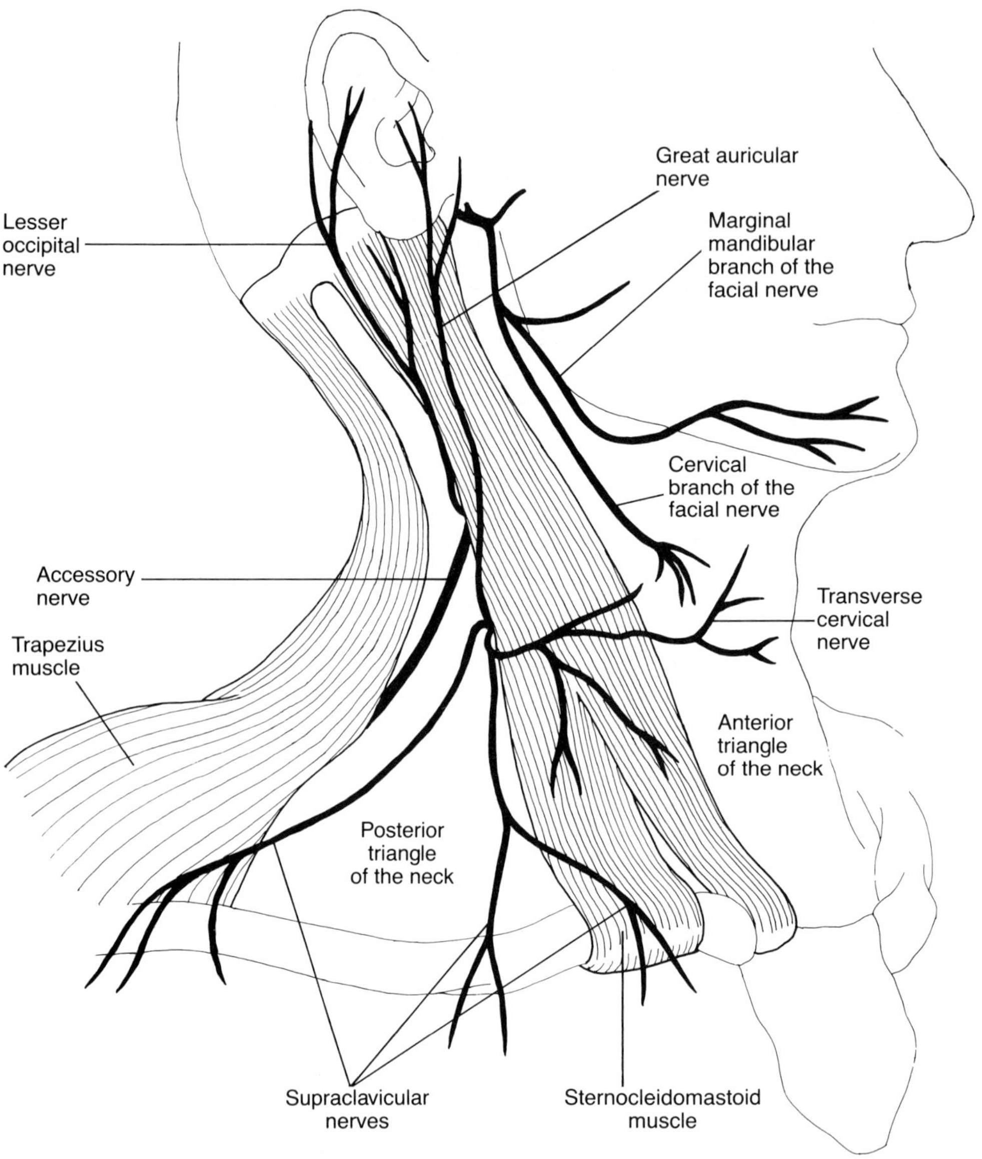

FIGURE 5–8. Anterior and posterior neck triangles showing nerve supply; note superficial location of accessory nerve near the trapezius and sternocleidomastoid muscles.

vided into two smaller triangles—the subclavian and the occipital triangle. The subclavian triangle is bordered by the clavicle, the sternocleidomastoid muscle and the inferior belly of the omohyoid muscle. The occipital triangle is bordered by the inferior belly of the omohyoid muscle, the sternocleidomastoid muscle, and the trapezius muscle.

The skin of the neck is quite thin and pliable and is well represented with hair follicles, sebaceous glands, and sweat glands. The pliability and mobility is in part related to a thin layer of looser areolar connective tissue known as the superficial cervical fascia. This fascia is continuous with the superficial fascia of the face. Within the anterior triangle is the platysma muscle, the only superficial muscle in this area, which originates from the fascia of the upper chest region and continues upward across the neck, crossing the mandible to insert into the skin and superficial tissue of the lower face. In addition to acting with other muscles as a depressor of the mouth, the platysma muscle also tenses the skin of the neck. Innervation of the platysma muscle is by the cervical branch of the facial nerve. This muscle has much more of a function in some animals than it does in man. The platysma is a very thin muscle that may decrease in thickness with age. The platysma muscle does cross the sternocleidomastoid to cover only the most inferior aspect of the occipital triangle. The platysma does not cover that portion of the posterior triangle containing the spinal accessory nerve. The sternocleidomastoid muscle arises from both the sternum and the proximal portion of the clavicle. For the most part, it is covered by the platysma as it passes obliquely across the neck to insert into the mastoid process.

Within the anterior triangle of the neck the hyoid bone is located at the second cervical vertebral level. This should be palpable in the midline just inferior to the chin. Just below the hyoid bone the prominence of thyroid cartilage is also palpable in the midline. Below the thyroid cartilage is the anterior lamina of the cricoid cartilage with rings of the trachea and the isthmus of the thyroid gland below.

The vascular supply to the skin and superficial areas of the neck is provided by penetrating branches from the external carotid artery as well as branches of the thyrocervical trunk. The anterior superficial venous system is located immediately deep to the platysma muscle, with drainage into the anterior jugular vein, which may be connected to the common facial vein by a small communicating vein. The external jugular vein drains the superficial area of the posterior cervical triangle.

The sensory innervation of the neck for the most part is derived from the cervical plexus. A number of nerves emerge into the neck at the midpoint of the sternocleidomastoid muscle along its posterior border (see Fig. 5–8). At this point, the transverse cervical nerves cross the sternocleidomastoid muscle horizontally to provide sensory supply to the midanterior cervical triangle. Inferior to the transverse cervical nerve, a series of supraclavicular nerves appear and pass downward to supply the skin of the anterior and posterior cervical triangles as well as the upper pectoral area. The lesser occipital nerve becomes visible at the posterior portion of the sternocleidomastoid muscle near its midpoint and runs upward, paralleling the posterior border of the sternocleidomastoid muscle to provide sensory supply to the posterior ear and mastoid area. The greater auricular nerve also arises at the midpoint and overlies the sternocleidomastoid muscle, running upward to provide sensory innervation to the lower portion of the ear.

In addition to the motor innervation of the platysma muscle from the cervical branch of the facial nerve, the marginal mandibular branch of the facial nerve frequently descends into the anterior triangle (submandibular triangle) of the neck as it parallels the mandible before innervating the muscles of the lower lip. While protected by the overlying superficial cervical fascia, the platysma muscle, and the skin, this nerve may be at risk during removal of tumors in this area via Mohs surgery. The nerve most frequently at risk in the posterior triangle is the spinal accessory nerve, which supplies the sternocleidomastoid and trapezius muscles (see Fig. 5–8). The nerve is protected by the sternocleidomastoid muscle but exits from its posterior border, entering the posterior triangle of the neck at the junction of the upper and middle third of the muscle. The nerve then passes in a very superficial location inferiorly and diagonally across the posterior cervical triangle before being protected by the anterior edge of the trapezius muscle. The accessory nerve is covered only by skin and superficial cervical fascia, and the nerve itself should be identified during surgical procedures in this area. Disruption of the nerve results in an inability to elevate the shoulder on the affected side.

The lymphatic system of the neck is formed by scattered lymph nodes that drain into the superficial and deep cervical lymphatic chains, associated with the external and internal jugular veins (Fig. 5–9). The submandibular and submental nodes receive lymph flow from above, with the submandibular region draining into the jugulodigastric node.

Knowledge of superficial anatomy of the neck allows the cervical plexus to be blocked by local anesthesia at the posterior midpoint of the sternocleidomastoid muscle, providing anesthesia to a wide area. Attention must be paid to nerves at risk during superficial neck surgery, which include the marginal mandibular branch of the facial nerve, the spinal accessory nerve, and the great auricular sensory nerve. The anterior and external jugular vein may be encountered frequently. Portions of the parotid and submandibular glands may be encountered where tumors extend more deeply. The

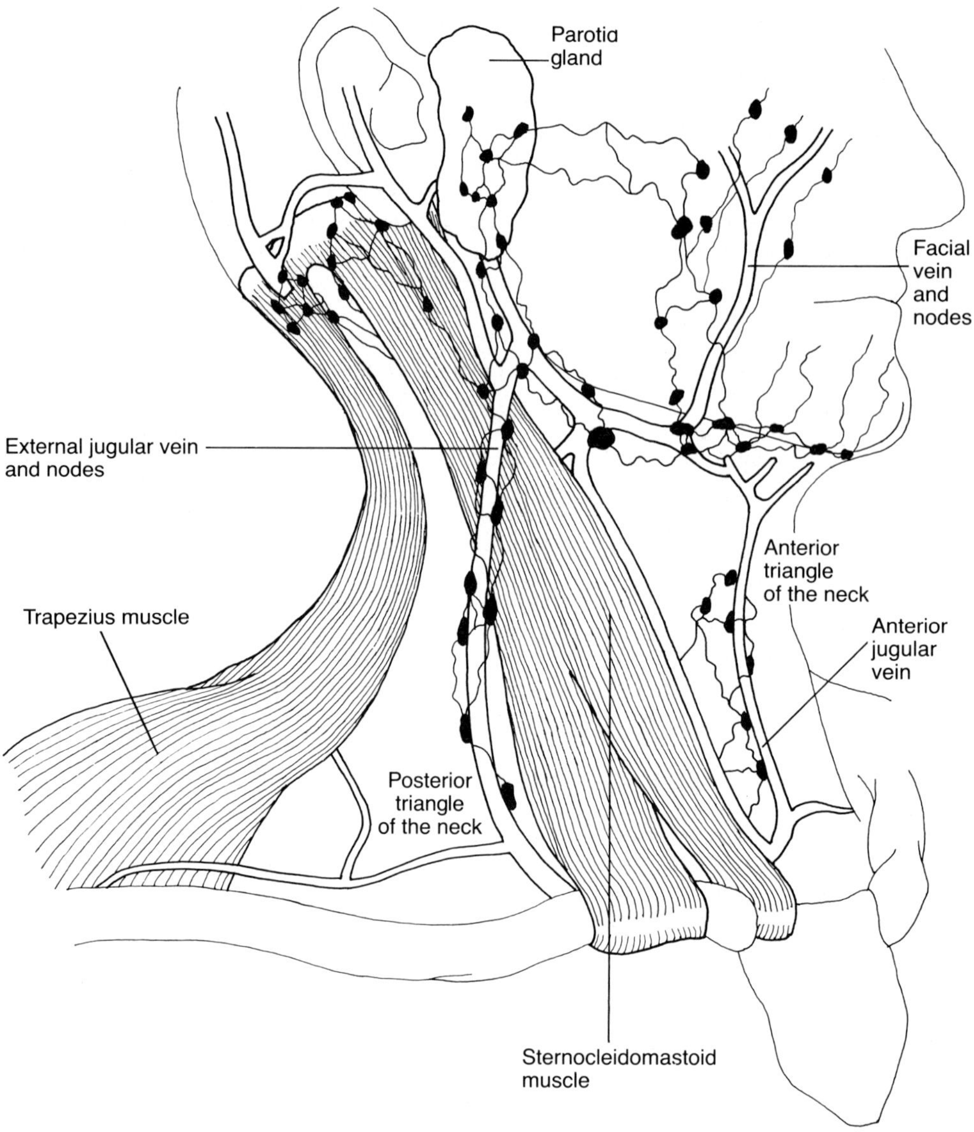

FIGURE 5–9. Lymphatic drainage of the face and neck.

platysma muscle provides excellent coverage of the anterior triangle of the neck, and all structures at risk would lie deep to the muscle. However, with time, the platysma may become extremely thin. It should be noted that the platysma never extends far enough in the posterior cervical triangle to protect the accessory nerve. Damage to the marginal mandibular branch of the facial nerve in the neck will significantly affect the function of the lower lip.

REFERENCES

1. Hollingshead WH: The Head and Neck. Anatomy for Surgeons, vol. 1, 3rd ed. New York: Harper and Row, 1982.
2. McCord CD: Oculoplastic Surgery, 2nd ed. Raven Press, 1987.
3. Lang PG, Osgothorpe JD: Mohs micrographic surgery of the head and neck: A multidisciplinary approach. Dermatol Clin North Am 7(4):609–843, 1989.
4. Yaremchuk YJ: Vascularized grafts for maxillofacial reconstruction. Clin Plast Surg 16(1):29–39, 1989.

CHAPTER 6

Local and Regional Block Anesthesia

George R. Mikhail, M.D., M.S.

With the advent and prevalence of the fresh tissue method of Mohs micrographic surgery, local anesthesia has become an essential part of the procedure. The administration of local anesthetics is in itself an art with numerous facets that are beyond the scope of this book. Those aspects that are practical and relevant to Mohs surgery are presented here. They are based on personal experience.

TYPES OF ANESTHETIC AGENTS

The local anesthetics most commonly used are listed in Table 6–1. They belong to one of two chemical structures: esters and amides. The maximum 24-hour dosage in dry weight and in solution is also indicated. Note that in case of hypersensitivity to one agent, cross-reactivity occurs to others that are chemically related (ester or amide). Of the drugs listed here, lidocaine appears to be the first choice of the majority of surgeons. It induces rapid onset of analgesia because it spreads quickly through the tissues. Its length of action is intermediate, one to two hours, but it can be increased 50% to 100% by the addition of epinephrine. The relatively newer amide agents, bupivacaine and etidocaine, have much longer durations of action, four to eight hours, but the onset of analgesia is very slow. They are useful for lengthy procedures.

Most local anesthetics are well tolerated with the recommended dosage. When toxicity occurs, it is usually related to the effects of the drugs on the central nervous and cardiovascular systems, and the severity is determined by the dose, rate of absorption, and the patient's medical condition. Inadvertent intravascular injection and allergy are important factors. For details on complications and precautions, see Chapters 8 and 9.

LOCAL INFILTRATION ANESTHESIA

Our experience, as well as that of others, has shown that lidocaine is both safe and effective. The 0.5% solution with 1:200,000 epinephrine is our routine. The addition of this small amount of vasoconstrictor greatly reduces intraoperative bleeding, appreciably prolongs the analgesia, and makes the anesthetized area visible due to blanching. With this combination, the onset of action is within 10 to 15 minutes and lasts 1½ to 2½ hours.

Local infiltration is adequate for excising small lesions and for obtaining biopsies. The method of administration and the precautions that apply in general dermatologic surgery also apply here. The minimum dose and concentration that are effective should be used, preferably in combination with epinephrine. Intra-

TABLE 6–1. Commonly Used Local Anesthetics

Generic Name	Proprietary Name	Chemical Derivation	Maximum 24-Hour Dosage	
			Dry Weight	*(Solution)*
bupivacaine	Marcaine	amide	0.18 gm	(15 ml 0.5%; 30 ml 0.25%)
etidocaine	Duranest	amide	0.3 gm	(30 ml 1%; 60 ml 0.5%)
lidocaine	Xylocaine	amide	0.5 gm	(50 ml 1%; 100 ml 0.5%)
mepivacaine	Carbocaine	amide	0.4 gm	(30 ml 1%; 60 ml 0.5%)
prilocaine	Citanest	amide	0.5 gm	(50 ml 1%; 100 ml 0.5%)
procaine	Novocaine	ester	1.0 gm	(50 ml 2%; 100 ml 1%)
tetracaine	Pontocaine	ester	0.1 gm	(50 ml 0.2%; 100 ml 0.1%)

vascular injection, direct injection into a nerve (in case of nerve block), and injection into an infected area are to be avoided.

FIELD BLOCK

In field block, analgesia is accomplished by circuminjecting the lesion with the anesthetic solution. This method is adequate for the majority of Mohs procedures. In the case of relatively small basal cell carcinomas on the nose or pinna, it is advantageous to elevate the skin by injecting some of the anesthetic between the skin and cartilage. This maneuver facilitates obtaining a good layer of tissue and minimizes the loss of cartilage.

REGIONAL BLOCK ANESTHESIA

There are certain conditions in which anesthesia is best achieved by regional block:

1. When prolonged anesthesia is required
2. When treating large lesions
3. When multiple procedures are to be done in the same area
4. In cases of inflamed or ulcerated lesions
5. In cases of melanoma or suspected melanoma
6. In squamous cell carcinoma
7. In lesions on appendageal parts of the body, e.g., the digits, nose, ear, or penis.

Regional anesthesia can be undertaken either by the technique of field block or nerve block. In the field block method, nerve conduction is interrupted by placing a wall of anesthetic between the operative site and the central nervous system. This can be accomplished by intracutaneous and subcutaneous infiltrations in the vicinity of the nerves that supply the operative site.

In nerve block, the nerve supplying a region is injected to produce a transient pharmacologic "section" of the nerve. The injection may be intraneural or, preferably, extraneural. Painful parasthesias are felt while the solution is being injected intraneurally. The pain is due to distention of the nerve and can be relieved by withdrawing the needle a millimeter or two. In extraneural injection, the anesthetic is deposited close to the nerve. It is adequate and safe.

The solutions used in block anesthesia are the same as those employed in local infiltration anesthesia. We have routinely used lidocaine for many years with only rare, but minor, toxic reactions. The rule in block anesthesia is not to exceed 500 mg of lidocaine. The dose may vary from a few milliliters up to 100 ml of 0.5% solution with or without 1:200,000 epinephrine, or up to 50 ml of the 1% solution with or without 1:100,000 epinephrine. The operative analgesia in regional block is established in 10 to 15 minutes and lasts 1 to 3 hours. Stronger concentrations of the anesthetic and solutions containing epinephrine give the longest duration. If the block proves unsatisfactory after allowing adequate time for the anesthesia to become established, reblocking should be undertaken. However, the total of the two doses should not exceed the maximum dosage for the drug used.

Block of the Scalp

An intradermal wheal is raised over the glabella and another over the occiput. Local infiltration is then carried out intradermally, subcutaneously, and intraperiosteally in a line extending

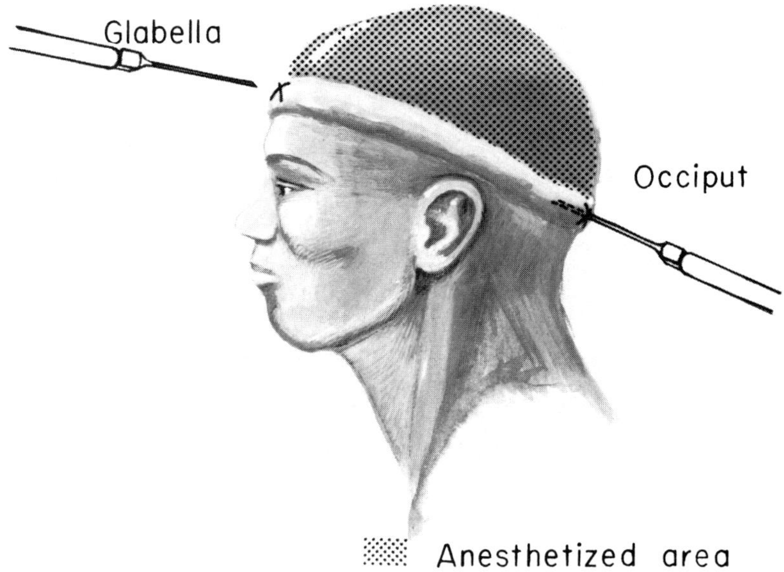

FIGURE 6–1. Block of the scalp resulting in "skull cap" analgesia.

from one wheal to the other until a wall of the injected anesthetic encircles the head. The temporal fossa should be carefully infiltrated because the nerves are situated deeply in relation to the muscles in this area. The total amount of lidocaine needed is variable but is usually about 30 to 50 ml. A "skull cap" type of analgesia is produced by this method (Fig. 6–1). Solutions containing epinephrine are indicated to control bleeding because a local anesthetic without the vasoconstrictor is readily absorbed from the richly vascular scalp and can result in toxic reactions.

Block of the Branches of the Ophthalmic Division of the Trigeminal Nerve

The supraorbital and the supratrochlear branches innervate the central part of the forehead and the frontal scalp. These are blocked by injecting the anesthetic solution along the upper margins of the orbits (Fig. 6–2).

The infraorbital nerve, the terminal branch of the maxillary nerve, emerges from the infraorbital canal through the infraorbital foramen. Here, it divides into branches that supply the skin of the lower eyelid, the lateral part of the nose and ala, the mucosa of the nasal vestibule, and the upper lip and its mucosa.

The infraorbital foramen is situated on the infraorbital ridge at approximately 2.5 cm (1 inch) from the midline of the face or 2.0 cm (¾ inch) lateral to the frontal process of the maxillary bone (the lateral surface of the nose). The foramen can be located by palpation and a mark made on the overlying skin. Another mark is placed 0.6 cm (¼ inch) below and slightly medial to the first mark in order to allow for the slant of the infraorbital canal and to permit easy entry into it. A skin wheal is made at the lower mark. Subcutaneous infiltra-

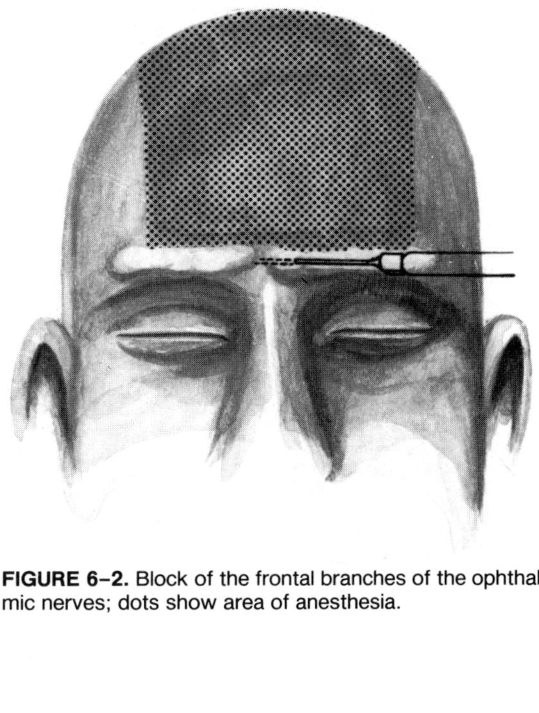

FIGURE 6–2. Block of the frontal branches of the ophthalmic nerves; dots show area of anesthesia.

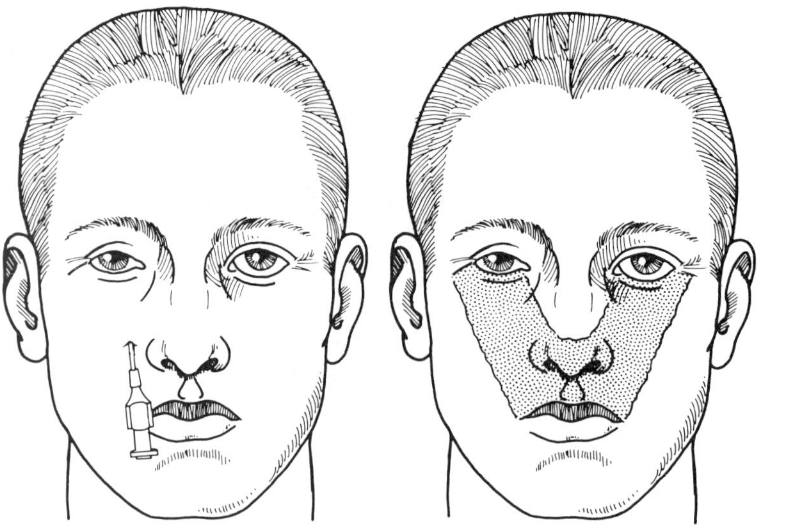

FIGURE 6–3. Block of the infraorbital nerve; dots show area of anesthesia.

tion is carried out along the line between the two markings, using approximately 1 to 2 ml of the anesthetic solution. A 4 cm (1½ inch), 22-gauge needle is then entered at the lower mark and advanced toward the infraorbital foramen until it strikes bone or elicits paraesthesia (sharp, electric-like sensations in the upper lip and ala nasi). Here, 2 to 3 ml of anesthetic solution are injected (Fig. 6–3). There is no need to insert the needle into the canal unless block of the anterior superior alveolar nerve (innervates the upper incisor and bicuspid teeth) is desired. It is inadvisable to insert the needle into the infraorbital canal since such injection may result in lesions of the nerves or injury to the contents of the orbit and may cause prolonged discomfort. If the lesion is near the midline, bilateral block has to be undertaken.

Digital Block

Each digit is supplied by four nerve branches—two dorsal and two palmar (or plantar) that run distally along the respective edge of the digit.

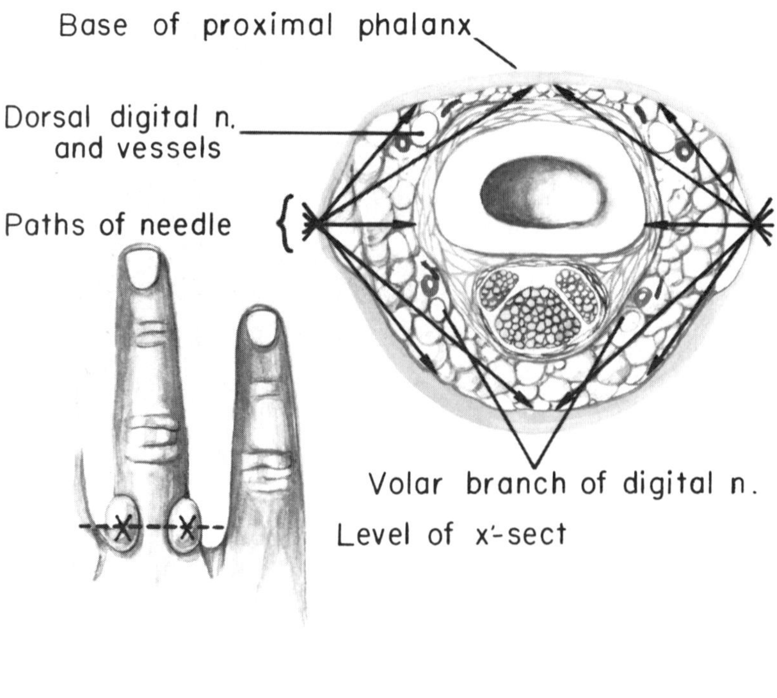

FIGURE 6–4. Digital block.

These nerves can be easily blocked at the base of the finger and toe.

Lidocaine can be used in 0.5% to 1% concentration. Whether solution ought to contain a vasoconstrictor is debatable. We have always used 1:200,000 epinephrine without complications. Skin wheals are raised in the interdigital folds, on each side of the base of the digit. Using a 25- or 30-gauge needle, a ring of anesthetic solution is then placed around the finger or toe from the skin to the bone by fanwise insertion of the needle from the points in the interdigital folds (Fig. 6–4). The amount needed is usually 3 to 4 ml. The total volume injected should not exceed 8 ml per digit in order to avoid gangrene by unduly compressing the vessels. Operating analgesia is established in about 15 minutes and lasts 1 to 3 hours.

Block of the Ears

The auricle is mainly innervated by the great auricular nerve, a branch of the cervical plexus. It supplies the whole of the medial (posterior) aspect of the pinna and the lower part of its lateral (anterior) aspect. The anterior superior part of the lateral surface of the pinna is innervated by the auriculotemporal nerve, a branch from the mandibular nerve (third branch of the trigeminal nerve), which runs up immediately anterior to the external auditory canal. The concha is innervated by the auricular branch of the vagus which lies immediately anterior to the mastoid process behind the external auditory meatus.

The entire pinna can be anesthetized by circuminjecting its base, as shown in Figure 6–5.

The great auricular and auricular branches of the vagus nerve are blocked by the injection of about 1 ml of anesthetic solution into three or four sites over the mastoid process. The auriculotemporal nerve is anesthetized by the injection of about 1 ml into the junction between the bony and cartilaginous parts of the anterior wall of the auditory canal.

Block of the Lips

The upper lip can be anesthetized by introducing the anesthetic solution through two wheals near the buccal commissure and directing the needles toward the ala nasi (Fig. 6–6A). Block of the lower lip can be achieved by injecting

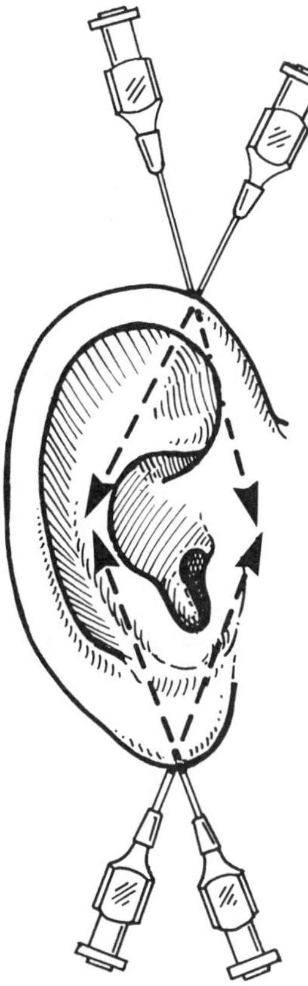

FIGURE 6–5. Block of the ear pinna.

from the middle line of the chin toward each buccal commissure (Fig. 6–6B).

Block of the Eyelids

Each eyelid can be anesthetized by means of field block through one needle insertion, as shown in Figure 6–7.

When the eyelid margin or the palpebral or bulbar conjunctiva is within the surgical area, instillation of 2 drops of 4% cocaine or 0.5% proparacaine hydrochloride (Alcaine, Ophthaine) is recommended. Cocaine has the advantage of a vasoconstricting action, but the record-keeping of its use, which is necessary to prevent its being taken away by former addicts, is cumbersome.

Anesthesia of the Male Genital Area

Excision of lesions on the scrotum and the skin of the penile shaft may be accomplished after

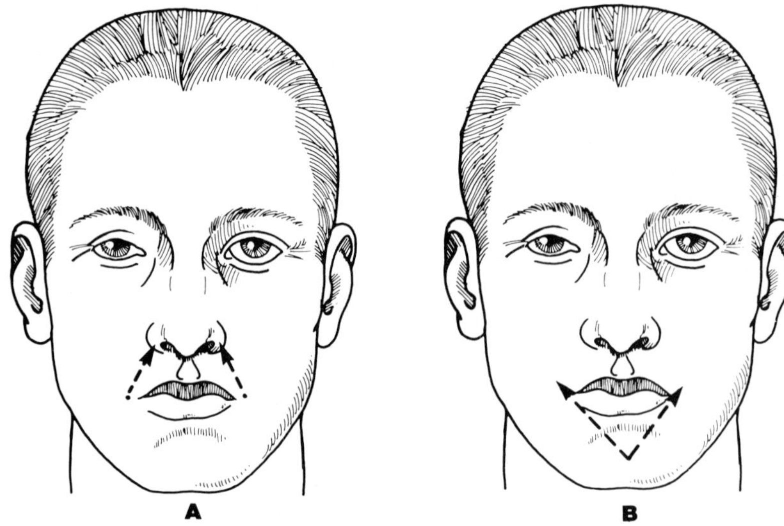

FIGURE 6–6. Block of the lips.

local infiltration, or by means of field block if the lesions are small. Regional block of the penis is required when lesions are numerous and when the glans penis, corpus spongiosum, corpora cavernosa, or frenulum are involved. Because of the anatomic innervation of the penis, block anesthesia requires a special procedure.

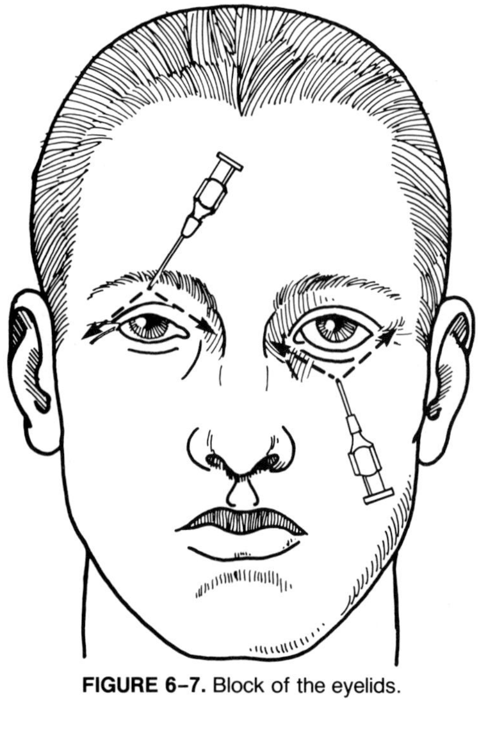

FIGURE 6–7. Block of the eyelids.

The penis is innervated by the right and left dorsal nerves, which are divisions of the pudendal nerves that originate from sacral regions (S2 to S4). The two nerves run distally along the dorsal aspect of the penis and give off smaller branches that innervate the ventral surface. This innervation supplies all superficial parts of the penis with the exception of the frenulum, which is supplied by branches that lie between the deep fascia (Buck's fascia) and the corpora cavernosa.

To undertake block anesthesia, the spines of the pubic bone are palpated. These two points are then connected by means of intradermal and subcutaneous infiltrations from the skin to the bone. Intradermal and subcutaneous infiltration is then carried out between each of the previous points and a third point at the median raphe of the scrotum at the base of the penis (Fig. 6–8A). Usually 10 ml or less of solution are needed for this maneuver.

The penis is then held in a vertical position and the anesthetic is injected fan-like from each of the three points at the base of the penis. The solution should reach the level between the deep fascia (Buck's fascia) and the corpora cavernosa (Fig. 6–8B). This last step requires the injection of 5 to 10 ml in order to anesthetize the frenulum. It may be omitted if the frenulum is not in the operative site. The total amount of lidocaine needed is, therefore, about 15 to 20 ml of 0.5% to 1% solution. Operating analgesia is established in about 15 minutes and lasts 1 to 3 hours. Stronger concentrations

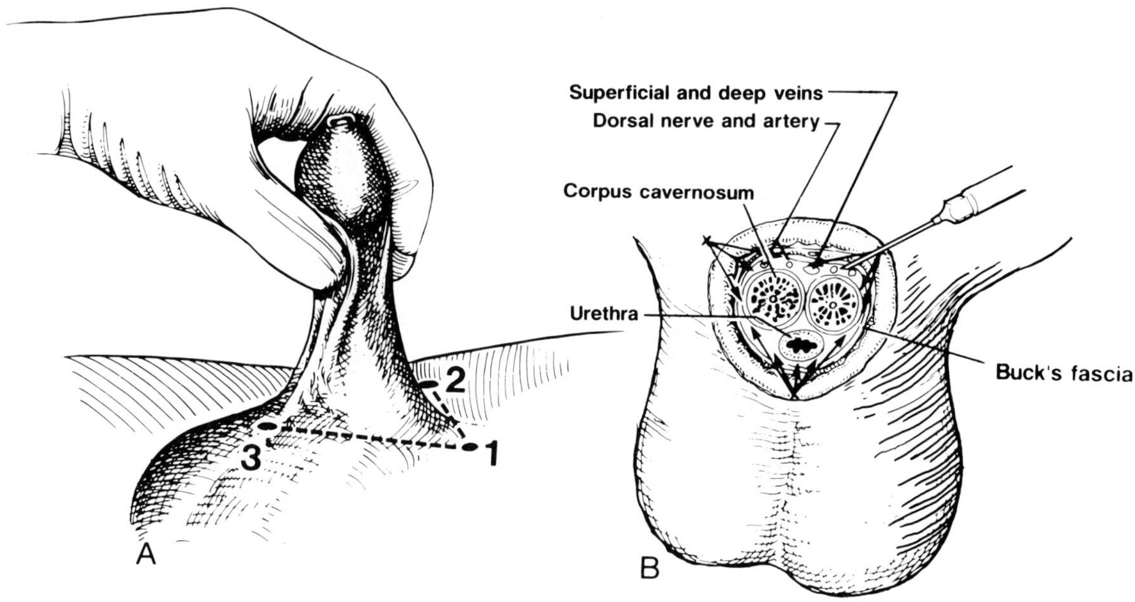

FIGURE 6–8. Block of the penis. (A) First step: ring of anesthetic around base. (B) Second step: infiltration of branches of the pudendal nerve underneath Buck's fascia.

and solutions containing epinephrine accomplish the longer limit. We routinely use 0.5% lidocaine with 1:200,000 epinephrine and have not experienced any adverse sequelae with this practice. It is convenient because it permits longer analgesia. Infiltration of the prepuce is to be avoided, since it has resulted in sloughing. Block of the penis is the method of choice.

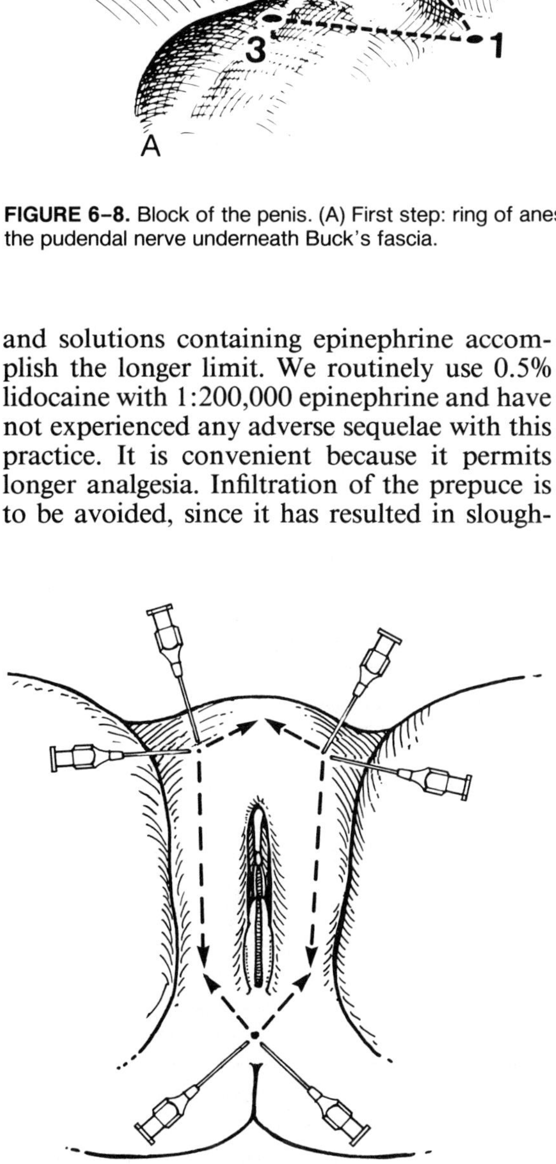

FIGURE 6–9. Block of the vulva by circuminjections.

Block of the Vulva

For obtaining biopsies and excising small benign growths or malignant neoplasms of the labia majora and minora, local infiltration or a field block may be used. The lesion is circuminjected with 0.5% lidocaine and 1:200,000 epinephrine. In the case of large or multiple lesions of the vulva, the solution can be injected in a circumferential fashion around the vulva after raising three or more wheals in the skin at the pubic eminences and the perineal body (Fig. 6–9).

REFERENCES

1. Adriani J: Labat's Regional Anesthesia, 4th ed. St. Louis: Warren H. Green, 1985.
2. Eriksson E (ed): Illustrated Handbook in Local Anesthesia, Chicago: Year-Book Medical Publishers, 1969.
3. Moore DC: Regional Block, 3rd ed. Springfield, Ill.: Charles C. Thomas, 1961.
4. Abadir A: Use of local anesthetics in dermatology, J Derm Surg Oncol 1:65–70, 1975.
5. Katz J: Regional Anesthesia. Norwalk, Conn. Appleton-Century-Crofts, 1985.

CHAPTER 7

Preoperative Evaluation of the Mohs Surgery Patient

Steven A. Proper, M.D.
Paul T. Rose, M.D.

The preoperative evaluation of the Mohs patient is outlined in this chapter. It is intended to serve as a simplified guide toward making the surgery as uneventful and safe as possible. The preoperative approach follows the conventional orderly clinical evaluation of a general surgical problem. The Mohs surgeon thoroughly investigates and documents the history, previous treatment, laboratory tests, gross appearance, and the histopathology of the skin cancer. A full discussion with the patient, and, if possible, the family is undertaken. The Mohs micrographic surgical technique is thoroughly explained including advantages, disadvantages, and possible complications. Other techniques should be discussed to inform the patient of alternative therapies.

Postoperative disposition including wound care is best planned at this time. Consultation with a reconstructive surgical specialist is initiated promptly if the Mohs surgeon anticipates that an extensive or high-risk postoperative wound will require major repair. An appointment should be scheduled so that the reconstructive surgeon may become familiar with the patient. If a more detailed examination of a particular organ system is required, such as the eye, ear, genitalia, or hands, the patient should be referred to the appropriate specialist.

As most of the patients are middle-aged or elderly, they are apt to be taking medications for cardiovascular conditions and other systemic diseases. Medical clearance for the forthcoming surgery should be obtained if the patient is at high risk for any complications.

HISTORY

Inquiries are made regarding the patient's general health, prior illnesses, hospitalizations, surgical procedures, and complications such as excessive bleeding and poor wound healing. Any history of skin cancer and treatment should be ascertained as well as a summary of the patient's dental history to disclose reactions to local anesthetics and coagulopathies.

Family History. The patient is questioned as to ancestry and genetic disorders, especially those that may relate to bleeding disorders or allergies.

Social History. When the patient is in a high-profile occupation or seems extremely vain, consider the possible effects that the surgery may have on both the physical appearance and the psyche. A consultation with a plastic surgeon and a mental health professional may be indicated.

Allergies. An essential part of the preoperative evaluation is to determine any factors that can affect the ultimate outcome of the surgery. Inquiries about allergies to antibiotics, antiseptics, tape, aspirin or aspirin-containing compounds, narcotics, and anesthetic agents must be clear and explicit. Furthermore, a detailed history of known allergies may be obtained from the family physician. Investigation should determine the specific anesthetic agent the patient may be allergic to and the type of reactions the patient has had in order to decide whether they were true allergies or adverse allergic reactions, e.g., nausea or vasovagal reaction. Palpitations may occur with epinephrine, and the patient may consider this an allergic reaction. In particular, we have found that patients confuse procaine (Novocaine) with lidocaine (Xylocaine).

Current Medications. Most elderly patients ingest multiple medications, the names of which they may not know. We encourage patients to carry a list of their medications, and when there is any doubt, an up-to-date list from the family and specialty physicians is obtained. Particular attention is paid to the use of anticoagulants, analgesics, antibiotics, antiarthritic medications, cardiac medications, respiratory medications, antidepressants, antihypertensives, steroids, tranquilizers, and antianxiety or sedative agents. Remember to inquire about over-the-counter products that may contain undesirable pharmacologic ingredients. Patients must be advised that aspirin and related products are dispensed in many different forms and may be part of medications which do not specifically state that they are aspirin-containing products (Fig. 7–1).

Review of Systems

Dermatologic. The patient is questioned about scars, wound healing, and keloid formation. Information regarding any prior radiation treatments to the skin of the head and neck for acne or tinea capitis should be elicited.

Cardiovascular. Assessment of the cardiovascular status of the Mohs surgery patient is essential because underlying heart disease is frequently encountered in the elderly. Inquiries about syncope, orthopnea, paroxysmal nocturnal dyspnea, chest pain, angina, valve disease, prosthetic valves, intermittent claudication, hypertension, palpitations, cyanosis, edema, hypertension, myocardial infarction, arrhythmias, pacemakers, bypass surgery, deep vein thrombophlebitis, and pulmonary embolism should be made.

Pulmonary. Although pulmonary complications are rare with Mohs surgery, they can arise in smokers and people who are over age 60, obese, or undergoing extended Mohs procedures. Pulmonary review should include questions relating to shortness of breath, chronic cough, asthma, emphysema, chronic obstructive pulmonary disease, and sarcoid.

Neurologic and Psychiatric. The neurologic and psychiatric review should note a history of seizures, cerebral vascular accidents, transient ischemic attacks, headaches, facial or other types of paralysis, paresthesias, tremors, insomnia, anxiety, psychiatric treatments, and hospitalization. Preoperative documentation of the disorders is helpful in deciding the type of anesthesia to use as well as to forewarn the Mohs surgeon of the operative risk to the patient. Special precautions can then be instituted to carry out the planned surgery more safely, including administering medications to circumvent headaches, seizures, and tremors.

Hematologic. Inquiries are made regarding easy bruising, excessive bleeding, the intake of any medications that may affect coagulation, specifically aspirin or sodium warfarin (Coumadin), epistaxis, anemia, hematologic diseases such as polycythemia vera, and platelet disorders such as von Willebrand's disease. It is important to ask whether there is a history of oncologic disease such as leukemia or lymphoma.

Ophthalmologic. Questions must be asked concerning the presence of glaucoma, changes in vision, or eye pain. The patient should also be questioned about the use of contact lenses, the presence of cataracts, excessive tearing, dryness of the eyes, and the date of the last eye examination. This is especially important in surgery on or near the eyelids.

Otolaryngologic. In cases where the ear or nose is involved, hearing loss, tinnitus, vertigo, otic discharge, ear infections, epistaxis, rhinitis, si-

MEDICATION PRECAUTIONS FOR MOHS SURGERY PATIENTS

These Instructions are to be Followed Before and After Your Surgery

For a two-week period prior to and after the scheduled date of your surgery, please do not take any medication that contains aspirin or aspirin-related products, such as ibuprofen (Motrin, Advil) as an ingredient. Aspirin has an effect on your blood's ability to clot and could increase your tendency to bleed at the time of surgery and during the postoperative period.

Please check the labels of all medications that you take, even those available without a prescription, to make sure you are not taking any aspirin or aspirin-like substances.

Please consult your physician before stopping any prescribed medication.

The following is a list of the more common medications and substances that can increase your tendency to bleed:

ADVIL	CHILDREN'S ASPIRIN	FELDENE	PHENAPHEN
ALCOHOL	CLINORIL	FIORINAL	QUAGESIC
ALKA SELTZER	CONGESPRIN	FOUR-WAY COLD TABS	ROBASISAL
ANACIN	COPE	IBUPROFEN	RUFIN
ANAPROX	CORICIDIN	INDOCIN	SINE OFF
ANAPROXN	COUMADIN	INDOMETHACIN	SINE AID
APC	DARVON	MECLOMEN	TRANDATE
5A.S.A.	DARVON WITH A.S.A.	MEDIPREN	TRENTAL
ASCODEEN	DOLOBID	MIDOL	TRIGESIC
ASCRIPTIN	DRISTAN	MOTRIN	TRILISATE
ASPIRIN	EASPRIN	NALFON	VANQUISH
BUFFERIN	ECOTRIN	NAPROSYN	VOLTAREN
BRUFEN	EMPIRIN	NORGESIC	ZACTRIN
CEPHALGESIC	EMPRAZIL	NUPRIN	ZORPRIN
CHERACOL CAPSULES	EXCEDRIN	PERCODAN	

If you are on any antirheumatoid, antiarthritic, circulation, or anticoagulant medication (e.g., Motrin, Naprosyn, Persantine, or Coumadin), please inform us.

If you need minor pain medication, please take acetaminophen (Tylenol) or another *nonaspirin* medication. Tylenol or Anacin-3 are available at your local pharmacy without a prescription and have comparable pain relief potential to that of aspirin. If you are allergic to acetaminophen (Tylenol) or unable to take it for other reasons, please notify us so that we might arrange for a suitable substitute.

FIGURE 7–1. Medication instructions for Mohs surgery patients.

nusitis, and changes in smell should be evaluated.

Physical Examination

Routine physical examination initially includes recording vital signs—pulse, respirations, temperature, and blood pressure. The examination should include a systematic evaluation of all organ systems with special attention to the regional lymph nodes.

Skin. The skin should be examined for any evidence of underlying dermatologic disease, e.g., candidiasis, psoriasis, herpes, infections, ecchymoses, scars, keloids, and any suspected malignant lesions. Scars may be a clue to prior surgeries, specifically cardiac and cosmetic, alerting the surgeon to a serious underlying medical condition or a demanding personality, respectively.

Eyes, Ears, Nose, and Throat. Complete evaluation of the eyelids and eyes in relevant instances, preferably by an ophthalmologist, is in order. Extraocular muscle movements should be tested as well as lacrimal function, if applicable. Particular note should be made of pupil size and shape as well as icteric sclerae or pale conjunctivae. All aspects of the auricular apparatus, including auditory function, are examined and tested, especially if it is the location of the lesion to be treated. Close attention should also be given to the postauricular sulcus and the ear canal. Nasal examination should include the nasal vestibule and palpation of the sinuses. The oral cavity should be inspected for signs of disease. With head and neck cancers palpation of the neck for suppleness and lymphadenopathy is important. Palpation of the thyroid and auscultation of the carotid arteries for bruits are recommended. When appropriate, consultation with an otolaryngologist should be obtained.

Lungs. Respiratory rate and abnormal breath sounds including crackles, rhonchi, or wheezes should be noted.

Heart. The surgeon should listen for significant murmurs and rhythm disturbances.

Neurologic Examination. A simple neurologic examination should assess the function of cranial nerves, especially the facial nerve.

ASSESSMENT OF OPERATIVE RISKS

The American Society of Anesthesiologists[1,2] classifies patients as follows:

- **Class I** Healthy—elective procedure
- **Class II** Mild to moderate systemic disease
- **Class III** Severe systemic disease—limited activities but not incapacitating illness.
- **Class IV** Life-threatening disease
- **Class V** Moribund, not expected to live without surgery

The majority of Mohs surgery patients fall into Class I or Class II status and do not experience significant operative morbidity. Since local rather than general anesthesia is employed, the operative risks of even Class III patients are greatly reduced. A discussion of the more significant preoperative considerations encountered by the Mohs surgeon is presented below.

Cardiac Disease

In general, the major cardiac risks are uncompensated congestive heart failure and myocardial infarction within the six months preceding surgery. It is advisable to have cardiac patients stabilized and appropriately treated prior to surgery. Medical clearance after appropriate evaluation by the Mohs surgeon should be obtained before surgery is undertaken in high-risk cardiac patients, especially if arrhythmias or prosthetic valves are present. Hypertension should be controlled before attempting even minor surgery. The small dose of epinephrine in the local anesthetic used in Mohs surgery should not present significant risk in patients with cardiac or hypertensive disease.

Caution should be used in patients who are on diuretics because of serum potassium changes. Alterations in serum potassium can precipitate or aggravate arrhythmias. A potassium level measurement is recommended in those patients who have not had a recent potassium level check or who have recently been placed on diuretics. Additionally, an electrocardiogram should be considered for patients who are over age 40 and who have not had a recent cardiogram.

Pacemakers present a special problem during the surgical procedure. Modern pacemakers are of the demand rather than the fixed-mode type. The demand type is sensitive to a prolonged electrocautery current. Short bursts of electrical current, however, are usually of no consequence as the pacemaker will revert to normal sensing upon discontinuance of the current.[3] Other techniques which permit the use of electrocautery include the use of a sterile magnet over the demand pacemaker, or the use of bipolar current. Nevertheless, the use of thermal cautery and vessel ligation are preferred in pacemaker patients.

Pulmonary Disease

Mohs micrographic surgery is generally performed under local anesthesia, and as such, there is very little risk of altering pulmonary function even in patients who are compromised. One should, however, be cautious in using analgesics and sedatives in these patients in order to avoid respiratory depression.

Asthmatic patients are at greater risk for respiratory compromise during surgery. Continuance of medication throughout the operative period is advisable. Familiarity with the use of the frequently prescribed asthmatic medications and their possible interactions with other drugs is highly recommended. In particular, caution must be exercised when administering epinephrine and other stimulants in the patient on aminophylline. Aminophylline is known to interact with erythromycin causing an increase in the serum concentration of aminophylline. Sympathomimetic bronchodilator drugs, e.g., epinephrine and ephedrine, can also increase the risk of cardiac arrhythmias in asthmatic patients. Chronic steroid therapy in these patients may necessitate an increased steroid dose prior to surgery to circumvent adrenal insufficiency.

Gastrointestinal Disease

Liver disease may lead to coagulopathies complicating the course of the Mohs surgery. Alcohol-induced cirrhosis contributes to increased bleeding because of an elevated prothrombin time. Chronic active hepatitis in an asymptomatic patient is a greater risk to the physician and staff rather than to himself or herself. A hepatitis B surface antigen test should be performed and, if positive, proper caution exercised with regard to risks to the surgical staff. Individuals involved in the surgical treatment of patients should be counseled about the advisability of receiving the hepatitis B recombinant vaccine. Although AIDS does not always present as a gastrointestinal problem, patients with a high suspicion of having AIDS constitute a special risk to the medical staff. Clinical and laboratory confirmation should be established so that proper precautions may be taken to protect the surgical team from exposure to the AIDS virus.

Renal Disease

Transplant patients are particularly susceptible to aggressive skin cancers while on immunosuppressive agents. Before treating these patients, it is recommended that the physician discuss the patient's problem with the nephrologist and transplant surgeon.

Endocrine Disease

Diabetes is the most common endocrine problem increasing surgical risk. The stress of surgery can cause an increase in the glucose level. Patients with glucose levels less than 300 mg/ml may be considered for Mohs micrographic surgery without significant operative risk, but higher levels are associated with greater risk of infection and poor wound healing. Diabetic patients on oral hypoglycemics are allowed to continue their oral dosage, while insulin-dependent patients undergoing Mohs surgery are requested to decrease food intake preoperatively and adjust their insulin dosage accordingly. Carbohydrate-containing snacks should be available in anticipation of the prolonged waiting period associated with the Mohs procedure. A fasting blood sugar report and a consultation with the patient's primary physician is judiciously recommended.

A history of chronic steroid use should alert the physician to the possibility of precipitating adrenal insufficiency during surgery. The administration of additional exogenous corticosteroids prior to the surgical procedure may be necessary.

Hematologic Disease

An anemic patient with hemoglobin less than 9 to 10 gm and a hematocrit less than 30 is a serious concern to the Mohs surgeon. Nevertheless, since Mohs micrographic surgery is usually associated with a minimal loss of blood, it is generally safe to operate on mildly anemic patients, particularly if preoperative coagulation screening tests are normal. The decision to discontinue anticoagulation medications, e.g., sodium warfarin, ibuprofen or aspirin, is advised at least 10 to 14 days prior to surgery.[4] In those patients who are taking sodium warfarin (Coumadin) for thromboembolic disease, the drug should be discontinued approximately 72 hours prior to surgery in order to allow for the prothrombin time to normalize. Dipyridamole (Persantine) is primarily a vasodilator but is capable of anticoagulation effects; consequently, patients are advised to discontinue its use 2 to 3 days prior to surgery. In all cases, the patient's primary physician should be consulted concerning any medication changes.

Antibiotic Prophylaxis

Transient bacteremia associated with skin surgery rarely occurs. Some physicians advocate the administration of antibiotic prophylaxis in patients with prosthetic valves or joints, rheumatic valve disease, and mitral valve prolapse as well as in those who are immunosuppressed. The standard regimen for endocarditis prophylaxis[5] is as follows: penicillin V—2 gm by mouth (PO) one hour before the procedure and 1 gm PO one hour after, or alternatively, penicillin G—2,000,000 units intravenously (IV) or intramuscularly (IM) 30 to 60 minutes before the procedure and 1,000,000 units IV or IM 6 hours later. For those patients allergic to penicillin, erythromycin may be given—1 gm PO one hour before the procedure, and 500 mg PO 6 hours later. These guidelines, however, have been advocated for dental procedures and, as yet, have not been established for cutaneous surgery. Consultation with the patient's family physician or cardiologist is strongly advised.

MISCELLANEOUS CONSIDERATIONS

Convenient transportation and accommodation arrangements are suggested for the Mohs surgical patient. Patients should not be allowed to leave the facility alone; arrangements must be made prior to the surgery to have the patient appropriately escorted home or to the hotel or hospital. Out-of-town patients are advised to remain in the city for several days postoperatively to receive optimal follow-up care. Convenient scheduling of the reconstructive surgery after the Mohs procedure will result in minimal delay, a more relaxed atmosphere, and increased patient comfort. Beverages, such as juices, and light snacks should be provided for the Mohs surgical patient while waiting for the histologic slides to be read.

Laboratory and Special Studies

As part of the routine work-up, the histopathologic slides of the lesion should be reviewed. Blood chemistries as well as complete blood count, prothrombin time, partial thromboplastin time, and urinalysis are performed when deemed appropriate, specifically when the patient is suspected of having coagulopathy or highly contagious disease, such as hepatitis or AIDS. Patients with a history of cardiac disease or those over age 40 should have a recent electrocardiogram reviewed. When the patient's disease appears to be extensive and bone invasion is suspected, computed tomography, magnetic resonance imaging, or other radiologic studies are in order.

Photographs

We recommend that photographs, both 35 mm and Polaroid, be taken of all lesions preoperatively and postoperatively (see Chapter 19). Photographs should also be taken to document any facial asymmetry that the patient may have prior to surgery. Permission to take photographs should be obtained in writing.

Preoperative Discussion and Informed Consent

Once the preoperative evaluation, history, and physical is obtained (Fig. 7–2), and the patient is considered to be a candidate for Mohs micrographic surgery, a discussion is again held with the patient and family (whenever possible) outlining the actual procedure and risks. A written preoperative informed consent is obtained at that time (Fig. 7–3). The patient is encouraged to ask any questions that may relate to the procedure and his or her disease. Preoperative verbal and written instructions relating to medications and any dietary restrictions are then given to the patient (Fig. 7–4).

Precautions and Contraindications to Surgery

Once the history and physical are completed, the Mohs surgeon may wish to speak to the patient's personal physician to discuss the proposed surgery and any current medical problems. The patient and family should be advised of any risk factors that may affect the surgery, complications that could occur, and adjunctive therapy needed to minimize operative risk.

Superficial cutaneous infection at the site of the lesion to be excised is not an absolute contraindication to surgery. The infection should be appropriately treated and cultured, whenever possible, prior to surgery.

There is no contraindication to Mohs micrographic surgery based solely on age. Caution should be used, however, in elderly patients with regard to their general health. In those

Presurgical and Anesthesia History and Physical.

Patient Name ____________ Pt. No. ______ Ht. ______ Wt. ______ Sex ____ Age ____

Diagnosis ____________________ Proposed Procedure ____________

Date of Interview ______________ Surgery Date ______________

1. History of disease: (To be completed by patient) Do you have or have you ever had any of the following:

Lung

Yes No

[ ] [ ] Bronchitis
[ ] [ ] Emphysema
[ ] [ ] Asthma
[ ] [ ] Chronic or A.M. cough

Vascular

[ ] [ ] High blood pressure
[ ] [ ] Heart attack
[ ] [ ] Heart murmur
[ ] [ ] Palpitation/irregular or fast heart beat
[ ] [ ] Heart disease or chest pain

Systemic

Yes No

[ ] [ ] Diabetes
[ ] [ ] Thyroid trouble
[ ] [ ] Kidney or bladder problems
[ ] [ ] Stomach or bowel problems
[ ] [ ] Hepatitis or jaundice
[ ] [ ] Convulsions or epilepsy
[ ] [ ] Fainting
[ ] [ ] Glaucoma
[ ] [ ] Alcoholism
[ ] [ ] Hepatitis B exposure
[ ] [ ] Aids or HIV exposure

A. Do you smoke? [ ] Yes [ ] No How much? ____________
B. (Women) Are you now pregnant? [ ] Yes [ ] No Expected date: ____________
C. Do you have bleeding tendencies? [ ] Yes [ ] No
D. Do you have any allergies? [ ] Yes [ ] No List ____________
E. Do you have any other disease, condition, or problem that we should know about? List: ____________
F. Have you ever had a blood transfusion? [ ] Yes [ ] No If yes, when? ____________

2. Drug History: (To be completed by nurse)

_____ Steroids
_____ Birth control pills
_____ Anticoagulants
_____ Aspirin
_____ Arthritic medications
_____ Tranquilizers
_____ Narcotics
_____ Cocaine
_____ Diabetic medication
_____ Thyroid medication
_____ Blood pressure medication
_____ Heart medication

List current medications: ____________

Nurse's signature: ____________

FIGURE 7–2. Presurgical and anesthesia history and physical.

3. Personal History: (To be completed by nurse)

A. Any physical limitations or special problems: ______
B. Prior surgery (within last 5 years): ______
C. Prior anesthesia date(s): ______ [ ] Local [ ] Regional [ ] General
D. Have you or your family ever had any unusual reaction to anesthesia, such as elevated temperature or difficulty in awakening? ______
E. Do you have dentures, loose teeth, capped, broken or missing teeth? [ ] Yes [ ] No
F. Do you have contact lenses? [ ] Yes [ ] No

4. Preoperative tests:

Chest x-ray ______ ECG ______ UA/SP. GR. ______ HGB/HCT ______ PT/PTT ______
Na^+ ______ K^+ ______ CO_2 ______ Cl^- ______ BUN ______ Glucose ______

5. Mental status: ______

Nurse's Signature: ______

6. Physical Examination: (To be completed by physician) B/P ______ T ______ P ______ R ______

HEENT ______

Neck ______

Pulmonary ______

Cardiac ______

Abdomen ______

Breast ______

Neuro ______

GU ______

Extremities ______

Skin ______

Medical clearance required? [ ] Yes [ ] No

Comments: ______

______

______ M.D.

I believe this patient will satisfactorily tolerate the proposed procedure using anesthesia.

______ M.D.

SURGICAL CONSENT

Patient: ______________________ No.: __________ Date: __________ Time: ____
I am scheduled for outpatient surgery at ______________________
on ______________, 19______ for ______________________

____

to be performed by Dr. ______________________ and/or such assistants as may be selected by him.

I have been informed, to my satisfaction, of the above-mentioned procedure(s), why it is necessary, the risks to my health if the condition remains untreated and what the procedure will entail.

I give my permission for the administration of presurgery medication and anesthesia (local or general) for outpatient surgery.

The advantages and disadvantages of outpatient surgery have been explained to me as well as the procedure which will be performed on me. I realize that following my operation, admission to a hospital might be advised. I agree to admission at ______________________, if in the opinion of my physician, such admission should be deemed advisable.

I also understand that during the course of the operation, unforeseen conditions may be revealed that necessitate an extension of the original procedure(s) or different procedure(s) than those planned. I authorize the above-named surgeon or his designee(s) to perform such surgical procedures as are necessary and desirable in the exercise of professional judgment.

I have been made aware that there are certain risks inherent to the performing of any surgical procedure such as loss of blood, infection, reactions to anesthesia, and the formation of thick or otherwise objectionable scars. Additionally, I acknowledge that the doctor has made no promises to me, oral or written, in connection with the operation. I recognize that every surgical procedure involves uncertainty and that no result can ever be guaranteed.

Following surgery, I will have a responsible adult drive me home as per previous arrangements. I realize that impairment of full mental alertness may persist for several hours following the administration of anesthesia, and I will avoid making decisions and taking part in activities that depend upon full concentration or judgment during that period.

I release the doctor from any responsibility that takes place as a natural complication of the procedure. I also realize that it is my responsibility to keep postoperative appointments. If I feel that any problems exist, such as bleeding or infection, or if I have any doubts, I am to contact the doctor as soon as possible.

For the purpose of advancing medical education, I consent to photographing and/or video recording of the operation provided my identity is not revealed by the pictures or descriptive text accompanying them. I consent to the disposal of any tissue which is removed in accordance with accustomed practice and procedure.

______________	______________________
Date	Patient or Guardian (Relationship)
______________	______________________
Witness	Physician

FIGURE 7–3. Surgical consent form.

PREOPERATIVE INSTRUCTIONS

1. Eat a light breakfast if you are scheduled before 12:00 noon. You may have decaffeinated coffee, juice, and toast.
2. Take your regularly prescribed medications, although aspirin and aspirin-containing medications (e.g., Alka Seltzer and decongestants) should *not* be taken for 10–14 days prior to surgery. Please check all medicine labels. If you are unsure, please call for instructions. Please bring your medications with you on the morning of surgery. Advise your physician of any over-the-counter medications that you regularly take.
3. We recommend a shower the evening or morning before surgery and freshly laundered clothes to help reduce the chances of you getting an infection. Wear a shirt or blouse that buttons up the front.
4. Do not apply make-up, cremes, or shaving lotion, etc., to the affected area.
5. A container for contact lens or dentures should be brought.
6. On the day of surgery, you must be accompanied by a family member or friend. Medicated patients will *not* be allowed to drive themselves home, and all patients must be escorted when leaving this office after surgery. If we need to call for your ride after the procedure, bring the names and phone numbers.
7. You will be here several hours on your surgery day.
8. Please call our office if you get sick between now and the time of your surgery.
9. Please call our office if you have any questions. Our phone number is listed below.
10. Take two multiple vitamin tablets each day for 7 days prior to surgery. These should contain vitamins A and C and zinc (e.g., Zbec or Centrum). Do *not* take vitamin E.
11. If you are allergic to any medications or have any sensitivities, please notify us immediately.
12. You will receive a phone call from this office concerning your scheduled surgery. If you do not receive this call at least 3 days prior to the scheduled procedure, please call our office and leave your name and number and our patient care coordinator will return your call.

FIGURE 7–4. Preoperative instructions.

who are severely debilitated, an alternative therapy may be considered if an extensive procedure may cause unfavorable sequelae.

There is no contraindication with regard to mental status changes. Patients who are disruptive or disoriented may require appropriate medication before Mohs micrographic surgery can be performed.

Pregnancy is not a contraindication to Mohs surgery since the surgery is performed under local anesthesia. However, in the present medicolegal climate, it may be wise to postpone surgery until after delivery.

Mohs micrographic surgery is an extremely safe procedure; however, medical complications can occur. The preoperative evaluation should be designed to detect factors that could lead to complications that hinder the surgical procedure and course of healing.

A frank and open discussion to fully inform the patient regarding the forthcoming Mohs surgery will establish a more comfortable and trusting rapport between the surgeon and the patient.

REFERENCES

1. Elliot DL, Tolle SW, Miller SH, et al.: Medical considerations in ambulatory surgery, Clin Plast Surg 10(2):295–308, 1983.
2. Dripps RD, Lamont A, Eckenhoff JE: The role of anesthesia in surgical mortality, JAMA 178:261–266, 1961.
3. Fullerton DA, Harken AH: Cardiac insufficiency. In Wilmore DW, et al. (eds): Care of the Surgical Patient, vol 2. New York: Scientific American, 1989, p. 7.
4. Davies DW, Steward DJ: Unexpected bleeding during operations: Role of acetylsalicylic acid, Can Anaesth Soc J 24:452–458, 1977.
5. Shulman ST, et al.: Prevention of bacterial endocarditis, Circulation 70:1123A, 1984.

CHAPTER 8

Medical Complications and the Mohs Surgery Patient

Steven A. Proper, M.D.
Paul T. Rose, M.D.

Dermatologic surgeons are familiar with surgical complications such as hemorrhage, infection, and nerve damage. However, medical complications occasionally occur. Nonhospital-based Mohs surgeons should be especially familiar with them.

Optimal treatment for medical complications begins with adequate preparation to deal with some acute emergencies which may occur intraoperatively and postoperatively. It is recommended that every office be staffed with a crash cart or emergency kit (e.g., Banyan Emergency Kit, obtainable from the Banyan International Corporation, Abilene, Texas 79604) and that office personnel be adequately trained in basic life support and, if possible, advanced cardiac life support (see Fig. 8–1). All members of the surgical and office staff should be acquainted with the phone number and procedures for obtaining local emergency personnel from the fire department or from a local emergency medical service (EMS) station or hospital. Early recognition of these medical complications is an integral part of the complete care of the surgical patient. In this chapter, some intraoperative medical complications, including their presentation, etiology, and immediate management, are briefly reviewed.

CARDIOVASCULAR SYSTEM

Angina

Angina pectoris may be associated with atherosclerosis, coronary artery spasm, platelet aggregation, or embolism. The Mohs patient with underlying cardiac disease may be at greater risk of angina in protracted and extensive procedures. Factors that increase the risk of precipitating an anginal attack include: (1) the use of epinephrine, which increases both heart rate and blood pressure, (2) the physical stress and anxiety of surgery, and (3) significant blood loss with hypovolemia. Patients at high risk for angina include those with hypertension, hyperlipoproteinemia, glucose intolerance, obesity, and hyperthyroidism.

The clinical presentation is usually that of substernal chest pain. The sensation of dull pressure, tightness, heaviness, sharp pain, or shortness of breath comes on suddenly and lasts from 30 seconds to 30 minutes. Diaphoresis, nausea, vomiting, and numbness may also accompany an attack. Occasionally, jaw, abdominal, and left arm pain may indicate an anginal attack or an acute myocardial infarction. The differential diagnosis includes intestinal gas, dysphagia, pulmonary hypertension,

ADVANCED CARDIAC LIFE SUPPORT

Guidelines for Asystole

If rhythm is unclear and possibly ventricular fibrillation (VF), defibrillate as for VF. If asystole is present[a]

↓

Continue CPR

↓

Establish IV access

↓

Epinephrine, 1:10,000, 0.5 to 1.0 mg IV push[b]

↓

Intubate when possible[c]

↓

Atropine, 1.0 mg IV push (Repeated in 5 minutes)

↓

(Consider bicarbonate)[d]

↓

Consider pacing

Asystole (cardiac standstill). This sequence was developed to assist in teaching how to treat a broad range of patients with asystole. Some patients may require care not specified herein. This algorithm should not be construed to prohibit such flexibility. Flow of algorithm presumes asystole is continuing.

[a]Asystole should be confirmed in two leads.

[b]Epinephrine should be repeated every five minutes.

[c]Intubation is preferable; if it can be accomplished simultaneously with other techniques, then the earlier the better. However, cardiopulmonary resuscitation (CPR) and use of epinephrine are more important initially if patient can be ventilated without intubation. (Endotracheal epinephrine may be used.)

[d]Value of sodium bicarbonate is questionable during cardiac arrest, and it is not recommended for the routine cardiac arrest sequence. Consideration of its use in a dose of 1 mEq/kg is appropriate at this point. Half of original dose may be repeated every 10 minutes if it is used.

Reproduced with permission from Sotelo-Albarran R, Atkins JM, Bloom RS, et al.: *Textbook of Advanced Cardiac Life Support.* Copyright 1987, American Heart Association.

FIGURE 8–1. Advanced cardiac life support: Sequence for asystole. (Reproduced with permission from *Textbook of Advanced Cardiac Life Support,* 1987. Copyright, American Heart Association.)

pulmonary emboli, pleurisy, pneumothorax, peptic ulcer disease, esophageal reflux, and visceral spasms of the esophagus or the pancreatic or gallbladder ducts. Immediate treatment should include supplemental oxygen and nitroglycerin sublingually, 0.3 to 0.6 mg given at 5-minute intervals. If the symptoms do not remit after two to three sublingual tablets of nitroglycerin, EMS should be notified and an intravenous (IV) line established, if possible.

Myocardial Infarction

Myocardial infarction (MI) may present as angina. The classical clinical presentation is often that of substernal chest pain lasting longer than 30 minutes. Pain radiating to the left arm or jaw, dyspnea, diaphoresis, nausea, and vomiting may also herald the occurrence of acute MI. Approximately 20% of myocardial infarctions are painless, especially in diabetic patients, and recognition can be established only if an electrocardiogram (ECG) monitor is functioning or cardiac enzymes are drawn post facto.[1] Other symptoms include a change in the previously stable pattern of the anginal pain, e.g., increase in severity, the occurrence of chest pain at rest for the first time, and chest pain unrelieved by nitroglycerin. Physical findings may include diaphoresis, pallor, crackles in the lower posterior lung bases, an S_4 gallop, and an apical systolic murmur.

Immediate management of the MI patient begins with nitroglycerin sublingually, 0.3 to 0.6 mg. If pain resolves quickly with nitroglycerin, infarction is unlikely. Caution should be exercised in administering nitroglycerin to patients who are hypotensive. Nasal oxygen should be administered at 2 to 4 liters per minute. Morphine sulfate is the drug of choice for analgesia in acute MI and is administered in small doses of 2 to 5 mg intravenously. It may be repeated at 5-minute intervals. Morphine has analgesic properties and increases venous capacitance, which reduces venous return and preload, thereby reducing systemic vascular resistance and ultimately diminishing myocardial work load. Pain is alleviated, anxiety decreases, excretion of catecholamines is diminished, and blood pressure is lowered. With administration of nitroglycerin and diuretics, hypotension may occur. The resultant hypotension should be treated with appropriate and cautious fluid administration and the patient repositioned with the head down and legs elevated. It is rarely necessary to use a pressor agent. Atropine may be used if bradycardia and hypotension occur concomitantly. Respiratory depression can occur with morphine, and naloxone (Narcan), 0.8 mg IV may be given as a narcotic antagonist. EMS and cardiology service should be called as soon as possible once MI is suspected.

Cardiac Arrhythmias

A detailed discussion of cardiac arrhythmias is beyond the scope of this book. Although most of the arrhythmias encountered in the Mohs surgical setting are not usually associated with significant morbidity, the physician should have a system in place to stabilize the patient and obtain emergency medical assistance.

Cardiopulmonary Resuscitation

Cardiopulmonary resuscitation (CPR), for the patient with cardiac arrest and life-threatening arrhythmias, should be familiar to any physician and staff who is performing surgery in the clinical office setting. In the Mohs surgery office setting, a witnessed arrest will be the rule rather than the exception, if it occurs, the pulse should be checked initially. If no pulse is present, a precordial thump should be delivered and an IV line started whenever possible. Ancillary personnel should be advised to notify EMS. While the IV line is being placed, CPR should be performed without interruption.

Initiation of CPR should be directed to the ABCs, i.e., establishment of an *a*irway, rescue *b*reathing, and attainment of an effective *c*irculation. The patient should be on a solid level surface. Any foreign obstructions should be manually cleared, and the American Heart Association's jaw-chin lift is utilized to prevent the tongue from blocking the airway. Either mouth-to-mouth or a ventilating bag (Ambu bag) should be used to deliver four full breaths initially into the patient's airway in order to maintain positive pressure and prevent airway collapse. Dentures should be left in place because they help form an airtight seal. Suction apparatus, if available, is helpful in case of vomiting. If an endotracheal tube is available, it should be placed to establish adequate ventilation. The carotid artery pulse should be checked intermittently. If no pulse is found, continue the orderly sequence of CPR and initiate chest compressions and ventilation. If an ECG monitor is present, it should be set up to monitor the patient as soon as possible. With two rescuers, a rate of 60 compressions per minute with one ventilation delivered for every five compressions can be established. With one rescuer, the rate should be 80 compressions per minute with two ventilations administered every 15 compressions. The carotid pulse should be monitored to establish the effectiveness of cardiopulmonary resuscitation. Pupils should be checked for reactivity as an indication of adequate oxygenation. An intravenous access line and ECG monitoring should now be secured. As soon as possible, 100% oxygen should be administered; the ventilating bag mask provides an excellent administration technique for supplemental oxygen. Continue uninterrupted CPR until the EMS arrives.

If the physician is familiar with advanced cardiac life support (ACLS) techniques and the appropriate equipment is available, the established therapeutic guidelines should be followed (Fig. 8–1).[2]

Congestive Heart Failure

Congestive heart failure is caused by the inability of the myocardium to adequately perfuse oxygenated blood to meet the metabolic requirements of the body. The Mohs surgeon may observe congestive heart failure in the elderly. Patients complain of dyspnea on exertion, orthopnea due to the increased venous return in the recumbent position, and paroxysmal nocturnal dyspnea.

On physical examination, the physician observes tachypnea, tachycardia, and venous distention of the jugular veins. Crackles and wheezing may be present (cardiac asthma). On cardiac auscultation, there may also be an S_3 gallop, cardiac murmur, and paradoxical splitting of the S_2 heart sound. Right ventricular failure is characterized by peripheral edema, hepatosplenomegaly, and hepatojugular reflux.

Treatment is based on removing the excess fluids with diuretics, providing adequate oxygenation with supplemental oxygen, and the use of vasodilators. The treatment is best performed in a hospital setting, but the Mohs surgeon may have to initiate treatment in the office.

Pulmonary Edema

Pulmonary edema is associated with severe left ventricular dysfunction manifested by marked dyspnea. On auscultation, moist crackles are apparent with an increase in the pulmonary second sound and often an S_3 gallop.

Treatment should begin with oxygen at 1 to 2 liters per minute by mask or nasal prongs. The patient should be placed in a semi-Fowler's position and an IV provided through which the patient should be given 40 to 100 mg of furosemide (Lasix). In the emergency setting, morphine 2 to 4 mg IV may also be administered. The patient should be hospitalized as soon as possible.

Hypertension and Hypertensive Crisis

Many patients suffer from hypertension. This is especially so in the middle-aged and elderly who comprise the majority of Mohs surgery patients. Hypertension is commonly divided into four categories: mild or moderate, severe, accelerated, and acute hypertensive crisis. Moderate and severe hypertension are very often easily treated with oral medications and do not usually require hospitalization. The Mohs surgeon may find it beneficial to delay surgery until the patient's blood pressure can be controlled.

Hypotension

Hypotension may be due to blood loss, vagal stimulation, decreased cardiac output, congestive heart failure, and endocrine or metabolic disorders such as adrenal deficiency or dehydration. Similarly, drugs either taken by the patient or provided by the physician for sedation and pain management may contribute to hypotension. Clinically, patients may feel weak, faint, and diaphoretic. At times they may experience shortness of breath. The physician is advised to seek out the appropriate cause of the hypotension and treat accordingly. For example, simple dehydration is treated with 5% dextrose in water with 0.45% or 0.9% saline.

Syncope

Syncope is the temporary loss of consciousness due to a reduction in cerebral perfusion. The etiology of syncope may be cardiac related, cerebrovascular, or most commonly, vasovagal. Vasovagal episodes of syncope relate to reduced venous return and are evident with Valsalva's maneuver, such as during coughing, defecation, or micturition. Vasovagal syncope may occur with external stimuli such as psychophysiologic events (e.g., the sight of blood, the stress of a surgical procedure, or other emotional factors). Clinically, the patient may experience weakness, light-headedness, nausea, vomiting, pallor, and diaphoresis. Patients who experience vasovagal syncope have dilated pupils upon loss of consciousness as well as bradycardia and hypotension. Seizure-like activity may occasionally be seen, but this is brief and usually without a postictal state.

For vasovagal syncope, the patient should be placed in the supine position with legs elevated. Ammonia salts may be useful, and the patient should be provided with oxygen, if necessary, and reassured.

PULMONARY AND RESPIRATORY SYSTEM

Aspiration. Aspiration may be associated with nausea or vomiting which may be secondary to anxiety or due to medication reactions, e.g., analgesics. Aspiration can also occur with seizures. Aspiration is most likely to occur when the patient is sedated. Crackles, rhonchi, wheezing, coughing, and dyspnea may all be present. If the patient is supine, the physician must make sure that the head is turned to the side to avoid further aspiration and to clear the airway of any debris. Concomitantly, the physician may have to use suction to remove the aspirated debris. The patient should be given oxygen 5 to 10 liters per minute by nasal prongs or Venturi mask and hospitalized, but if the respiratory status is severely compromised, intubation may be required.

Asthma. Asthma may be caused by extrinsic or intrinsic factors that lead to bronchial spasm and increased secretion of mucus. This further leads to airway obstruction and air trapping. Treatment begins with oxygen supplied at 2 to 4 liters per minute via nasal prongs or Venturi mask. The Venturi mask may have to be used when up to 40% inspired flow of oxygen (FIO_2) is needed. If the patient becomes obtunded, intubation is required. Once an airway is established, an IV line should also be placed and the patient hospitalized.

Chronic Obstructive Pulmonary Disease. Patients with chronic obstructive pulmonary disease (COPD) who undergo Mohs micrographic surgery may have exacerbation of their disease from the stress of the surgical procedure or may have difficulty with the body positioning required for the surgery. These patients have decreased lung volume caused by loss of lung parenchyma or decreased lung compliance. There are essentially two types of COPD patients: "blue bloaters," who have chronic bronchitis and often peripheral edema, and "pink puffers," who have emphysema and appear thin and malnourished. To compensate for hypoxia and chronic shortness of breath, pink puffers will often purse their lips and breathe with the use of accessory muscles.

Initially, oxygen should be provided by nasal prongs at 1 to 2 liters per minute or a Venturi mask at 24% to 28%. It is imperative to avoid decreasing the hypoxic drive by providing oxygen at too high a concentration. At times it may be necessary to have suction available to clear the airway, and bronchodilators, such as aminophylline, may be needed.

Pulmonary Embolism. Patients undergoing Mohs surgery may be at risk of pulmonary embolism in prolonged procedures when they have underlying risk factors. The risk factors include obesity, hematologic disease (e.g., polycythemia), heart disease (e.g., atrial fibrillation), and congestive heart failure. Patients with a prior history of deep vein thrombosis, pulmonary embolism, thrombophlebitis, varicosities, neoplastic pancreatic disease, and trauma to the lower extremities are at increased risk.

Once a pulmonary embolism is suspected, the patient should be given oxygen at 5 to 10 liters per minute and kept comfortable. The physician should arrange for immediate hospitalization.

Hyperventilation. Patients who experience hyperventilation often complain of anxiety and sudden onset of shortness of breath, and may experience paresthesias. Psychogenic hyperventilation must be differentiated from true pathologic dyspnea. With psychogenic hyperventilation, there is improvement with exercise, and the patient can often be calmed down enough to allow for speech. The treatment for hyperventilation is primarily reassurance and encouraging the patient to breath into a closed system, i.e., a rebreathing bag, to raise the carbon dioxide level.

NEUROLOGIC SYSTEM

Seizures. Seizures can occur during any surgical procedure and may have multiple etiologies, including primary neurologic disease (e.g., brain lesions), cerebrovascular accidents, meningitis, or encephalitis. Secondary causes include metabolic diseases, such as hypoglycemia, and alcoholism. The vast majority of seizures cease over a 30- to 90-second period and is usually of the grand mal type.

The initial treatment is to maintain the airway. Clinicians are cautioned not to insert a tongue blade through clenched teeth as this may cause breakage of teeth. One should consider placing an intravenous line. If the seizure ceases no further treatment is required except to stabilize the patient and consider neurologic evaluation.

Cerebrovascular Accidents. Cerebrovascular accidents (CVA) are characterized by a neurologic deficit that lasts more than 24 hours and involves a focal cerebrovascular area. Cerebrovascular accidents are usually acute and occur in two forms, thrombosis or embolism.

Patients experiencing CVA often have a history of transient ischemic attacks. Thromboembolic-induced strokes evolve over hours to days and the neurologic deficit begins as a minimal dysfunction which then progresses. Patients with arteriosclerotic heart disease, hypertension, and diabetes are at risk for this type of stroke. The physician should attempt to stabilize the patient and make appropriate arrangements for hospitalization and neurologic evaluation.

Transient Ischemic Attacks. Transient ischemic attacks (TIAs) occur suddenly causing a neurologic deficit that lasts less than 24 hours. The etiology may relate to carotid or vertebrobasilar disease, cardiac disease, hematologic disease, or mechanical problems, such as osteophyte formation impinging on vessels. Often patients are over age 40, which places them in the group most likely to require Mohs surgery. TIAs may occur either during the surgical procedure or postoperatively. Treatment of TIA requires that the patient be appropriately oxygenated and vital signs stabilized. A neurologic consultation should be sought, and hospitalization may be required.

Antianxiety Agents. Anxiety is a common problem associated with surgical procedures. Many patients are apprehensive at the prospect of undergoing surgery, and at times, it may be useful to provide patients with antianxiety pharmaceutical therapy. The common classification of antianxiety agents include the benzodiazepines, carbamates, barbiturates, and antihistamines. Benzodiazepines and carbamates produce a mild degree of sedation without impairing mental alertness or inhibiting psychomotor function.

Diazepam. Diazepam (Valium) works as an antianxiety agent by increasing inhibition and blocking cortical and limbic excitement by gamma aminobutyric acid. Diazepam has an onset of action within 30 to 60 minutes of an oral dose and the peak action is 1 to 2 hours. It has a half life of 20 to 50 hours.[3] As with other benzodiazepines, diazepam is contraindicated for patients with acute narrow-angle glaucoma or untreated open-angle glaucoma. It has interactions similar to other benzodiazepines and specifically may interact with digoxin causing decreased clearance. The metabolism of diazepam can be impaired by oral contraceptives and can decrease the therapeutic effects of levodopa. The usual dosage is 2 to 10 mg by mouth, intramuscularly, or intravenously. With large doses, cardiovascular collapse as well as respiratory depression can occur. Anexate, a benzodiazepine antagonist, unfortunately, is not available in the United States.[4] It is used at 0.5 to 0.6 mg up to 1 mg IV.

ENDOCRINE AND METABOLIC PROBLEMS

Obesity. Obesity is a significant risk factor in surgical procedures. The increased weight that the obese patient carries produces an increased myocardial work load. Decreased respiratory function with diminished vital capacity leads to hypoxia and hypercapnia (alveolar hypoventilation). Additionally, obese individuals may be difficult to maneuver into appropriate positioning on the surgical table. These patients should be monitored with regard to cardiac status and vital signs. Oxygen may be required if the patient has difficulty breathing while in a supine position.

Hypoglycemia. Hypoglycemia is defined as a plasma glucose of less than 50 mg/dl. In most instances, it is associated with either an excess of exogenous or endogenous insulin. It may, likewise, occur in the setting of excessive ethanol ingestion and, rarely, may be seen in patients with disorders such as Addison's disease and hypopituitarism. Hypoglycemia may also be associated with hepatic failure and dialysis for renal failure. Clinically, patients may demonstrate anxiety, tremor, palpitations, paresthesias, or changes in mental status and complain of hunger. On physical examination, there is tachycardia, but this may not be manifested if the patient is on a beta-blocker. Severe hypoglycemia can result in seizures and coma.

After confirmation of hypoglycemia, administration of readily usable glucose intravenously or sublingually is the treatment of choice. The Mohs surgeon should consider hospitalization even in cases in which the hypoglycemic episode is uncomplicated.

Thyroid Storm. Thyroid storm occurs with excessive release of thyroxine and usually occurs in a hyperthyroid patient who is undiagnosed or inadequately treated. Thyroid storm may be precipitated by stress, such as a surgical procedure, or infection. Clinically, patients may complain of fever, rapid heart beat, palpitations, anxiety, weakness, nausea, and vomiting. A goiter may be present, and the physician may note tremors, tachycardia, hypertension, and cardiac arrhythmias. The patient with thyroid storm requires immediate hospitalization.

Adrenal Insufficiency. Adrenal insufficiency occurs when there is an inadequate production of corticosteroids, usually associated with adrenal gland dysfunction, administration of exogenous corticosteroids, or hypothalamic-pituitary disease. Addisonian crisis may be caused by stress associated with infections, surgery, or hemorrhage. Patients may complain of general weakness, nausea, and vomiting. Clues to the diagnosis include hyperpigmentation at the palmar creases, buccal mucosa, and perioral areas. Addisonian crisis is accompanied by circulatory collapse, dehydration, nausea, vomiting, and fever. Laboratory data may reveal hyponatremia, hyperkalemia, azotemia, hypoglycemia, and a normocytic anemia. Immediate treatment consists of the administration of intravenous hydrocortisone sodium succinate (SoluCortef). Immediate hospitalization may be required.

Diabetes. Diabetes is commonly encountered in the elderly population by the Mohs surgeon. Specifically, the surgeon should be familiar with the factors that exacerbate the patient's diabetic condition in the Mohs operative setting, including anxiety and stress of surgery. In addition, the surgeon should be familiar with the side effects of oral hypoglycemic drugs.

DERMATOLOGIC AND IMMUNOLOGIC PROBLEMS

Anaphylaxis

Anaphylaxis is a profound allergic reaction that usually occurs within a short time of the patient receiving substances, usually parenterally. The medication is usually a protein, polypeptide, polysaccharide, or even an anesthetic agent or antibiotic. Anaphylaxis is usually a Type I immunologic reaction accompanied by the sudden release of histamine, serotonin, acetylcholine, various enzymes, and cell mediators. Clinically, the patient may complain of pruritus, rhinitis, anxiety, and flushing. Urticaria usually occurs and may be generalized. In extreme cases, there may be angioedema, cough, bronchial spasm, wheezing, cyanosis, and choking. Nausea and vomiting may accompany the reaction. Hypotension may occur leading to unconsciousness.

The treatment of anaphylaxis consists of placing the patient, if conscious, in a comfortable position. If unconscious, the patient is placed in a recumbent position with legs elevated. It is imperative that an airway be maintained and oxygen provided up to 10 liters per minute. In rare instances, intubation or even cricothyrotomy may be required. Epinephrine 1:1,000 should be administered 0.3 to 1 mg subcutaneously and repeated every 5 to 10 minutes if needed. In severe anaphylactic reactions, the physician should consider the administration of 0.1 to 0.3 mg of 1:1,000 epinephrine diluted in 9 ml of normal saline administered IV over 3 to 5 minutes. This may be repeated every 5 to 10 minutes. A continuous infusion can be set up with 1 ml of epinephrine 1:1,000 and 250 ml of 5% dextrose in water to yield a concentration of 4 μg/ml. This can be infused at 1 μg per minute and increased up to 4 μg per minute if needed. It is important to maintain the IV line and hydrate the patient with 5% dextrose in water with 0.45% normal saline. Diphenhydramine (Benadryl), 50 mg IV, should be administered as soon as possible. Steroids such as hydrocortisone sodium succinate (SoluCortef), 100 to 250 mg IV, or methylprednisolone sodium succinate (Solu-Medrol), 50 to 100 mg IV, may be given and repeated every 1 to 4 hours. In cases of severe wheezing, aminophylline can be administered with a loading dose of 5 to 7 mg/kg and a maintenance dose similarly administered, as in asthma or bronchial spasm. While measures are being taken to stabilize the patient, the staff should prepare to have the patient transferred to the hospital.

Urticaria and Angioedema

The onset of acute urticaria is sudden, occurring within minutes of the inciting agent, but can be delayed 24 to 48 hours. Angioedema involves swelling of the subcutaneous or submucosal tissues, usually with pruritus, lasting longer than 24 hours. The pathogenesis may be immunologic or nonimmunologic.

In the setting of Mohs surgery, most episodes of urticaria and angioedema relate directly to the use of medications or substances in the preoperative period or during surgery. In particular, one should suspect drugs such as penicillin, morphine, codeine, aspirin, or indomethacin as well as locally applied agents such as bacitracin or Neosporin.

Although urticaria and angioedema may not progress to an anaphylactic reaction, the physician must be prepared for such a possibility. In general, patients should be treated with epinephrine 0.5 ml of 1:1,000 subcutaneously. This may be repeated in 30 to 60 minutes. An antihistamine, such as diphenhydramine (Benadryl), 50 mg intramuscularly, should be given.

Contact and Irritant Dermatitis

Contact and irritant dermatitis are commonly encountered in the surgical patient and are usually due to a reaction to adhesive tape or topical antibiotic preparations applied to wound sites. The reaction must be differentiated from infection, i.e., impetigo. Most often, reactions follow the application pattern of the tape, ointment, or cream. There is no streaking as seen in cellulitis with lymphangitis, and the area is not usually tender. Treatment is based on elimination of the inciting agent. Patients are given topical steroids, and if there is any doubt about the etiology, they may be placed on systemic antibiotic therapy. Most commonly applied topical antibiotics include bacitracin, polymyxin, neomycin, and gentamicin. It should be remembered that bacitracin can produce anaphylactic shock, and that bacitracin and neomycin can co-react to cause allergic reactions. Gentamicin cross-reacts with neomycin. The administration of cross-reacting drugs, e.g., streptomycin in a neomycin-sensitive person, can produce a severe systemic eczematous dermatitis.[5]

OPHTHALMIC PROBLEMS

Glaucoma. The physician should be aware of the presence of glaucoma and avoid the use of epinephrine around the eye. The authors are aware of a case where a patient with undiagnosed glaucoma or subclinical glaucoma was injected with lidocaine and epinephrine in the periorbital area and subsequently developed acute glaucoma. Acute glaucoma is an ophthalmologic emergency, and as such, the patient should be referred immediately to an ophthalmologist.

ADVERSE REACTIONS TO LOCAL ANESTHETICS

Local anesthetics are divided primarily into amides, esters, and miscellaneous agents. Amides are metabolized in the liver and include drugs such as lidocaine; esters include drugs such as benzocaine and tetracaine.

Lidocaine. Lidocaine is administered at 0.5% to 2% solution with or without epinephrine. It has a rapid onset of action and has a duration of about 1 to 2 hours. The maximum dosage is approximately 300 to 500 mg when used in association with epinephrine. Epinephrine may be premixed with local anesthetics to provide vasoconstriction. Epinephrine, however, adds to the pain of injection because it must be buffered to a pH of 3 to 4.5 to allow for storage of the premixed solution. This acidity can be overcome by adding sodium bicarbonate as a buffer to neutralize the acidic pH before injection.

Toxicity can occur when the dosage is inappropriately high or when there is a decrease in liver clearance because of changes in hepatic blood flow or hepatic extraction. Congestive heart failure and cirrhosis can raise the blood level of lidocaine. Most of the toxic reactions that occur with local administration of lidocaine are due to inadvertent intravascular injection. At 4 to 6 μg per ml, serum lidocaine toxicity is usually manifested as an initial period of excitement, light-headedness, apprehension, disorientation, or euphoria. Patients may complain of a bitter taste and may experience tinnitus, chills, nausea, or vomiting. Convulsions may occur at a level of 8 to 12 μg/ml, but usually, a prodrome of slurred speech and tremor occurs first. Patients may become comatose, areflexive, and apneic. At 20 to 25 μg per ml, circulatory collapse can occur with myocardial depression and vasodilatation. Treatment requires the use of vasopressors, CPR, and appropriate therapeutic measures for circulatory collapse. If seizures occur, diazepam may be administered at 0.1 mg per kg IV.[6]

Prilocaine. Prilocaine has a duration of 1½ to 3 hours and a maximal dose of 300 mg without epinephrine (500 mg with epinephrine). Prilocaine is metabolized to O-toluidine, which can cause methemoglobinemia. Methemoglobinemia is treated with methylene blue, 1 mg/kg IV.

Mepivacaine. Mepivacaine is utilized at a dosage of 0.25% to 0.5% and has a slower onset and longer duration of action than prilocaine, lasting 4 to 8 hours. The maximal dose is 175 mg without epinephrine and 250 mg with epinephrine.

Etidocaine. Etidocaine is utilized as a solution of 0.5% to 1%. It has a slow onset and duration of action lasting 4 to 8 hours. Maximal dose is 200 mg without epinephrine and 300 mg with epinephrine. It can produce marked motor block without drowsiness at toxic blood levels. Etidocaine and bupivacaine are two to four times as potent as lidocaine and can produce seizures at blood levels of approximately one-quarter that of lidocaine.

Procaine. Procaine (Novocaine) is utilized as a 1% solution. It has a slow onset and short duration of action lasting 30 to 45 minutes. The maximum dosage is 500 to 1,000 mg. Procaine can be used for patients who have a history of malignant hyperthermia. This drug is rapidly metabolized and can cause allergic reactions in patients sensitive to para-aminobenzoic acid (PABA) and paraphenylenediamine.

Apart from local allergic reactions, procaine and other ester anesthetics can cause anaphylaxis and urticaria. These reactions may also be caused by the paraben and sulfa preservatives in the anesthetic agents. To avoid allergic reactions, alternative classes of local anesthetics may be substituted or, for a superficial surgery, the use of diphenhydramine (Benadryl) intradermally, an analgesic in preservative-free saline, saline alone, or a topical refrigerant is advised.

REFERENCES

1. Ferri FF: Practical Guide to the Care of the Medical Patient. St. Louis: C. V. Mosby, 1987, pp 94–102.
2. Sotelo-Albarran R, Atkins JM, Bloom RS, et al.: Textbook of Advanced Cardiac Life Support. American Heart Association, 1987, pp 235–248.
3. Blake GJ (ed): Physician's 1989 Drug Handbook. Springhouse, PA: Springhouse Corporation, pp 315–317.
4. Malamed SF: Sedation—A Guide to Patient Management, 2nd ed. St. Louis: C. V. Mosby, 1987, p 372.
5. Fisher AA: Contact Dermatitis, 3rd ed. Philadelphia: Lea & Febiger, 1986, pp 195–210.
6. Elliot DL, Tolle SW, Miller SH: Medical considerations in ambulatory surgery, Clin Plast Surg 10(2):295–308, 1983.

CHAPTER 9

Surgical Complications

Paul O. Larson, M.D.

Surgical complications are adverse events not essential to the surgical treatment. Complications include, but are not limited to, bleeding, hematoma, infections, wound dehiscence, disfiguring scars, and keloids. Unfortunately, surgical complications cannot be completely eliminated, although every effort should be made to anticipate and avoid them. Each complication, major or minor, should be critically reviewed and steps taken to eliminate them. In this chapter, we review common surgical complications and discuss methods of prevention and treatment.

PREOPERATIVE MEASURES

Preoperative medical evaluation and orders are covered in Chapter 7. Several points, however, are particularly important in minimizing surgical complications. Patients should be instructed to stop all aspirin- and ibuprofen-containing products 1 week prior to surgery to help prevent operative and postoperative bleeding.[1] The patients should consult their physicians prior to stopping any other anticoagulants.

Preoperative Antibiotics

Transient septicemia has been demonstrated following minor skin surgery by Halprin and colleagues[2] and Sabetta and Zitelli.[3] For this reason, patients with artificial heart valves or valve disease should be treated with prophylactic antibiotics.[4,5] Opinion varies as to whether patients with prolapse of the mitral valve or those with artificial hips and other orthopedic prostheses should be treated with prophylactic antibiotics. Documented risk or benefit data for prophylactic antibiotics under these circumstances is lacking.

INTRAOPERATIVE COMPLICATIONS

Complications resulting from Mohs surgery are few and usually minor. There are no published reports indicating the exact frequency. Severe, life-threatening situations do occur but are apparently rare.

Reactions to Local Anesthetics

Local anesthetics are infrequently associated with complications. The severity of adverse effects, however, is potentially so great that all surgeons using local anesthetics must know how to deal with them (see Chapter 8).

Bleeding

Bleeding is a part of all dermatologic surgery procedures. Bleeding cannot be considered a complication unless it is uncontrolled or results in hematoma. Small-vessel bleeding is routinely handled by pressure, spot electrofulguration, or hemostatic agents. Bleeding from larger vessels can usually be controlled by clamping with a hemostat and suture-ligating the vessel. If small arteries and veins are partially transected, the transection should be completed to allow the vessels to constrict and retract. The severed ends of the vessel are visualized and ligated. Excessive intraoperative bleeding may result from coagulation disorders. In patients with a history of bleeding problems, a complete blood count, platelet count, prothrombin time, partial thromboplastin time, and capillary bleeding test should be performed. If these are normal, significant bleeding is unlikely. Persistent bleeding can generally be handled by using a combination of electrofulguration and/or pressure. Other hemostatic agents that may be of help include absorbable gelatin sponges (Gelfoam), oxidized cellulose (Oxycel or Surgicel), microfibrillar collagen, or thrombin.[5]

Postoperative hemorrhage occurring after the surgical procedure is completed may result from relaxation of the arterioles after the effect of epinephrine has worn off, bleeding from insecurely ligated vessels, or as a result of a clot or crust retraction. Minor hemorrhage can usually be treated by having the patient hold firm pressure over the bleeding site for 5 to 7 minutes, resisting the temptation to "peek." If this is not effective, the patient should be reevaluated. Meticulous hemostasis, proper use of hemostatic agents, and pressure will usually prevent hemorrhage.

Nerve Injury

Injury to small terminal sensory nerves at surgical sites is unavoidable. Small terminal nerves generally regenerate without problems. During the period of regeneration, the patient may complain of anesthesia, hyperesthesia, itching, burning, or transient pain. The symptoms gradually subside over a period of 3 to 12 months. Neuroma formation may infrequently cause persistent pain at the site of nerve transection.

Transection of major nerves should be avoided if possible. Cancers may follow nerves, however, as the path of least resistance.[6,7] Preserving a nerve under these circumstances may invite further tracking along the nerve, resulting in major or unresectable disease. Janecka[8] recommends aggressive investigation of the entire length of the facial nerve in patients with progressive, unexplained facial nerve weakness. Mohs surgery allows examination of perineural tissue with the greatest likelihood of preserving normal areas of the nerve. If major nerves (e.g., the facial nerve) must be transected, every effort must be made to restore function. The patient should be seen in conjunction with a plastic surgeon to consider nerve grafting, a nerve crossover procedure, or muscle transfers.[8] Grafting of the nerves should ideally take place within 2 to 3 days of the nerve transection.

Surgical Mishaps

Injuries from mishaps may occur with any surgery. "Murphy's law" also applies to Mohs surgery; if you can think of a possible mishap, it will eventually happen. The best way to avoid mishaps is to anticipate all possible problems and structure the surgery to avoid them. Simple measures can be taken to protect both the safety of the patient and the surgical staff. With conscious patients, injury due to unanticipated movement is possible. An assistant should always maintain control of the patient during treatment. This may require only a light stabilizing pressure. The surgeon's hand or finger should be braced on the patient so that if the patient moves, the surgeon's hand and scalpel will be pushed away (Fig. 9–1). Patients who have difficulty in cooperating may have to be treated while under a general anesthetic in order to treat them safely.

Injury to the patient and surgical staff may occur from inadvertent scalpel or needle sticks. All instruments must be exchanged away from the patient, i.e., not over the patient's face, where a poor exchange may injure the patient. A simple, secure method of instrument transfer is illustrated in Figure 9–2. This method can be easily learned by all assistants.

POSTOPERATIVE COMPLICATIONS

Hematoma

Hematoma, the circumscribed accumulations of blood at surgical sites, is one of the more frequent complications of skin surgery. Hematomas usually form within several hours to several days after surgery and present as painful, expanding masses. Small hematomas around noncritical organs are usually absorbed without problems. Large hematomas may compro-

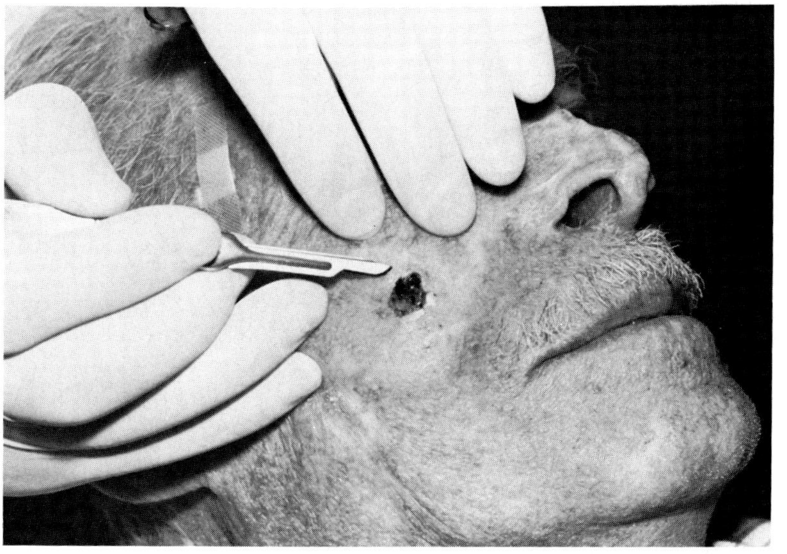

FIGURE 9–1. Surgeon's hand is braced so that unexpected movement will push the scalpel away from the patient.

mise vital structures, become infected, cause the loss of flaps or grafts, or eventually organize and calcify.[9]

Meticulous hemostasis must be practiced to prevent the formation of hematomas. Undermined skin edges must be examined by lifting and retracting the skin so that bleeding points can be visualized and electrofulgurated. Bleeding from arteries and large veins must be treated with suture ligature. Thrombin solution (100 to 1,000 units/ml) may be used if controlled capillary bleeding persists. Wounds to be grafted may be routinely treated with thrombin solution to prevent hematoma formation. In wounds in which hemostasis is difficult and fragile, a Penrose drain may be placed to facilitate drainage. Closed suction drainage with minidrains may also be used (Fig. 9–3). A step easily overlooked but extremely important is to apply pressure to the wound immediately after surgery. Pressure (up to 30 mmHg) can be maintained by applying a well-designed pressure dressing.[10] Stents are used to maintain pressure over skin grafts[11] or flaps. Superficial wounds that bleed persistently may be best left to heal by second intention. Aspirin or other blood thinners should be prohibited unless specifically prescribed by the patient's physician. The patient should be told to call if there is a persistent, distending pain that would suggest hematoma formation.

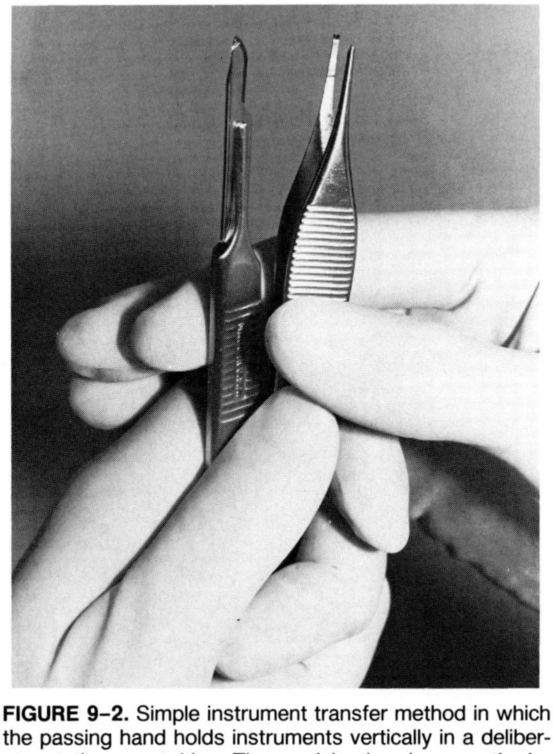

FIGURE 9–2. Simple instrument transfer method in which the passing hand holds instruments vertically in a deliberate, stationary position. The receiving hand grasps the instruments only after they have reached the stationary position.

The treatment of a hematoma depends on its size.[9] Very small hematomas mobilize and resolve without treatment. Larger hematomas or hematomas around vital structures should be drained. Large hematomas may serve as media for infection, prolong the healing process, alter or threaten vital structures, or result in hypertrophic scars or even organized calcified tumors. Hematomas occurring in the

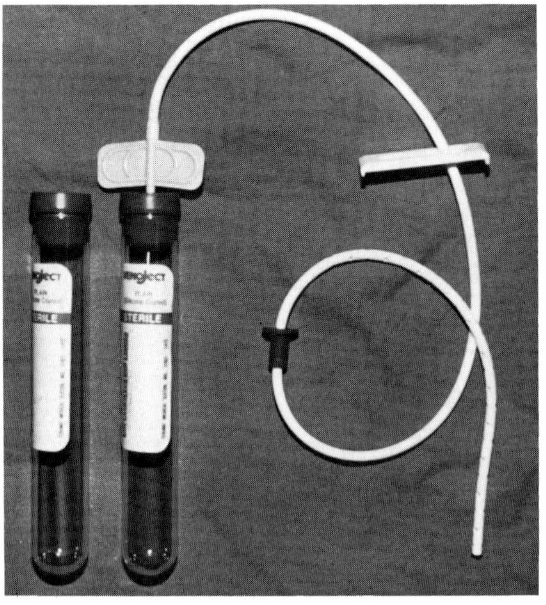

FIGURE 9–3. Mini-drain with vacuum tube used to facilitate blood drainage in primary closure or under flap.

immediate postoperative period should be drained and explored in order to stop the source of bleeding.

Postoperative Bleeding

The situation in postoperative bleeding is much the same as in the case of hematomas. Meticulous intraoperative hemostasis along with the judicious use of hemostatic agents and pressure is important to prevent bleeding. Most bleeding following superficial surgery is harmless but is dramatic and distressing to the patient. The patient should be told in advance of the possibility of bleeding and instructed on how to control it. This can routinely be done by the nursing staff at the time wound care instructions are given. Direct pressure should be applied to the site of hemorrhage and pressure maintained for 7 minutes without "peeking" to allow the completion of the clotting. If the patient experiences further bleeding, medical care should be sought.

Seroma

A seroma is the postoperative accumulation of serum under skin grafts or flaps.[12,13] Seromas form where serum accumulation is greater than the rate of its mobilization. Pressure is commonly applied via stents to prevent seroma from forming under grafts. Since seromas provide excellent culture media, and separate grafts from the wound bed, they should be drained.

Wound Dehiscence

Dehiscence is the separation of closed wound edges after sutures are removed.[9] Dehiscence may result from incomplete coaptation of the skin edges or necrosis of devitalized skin edges from trauma, excessive tension, or rough handling. In addition, hematoma formation, infection, or deficient wound healing from a metabolic problem can be factors. Meticulous attention to surgical detail is very important in preventing this event. Hemostasis must be complete, tissue handling must be gentle, and coaptation of wound edges must be precise. At the time of suture removal, proper judgment must be used to determine if the sutures are ready to be removed. It is best to partially remove them if the wound edges have not fused completely. The remaining sutures can be removed 3 to 7 days later. The wound should not be spread laterally when removing the sutures. Steri-Strips may be applied to give additional wound reinforcement. If wounds dehisce within 12 to 24 hours because the sutures unravel, the wound may be irrigated and resutured. If the dehiscence occurs later, it is best to allow the wound to heal by second intention.

Flap Necrosis and Graft Failure

Flap necrosis is generally related to faulty flap design. Excess stretching of the flap compromises microcirculation.[14] The flap must be designed to allow draping of the rotated skin into the defect without excess tension. If wounds cannot be closed without causing excessive tension, they may be partially closed, allowing a portion to heal by second intention. Skin grafts most frequently fail because of hematoma or infection (Fig. 9–4). Inadequate apposition of the graft to the wound bed, sheering motion, and seroma formation are other causes of failure. Prophylactic antibiotics may be used to help prevent wound infections. Stents are used over skin grafts, and occasionally over flaps, to prevent sheering motion and seroma. Stents

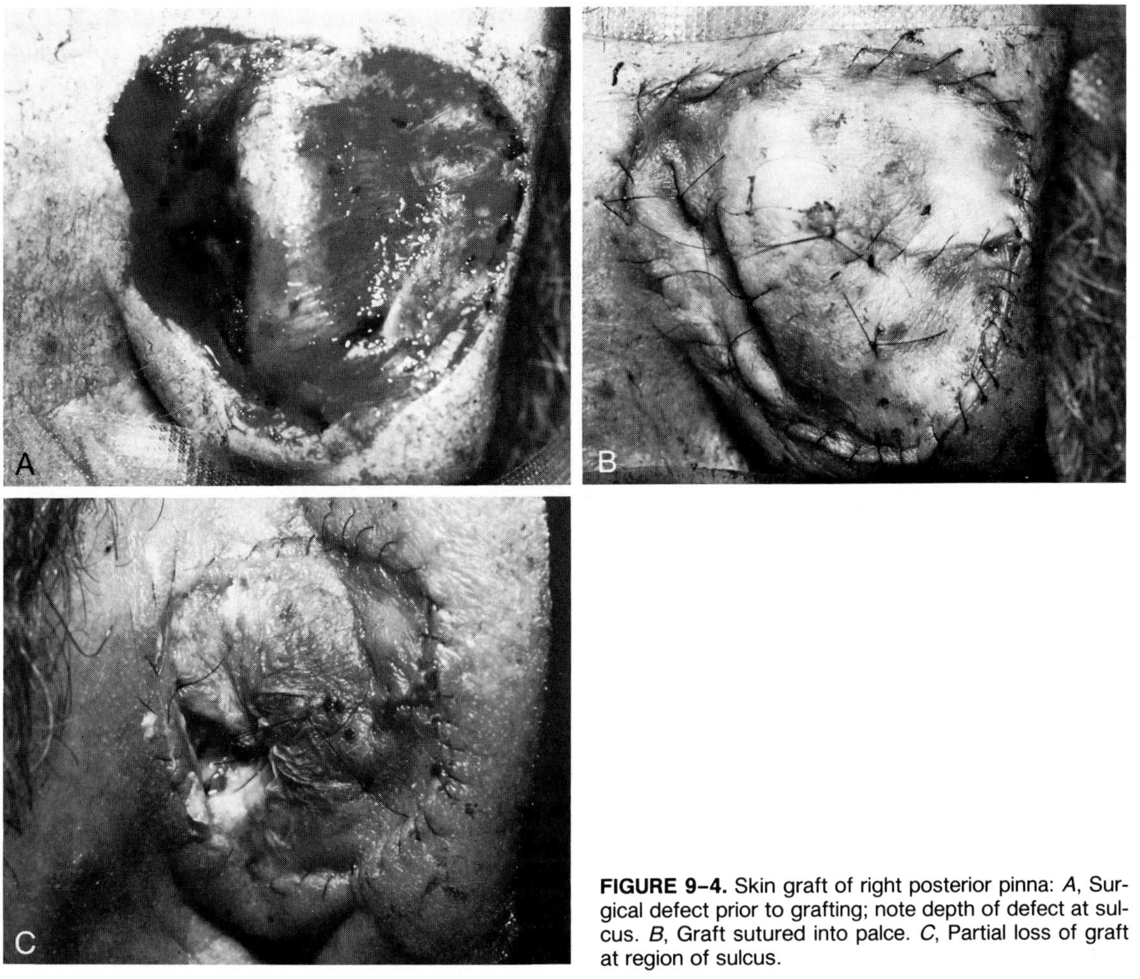

FIGURE 9-4. Skin graft of right posterior pinna: *A*, Surgical defect prior to grafting; note depth of defect at sulcus. *B*, Graft sutured into palce. *C*, Partial loss of graft at region of sulcus.

should be left undisturbed for 1 week before examining the repair.

Infection

Infected wounds become inflamed, tender, erythematous, and purulent. The patient may also become febrile. Most significant wound infections are caused by *Staphylococcus* and *Streptococcus* species. Infection after Mohs surgery is surprisingly infrequent. One would think that wounds left to heal by second intention would frequently become infected, but the reverse is true. Wounds closed over sequestered areas of devitalized tissue are more likely to become infected. Infected wounds must be drained in order to prevent abscess formation or spreading cellulitis. An iodoform gauze may be placed in an infected wound to assure continued drainage. The patient should be started on dicloxacillin sodium (or erythromycin if allergic to penicillin) while bacterial culture and sensitivity tests are pending.

Osteomyelitis is an uncommon occurrence following Mohs surgery.[15] Considering the frequency of bone manipulation in Mohs surgery, it is surprisng that infection is not more common. Healing by second intention allows for open drainage, which rarely results in osteomyelitis. Treatment of osteomyelitis consists of open drainage and appropriate antibiotics.

Other opportunistic infections have not been reported in Mohs surgery but remain a possibility, as in any other surgical procedure. An often overlooked potential complication is tetanus. Since tetanus is preventable, it is reasonable to check for immunization on a routine questionnaire.

Contact Dermatitis

Allergies, including contact dermatitis, should be screened for on a routine questionnaire. Although contact allergy is generally localized, it may become generalized and severe. Delayed hypersensitivity with first exposure develops about 1 week after exposure to the allergen. Contact dermatitis in an already sensitized patient may occur within 48 to 72 hours. Potential allergens include neomycin, bacitracin, polymyxin, tape, or hemostatic agents (Fig. 9–5). All nonessential agents must be stopped until the etiology of the allergy is clear.[16,17]

Excessive Granulation

Excessive granulation, or "proud flesh," occurs in the early healing phases after Mohs surgery when defects are left to heal by second intention. If the granulations become excessively elevated, they may interfere with wound healing. This occurs most frequently in wounds that are occluded and become macerated. If not too protuberant, the excessive granulation can be treated by instructing the patient to dry the wound. The wound is cleaned in the usual fashion, air-dried or dried with a hair dryer, a drying antiseptic applied, e.g., merbromine (Mercurochrome) or polymyxin B sulfate and bacitracin zinc (Polysporin) spray, and covered with a loose dressing. With simple instructions, patients become very adept at knowing when wounds are too wet or too dry. If granulation becomes excessive, it can be cauterized with the silver nitrate stick, or curetted.[18] It is important to cauterize only the granulation tissue and not the epithelializing tissue at the margins because this delays the healing.

Keloids and Hypertrophic Scars

Keloids and hypertrophic scars are a bane to all surgeons. A hypertrophic scar forms excess, dense, fibrous scar tissue that eventually involutes, while a keloid persists or increases with time.[19] Infrequently, keloids may become massive and disfiguring. Hypertrophic scars occur more frequently on convex surfaces or areas subjected to continuous tension, such as the posterior arms or shoulders, or on the sternum. Keloids are more frequent among blacks and may occur in areas of tension but also on other areas such as the ear lobe or nape. It is difficult to prevent keloids or hypertrophic scars.[20] Identifying high-risk patients and discussing the possibility of keloids and hypertrophic scars with them prior to surgery is very helpful. Meticulous surgery, minimal destruction of tissues, hemostasis, closure of wound edges without tension, and intralesional injection of steroids may all help prevent hypertrophic scars

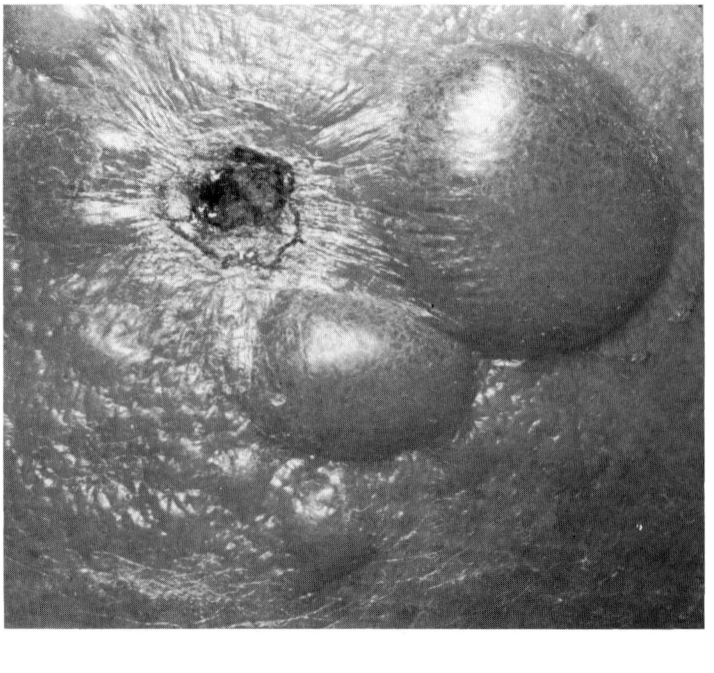

FIGURE 9–5. Contact dermatitis at minor excision site secondary to oxidized cellulose used for hemostasis.

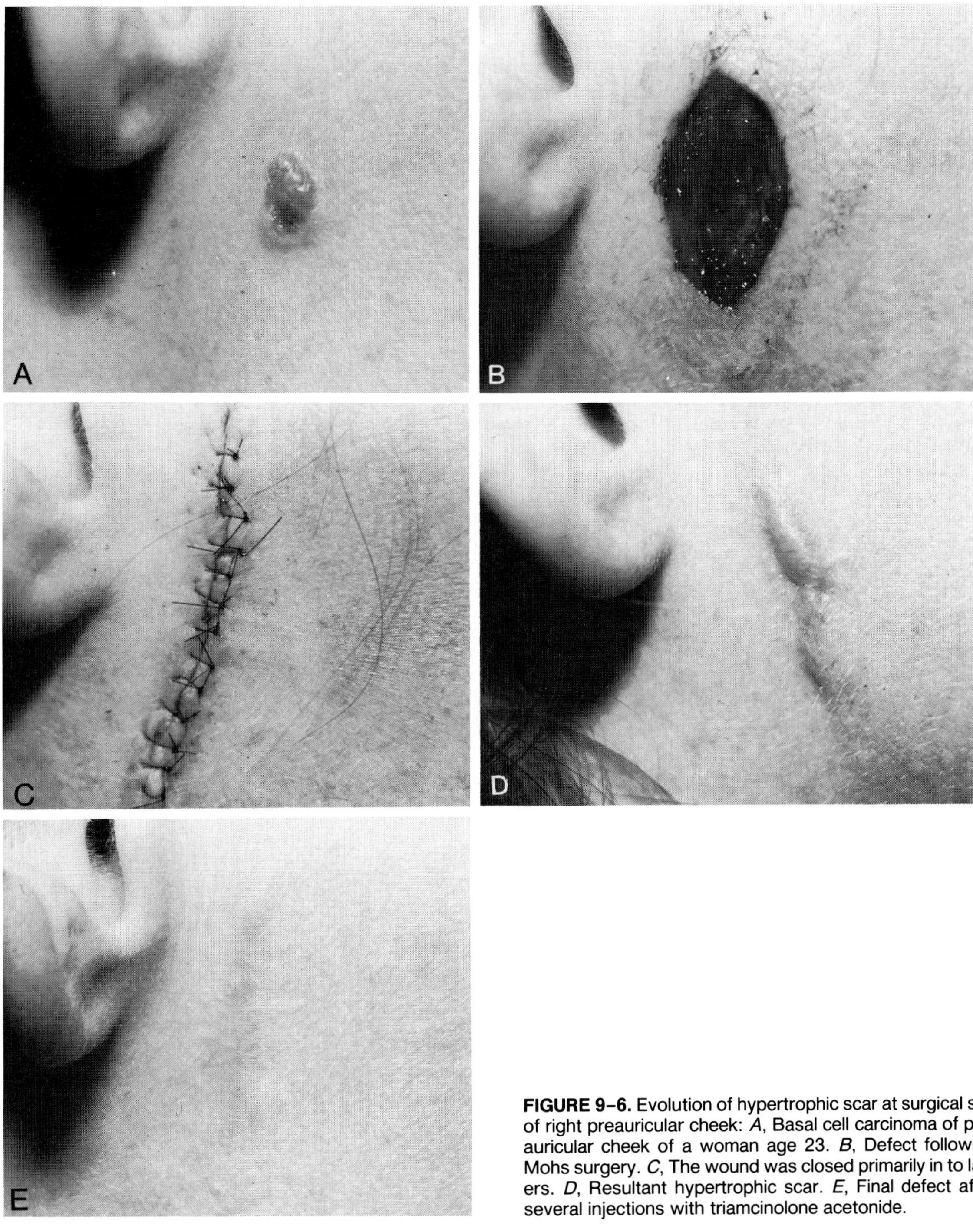

FIGURE 9–6. Evolution of hypertrophic scar at surgical site of right preauricular cheek: *A*, Basal cell carcinoma of preauricular cheek of a woman age 23. *B*, Defect following Mohs surgery. *C*, The wound was closed primarily in to layers. *D*, Resultant hypertrophic scar. *E*, Final defect after several injections with triamcinolone acetonide.

or keloids. Despite these measures, keloids and hypertrophic scars form in certain individuals. Keloids may be treated with intralesional steroids, topical steroids, pressure, and reexcision, all with varying degrees of success or failure. Hypertrophic scars will flatten with time (Fig. 9–6).

Scar is a repair process that occurs following all surgical procedures. The scar restores tissue strength and integrity to the injured skin.[21]

However, excessive scar tissue may interfere with normal function and may be disfiguring, painful, unsightly, and distressing to the patient. Mohs surgery has undergone criticism for years from some medical groups because of the scars that result from surgery. This is often a misunderstanding of the role of Mohs surgery that deals with tumor extirpation, not wound repair. Another misunderstanding is that Mohs surgery often leaves too large a hole, which may be hard to repair. With Mohs surgery, the size of the defect is dictated by the size of the cancer. Therefore, the idea that Mohs surgery causes too large a defect is a result of ignorance of skin cancers and their potential for inapparent actual extent.

Steps should be taken to minimize scar formation in Mohs surgery wounds. This requires a great deal of experience and judgment. Wounds that result from the primary excision of skin cancers which can be easily closed, should be closed. Although there may be great pressure to do so, not all wounds should be closed primarily. Small, superficial wounds in concave areas often heal better by second intention. Defects at the site of multiple recurrences of skin cancers should usually be left to heal by second intention, delaying repair for 6 to 12 months. Wounds that may entail considerable functional or cosmetic deficiency should be closed in an uncomplicated fashion, a final cosmetic repair being delayed for an appropriate period of time. Defects requiring major reconstruction should be covered with a skin graft to prevent skin contracture, with the major repair delayed for 6 to 12 months to allow for tumor surveillance.

The possibility of scar tissue should be dealt with in a frank and direct way with the patient. A plan of action should be discussed in the event that an unacceptable scar occurs. Irregularity of wounds can often be easily dealt with by curettement or spot dermabrasion of the margins. Areas of tension may be relieved by placing a relaxing Z-plasty. Tissue protrusions may be removed by simple excision and excessive fat may be excised (Fig. 9–7). Violaceous or red coloring during the immediate postoperative period may be covered with Blenderm or Dermablend. Early referral to a plastic sur-

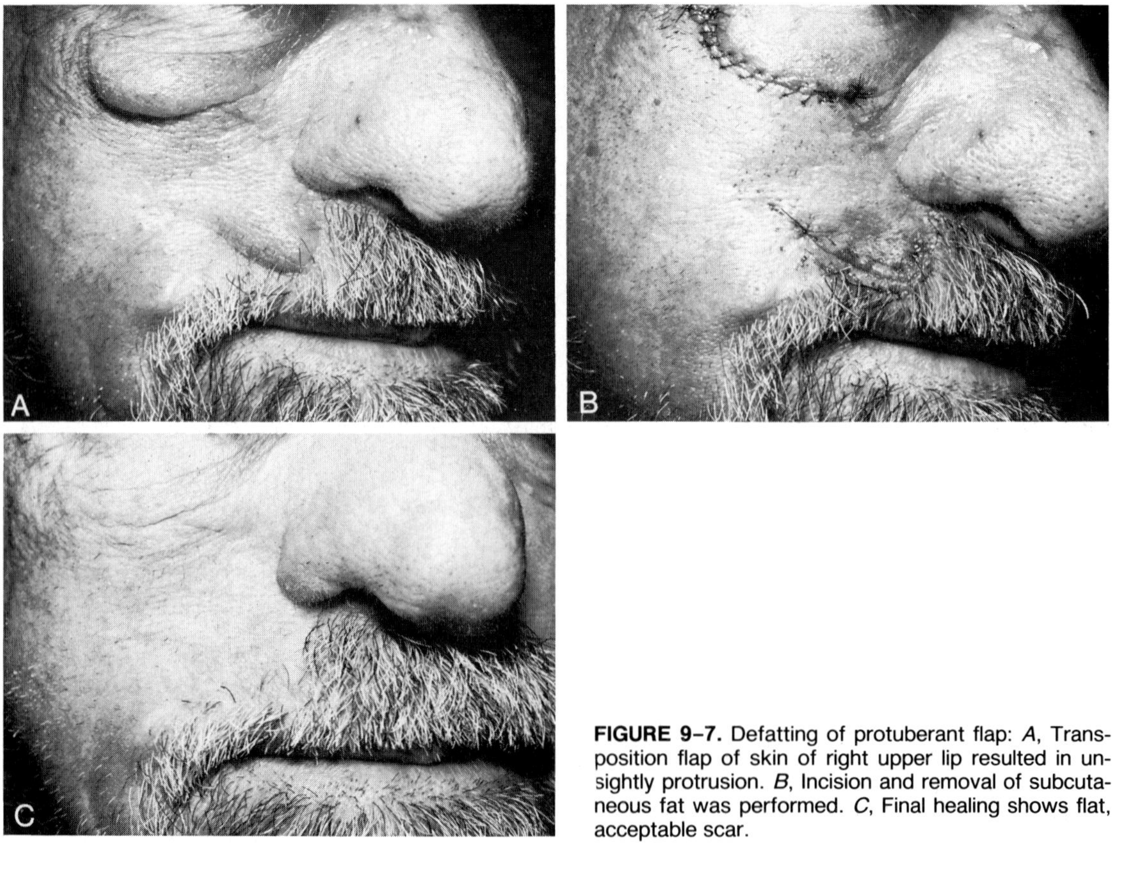

FIGURE 9–7. Defatting of protuberant flap: *A*, Transposition flap of skin of right upper lip resulted in unsightly protrusion. *B*, Incision and removal of subcutaneous fat was performed. *C*, Final healing shows flat, acceptable scar.

geon, otolaryngologist or other specialists should be done when appropriate and indicated.

Hyperpigmentation and Hypopigmentation

Pigment changes at the surgical scar can be distressing to the patient.[22] Hypopigmentation is more common in fair-skinned patients and is generally well covered with cosmetics, such as Blenderm or Dermablend. Preventing a tan by the use of sunscreens reduces the contrast between normal or more deeply pigmented skin and the hypopigmented scar. Hyperpigmentation around a surgical site is more likely to occur in dark-skinned individuals. These patients should be advised to use sunscreens regularly at the surgical site to prevent hyperpigmentation. Treatment with bleaching agents has not been particularly successful in our experience.

COMPLICATIONS BY SITE

Eye

The eye is perhaps the most critical of all the special organs treated by Mohs surgeons. Surgery around the eye, as with all other types of

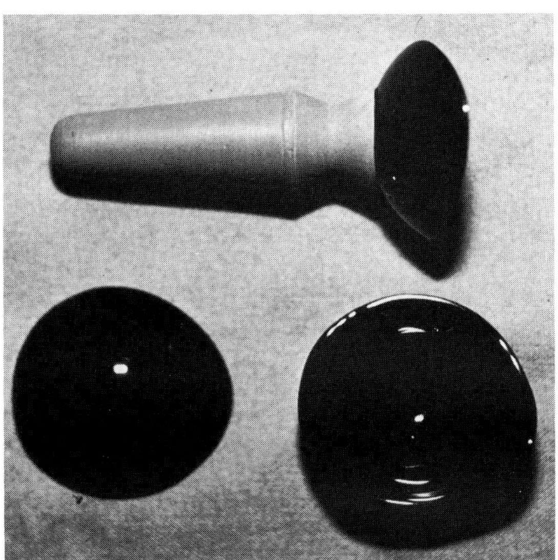

FIGURE 9–8. Eye shields used to protect cornea during periocular surgery; rubber suction device facilitates placement and removal.

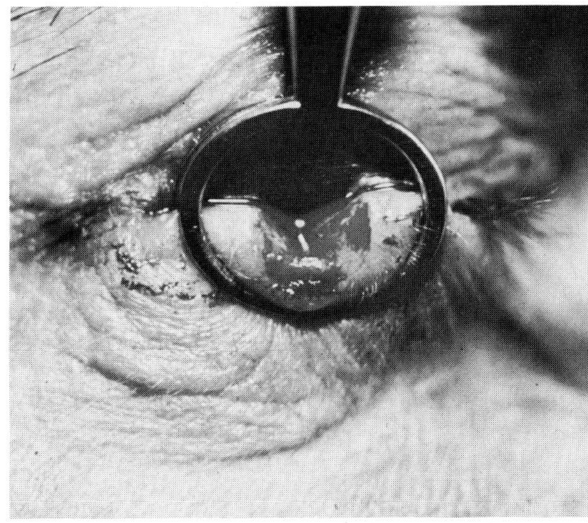

FIGURE 9–9. Chalazion clamp facilitates secure bloodless grasp of the eyelids.

surgery, should be done in a deliberate, coordinated fashion to prevent surgical mishaps. Movements should be deliberate and controlled and the operating routine should be well established. Movement behind the operator or assistants should be prohibited to prevent bumped elbows. The cornea must be protected during periocular surgery. This may be done by having the patient close the eye, holding the lid closed, or taping the lids closed during a periocular procedure. An eye shield (Fig. 9–8) or chalazion clamp (Fig. 9–9) can also be used for secure protection. Topical anesthesia is required when ocular shields or chalazion clamps are used. As ocular anesthesia interferes with the normal protective reflexes, the eye should be patched until normal corneal sensation is restored.

The lacrimal drainage system can be injured during periocular surgery. Because skin cancer will take the path of least resistance, e.g., tear ducts, injury to this system may be unavoidable in extirpating the tumor.[23] Strictly speaking, such injury should not be called a complication if it is unavoidable. Dr. Mohs has approached these injuries to the lacrimal system in a simple fashion.[24,25] If defects are in the convexity of the inner canthus with little tendency to cause ectropion, Dr. Mohs allows them to heal by second intention. Tearing usually is not a problem, and cosmesis is generally excellent. If complications develop, the patient is referred to an oculoplastic surgeon for repair. Steps must be taken to prevent unnecessary injury to the lacrimal system. Tear ducts may be cannulated prior to excision of cancers near the lacrimal puncta.[26] If the tear ducts are severed during surgery, they may be cannulated postoperatively to preserve the remaining system.[27] Repair of the tear ducts is highly specialized and requires the expertise of an oculoplastic surgeon.

Ectropion is the eversion of the lower eyelid and may occur after Mohs surgery of the eyelids (Fig. 9–10), resulting in exposure and inflammation of the palpebral conjunctiva.[23] The patient may also complain of chronic tearing, especially when exposed to wind. This is because the puncta are not properly apposed to the globe, causing incontinuity of the tear drainage system. Surgical defects of the lower eyelid and upper cheek should be managed in a fashion that avoids ectropion. Small wounds may be left to heal by second intention. Larger wounds may require primary closure, flaps, or grafts. In closing a wound primarily, vertical, downward traction of the lower eyelid can be converted to an upward push by closing in a vertical fashion. Flaps and grafts on the lower eyelid should be slightly overcorrected in order to push the eyelid into apposition with the globe. Correction of ectropion should be done by the oculoplastic surgeon.

Corneal abrasions can result from superficial trauma to the cornea from surgical mishaps, incorrect bandaging, or self-induced trauma to the cornea while the cornea is anesthetized. Cornea abrasions may be extremely painful. To prevent corneal abrasions, eye patches should be applied with the lids fully closed,[28] periocular bandages must not rub the cornea, and periocular suture material must be left long and the tails taped or sutured away from the eye. Abrasions are usually treated with topical antibiotics, mydriatic agents, eye patches, pain medications, and close follow-up with an ophthalmologist.

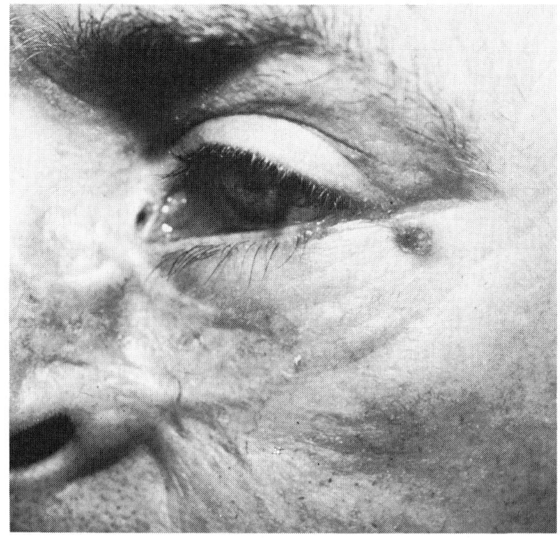

FIGURE 9–10. Postoperative ectropion following Mohs surgery of left lower eyelid in patient with extensive basal cell carcinoma.

Exposure keratitis is due to corneal irritation by excessive drying, which may occur after paralysis of the eyelid muscles or from injury to or extensive loss of the eyelid. Constant drying of the cornea produces scarring, which may lead to loss of vision. Exposure keratitis is a preventable complication. Patients with eyelid paralysis or lid injury must be instructed to keep the eye lubricated, blink the eye manually, if necessary, and close or tape the eyelids shut at night. A temporary tarsorrhaphy[29] may be necessary to protect the cornea when there is extensive loss of the eyelid. The cornea may also be protected by using clear plastic moisture chambers, e.g., Guibor Bubble or Pro-ophta (Pro-ophta adhesive eye dressing with transparent shield, Selomas Inc., Wilmington, DE),[28] as shown in Figure 9–11.

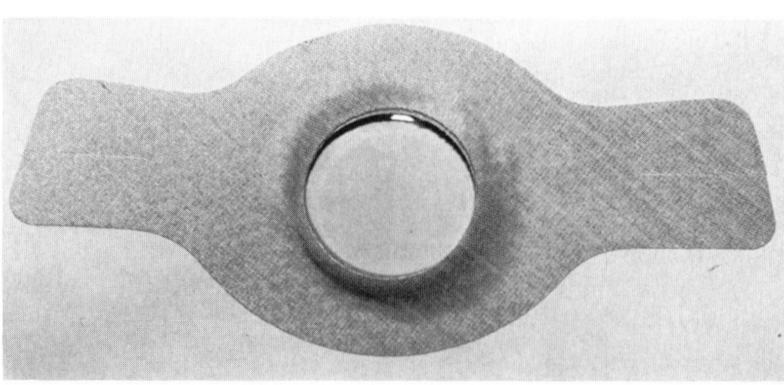

FIGURE 9–11. Pro-ophta moisture chamber used to prevent exposure keratitis.

Nose

Nasal complications are primarily related to scarring. Extensive excision may result in twisting and deformity of the nose. Healing by second intention may result in stenosis and fixed reduction of the nasal air passage. Stenosis may be prevented or treated by flap repair or grafting. Trap-dooring causes reduced air flow through a nostril during inspiration as a result of collapse of the ala. Trap-door defects may be repaired by surgically stabilizing the ala. Major reconstruction of nasal defects requires the care of a highly specialized otolaryngologist or plastic surgeon.

Ear

Infections have already been mentioned as a complication of Mohs surgery, but ear infections merit special mention. Chondritis of the external canal is a difficult problem to manage. In addition to possible infections with the usual gram-positive organisms, the ear may become infected with *Pseudomonas aeruginosa* (Fig. 9–12), which is very difficult to control and, until the recent advent of ciprofloxacin hydrochloride, required hospitalization for intravenous antibiotic treatment. Wide incision and drainage of the external canal is necessary to treat aggressive bacterial chondritis. A rare complication of ear infections is malignant otitis, which dissects cranially along the cartilaginous canal and may be fatal.[30]

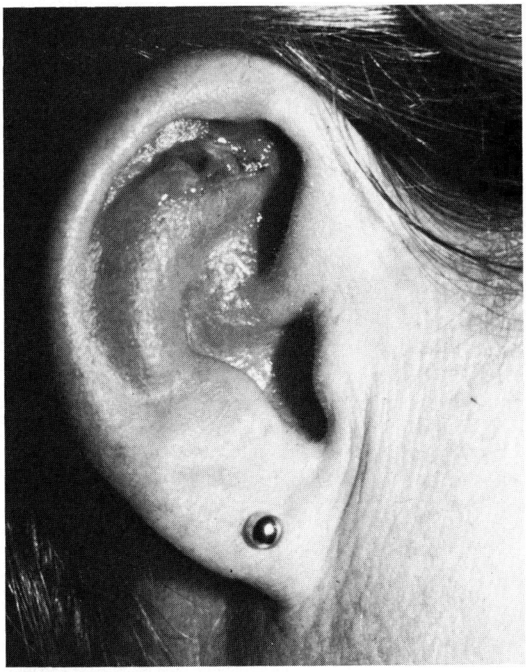

FIGURE 9–12. Chondritis secondary to *Pseudomonas aeruginosa* treated successfully with open drainage and intravenous antibiotics (treated before the availability of ciprofloxacin hydrochloride).

Preventing infections of the external ear should be stressed. The surgical defect over exposed cartilage should be closed if possible. If the wound is left to heal by second intention, cartilage that is not protected by viable perichondrium should be excised. Wounds should be checked regularly and exposed cartilage removed until healing is assured. The high cost of ciprofloxacin hydrochloride makes its use impractical for routine prophylaxis except in high-risk patients.

Other postoperative complications of the ear include deformity and stenosis of the external canal.[31] These problems may be avoided by stabilizing the ear with flaps, grafts, or stents.[32]

Fingers and Toes

Mohs surgery for the treatment of cancers of fingers and toes is uncommon. The urgency for treatment, however, may be greater since cancers at these areas are more commonly squamous cell carcinomas or melanomas. A major complication of deep wounds of the digits is the possibility of a septic tenosynovitis.[33] These infections can rapidly ascend along the tendons and result in extensive and serious limb infections. Although there are no reported cases of tenosynovitis following Mohs surgery, this should be considered when dealing with digital excisions. Surgical wounds should be closed, if possible, and the patient started on prophylactic antibiotics. In addition, rupture of the tendon has been reported following Mohs surgery.[34] Since management of tendon repairs of the fingers and toes is very specialized, it is appropriate to treat these patients in conjunction with a hand or foot surgeon.

Penis

Complications following Mohs surgery of the penis depend on the location and depth of the excision. However, in patients who would have been treated with penectomy, these complications often seem less severe.

Bleeding is one of the most distressing and common complications of penile surgery. Bleeding from the cavernous blood vessels can be very difficult to control. Although a tourniquet can be applied to the base of the penis, good results can be obtained by using a large chalazion clamp. We have also found that pressure with the broad, thermally heated blade of a Shaw scalpel (Oximetrix Inc., Mountain View, CA) provides excellent hemostasis. Other potential early complications following penile surgery include phimosis, paraphimosis, and urinary obstruction. If the foreskin remains intact and retracted after surgery (paraphimosis), swelling may constrict the blood supply to the glans and result in necrosis. If the foreskin cannot be pulled distally over the glans, immediate surgical release of the constriction is required. Also, if surgery of the penis results in severe swelling and urinary obstruction, immediate catheterization is necessary. Mohs surgery using the fixed tissue technique provides an excellent way to excise cancers of the penis in a bloodless field.[35]

Stricture is the most common complication when the urethra is involved and can generally be controlled with dilatation. Urethral perforations are not uncommon with deep Mohs excisions. Urethral perforations should not be called a complication of Mohs surgery when necessary for the complete extirpation of cancer. It is best to observe for recurrence for a period of 6 to 12 months prior to reconstructive surgery. Other potential complications include angulation of the penis with deviation of the urinary stream and painful intercourse. This requires follow-up with a urology service.

Vulva

Mohs surgeons are occasionally called on to excise superficial cancers of the distal vulva. These tumors may track into the urethral canal, introitus, or vagina. Potential complications include urinary incontinence, stenosis of the urethra, stenosis of the vagina, and dyspareunia.[36,37] These complications are best handled by a gynecologist.

Anal

Anal cancers are occasionally treated by Mohs surgeons and most frequently include Bowen's disease or Paget's disease. The tumor may be extensive and track into the anal canal. Contraction of wounds left to heal by second intention is the most common cause of complications. Stenosis results in rectal pain and constipation. Stenosis can be treated by dilatation or by surgery to relax the stenosis.[38]

RECURRENCES

Recurrence of skin cancer after excision is a complication of all cancer treatments, including Mohs surgery (Table 9–1). No method of treatment can guarantee a 100% cure. Mohs surgery, however, can provide the most certain method available for extirpation of the tumor.[39] Davidson and colleagues[40] estimated that standard microscopic examination of tumor examines less than 1% of the entire margin. In Mohs surgery 100% of the tumor margins are examined. Recurrences, however, may still occur for reasons listed in Table 9–1.

Despite the list of potential errors, the recurrence rate following Mohs surgery is very low. There are several ways to help reduce recurrences. Previously treated cancers may have multiple foci of tumor. Wagner and Cottel[41] demonstrated that 50% of recurrent basal cell carcinoma treated initially with electrodesiccation and curettage (EDC) contained multiple foci of cancer. In order to assure a cure, it is safest to excise the recurrent cancer plus any scar from previous treatment. A second consideration deals with intraoperative spread of cancer. Basal cell carcinomas have fastidious requirements for growth, and implantation of tumor from the syringe or other instruments is considered very unlikely. This becomes a distinct possibility though with squamous cell car-

TABLE 9–1. Causes of Recurrence Following Mohs Surgery

Physiologic causes:
- Primary tumor is multifocal
- Previous treatment left multiple unresected foci
- Metastatic tumor
- Surface seeding of tumor during surgery
- Needle implantation of tumor[42]
- New primary tumor as a result of field effect may appear to be a recurrence

Technical errors in performing Mohs surgery:
- Excising and marking tissue
- Mapping
- Tissue processing
- Interpretation and map notations
- Reexcising

cinoma[42] or malignant melanoma. Injections should be outside the cancer, not through it. In addition, instruments should be wiped clean or exchanged during the procedure. Wound beds of freshly excised squamous cell carcinoma and malignant melanoma may be cauterized with dichloracetic acid. There is little or no possibility of implanting cancers when using the fixed tissue technique.

Another major consideration to be gleaned from Table 9–1 is an appreciation of potential error in performing Mohs surgery. It is important to set up routine procedures for marking, mapping, processing, and reexcision of tumors, and alter these routines as little as possible. Simple Mohs excisions are not difficult, but for the occasional Mohs surgeon, it may be hard to establish this strict routine.

APPROACH TO THE PATIENT WITH SURGICAL COMPLICATIONS

Surgical complications are adverse events not essential to the surgical treatment. Unfortunately, patients often view undesirable results as complications resulting from physician error. Under most circumstances, this is not true. For example, if a cancer invades the nose and requires extensive excision, a patient may tend to view the resulting defect as a complication rather than a necessity. An undesirable defect is not the same as a surgical complication.

One of the more difficult jobs in medicine is dealing with patients who do experience surgical complications. Such situations are embarrassing and humiliating to the physician and cause anger and frustration to the patient. It is very important in dealing with surgical complications or with undesirable results to be straightforward and forthright with the patient. The patient should know that there is no repeated surgery without risk. The patient should willingly agree to surgery and know the consequences of treating and not treating the cancer. If complications arise, the patient should be informed of these complications as soon as possible. Rather than be defensive about complications, the Mohs surgeon should become a patient advocate and work to resolve these problems. Appropriate consultations should be made, and records should be well documented.

In summary, surgical complications are a possibility with all types of surgery, including Mohs surgery. Careful attention to detail can be very helpful in preventing and treating those complications. The multidisciplinary approach in dealing with potential or developing problems should be encouraged.

REFERENCES

1. Salasche SJ: Acute surgical complications: Cause, prevention, and treatment. J Am Acad Dermatol 15:1163–1185, 1986.
2. Halpern AC, Leyden JJ, Dzubow LM, McGinley KF: The incidence of bacteremia in skin surgery of the head and neck. J Am Acad Dermatol 19:112–116, 1988.
3. Sabetta, JB, Zitelli JA: The incidence of bacteremia during skin surgery. Arch Dermatol 123:213–215, 1987.
4. Sebben JE: Prophylactic antibiotics in cutaneous surgery. J Dermatol Surg Oncol 11:901–906, 1985.
5. Wagner RF Jr, Grande DJ, Feingold DS: Antibiotic prophylaxis against bacterial endocarditis in patients undergoing dermatologic surgery. Arch Dermatol 122:789–801, 1986.
6. Larson PO: Topical hemostatic agents for dermatologic surgery. J Dermatol Surg Oncol 14:623–632, 1988.
7. Cottel WI: Perineural invasion by squamous cell carcinoma. J Dermatol Surg Oncol 8:589–600, 1982.
8. Hanke CW, Wolf RL, Hochman SA, Obrian JJ: Chemosurgerical reports: Perineural spread of basal cell carcinomas. J Dermatol Surg Oncol 9:742–747, 1983.
9. Janecka IP, Conley J: Primary neoplasms of the facial nerve. Plast Reconstr Surg 79:177–185, 1987.
10. Smith F: A rational management of skin grafts. Surg Gynecol Obstet 42:556–562, 1926.
11. Larson PO: Foam rubber stents for skin grafts. J Dermatol Surg Oncol (in press, 1990).
12. Baran R, Juhlin L, Brun P: Bullae in skin grafts. Br J Dermatol 111:221–225, 1984.
13. Koyama H, Isshiki N, Noda R, Nishimura R: Long-term survival of a free split-thickness skin graft on a large seroma. Plast Reconstr Surg 79:109–113, 1987.
14. Rudolph R, Hunt TK: Healing in compromised tissues. In Rudolph R (ed): Problems in Aesthetic Surgery. St. Louis: C. V. Mosby, 1986, p 65.
15. Snyder PA, Alper JC, Albom MJ: Osteomyelitis complicating Mohs' chemosurgery. J Am Acad Dermatol 11:513–516, 1984.
16. Kuwada GT, Dockery GL: Contact dermatitis. A review. Clin Podiatr Med Surg 3:551–561, 1986.
17. Snyder RJ: Contact dermatitis as a surgical complication. J Foot Surg 21:153–155, 1982.
18. Bennett RG: Problems associated with cutaneous surgery. In Fundamentals of Cutaneous Surgery. St. Louis: C. V. Mosby, 1988, pp 498–501.
19. Brown LA Jr, Pierce HE: Keloids: Scar revision. J Dermatol Surg Oncol 12:51–56, 1986.
20. Pollack SV: Wound healing: A Review, IV: Systemic medications affecting wound healing. J Dermatol Surg Oncol 8:667–672, 1982.
21. Goslen JB: Physiology of wound healing and scar formation. In Thomas JR, Holt GR (eds): Facial Scars: Incision, Revision and Camouflage. St. Louis: C. V. Mosby, 1989, p 10.

22. Ship AG, Weiss PR: Pigmentation after dermabrasion: An avoidable complication. Plast Reconstr Surg 75:528–532, 1985.
23. Baylis HI, Cies WA: Complications of Mohs' chemosurgical excision of eyelid and canthal tumors. Am J Ophthalmol 80:116–122, 1975.
24. Mohs FE: Micrographic surgery for the microscopically controlled excision of eyelid cancers. Arch Ophthalmol 104:901–909, 1986.
25. Fox SA: Repair of nasocanthal malignant neoplasms. Combined laissez-faire and chemosurgery techniques. Arch Ophthalmol 94:278–280, 1976.
26. Robinson JK: Prevention of intraoperative trauma to the lacrimal system. J Dermatol Surg Oncol 9:802–804, 1983.
27. Dortzbach RK, Angrist RA: Silicone intubation for lacerated lacrimal canaliculi. Ophthalmic Surg 16:639–642, 1985.
28. Whitaker DC, Goldstein GD, Birkby CS, Nerad JA: Postoperative techniques for corneal protection in Mohs micrographic surgery. J Dermatol Surg Oncol 14:951–955, 1988.
29. Pakarien M, Tervo T, Tarkkanen A: Tarsorrhaphy in the treatment of persistent corneal lesions. Acta Ophthalmol (Suppl.) 182:69–73, 1987.
30. Rubin J, Yu VL: Malignant external otitis: Insights into pathogenesis, clinical manifestations, diagnosis and therapy. Am J Med 85:391–398, 1988.
31. Buecker JW, Phelan JT: Carcinoma of the external auditory canal: Removal and prevention of stenosis. J Dermatol Surg Oncol 12:598–600, 1986.
32. Larson PO: Stenosis of the external ear canal: Prevention using hydroxylated polyvinyl acetal wicks. J Dermatol Surg Oncol 13:1121–1123, 1987.
33. Monstrey SJ, van der Werken C, Kauer JM, Goris RJ: Tendon sheath infections of the hand. Neth J Surg 37:174–178, 1985.
34. Gaspari AA, d'Aubermont PC, Bennett RG: Delayed extensor tendon rupture: A complication of Mohs surgery. J Dermatol Surg Oncol 10:721–723, 1984.
35. Mohs FE: Chemosurgery: Micrographically controlled surgery for skin cancer. Springfield, IL: Charles C Thomas, 1978.
36. Abell DA: Simple vulvectomy: A 10-year review. Aust NZ J Obstet Gynaecol 13:8–14, 1973.
37. Kadar N, Nelson JH Jr: Sling operation for total incontinence following radical vulvectomy. Obstet Gynecol 64:858–878, 1984.
38. Larson PO: Skin cancers in the perianal and rectal areas treated by Mohs micrographic surgery. In Bennett RG, Albom M (eds): Mohs Micrographic Surgery for Skin Cancer, St. Louis: C. V. Mosby (in press).
39. Rowe DE, Carroll RJ, Day CL Jr: Mohs surgery is the treatment of choice for recurrent (previously treated) basal cell carcinoma. J Dermatol Surg Oncol 15:424–431, 1989.
40. Davidson TM, Haghighi P, Astarita R, et al.: Microscopically oriented histologic surgery for head and neck mucosal cancer. Cancer 60:1856–1861, 1987.
41. Wagner RF Jr, Cottel WI: Multifocal recurrent basal cell carcinoma following primary tumor treatment by electrodesiccation and curettage. J Am Acad Dermatol 17:1047–1049, 1987.
42. Salzman RS, Bennett RG, Fleischer AS: Cutaneous implantation metastasis complicating a superficial temporal-middle cerebral artery anastomosis. Neurosurgery 11:268–270, 1982.

CHAPTER 10

Wound Dressings for Mohs Micrographic Surgery

George B. Winton, M.D.

The Mohs micrographic surgeon utilizes wound dressings in much the same manner as any dermatologic or plastic and reconstructive surgeon with three exceptions. First, because skin cancers involving critical anatomic structures, such as the eyelids, nose and ears, are commonly referred to the Mohs surgeon, he or she will frequently have to design a dressing for an awkward anatomic site. Second, Mohs surgeons utilize second intention healing in a small but significant portion of their cases, and the nuances of this type of wound care must be mastered. Mohs surgeons have been slow to adopt the new biosynthetic dressings and still prefer to use standard materials such as gauze and tape. Therefore, this chapter emphasizes the principles of moist wound healing using standard, inexpensive materials. Although the design of a clever, functional dressing for any anatomic site is limited only by the imagination of the surgeon, examples will be given for each area where difficulty is commonly encountered.

FUNCTIONS OF A WOUND DRESSING

An adequate wound dressing should perform several functions. It should protect the wound from external contamination, cushion the wound against trauma, and limit motion in the surrounding tissues by acting as a splint. The dressing should also provide an environment that is conducive to healing. This environment can be enhanced if the dressing maintains tissue hydration, wicks away exudate, and provides a tamponade effect to aid in hemostasis. It is also important that the dressing not adhere or stick to the wound, so the newly formed epithelium is not disturbed during dressing changes.[1]

PRINCIPLES OF WOUND CARE

The benefits of moist wound healing are now well established,[2–6] and can be achieved with standard dressing materials if patient and physician follow three simples rules: keep the wound clean, keep it moist, and keep it covered.[1] Wound exudate is a growth medium for bacteria and should therefore be removed from the wound at each dressing change or whenever it accumulates, usually daily. This task is easily accomplished with peroxide-soaked cotton-tipped applicators. Wounds can be kept moist both by the daily use of an antibiotic ointment and a sufficiently occlusive standard dressing. The heavy-pressure dressing applied postoperatively can usually be changed to a lighter cover after 24 hours. Sutured defects should be dressed for at least the first 48 hours until reepithelialization is complete.[7,8] Granulating wounds should remain dressed until reepithelialization is complete and there is no further tendency for the wound to form crusts. While daily changes are the norm, wounds with minimal exudate can be changed less frequently. On the other hand, any dressing that has become wet or soiled can no longer perform its function and should be changed at once.

LAYERS OF A STANDARD DRESSING

One can facilitate the design of a wound dressing by considering a composite of five layers.[1] Although there is some overlap, most dressing materials are designed to serve in a particular layer of the dressing (Table 10–1).

Ointment Layer

The first layer is the hydrating or ointment layer and consists of a thin film of antibiotic ointment of the surgeon's choice. The purpose of this layer is to maintain tissue hydration and provide an antibacterial effect. Commonly used ointments include polymyxin B sulfate and bacitracin (Polysporin); polymyxin B sulfate, bacitracin zinc, and neomycin sulfate (Neosporin); erythromycin (Ilotycin); and plain bacitracin. All of these ointments protect against colonization by organisms commonly encountered in cutaneous wounds. One of them, Neosporin, was found to significantly accelerate wound reepithelialization; however, when the ingredients were tested separately, it was determined that bacitracin zinc was responsible for the effect.[9] In clinical use, the other ointments also appear to serve well in this regard. Perhaps the most common problem with any antibiotic ointment is contact allergy. Should a patient be unable to tolerate any of them, plain white petrolatum or Eucerin may be substituted. Of these, Eucerin has been shown to promote more rapid reepithelialization.[10,11]

TABLE 10–1. Layers of a Wound Dressing

Layer	Material
Ointment	Bacitracin, Neosporin, Polysporin, Ilotycin, Eucerin, and white petrolatum.
Contact layer	Nonadherent pads (Telfa, Release, White Cross, and N-terface); packing gauze (Xeroform, Xeroflo, and Vaseline); povidone-iodine (Betadine) gauze; and Aquaphor Gauze.
Absorbent layer	Dry gauze pads and cotton balls.
Contouring layer	Dental rolls and gauze pads
Securing layer	Tape, sterile tape strips, gauze rolls, tubular gauze, and elastic bandages

Modified from Winton GB, Salasche SJ: Wound dressings for dermatologic surgery. Journal of the American Academy of Dermatology, 13:1026–1044, 1985.

Contact Layer

Perhaps the most important layer of a dressing is the contact layer because it actually touches the wound. This layer should be nonadherent so that it can be removed from the healing wound without disturbing newly formed epithelium. It should also be porous so that exudate may be wicked through it to the more absorbent layers of the dressing.

Materials used in this layer include nonadherent pads (e.g., White Cross, Telfa, and Release), petrolatum gauze (Vaseline, Adaptic), medicated petrolatum gauze (Xeroform, Xeroflo), Aquaphor Gauze, and even polyethylene oxide hydrogels (Vigilon) with at least one film backing removed. A material that epitomizes the favorable properties of the contact layer is N-terface, a high-density plastic in a monofilament-woven membrane.[12] This material is superbly nonadherent and readily allows exudate to pass through.

Absorbent Layer

The third layer of the dressing is the absorbent layer. This layer consists of dry gauze pads or cotton balls that function to wick exudate away from the wound so that maceration and bacterial colonization can be minimized.

Contouring Layer

The contouring layer is the portion of the dressing that fills in anatomic depressions or supports protruding structures, such as the ear. Fluffed gauze pads and gauze dental rolls are useful for this purpose.

Securing Layer

The securing layer fastens the dressing to the patient. In most cases, adhesive tape is used.

Many kinds of surgical tape are available, most of which are hypoallergenic. On relatively broad expanses of skin such as the back or extremities, wide 1-inch or 2-inch, relatively inelastic, plasticized tape (e.g., Transpore or Dermiclear) works well. In more confined areas with awkward curves, a ½-inch, somewhat elastic, flexible tape such as Dermiform works better. If additional pressure is desired on a wound, the elasticity of Microfoam can be useful. Finally, light-weight paper tapes (e.g., Dermalite II, Scanpore, or Micropore) are rarely irritating to the skin and are useful in applying a thin Telfa dressing to a granulating wound repeatedly over many weeks.

Other materials used in the securing layer include gauze rolls (Kling or Kerlix), tubular gauze (X-span), and elastic bandages (Coban or Ace). Tubular gauze is particularly useful on the scalp and cheeks and may substitute nicely for gauze rolls in a multitude of situations.

Although there are five recognizable layers of wound dressings, not every wound requires all of them. The contouring layer is not required for wounds in flat areas. If during the late stages of wound healing, minimal exudate is present, the absorbent layer may be omitted as well. Some surgeons prefer to use dressings on sutured facial wounds only until hemostasis is assured and the epithelial bridge is restored.[8] After 48 hours, only an antibiotic ointment is applied several times daily. Wounds treated in this manner should not be located in anatomic areas where the patient may cause a disturbance during sleep, e.g., the external ear and posterior scalp.

TEMPORARY DRESSINGS

Dressings Between Stages of Mohs Surgery

Normally, the elapsed time between stages of a Mohs procedure is an hour or less. During this period, the operative site must remain moist, and hemostasis must be maintained. A temporary dressing consisting of a nonadherent pad and dry gauze taped to the wound is sufficient. Ointments are not used on the wound during these brief periods for two reasons. First, they tend to obscure the field when surgery recommences, and second, if a skin graft is ultimately planned, they tend to interfere with the graft take.[13] If surgery is interrupted for a longer period of time (e.g., overnight), then the benefits of placing an antibiotic ointment on the wound outweigh these minor disadvantages.

Dressings for Delayed Repair

From time to time, proper surgical management of a cutaneous malignancy will dictate a delay in the repair of the wound following complete tumor extirpation. For example, Mohs surgery may be completed late in the afternoon and reconstructive surgery scheduled for the following morning. Or perhaps a case begun in the office has proved to be more complex than originally thought and must be continued in an operating room following a thorough radiographic evaluation of the site. These cases are usually among the more difficult and frequently involve critical anatomic structures. If a standard dressing does not suit the situation, then some improvisation is in order. Figure 10–1 demonstrates a large defect on the lower lip following removal of a squamous cell carcinoma. Reconstructive surgery was scheduled for the following morning. To get the patient through the night, antibiotic ointment was applied on a roll of petrolatum-impregnated gauze and sewn into the wound. The patient was able to eat a liquid diet that evening without difficulty.

Epigard and Cutinova Plus are two new dressing materials that have a foam rubber inner surface.[14,15] When the foam is placed against the wound, all exudate is absorbed by the sponge and neatly cleaned away with the old dressing at each change. Such dressings, changed every 1 to 3 days are excellent for maintaining the freshness of wound edges when repair must be delayed.

DRESSINGS FOR SECOND INTENTION HEALING

Standard Materials

For many years, Mohs surgeons have used standard materials to dress wounds that are left to heal by second intention. A typical dressing consists of ointment, nonadherent pad, gauze pad, or cotton balls and tape. Deep wounds may require more material to fill the cavity, and one of the medicated petrolatum dressings can be substituted for the nonadherent pad. If the petrolatum dressing tends to adhere to the

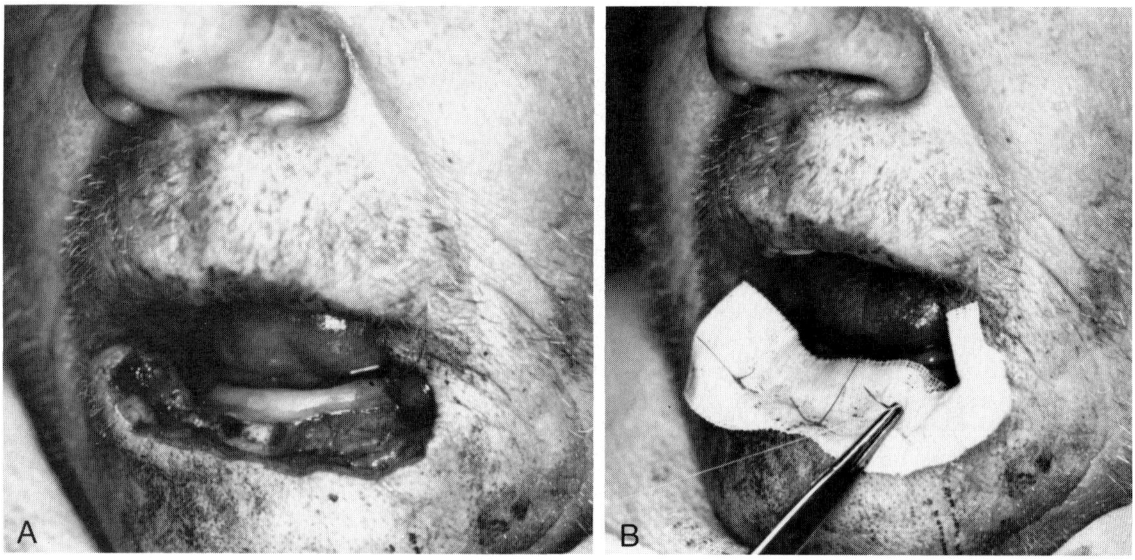

FIGURE 10–1. *A*, A large defect in the lower lip after Mohs surgery for a squamous cell carcinoma. *B*, A temporary dressing was made from Xeroform gauze which was sutured into the wound. This dressing could be comfortably worn for a brief period until reconstructive surgery was performed.

base of the wound, a layer of N-terface can be placed in first. The presence of this extra layer makes the dressing less adherent and dressing changes less painful. The original layer of N-terface can remain in the wound for 3 or 4 days while the outer layers are changed and the wound is cleaned regularly. If the N-terface is not removed by the 4th day, it may become imbedded in granulation tissue. When granulation tissue fills the wound cavity almost to the level of the surrounding skin and there is minimal exudation, the dressing can be simplified. At this point, ointment, nonadherent pad, and tape, changed daily, are sufficient.

Most patients, with the assistance of a family member, can handle the regimen of care for granulating wounds. During the early exudative phase of healing, wound cleaning and dressing changes may need to be performed twice a day. By the 2nd week, a daily routine is usually adequate. The importance of débriding all crusts, either with a cotton-tipped applicator and peroxide or with a sterile forceps, should be emphasized to the patient. A weekly débridement at the surgeon's office is also in order.

Biosynthetic Dressings

A plethora of biosynthetic dressing materials is now available for use. These dressings are reported to reduce pain and swelling and speed healing, especially in full-thickness wounds healing by granulation.[16] Mohs surgeons have been slow to adopt these products for several reasons. First, bacterial colonization can be increased under these semipermeable membranes.[17] Although colonization is rarely a problem in granulating wounds, sutured, full-thickness defects provide an entry for bacteria into deeper, enclosed spaces. Silent infections beneath film dressings have been reported in sutured wounds left covered for several days.[18] Furthermore, in a study of polyethylene oxide gel occlusive dressings on sutured wounds, 25% of the control wounds covered with the dressing alone without antibiotic ointment became infected.[19] None of these wounds treated with the dressing and an antibacterial substance became infected, and this infection rate is in marked contrast to the usual infection rate of no more than 1% seen in office-based cutaneous surgery.[20] A synthetic dressing placed on a sutured wound postoperatively might be removed at 24 hours in order to inspect for hemorrhage or hematoma. If these dressings must be replaced once or twice over a 5-day period until the sutures are removed, cost-effectiveness will be negated.

There are three additional difficulties in using synthetic dressings on wounds that heal by second intention. First, the sites where granulation provides the best cosmetic results and where it is most likely to be used are located in concave areas on the head,[21] such as the concha of the ear, the alar groove, and the postauricular sulcus, where it is difficult to apply such dressings. Second, film dressings are not designed to be used on wounds with heavy exudate. Mohs wounds exude a great deal during the first week and usually require frequent dressing changes. Finally, certain of the film dressings adhere to newly formed epithelium and may strip it away during dressing changes, thus delaying healing.[22]

Despite these difficulties, a recent study found significantly faster healing, better patient acceptance, and improved cosmesis in granulating Mohs wounds treated with a transparent film dressing when compared with a control dressing of Polysporin ointment and dry gauze.[23] This study can be criticized for its use of a suboptimal, standard dressing in the control wounds, namely, the omission of an adequate contact layer. Had a nonadherent pad been added to the control dressing, it is likely that greater occlusion could have been achieved, and stripping or desiccation of newly formed epithelium could have been prevented.

A new and interesting development in the use of biosynthetic dressings was discovered by

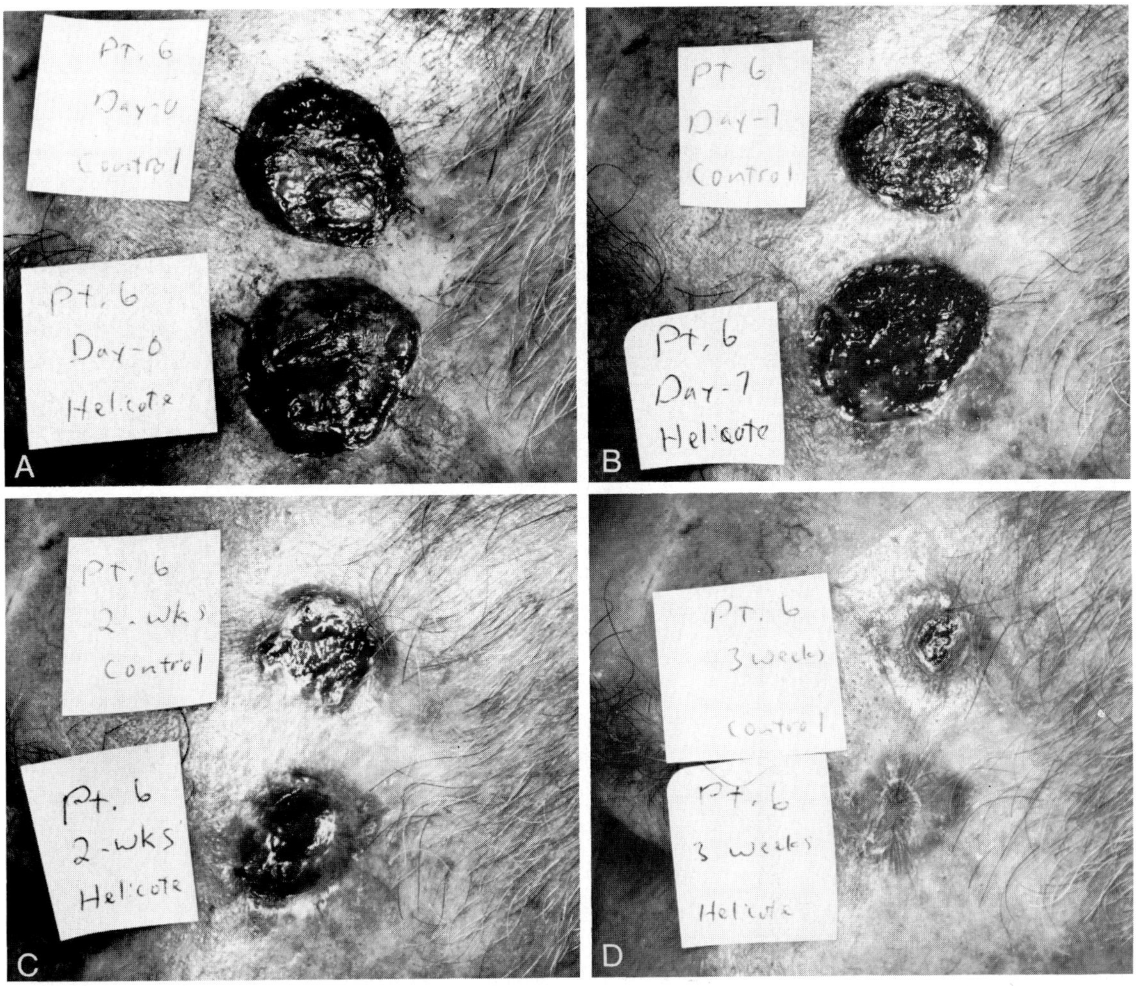

FIGURE 10–2. *A*, A Helicote study patient had two adjacent basal cell carcinomas removed by Mohs surgery. The wounds were similar in size and depth. The upper control wound was dressed each day with bacitracin, Telfa, dry gauze, and tape. The lower test wound had a Helicote dressing sutured into place and covered with a dry gauze pad. No daily care was given. *B*, At one week, the film backing was removed from the Helicote dressing. From this point onward, both wounds received a daily application of bacitracin and a Telfa dressing. *C*, By the second week, the test wound was two-thirds healed, while the control wound was only half healed. *D*, By the third week, the Helicote wound was healed; the control wound required another 5 days to completely reepithelialize.

Eaglstein and colleagues[24] who found that a window of opportunity exists between the 2nd and 24th hour after wounding when the continuous application of the dressing promotes more rapid healing. Wounds dressed too late, especially after the 6th hour, achieve suboptimal healing, while continued use of the dressing beyond 24 hours is of limited benefit. Armed with this information, the most cost-effective utilization of these dressings is demonstrated.

Collagen Matrix Dressings

Helicote is an acellular sponge composed of purified bovine tendon type I collagen laminated to a film membrane. It is currently in clinical trials for use as a dressing for granulating wounds. In animal experiments[25] and initial tests in humans,[26] these sponges were shown to decrease wound contraction and speed reepithelialization. However, these effects are not of large magnitude. Figure 10–2 shows a patient from one of the study centers who serendipitously had two skin cancers removed from the left temple providing a test site and an adjacent control site. At 3 weeks, the Helicote-treated site was completely reepithelialized while the control site dressed with bacitracin and Telfa required an additional 5 days. The clinical appearance of the wounds was similar. There was at most a 10% to 15% reduction in wound contraction.

The chief advantage of this dressing is not the effect on wound-healing parameters but the simplification of wound care. The dressing is sutured into the wound and covered with dry gauze immediately after surgery. No care is required during the first week. On the 7th day, sutures are removed, the membrane backing is stripped away, and any collagen that was not incorporated into the base of the wound is trimmed. A dressing of ointment on a nonadherent pad is then used until healing is complete. Thus, during the early exudative stage of

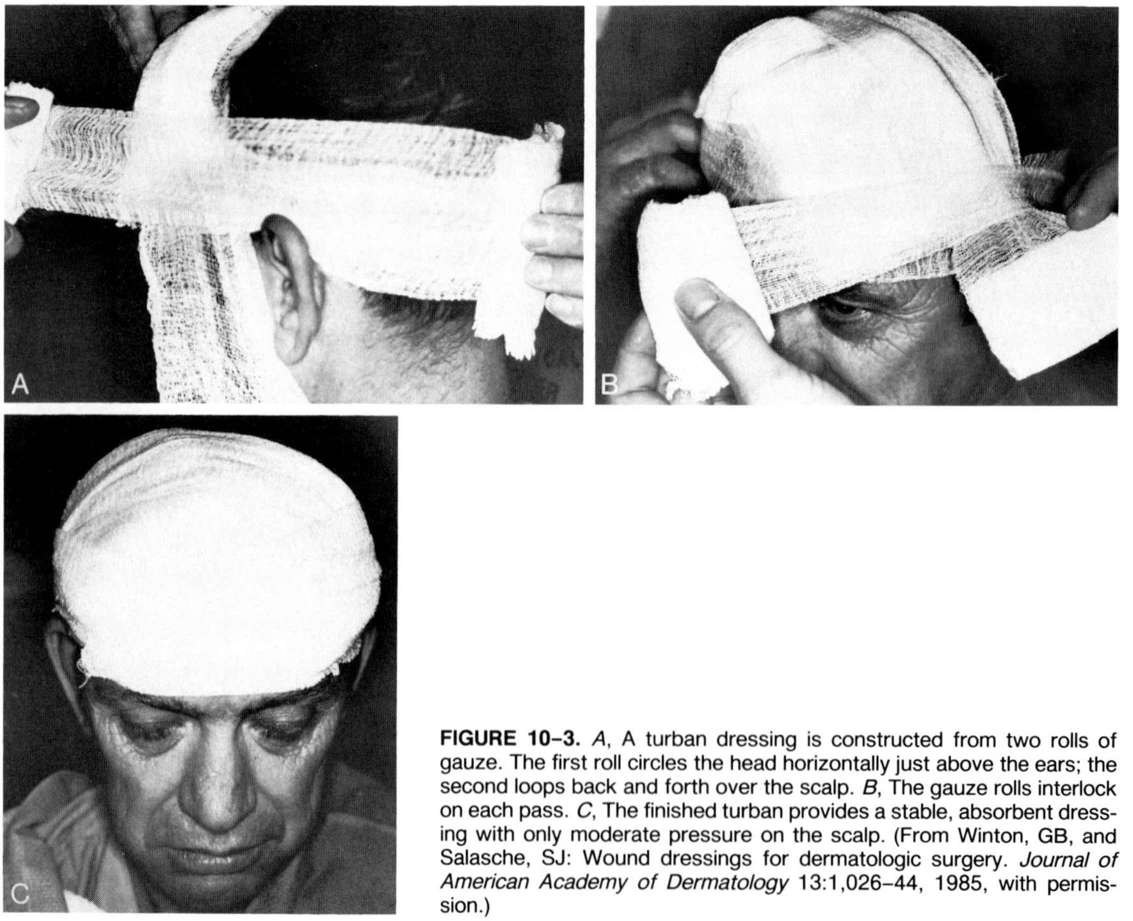

FIGURE 10–3. *A*, A turban dressing is constructed from two rolls of gauze. The first roll circles the head horizontally just above the ears; the second loops back and forth over the scalp. *B*, The gauze rolls interlock on each pass. *C*, The finished turban provides a stable, absorbent dressing with only moderate pressure on the scalp. (From Winton, GB, and Salasche, SJ: Wound dressings for dermatologic surgery. *Journal of American Academy of Dermatology* 13:1,026–44, 1985, with permission.)

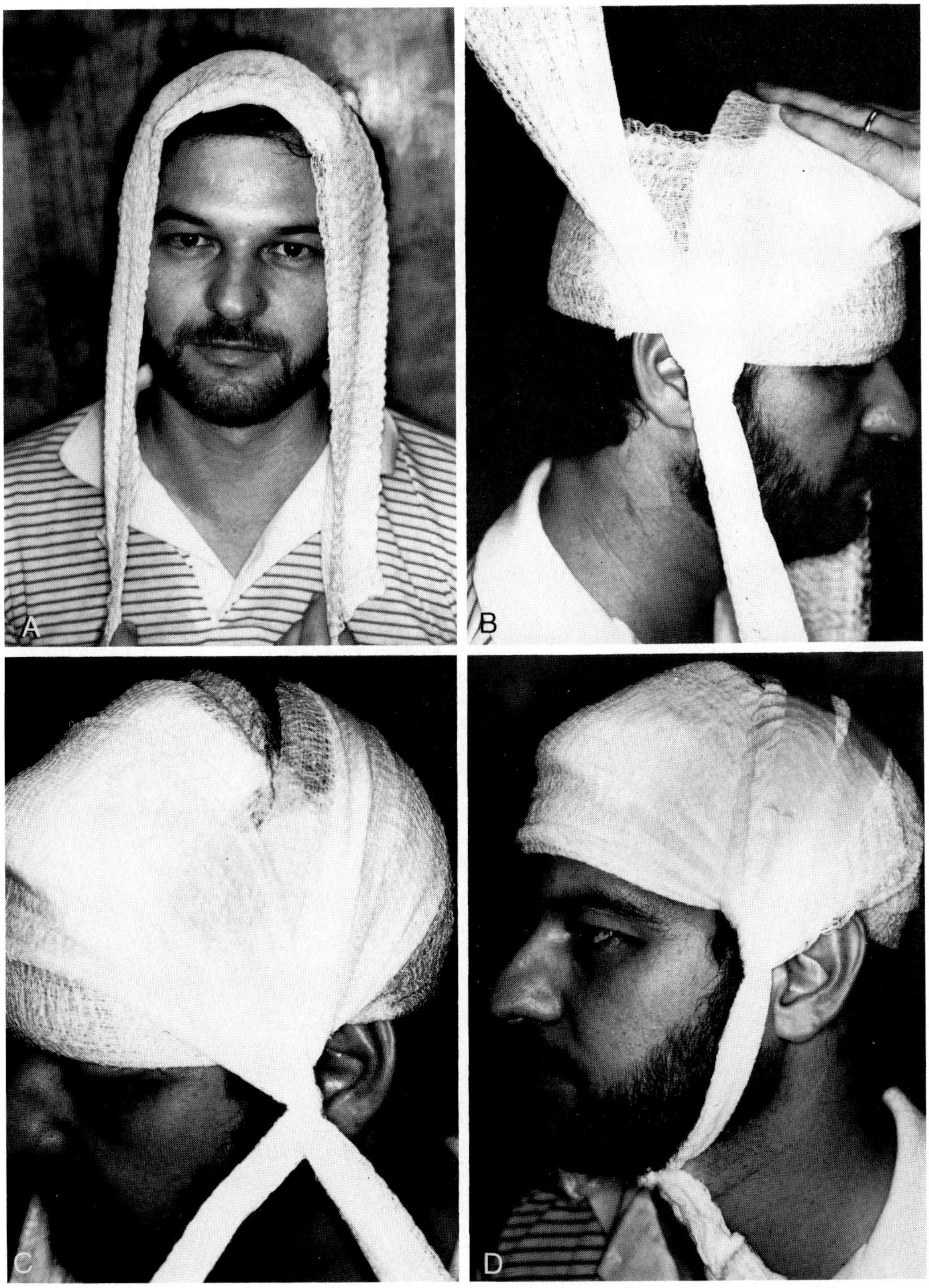

FIGURE 10–4. *A*, A modified Russian dressing is begun by cutting an anchoring piece which is placed over the head and held by the patient. *B*, A gauze roll is used to construct the head dressing. *C*, The gauze roll loops around alternating arms of the anchoring piece on each pass. *D*, The finished dressing is secured by knotting the anchoring piece under the chin. (From Winton, GB, and Salasche, SJ: Wound dressings for dermatologic surgery. *Journal of American Academy of Dermatology* 13:1,026–44, 1985, with permission.)

healing, when twice daily wound care is the rule, a Helicote dressing needs no attention.

Although Helicote is not yet available, Helistat,[27] an identical sponge without a film backing, is licensed as a hemostatic device (Collatech Corporation, 105 Morgan Drive, Plainsboro, NY 08536). It can be held in place with an occlusive dressing of the surgeon's choice for 5 to 7 days. Care of the wound after this period is similar to that described for Helicote.

DRESSINGS FOR VARIOUS ANATOMIC AREAS

Flat, Glabrous Skin

The basic dressing for flat, glabrous skin consists of an antibiotic ointment, a nonadherent pad, dry gauze, and tape. If pressure is desired, an elastic tape such as Microfoam is helpful. If there is no exudate, the dry gauze can be omitted.

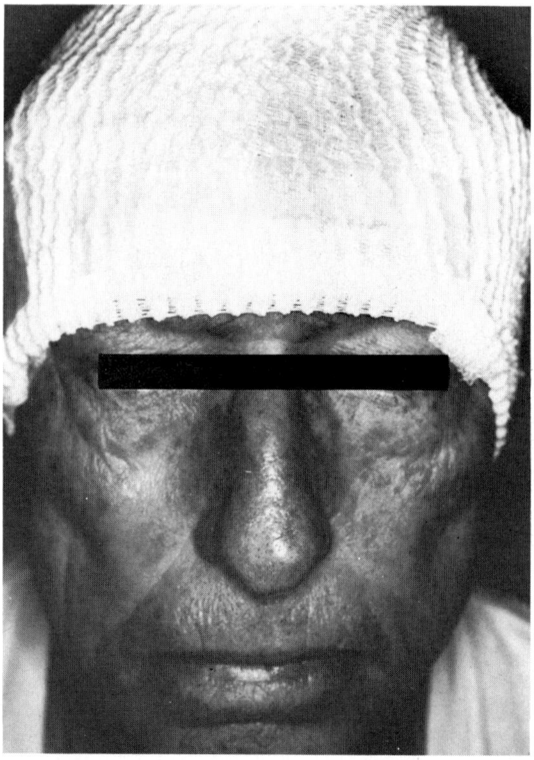

FIGURE 10–5. A satisfactory head dressing can also be made from number six tubular gauze. A knot is placed in one end of a 12 to 15″ piece and it is drawn over the head like a stocking cap.

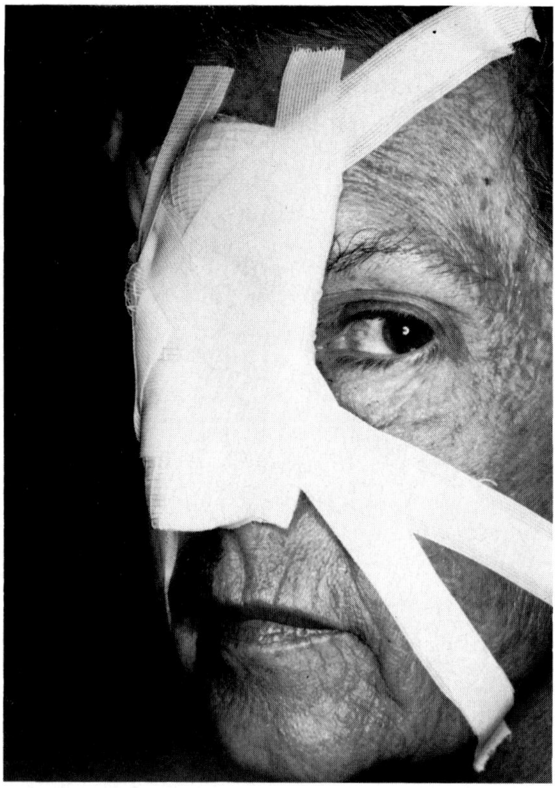

FIGURE 10–6. A dressing on the nose demonstrates a secure method of taping utilizing all available anchoring points.

Dressings for the Scalp

Turban Dressing. A simple turban dressing (Fig. 10–3) is useful for scalp wounds that require only mild pressure. It is usually constructed with two gauze rolls. First, the wound is covered with ointment, a nonadherent pad, and dry gauze. The first gauze roll is then wrapped horizontally around the scalp just above the ears, while the second roll loops back and forth over the crown and vertex of the scalp passing under the wraps of the first roll. The ends of each roll are secured wtih tape to complete the dressing.

Modified Russian Scalp Dressing. To apply more pressure to incisional wounds on the scalp and to better assure that a dressing does not fall off during sleep, a turban modified from Russian Army bandaging techniques[28] can be used (Fig. 10–4). After applying the usual underlayers to the wound, an anchoring piece made from 25 to 30 inches of Kerlix or

Kling gauze is draped over the scalp. The remainder of the gauze roll is then used to form a turban. On each pass over the scalp, the gauze roll interlocks with alternating arms of the anchoring piece. The free end of the roll is taped securely, and the anchoring piece is fastened under the chin. This head dressing is more secure, requires no tape on the skin, and provides more pressure to wounds near the crown or vertex of the scalp.

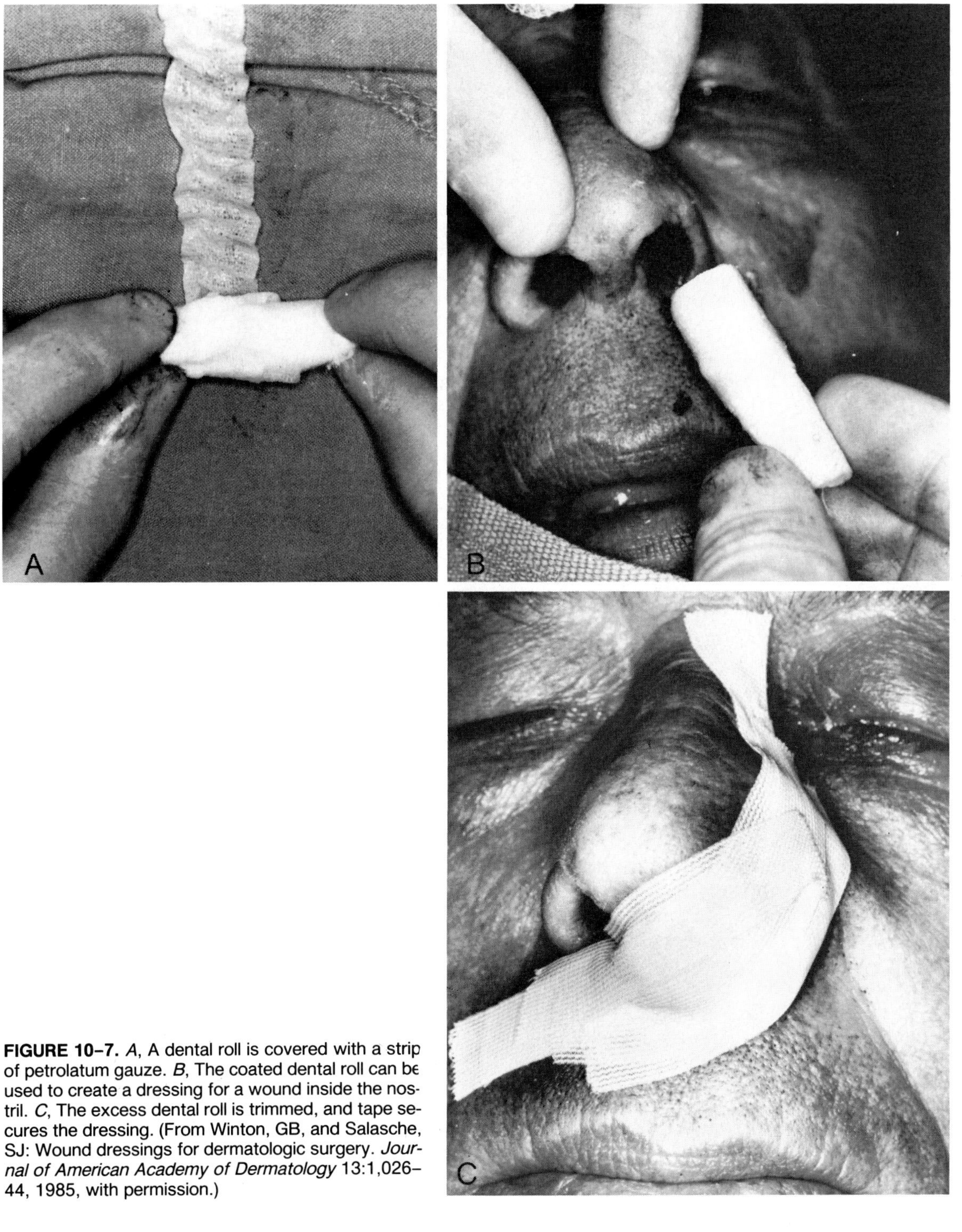

FIGURE 10–7. *A*, A dental roll is covered with a strip of petrolatum gauze. *B*, The coated dental roll can be used to create a dressing for a wound inside the nostril. *C*, The excess dental roll is trimmed, and tape secures the dressing. (From Winton, GB, and Salasche, SJ: Wound dressings for dermatologic surgery. *Journal of American Academy of Dermatology* 13:1,026–44, 1985, with permission.)

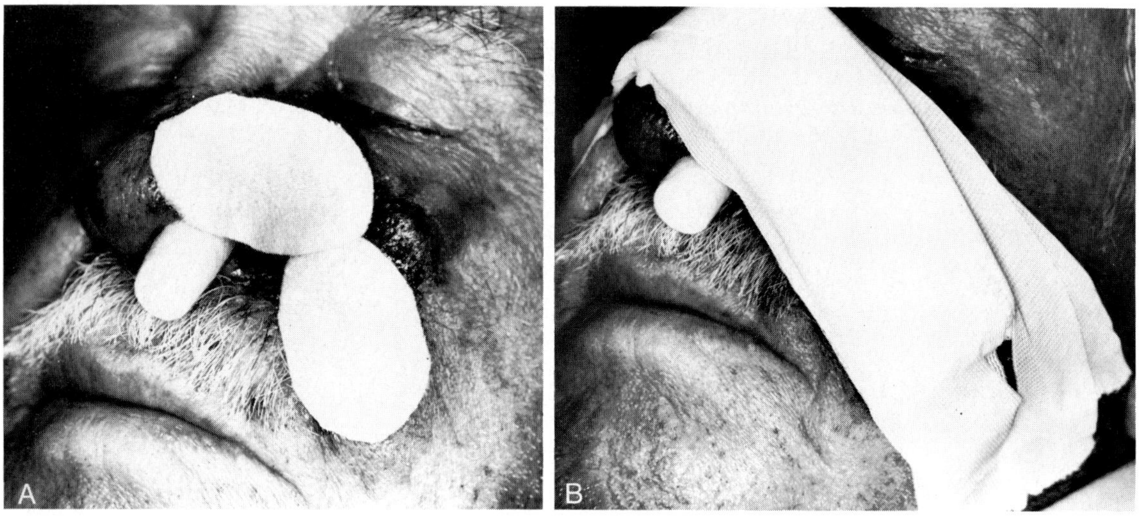

FIGURE 10–8. *A*, If a dressing on the nose tends to collapse the nostril, counterpressure can be supplied by inserting a dental roll. *B*, The dental roll can remain in place as part of the dressing.

Stockinette Dressing. If one wishes to avoid cumbersome turban dressings on the scalp, a simple stockinette dressing can be constructed with tubular gauze (Fig. 10–5) or even women's hosiery.[29] A 10- to 15-inch length of number 6 (scalp size) tubular gauze, e.g., X-span, is knotted at one end and pulled over the head and underlayers of the dressing like a stocking cap. The size is adjusted by folding the stocking one or more times at the temples and forehead, making sure to snug it securely over the wound but avoiding pressure on the ears.

Dressings for the Nose

A standard dressing can be easily secured to the nose by cutting all dressing materials to a size and shape just large enough to accomplish the task at hand (Fig. 10–6). These materials must then be taped in at least three directions to utilize all available anchoring points. A horizontal piece of tape is usually applied first. Additional pieces of tape are placed diagonally forming an *X* at the glabella. A common error is using pieces of tape that are too short or too wide. Half-inch Dermiform tape works well. The tape should be cut long enough to utilize all available nonhairy skin and may reach the tragus of the ears, mandible, and frontal hairline.

Small, gauze cylinders called dental rolls are useful for certain nasal wounds. If a wound has been created inside a nostril, a dental roll can be covered with petrolatum gauze, coated with an antibiotic ointment and inserted into the nostril (Fig. 10–7). A small piece of tape secures this dressing. On the other hand, certain wounds on the exterior of the nose near the alar rim can be difficult to dress because of the tendency of the nostril to collapse when external pressure is applied. A dental roll placed inside the nostril creates the requisite counterpressure in this situation (Fig. 10–8).

Dressings for the Ears

Small wounds on the external ear near the helical rim can frequently be bandaged with a

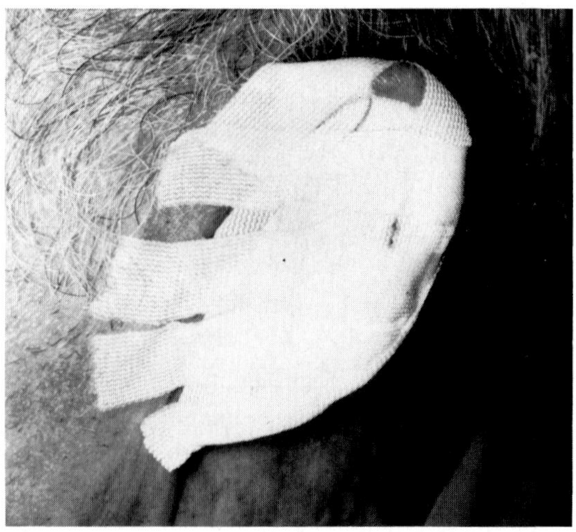

FIGURE 10–9. Small wounds on the external ear can sometimes be dressed with a bandage confined to the ear itself, taped in place with short, narrow strips of tape.

small dressing confined to the pinna (Fig. 10–9). The key to success is using many short pieces of ½-inch tape in the securing layer.

Larger wounds on the ears and periauricular skin are best managed with a head wrap dressing used by otolaryngologists following mastoid surgery[27] (Fig. 10–10). After ointment and contact layer are applied to the wound, the ear is contoured anteriorly and posteriorly with fluffed dry gauze. Next, two 8-inch pieces of a gauze roll are laid across the eyes. To avoid covering the contralateral ear, a twist is placed in the wrap each time as it passes just above the pinna. When the wrap is in place, the strips laid across the eyes are tied securely, pulling the dressing out of the patient's line of vision and securing the free end of the wrap. Tension in the dressing can also be adjusted as these strips are tied.

Dressings for the Cheeks

Utilization of tape in the securing layer of dressings on the cheeks and chin is frequently unsatisfactory because motion caused by talk-

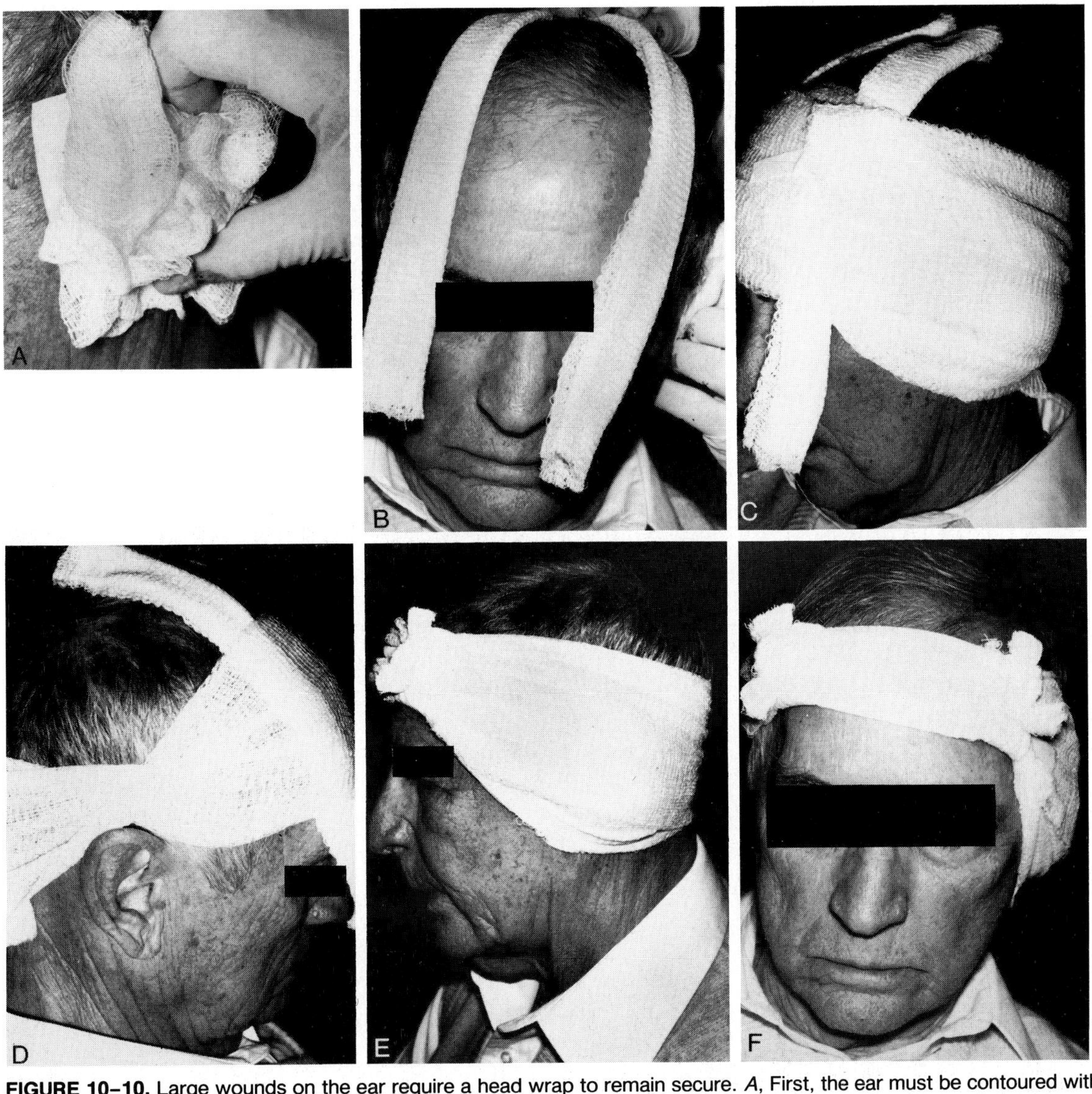

FIGURE 10–10. Large wounds on the ear require a head wrap to remain secure. *A*, First, the ear must be contoured with fluffed, dry gauze both anteriorly and posteriorly. *B*, Two gauze strips are laid over the forehead and eyes. *C*, A gauze roll is used to construct the dressing. *D*, The contralateral ear is left uncovered by twisting the roll as it passes. *E*, The dressing is adjusted by tying the two forehead strips so that visibility is not impeded. *F*, The final dressing is tidy and secure.

ing or eating may dislodge the dressing. A more satisfactory solution is to use tubular gauze instead of or in addition to the tape (Fig. 10–11).

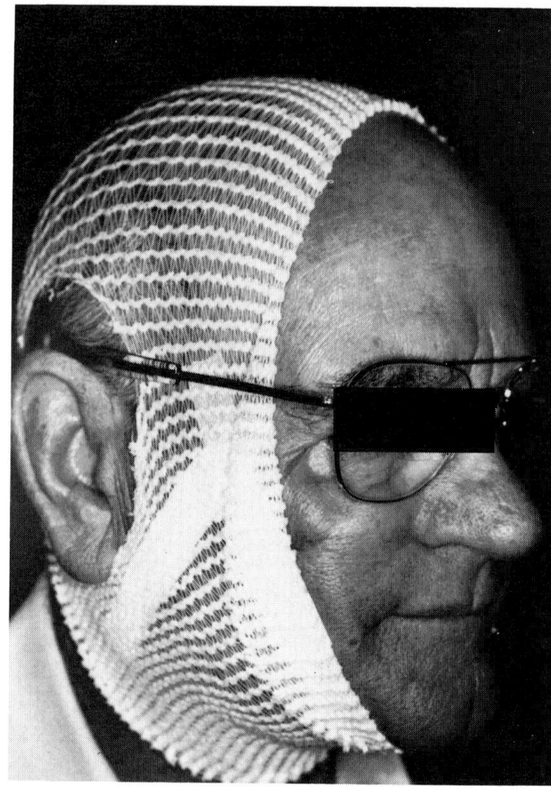

FIGURE 10–11. Tubular gauze secures dressings to the cheek in a satisfactory manner.

Dressings for the Eyelids and Medial Canthus

Small incisional wounds on the eyelids or in the periorbital tissues can sometimes be left to heal with only a coating of antibiotic ointment. Larger wounds and wounds awaiting occuloplastic reconstruction are best managed with an eye patch. Before placing an eye patch, the globe is protected by applying a thin coat of ophthalmic antibiotic ointment. It may then be useful to cover the closed eye first with a thin, smooth plastic film before taping a gauze eye patch in place.[30] The plastic film will inhibit evaporation of moisture from the wound and from the eye, and it will not cause corneal irritation should the patient inadvertently open the eye while wearing the patch. An eye patch should not remain in place continuously for longer than 24 hours without checking the eye for signs of irritation or infection and replenishing the antibiotic ointment.

Should so much tissue be sacrificed during Mohs surgery that the patient cannot close the eye, a temporary tarsorrhaphy suture should be placed. If a suture cannot be placed, the eye may be protected with a Guibor Bubble (Concept, Inc., 11311 Concept Blvd., Largo, FLA 34643).[30] This clear plastic moisture chamber

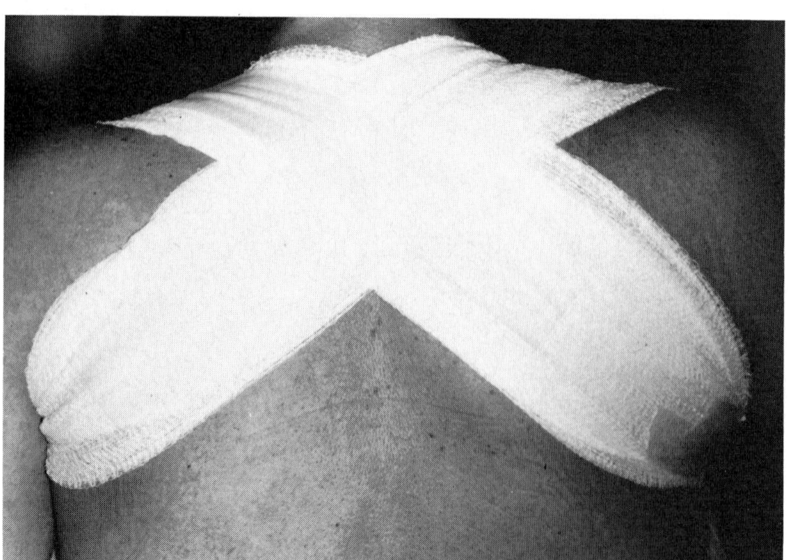

FIGURE 10–12. One or both axillae can be dressed with an elastic gauze roll applied in a figure-of-eight fashion.

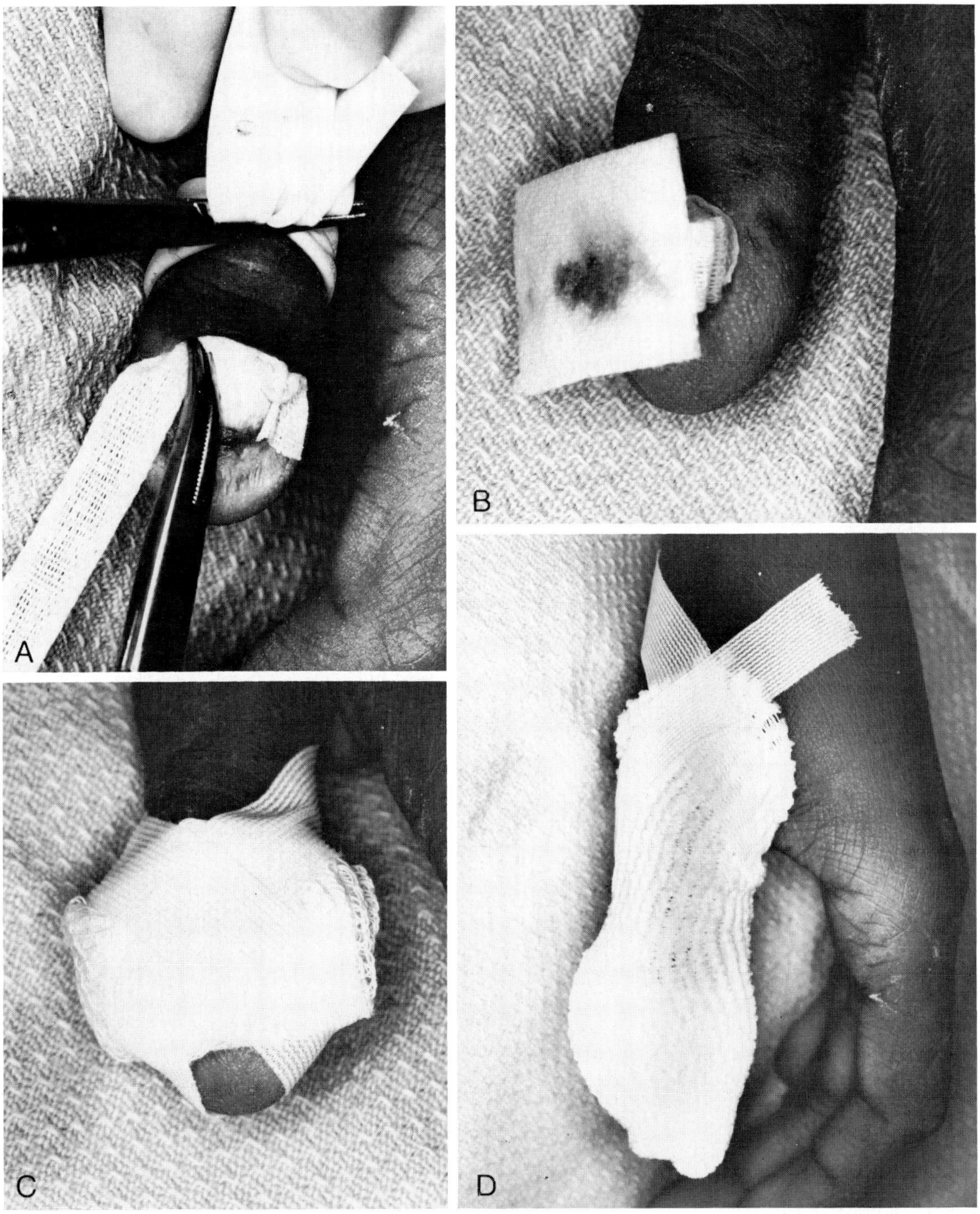

FIGURE 10-13. *A*, If surgery on a digit involves nail avulsion, hemostasis can be achieved by packing saline-soaked, iodoform gauze under the nailfolds. *B*, A nonadherent pad is added. *C*, A dry gauze pad is loosely taped in place. *D*, A length of small diameter tubular gauze provides both pressure and security. (From Winton, GB, and Salasche, SJ: Wound dressings for dermatologic surgery. *Journal of American Academy of Dermatology* 13:1026–44, 1985, with permission.)

is taped in place at the orbital rim after ointment has been applied to the globe. When secured in an airtight fashion, the chamber will quickly fog, demonstrating an adequate seal. It may be worn 12 hours or more as long as the seal is maintained.

Dressings for the Arms and Legs

Circumferential taping of dressings on the extremities can lead to vascular compromise, while vertical taping is rarely effective in securing a dressing to the skin. To avoid these problems, dressings can either be secured with diagonal taping or with tubular gauze of a suitable diameter.

The axilla is another problem area for achieving a secure dressing. Tape rarely works well because it is too rigid to allow comfortable motion in this area. To provide both security and flexibility, an axillary dressing can be achieved with a flexible gauze roll, such as Kerlix, wrapped in a figure-of-eight fashion across the back and around the contralateral shoulder and axilla (Fig. 10–12).

Dressings for the Hands, Feet, and Digits

A standard first-aid hand or foot wrap made from a gauze roll works well in these areas; tubular gauze is a handy substitute.

Tubular gauze in the smallest available size is commonly used to secure dressings on the digits (Fig. 10–13). If surgery has involved the removal of a nail, iodoform gauze moistened in saline can be packed under the nailfolds to aid in hemostasis. Antibiotic ointment, a small nonadherent pad, and a small dry gauze pad are loosely taped in place, avoiding constriction of vasculature. The tubular gauze then provides final security and pressure for the wound.

CONCLUSION

Wound dressings for Mohs surgery can be constructed of simple, inexpensive materials as long as the principles of moist wound care are followed. A dressing created in the office should not only be functional but also esthetically pleasing.

REFERENCES

1. Winton GB, Salasche SJ: Wound dressings for dermatologic surgery. J Am Acad Dermatol 13:1026–1044, 1985.
2. Hinman CD, Maibach H: Effect of air exposure and occlusion on experimental human skin wounds. Nature 200:377–378, 1963.
3. Harris DR: Healing of the surgical wound. J Am Acad Dermatol 1:208–215, 1979.
4. Winter G: Epidermal regeneration studied in the domestic pig. In Maibach H, Rovee D (eds): Epidermal Wound Healing. Chicago: Year Book Medical Publishers, 1976, pp 71–112.
5. Linsky C, Rovee D, Dow T: Effect of dressings on wound inflammation and scar tissue. In Dineen P, Hildick-Smith G (eds): The Surgical Wound. Philadelphia: Lea & Febiger, 1981, pp 191–205.
6. Geronemus RG, Robins P: The effect of two new dressings on epidermal wound healing. J Dermatol Surg Oncol 8:850–852, 1982.
7. Salasche SJ: Acute surgical complications: Cause, prevention, and treatment. J Am Acad Dermatol 15:1163–1185, 1986.
8. Eaglstein WH: Current wound management: A symposium. Clin Dermatol 2(3):134–142, 1984.
9. Eaglstein WH, Mertz PM, Alvarez OM: Effect of topically applied agents on healing wounds. Clin Dermatol 2(3):112–115, 1984.
10. Eaglstein WH, Mertz PM: "Inert" vehicles do affect wound healing. J Invest Dermatol 74:90–91, 1980.
11. Goslen JB: Wound healing for the dermatologic surgeon. J Dermatol Surg Oncol 14:959–972, 1988.
12. Salasche SJ, Winton GB: Clinical evaluation of a nonadhering wound dressing. J Dermatol Surg Oncol 12:1220–1222, 1986.
13. Salasche SJ, Feldman BD: Skin grafting: Perioperative technique and management. J Dermatol Surg Oncol 13:863–869, 1987.
14. Roth RR, Winton GB: A synthetic skin substitute as a temporary dressing in Mohs Surgery. J Dermatol Surg Oncol 15:670–672, 1989.
15. LaPiana FG: Epigard in the management of eyelid neoplasms. Ophthalmic Surg 12:744–746, 1981.
16. Eaglstein WH: Experiences with biosynthetic dressings. J Am Acad Dermatol 12:434–440, 1985.
17. Mertz PM, Eaglstein WH: The effect of a semi-occlusive dressing on the microbial population in superficial wounds. Arch Surg 119:287–289, 1984.
18. Field LM: Letter to the Editor. J Dermatol Surg Oncol 7:597, 1981.
19. Mandy SH: Evaluation of a new providone-iodine-impregnated polyethylene oxide gel occlusive dressing. J Am Acad Dermatol 13:655–659, 1985.
20. Whitaker DC, Grande DJ, Johnson SS: Wound infection rate in dermatologic surgery. J Dermatol Surg Oncol 14:525–528, 1988.
21. Zitelli JA: Secondary intention healing: an alternative to surgical repair. Clin Dermatol 2(3):92–106, 1984.
22. Zitelli JA: Delayed wound healing with adhesive wound dressings. J Dermatol Surg Oncol 10:709–710, 1984.
23. Hien NT, Prawer SE, Katz HI: Facilitated wound healing using transparent film dressing following Mohs micrographic surgery. Arch Dermatol 124:903–906, 1988.
24. Eaglstein WH, Davis SC, Muhle AL, Mertz PM: Optimal use of an occlusive dressing to enhance healing,

effect of delayed application and early removal of wound healing. Arch Dermatol 124:392–395, 1988.
25. Leipziger LS, Glushko V, DiBernardo B, et al.: Dermal wound repair: Role of collagen matrix implants and synthetic polymer dressings. J Am Acad Dermatol 12:409–419, 1985.
26. Zitelli J: Wound healing for the clinician. Adv Dermatol 2:243–268, 1987.
27. Salasche SJ, Winton GB, Adnot J: Surgical pearls. Dermatol Clin 7(1): 75–110, 1989.
28. Lobovits PE, Dzubow LM: A pressure dressing on the scalp by a modified Russian technique. J Dermatol Surg Oncol 6:259–263, 1980.
29. Robinson JK: An effective pressure dressing on the scalp that is easily made and cosmetically acceptable. J Dermatol Surg Oncol 7:607, 1981.
30. Whitaker DC, Goldstein GD, Birkby CS, Nerad JA: Postoperative techniques for corneal protection in Mohs micrographic surgery. J Dermatol Surg Oncol 14:951–955, 1988.

CHAPTER 11

Wound Healing

Mark R. Balle, M.D.
George R. Mikhail, M.D., M.S.

This section deals with practical aspects of the healing of defects following Mohs surgery in an outpatient setting. The indications for methods that may be applied in wound management for selected areas are also outlined. Reconstruction of the defects is not within the scope of this book.

Defects following Mohs surgery can be managed in several ways: primary closure (side-to-side closure), partial closure, flaps or grafts, or healing by second intention. Immediate closure decreases morbidity time, prevents the danger of secondary hemorrhage, and minimizes the chances of wound infection.

Many Mohs surgery wounds heal well by second intention. Certain areas heal particularly well with acceptable cosmetic results, depending on the size and site of the wound. Sites where good function and cosmesis may be obtained by second intention include the scalp, forehead, temples, canthi, eyelids, root of the nose, and the nasolabial folds. The main indications for allowing healing by second intention in our experience are:

1. After removal of recurrent lesions in order to detect early recurrence by avoiding burying tumor elements under a flap or a graft. Recurrent lesions are more likely to recur than primarily treated lesions.[1] This is particularly important when treating young patients.[2]
2. When the anatomic defect is expected to heal satisfactorily with good function and reasonable cosmesis.
3. When immediate repair cannot be easily undertaken because of the unusual size and site of the wound.
4. In areas where recurrences are common, such as the scalp and ears, and when the defect is small and distortion of the pinna, for example, can be avoided.
5. In cases with a history of radiotherapy, especially in lesions on the nose.
6. When there is loss of a major part of the nose. Such cases usually need prostheses (see Chapter 18).

In all of the above situations, the needed repair can be deferred, preferably for 12 months. Examples of healing in selected areas are presented here.

A woman had an extensive defect following Mohs excision of a large basal cell carcinoma (BCC) that involved the occipital scalp and posterior auricular area (Fig. 11–1). Excellent cosmesis resulted following healing by second intention. An identical wound in the same area in another patient is shown for comparison (Fig. 11–2). This wound was repaired with a split-thickness skin graft because the patient did not have help for wound care. Naturally, this resulted in a shorter morbidity.

Figure 11–3 illustrates a patient with a defect following Mohs surgery, using the fixed tissue technique for a BCC of the forehead. Although the postoperative wound was extensive, it healed with excellent cosmesis. There was no displacement of the eyebrows because of the

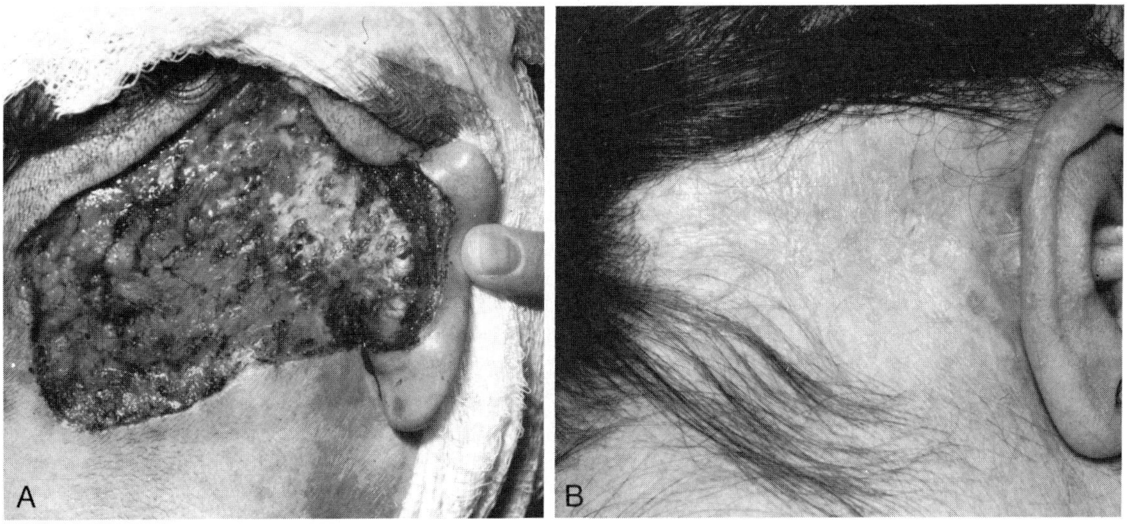

FIGURE 11–1. *A*, Defect following Mohs excision of a basal cell carcinoma on the occipital scalp and the posterior surface of the ear pinna. *B*, Result after healing by second intention.

central position of the defect. In the case shown in Figure 11–4, the patient had a large defect in the left temple area. The scar after healing by second intention was cosmetically acceptable. Figure 11–5 shows a patient with a large defect on the cheek following removal of a squamous cell carcinoma. The wound healed well by second intention with a final small scar despite the large size of the defect. This is usually the rule in elderly patients.

Wounds in the medial canthal area heal well provided they extend approximately equally above and below a line drawn between the medial canthi. Figure 11–6 illustrates this principle. The wound healed without ectropion. Wounds that have an appreciable portion of the defect below the intercanthal line as compared to the portion above it sometimes heal with acceptable results (Fig. 11–7); however, we usually advise immediate repair in such cases.

Some large defects of the lower eyelid can

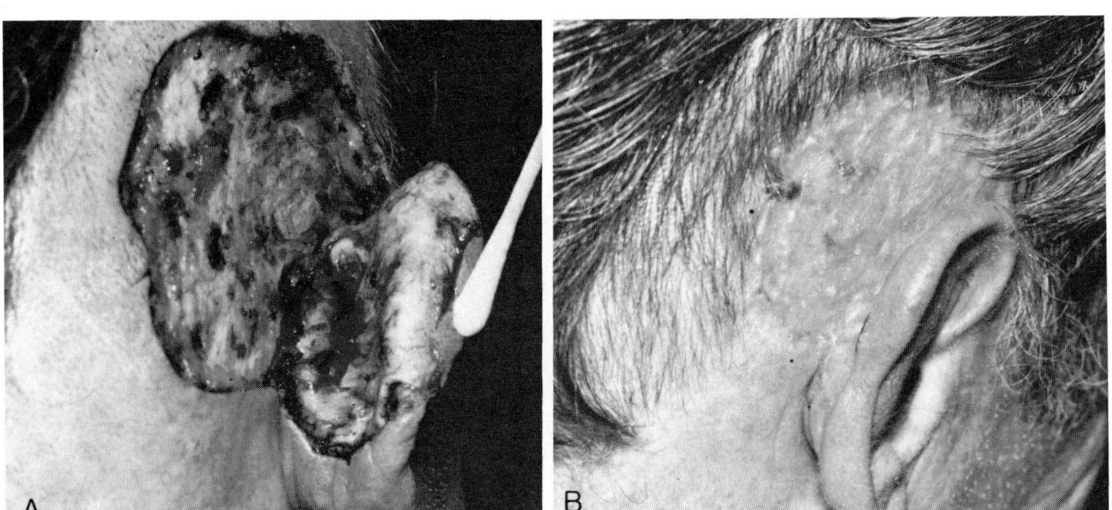

FIGURE 11–2. *A*, Defect after Mohs excision of a basal cell carcinoma almost identical in location and extent as that shown in Figure 11–1. *B*, Result after repair by split-thickness graft.

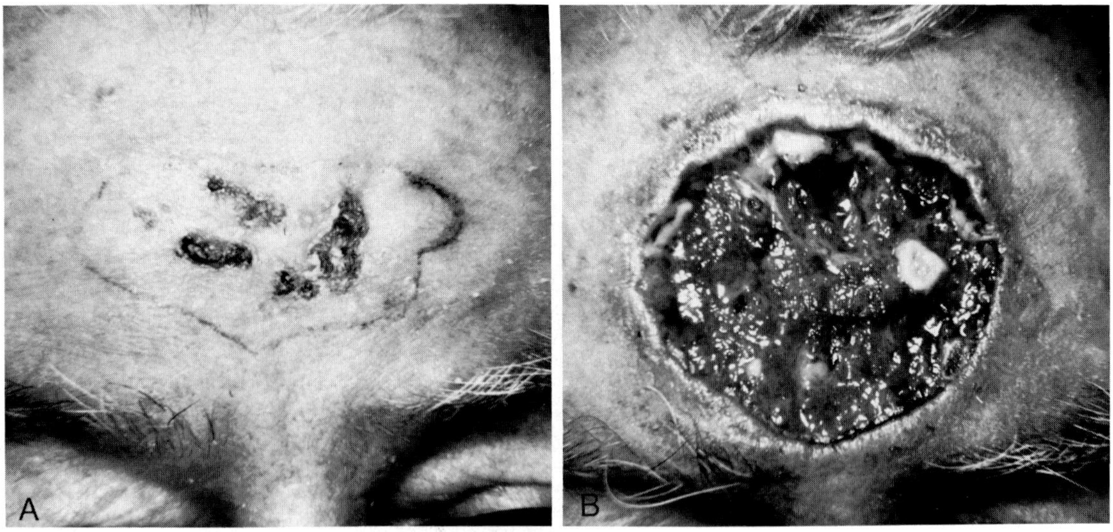

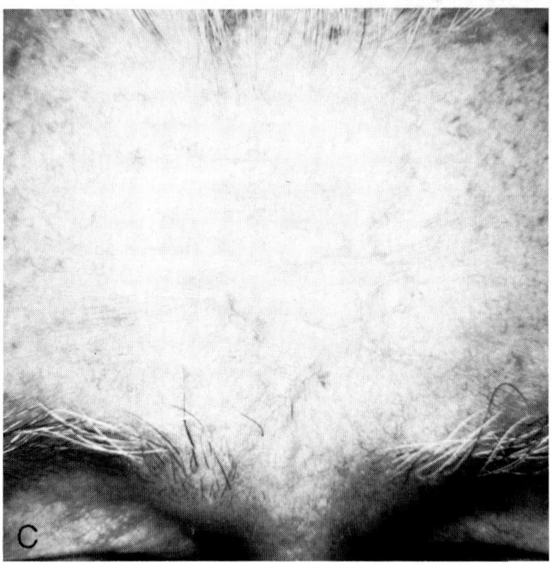

FIGURE 11–3. *A*, Basal cell carcinoma on the forehead. *B*, Defect following excision by Mohs fixed tissue technique. *C*, After healing by second intention; there was no displacement of the eyebrows.

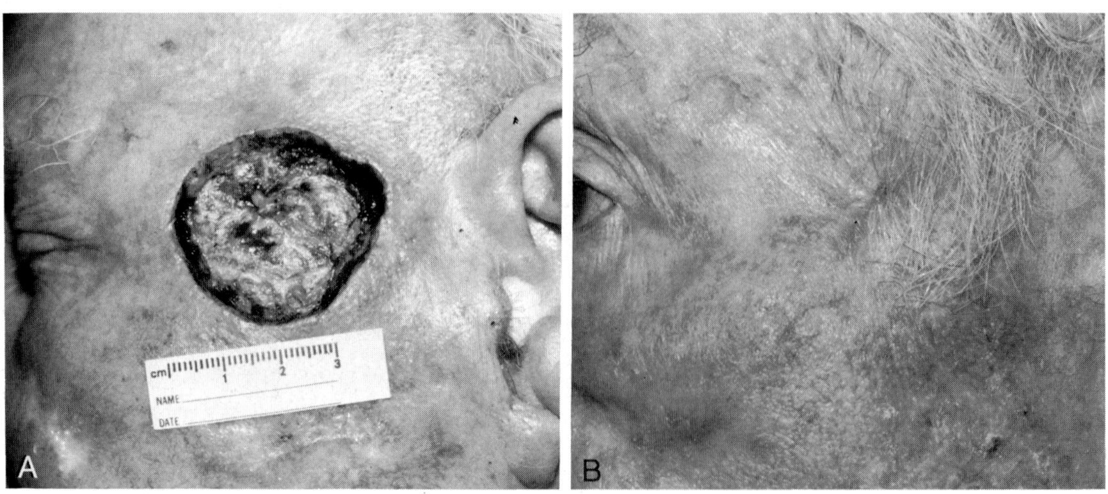

FIGURE 11–4. *A*, Defect in the left temple area after Mohs excision of a basal cell carcinoma. *B*, Result following healing by second intention.

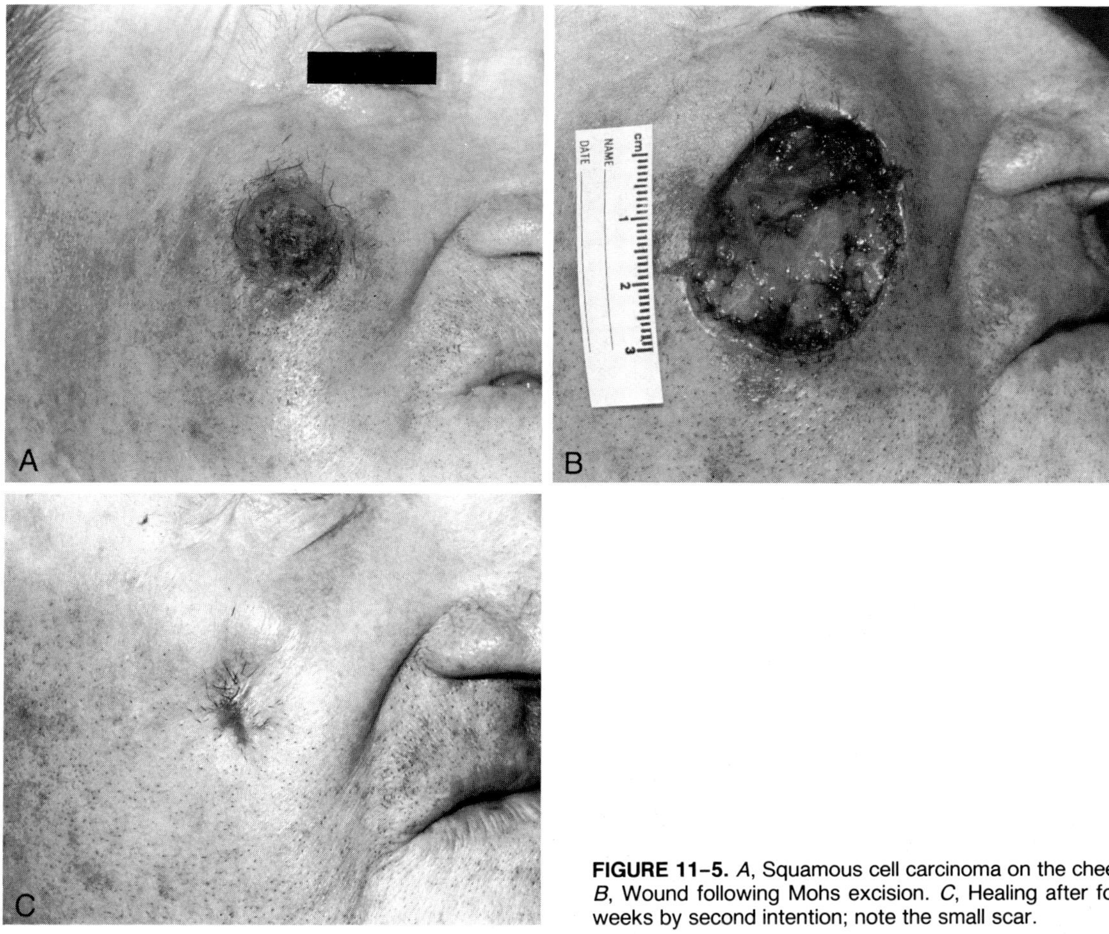

FIGURE 11–5. *A*, Squamous cell carcinoma on the cheek. *B*, Wound following Mohs excision. *C*, Healing after four weeks by second intention; note the small scar.

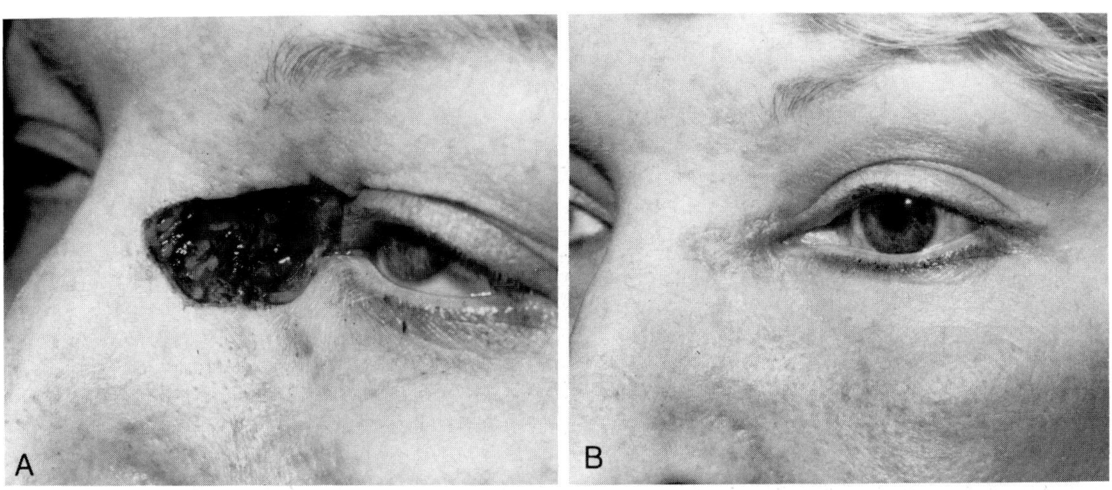

FIGURE 11–6. *A*, Defect following Mohs excision of a basal cell carcinoma in the medial canthal area. *B*, Result after healing by second intention; note acceptable cosmesis and function.

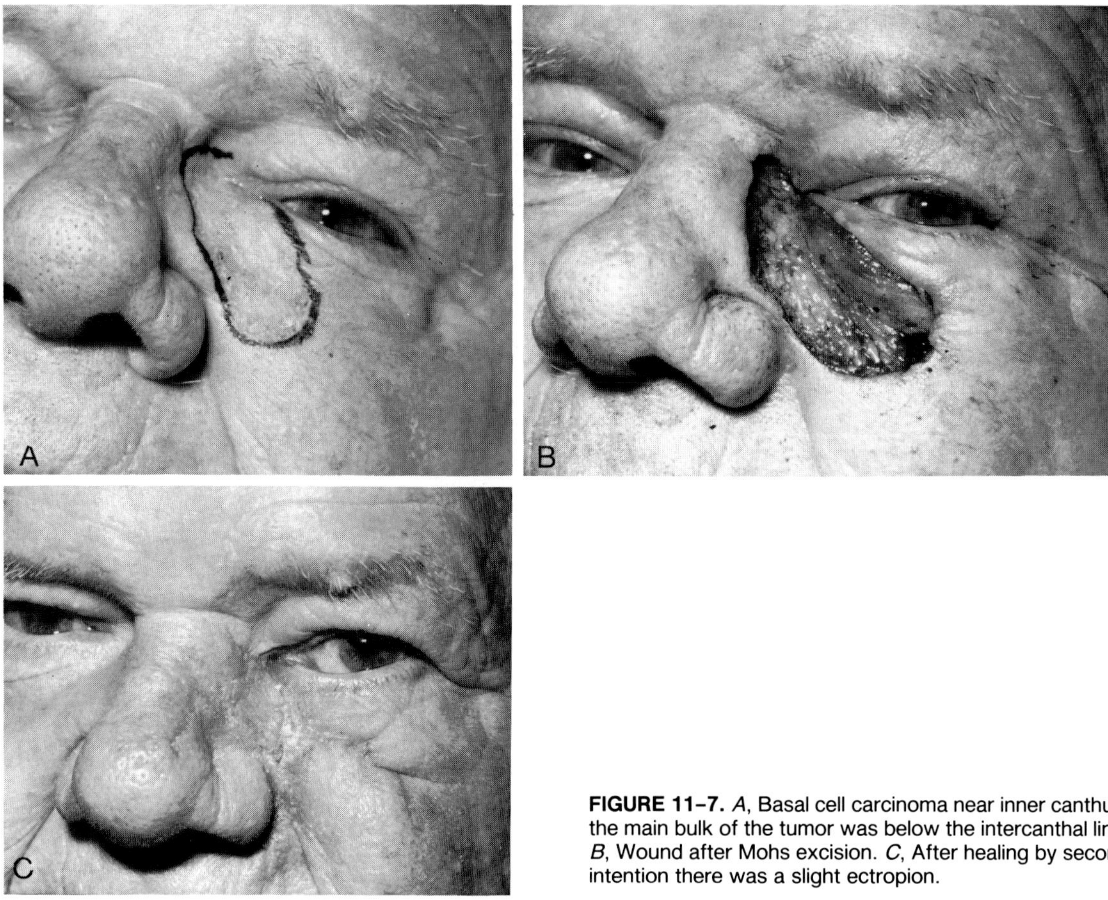

FIGURE 11–7. *A*, Basal cell carcinoma near inner canthus; the main bulk of the tumor was below the intercanthal line. *B*, Wound after Mohs excision. *C*, After healing by second intention there was a slight ectropion.

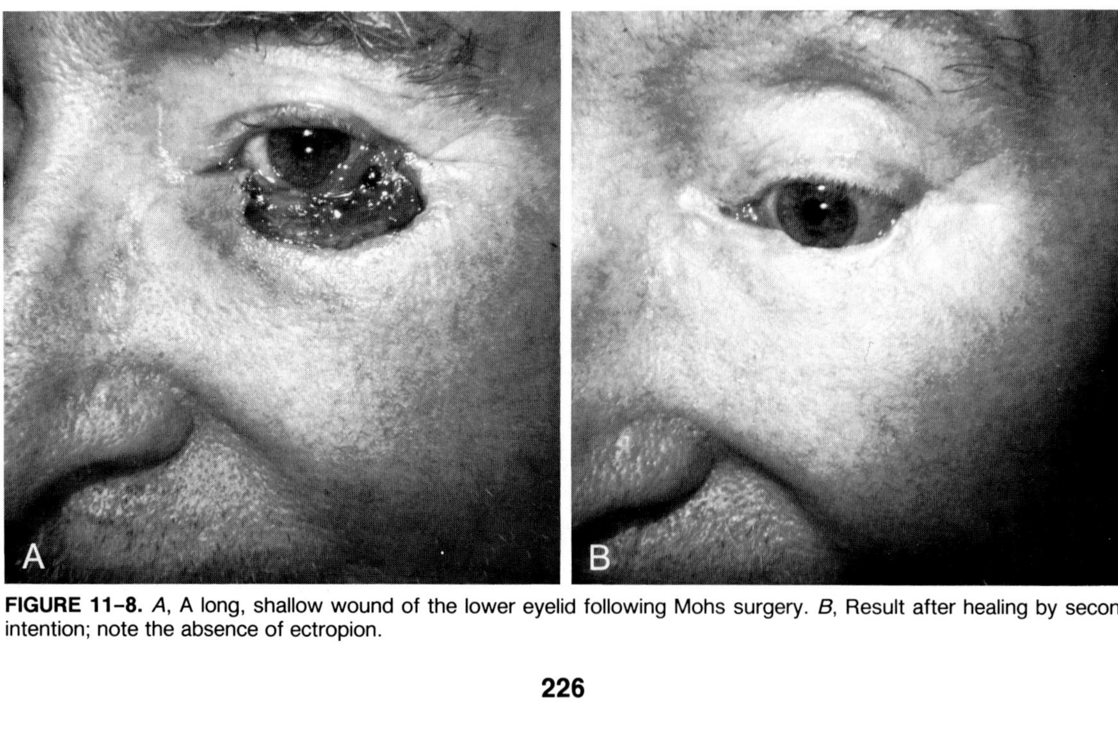

FIGURE 11–8. *A*, A long, shallow wound of the lower eyelid following Mohs surgery. *B*, Result after healing by second intention; note the absence of ectropion.

heal by second intention with very slight impairment of function and reasonably acceptable cosmesis. Defects of the lower eyelid that heal well by second intention are shallow and long, even when they encompass most of the eyelid margin (Fig. 11–8).

It is noteworthy that the conjunctiva, like other mucosal epithelium, regenerates much faster than the cutaneous epidermis,[3] and can therefore spread onto the lid margin by the time healing by second intention is complete (Fig. 11–9). This condition can clinically mimic a recurrent BCC to the uninitiated.

The next two cases illustrate healing by second intention on the nose. The first (Fig. 11–10) shows a wound after Mohs surgery for a BCC on the glabella and the root and bridge of the nose. Even though the wound was extensive, healing occurred without much distortion of the regional anatomy. The second patient

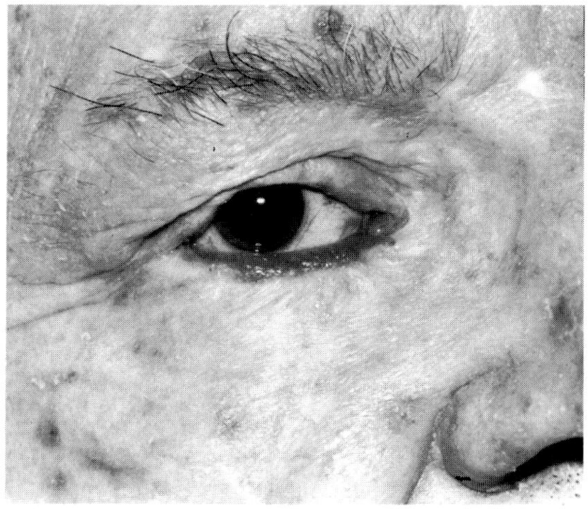

FIGURE 11–9. Wound of eyelid margin healed by second intention; note that the conjunctiva has spread onto the lid margin giving the impression of a recurrent basal cell carcinoma.

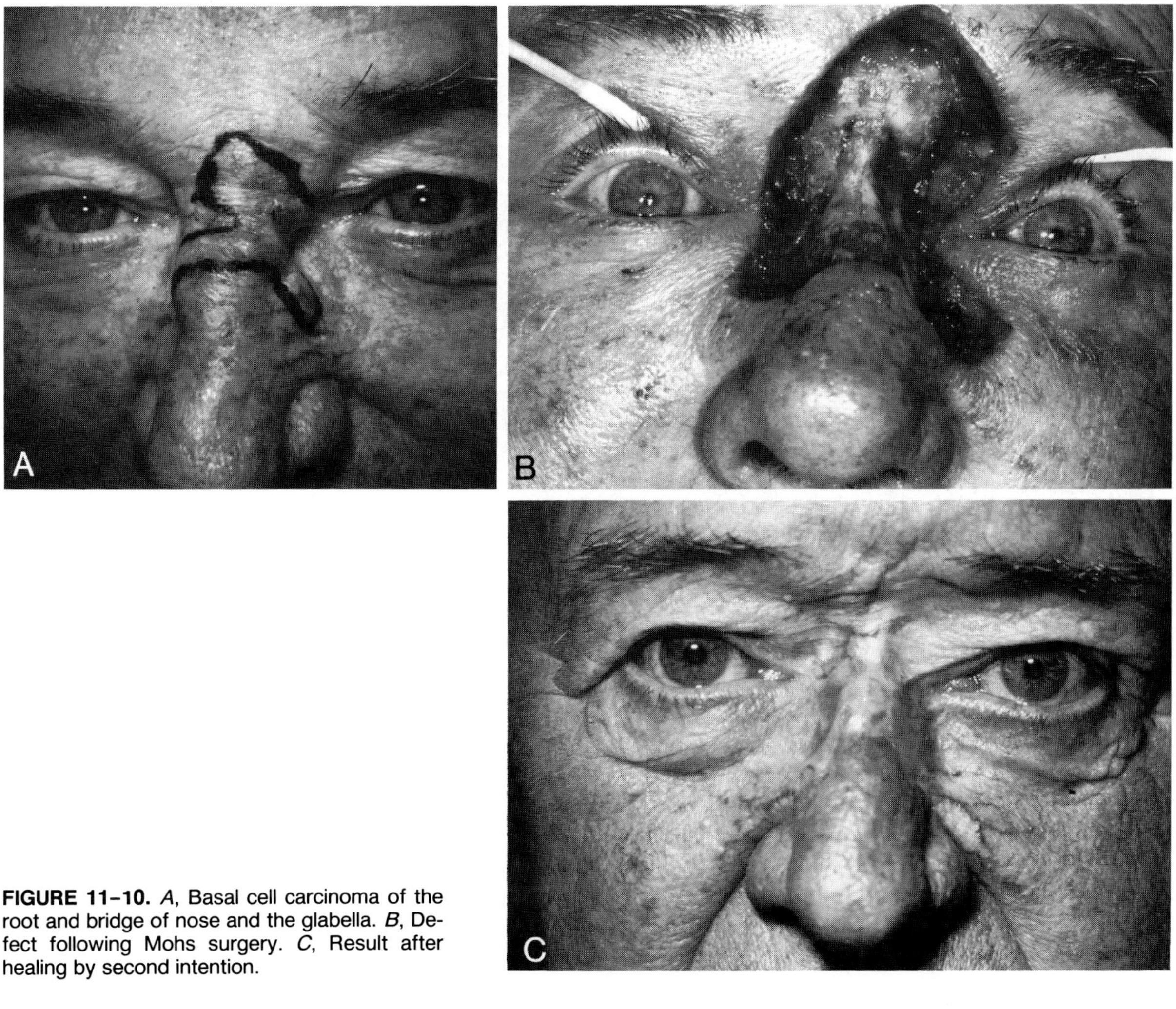

FIGURE 11–10. *A*, Basal cell carcinoma of the root and bridge of nose and the glabella. *B*, Defect following Mohs surgery. *C*, Result after healing by second intention.

(Fig. 11–11) had a basal cell carcinoma of the nose that after surgery resulted in a defect in the left tip and ala nasi. As the cartilage was spared, the wound healed with a slight distortion of the alar rim.

Even areas that often require immediate repair, such as the lip, can heal by second intention with reasonably satisfactory results. The patient in Figure 11–12 had a large defect of the upper lip that involved extensive portions of the cutaneous and mucosal surfaces of the lip following excision of a large BCC. The defect healed well by second intention, resulting in a scar that could be revised for optimal cosmesis.

There are many elegant ways to reconstruct wound defects using skin flaps. Whenever possible, the technique best suited to optimize the cosmetic result should be used. For a discussion of the design and use of skin flaps and grafts, the reader is referred to textbooks devoted to these topics. There are several main indications for immediate repair of wounds:

1. To retain function. Eyelid defects should be repaired when healing by second intention is expected to result in ectropion or inadequate protection of the eyeball. Wounds that result in a fistula through a cheek should be repaired.

2. To decrease morbidity time in debilitated patients and in those who cannot be assisted with dressing changes.

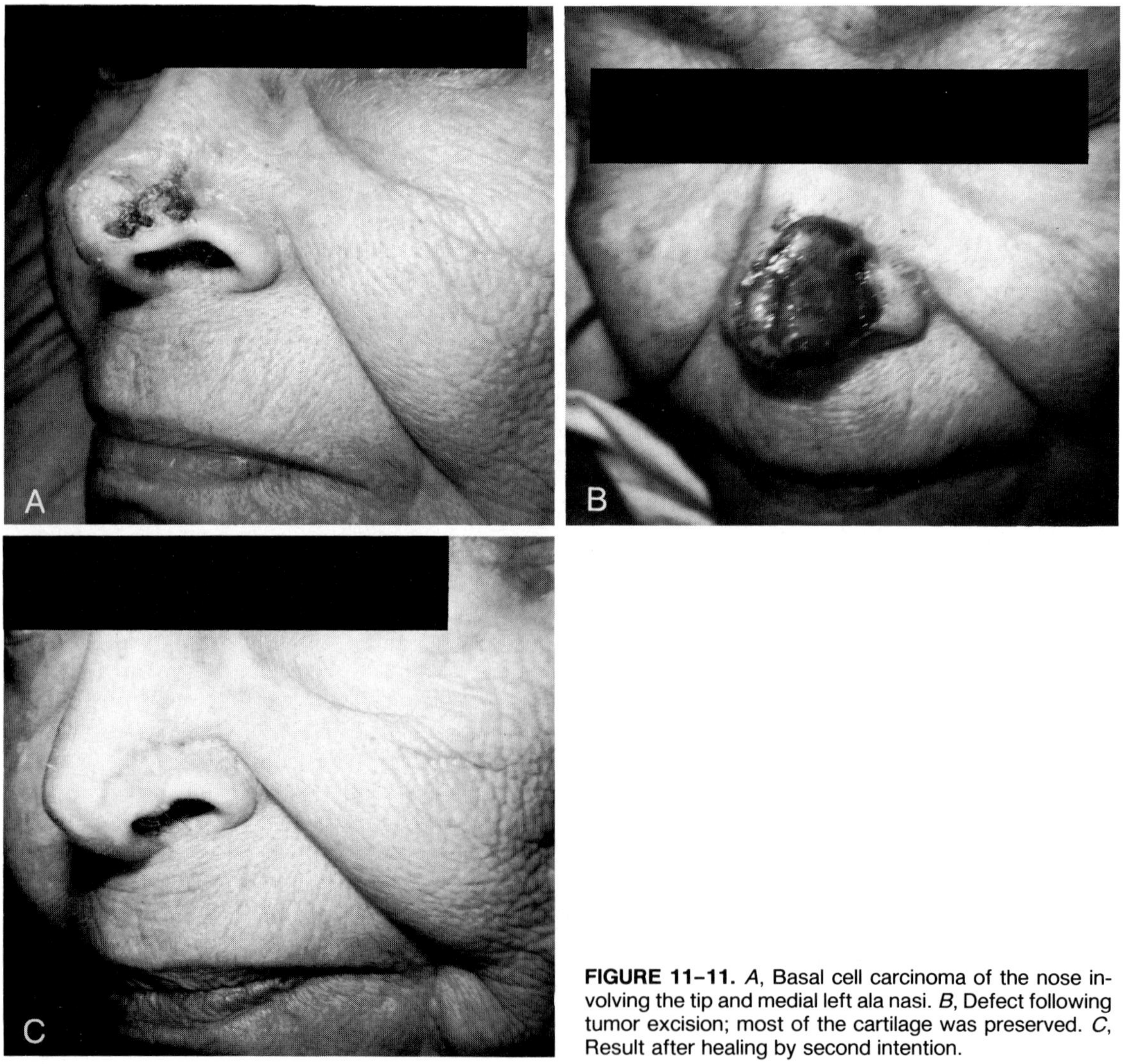

FIGURE 11–11. *A*, Basal cell carcinoma of the nose involving the tip and medial left ala nasi. *B*, Defect following tumor excision; most of the cartilage was preserved. *C*, Result after healing by second intention.

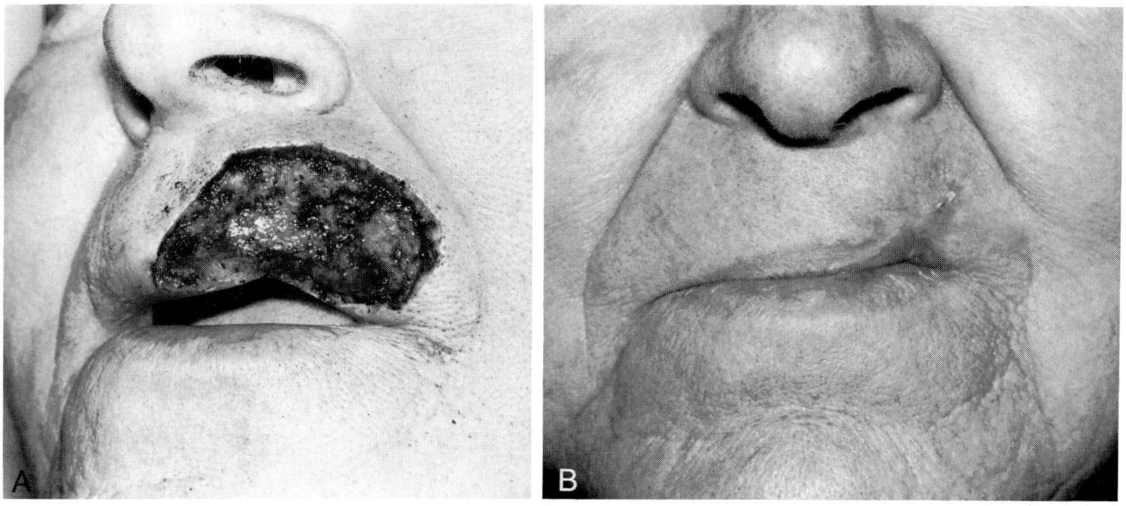

FIGURE 11–12. *A*, Large defect of upper lip that included skin and mucosa. *B*, Result 3½ months later. Note minimal scar and function; the scar can now be revised.

3. To avoid secondary hemorrhage when large arteries, e.g., the superficial temporal artery, are exposed.

4. To prevent stenosis of the external auditory meatus and ear canal.

5. To prevent undue disfigurement, e.g., distortion of the contour of the pinna of the ear or the lips. Large wounds above an eyebrow, where healing by second intention would result in upward displacement of the eyebrow, and defects on the nose that are expected to result in distortion of the nose and nasal vestibule if left to heal by second intention should also be repaired.

6. To perform skin grafts, if necessary, e.g., when the skull is exposed more than 2.5 cm.

A patient with an extensive BCC on the left forehead and temple (Fig. 11–13) was left with a large defect. A graft was used to close the

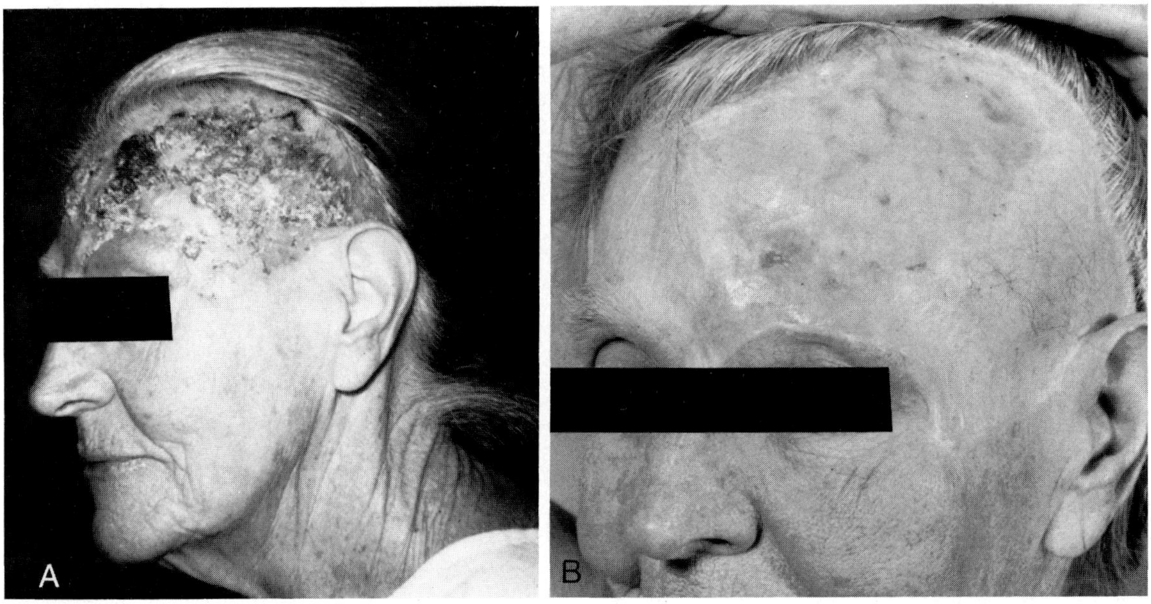

FIGURE 11–13. *A*, Patient with extensive basal cell carcinoma of the forehead and temple. *B*, Five years after repair by a split-thickness graft.

wound with a good functional result. Less extensive bone exposure justifies early repair in elderly people who do not have the help needed for the care of a granulating wound. The same applies to wounds in debilitated patients.

As mentioned above, it is important to repair defects that may result in stenosis of the external auditory meatus and ear canal. A BCC was removed from the patient in Figure 11–14 that resulted in an extensive defect that surrounded the external auditory meatus. The wound was grafted; however, stenosis of the meatus and canal occurred and the pinna was distorted. Subsequent revision and dilatation of the canal restored patency. This is especially important in people who wear hearing aids. The patient in Figure 11–15 had an extensive BCC of the concha and preauricular area that resulted in a large defect that surrounded the auditory meatus. Grafting the defect in the ear canal retained its patency. In another case (Fig. 11–16), the patient had a BCC removed from the ear that resulted in a defect equally distributed around the external auditory meatus.

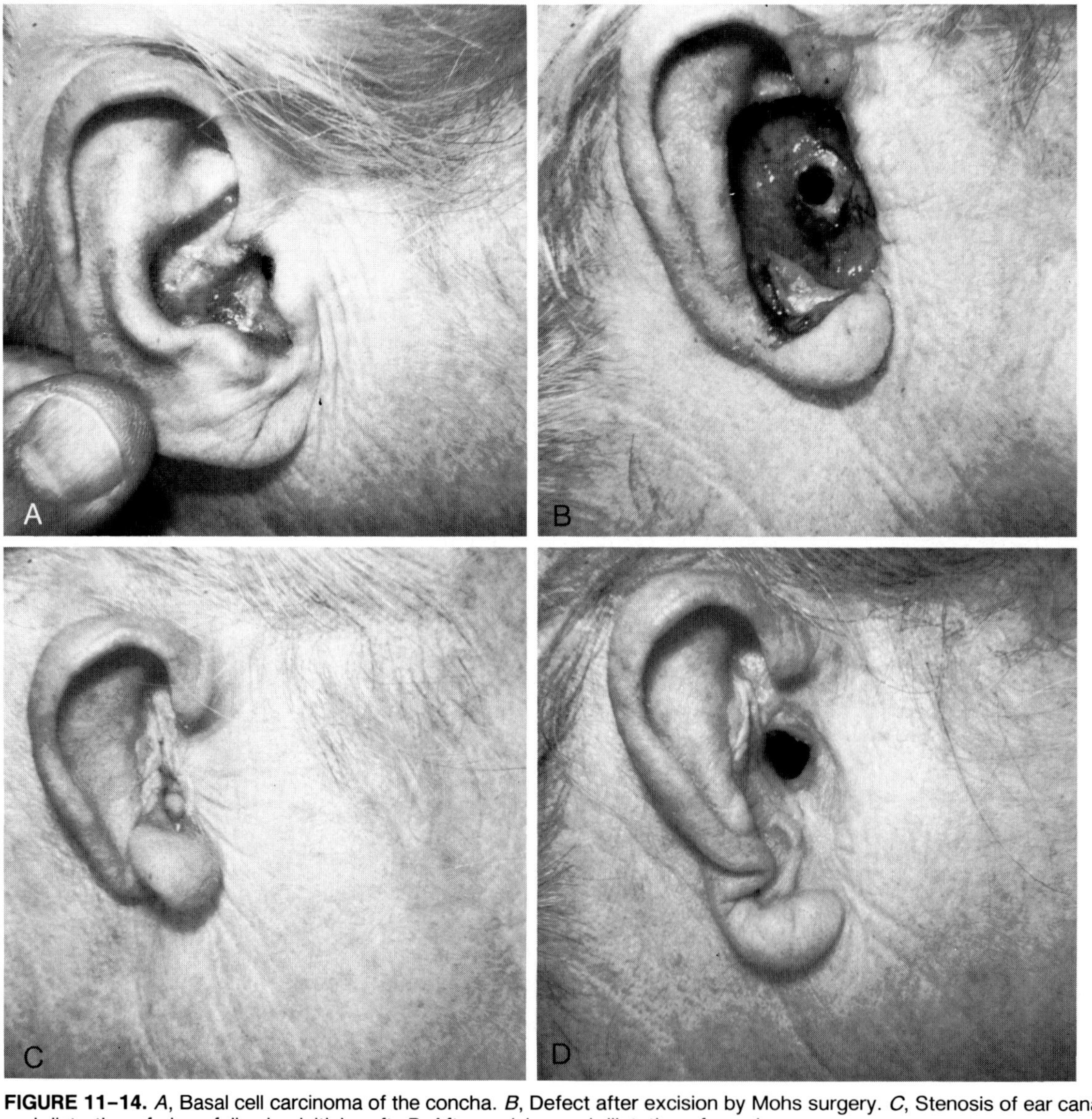

FIGURE 11–14. *A*, Basal cell carcinoma of the concha. *B*, Defect after excision by Mohs surgery. *C*, Stenosis of ear canal and distortion of pinna following initial graft. *D*, After revision and dilatation of canal.

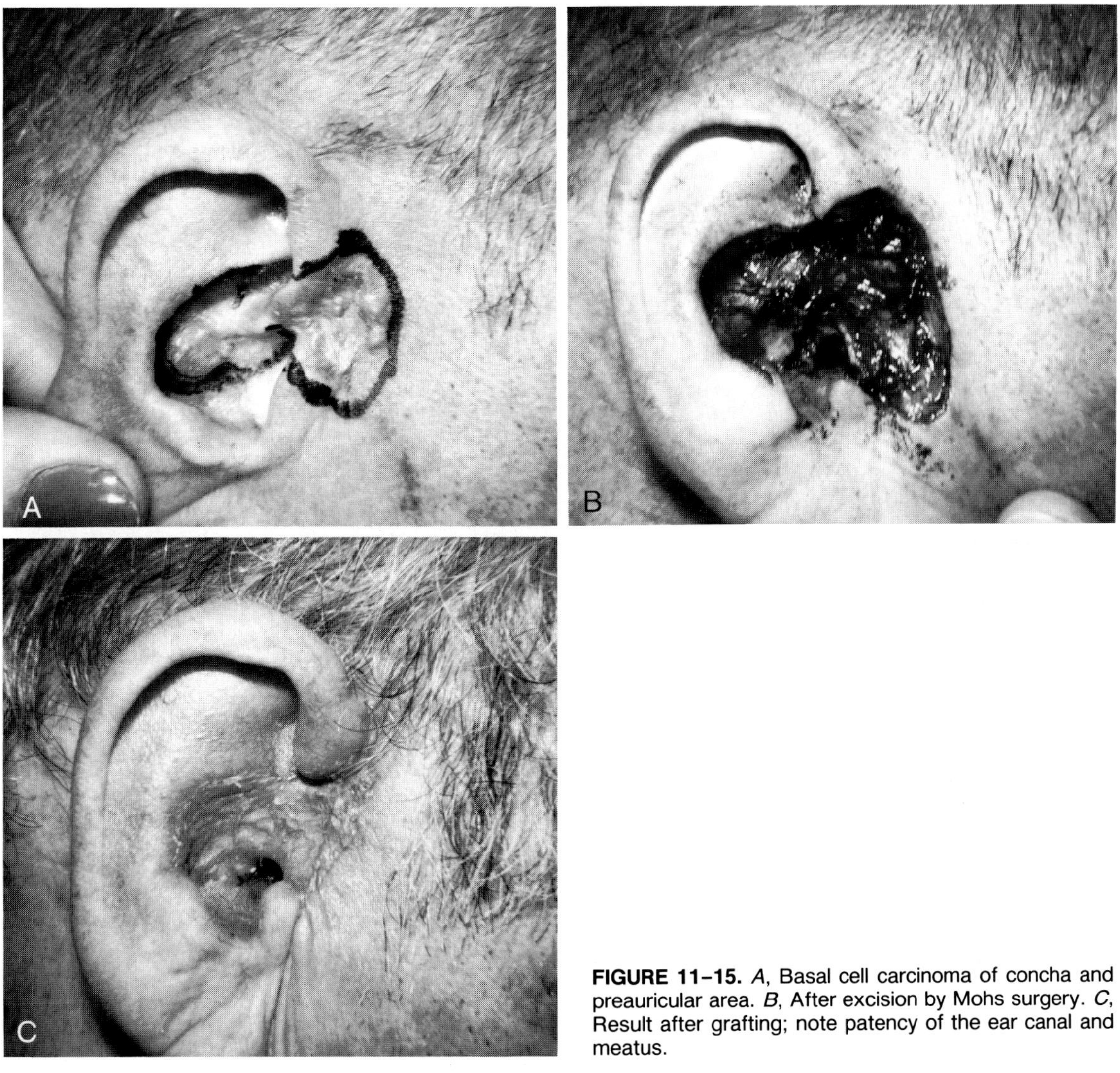

FIGURE 11–15. *A*, Basal cell carcinoma of concha and preauricular area. *B*, After excision by Mohs surgery. *C*, Result after grafting; note patency of the ear canal and meatus.

Healing by second intention, in this case, left a patent canal due to equal contraction of the wound around and away from the auditory canal.

In some defects of the pinna, sufficient cartilage is saved and can be left to heal by second intention. A method originally suggested by Latenser recommends making multiple perforations with a 3 mm skin punch through the remaining cartilage at the wound base in order to provide granulation tissue from the posterior connective tissue and expedite healing.[4] The patient in Figure 11–17 had a BCC removed that resulted in a defect of the antihelix. The wound healed by second intention with minimal distortion after applying this technique.

When removal of a tumor results in a defect of the pinna with extensive loss of cartilage, early repair is indicated. A patient following removal of a BCC on the antihelix of the ear was left with significant loss of cartilage (Fig. 11–18). The wound was left to heal by second intention. This resulted in collapse of the pinna. Early repair is recommended in such cases.

Partial closure can be useful in repairing some defects that involve the pinna. The patient in Figure 11–19 had a recurrent BCC that upon removal resulted in a defect in the infraauricular area and loss of the earlobe. The re-

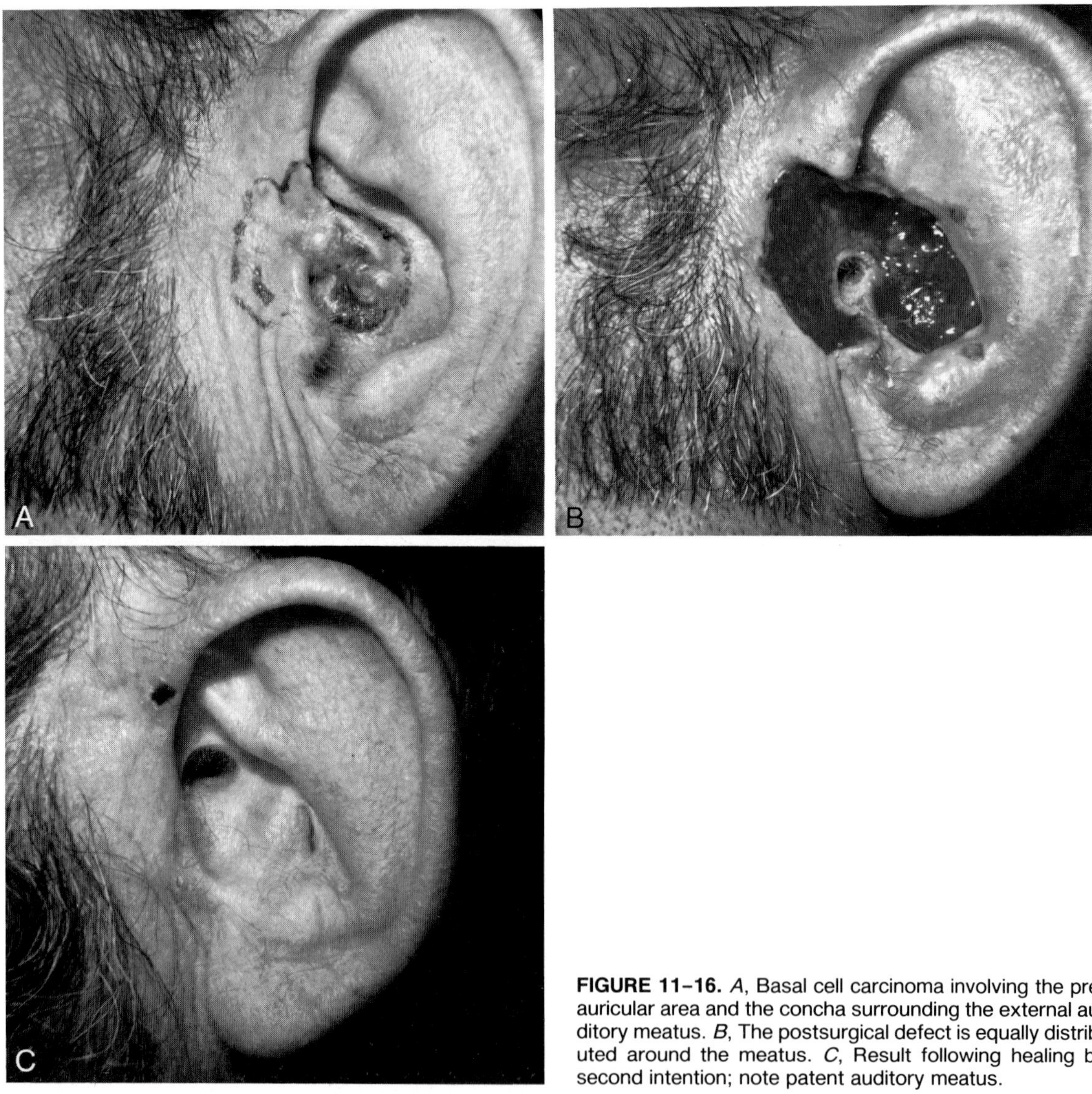

FIGURE 11–16. *A*, Basal cell carcinoma involving the preauricular area and the concha surrounding the external auditory meatus. *B*, The postsurgical defect is equally distributed around the meatus. *C*, Result following healing by second intention; note patent auditory meatus.

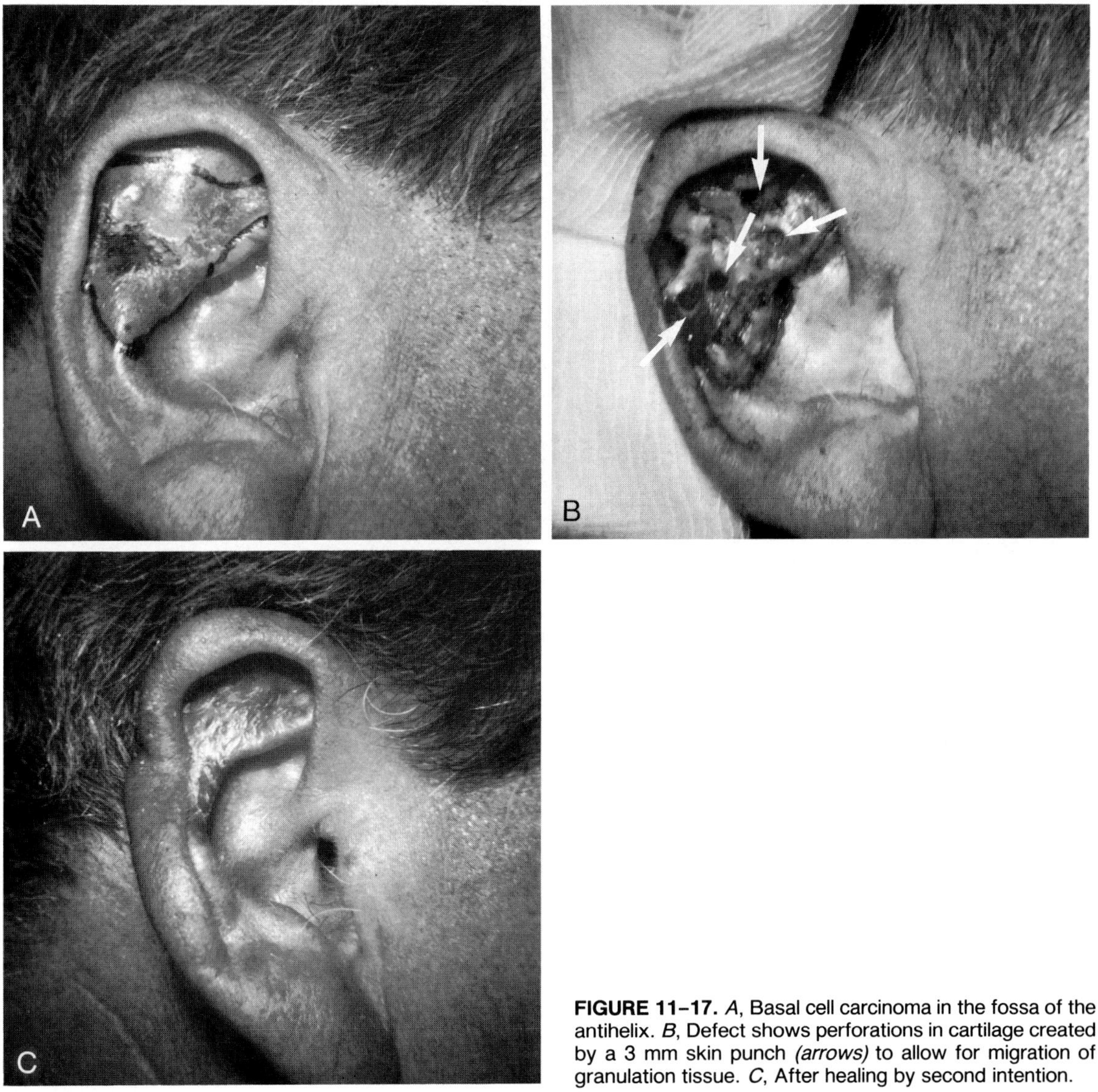

FIGURE 11–17. *A*, Basal cell carcinoma in the fossa of the antihelix. *B*, Defect shows perforations in cartilage created by a 3 mm skin punch *(arrows)* to allow for migration of granulation tissue. *C*, After healing by second intention.

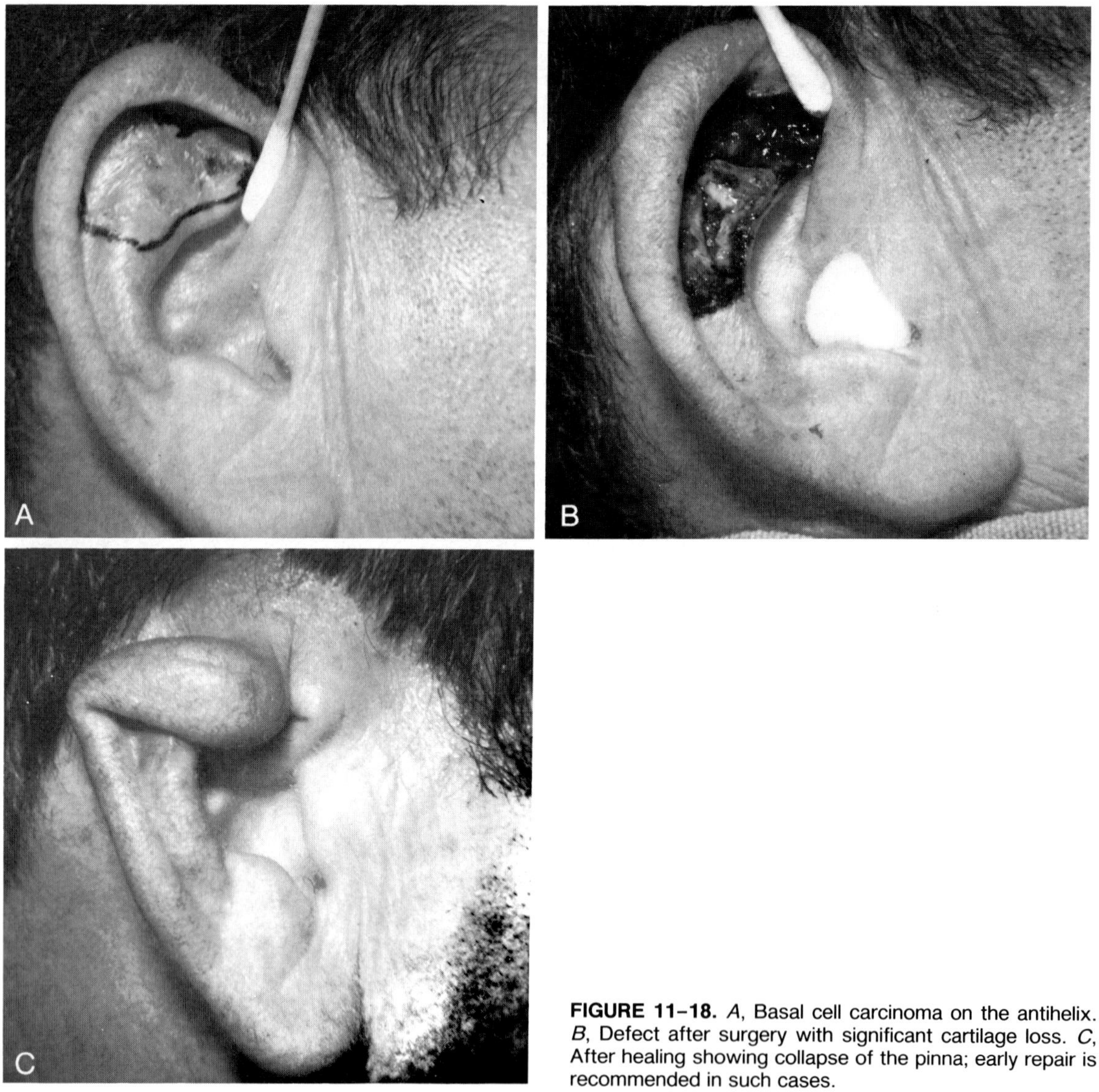

FIGURE 11–18. *A*, Basal cell carcinoma on the antihelix. *B*, Defect after surgery with significant cartilage loss. *C*, After healing showing collapse of the pinna; early repair is recommended in such cases.

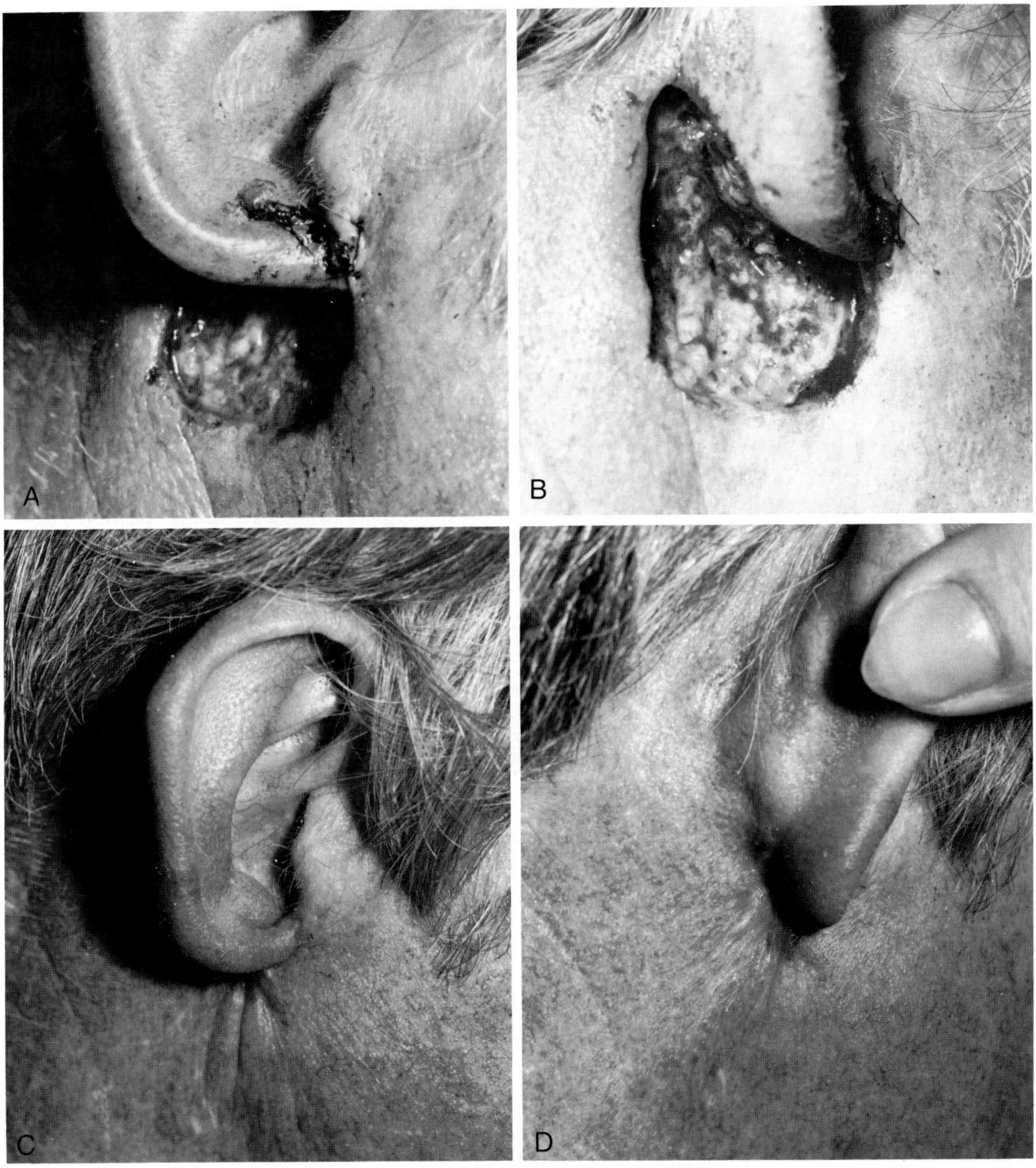

FIGURE 11–19. *A*, Partial closure after removal of a tumor that involved the lobe of the ear and the infra-auricular area; the base of the lobe was sutured to the anterior margin of the wound. *B*, Posterior view of *A*. *C*, Result after healing of remaining wound by second intention. *D*, Posterior view of *C*.

maining inferior tip of the pinna was sutured anteriorly to recreate the appearance of an earlobe. The remainder of the wound was left to heal by second intention. The patient had an acceptable result.

If a patient wears eyeglasses, and the majority of our patients do, the preservation of a portion of the ear serves an important function, a rest for the glasses. The patient in Figure 11–20 had a BCC that involved the helix and antihelix of the right ear that required extensive removal of cartilage in both areas. The remain-

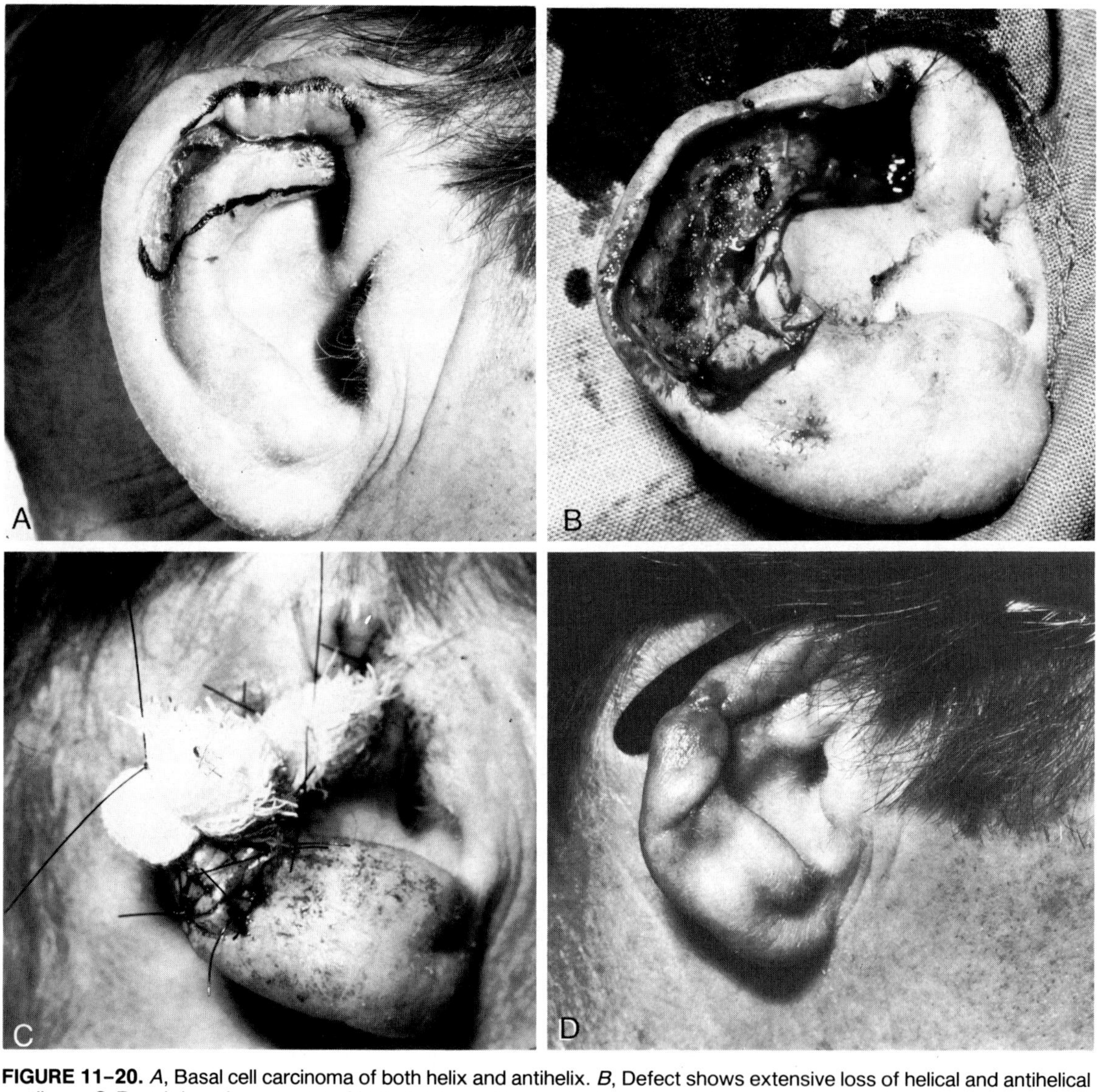

FIGURE 11–20. *A*, Basal cell carcinoma of both helix and antihelix. *B*, Defect shows extensive loss of helical and antihelical cartilage. *C*, Repair by advancement of helical skin. *D*, Newly created helical ridge supporting eyeglasses.

ing helical skin was sutured to that of the antihelix to form a "helical ridge," which provided enough support for the eyeglasses.

REFERENCES

1. Menn H, Robins P, Kopf A, Bart R: The recurrent basal cell epitheliomas. Arch Dermatol 103:628–631, 1971.
2. Robins P, Albom MJ: Recurrent basal cell carcinomas in young women. J Dermatol Surg 1:49–51, 1975.
3. Mackenzie HC, Binnie WH: Recent advances in oral surgery research. J Oral Pathol 12:389–412, 1983.
4. Mohs FE: Chemosurgery: Microscopically Controlled Surgery for Skin Cancer. Springfield, Ill.: Charles C. Thomas, 1978, p 87.

CHAPTER 12

Cancers of the Genitalia and the Perineum

George R. Mikhail, M.D., M.S.

Mohs micrographic surgery is assuming an important role in the treatment of malignancies on the genitals. The results obtained have been gratifying and well appreciated by the urologists we have interacted with and by the patients treated.

ANATOMIC CONSIDERATIONS

The surface of the genital area is made up of two different types of epithelium. Besides the skin covering, which contains hairs and sweat glands, mucosal epithelium that is devoid of horny layer and adnexal structures is present on the glans penis and the inner surface of the foreskin of the uncircumcised man and on the labia minor, the vestibule, and the clitoris in women. Recognition of these anatomic characteristics is important in the management of malignancies that develop in these areas.

Figure 12–1 depicts the surgical anatomy of the anterior part of the penis, as seen in a sagittal section. The superficial anatomy of the perineal region in the woman is shown in Figure 12–2.

The lymph vessels of the scrotal and penile skin and prepuce drain into the superficial inguinal lymph nodes. The glans, corpora cavernosa, and part of the urethra also drain into the deep inguinal glands bilaterally. However, some lymph vessels pass directly to the external iliac nodes. In the case of the female pudenda, the lymph vessels from the labia majora, the labia minora, and the lower third of the vagina drain into the superficial inguinal lymph nodes. Therefore, detection of local lymph node metastases from the external genitalia can be easily determined by simple clinical examination.

The nerve supply of the male and female external genital organs is derived from the pudendal nerves in the sacral area (S2 to S4). The penis is innervated by a right and left dorsal nerve that run along the dorsal surface of the penis and give off smaller branches that extend to the ventral surface. The frenulum is innervated by branches situated between the deep fascia (Buck's fascia) and the corpora cavernosa. In addition to the pudendal nerve supply, the vulva contains Meissner's corpuscles that are especially numerous in the clitoris. Pacini's corpuscles are also present in the clitoris and labia majora.[1]

REGIONAL BLOCK ANESTHESIA

Regional block anesthesia of the penis is achieved by injecting local anesthetic (we use 1% lidocaine) around and encircling the root of the penis. However, when the frenulum is in the surgical field, additional anesthetic has to be introduced between Buck's fascia in the perineum and the corpora cavernosa. A total of 10 to 20 ml of the lidocaine solution should suffice

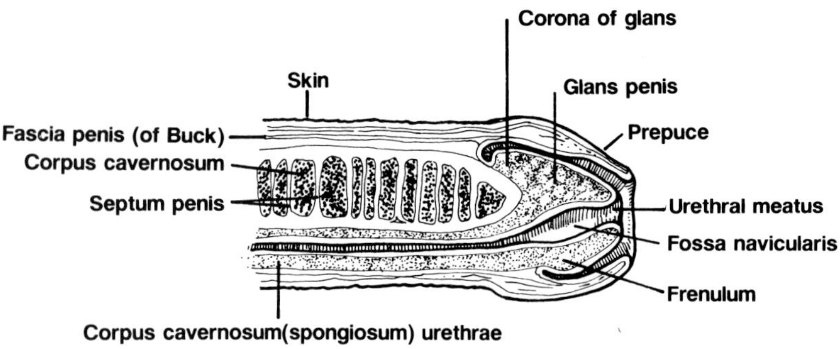

FIGURE 12–1. Surgical anatomy of the penis in a sagittal section.

for the entire procedure. Operative analgesia is established in about 10 to 15 minutes and lasts 1 to 3 hours. In the case of small lesions, analgesia can be simply achieved by injecting small amounts of the anesthetic into the involved area. This is particularly useful when the lesion is on the frenulum.

Block anesthesia of the female external genitalia requires that the clitoris be separately anesthetized if it is in the area of the surgery (see Chapter 6).

CLINICAL CONSIDERATIONS

The clinical features of malignant and premalignant lesions of the external genitalia can be protean. The presentation may appear quite banal or may simulate a benign condition so closely that incorrect diagnoses might easily be made. Remember that many skin diseases, including malignancies, that occur in the genital region may closely resemble one another; therefore, it is important to identify the lesion under consideration by histopathologic examination, particularly if malignancies are to be detected and treated as early as possible.

Biopsy material is most adequate and informative when obtained through an excisional or elliptic, incisional biopsy. However, deep shave biopsies and even punch biopsies can be helpful if subcutaneous tissue is included in the material. The biopsy wounds may be sutured or, in the case of shave biopsies, may be left to heal by second intention.

Benign tumors of the genitalia are relatively uncommon and usually not much of a problem. They include, among other entities, epithelial cysts, angiomas, Fordyce's angiokeratoma, fibromas, neuromas, myomas, lipomas, and molluscum contagiosum.

Although condyloma acuminatum, or venereal wart, is a benign lesion, it deserves special mention. It presents little difficulty in di-

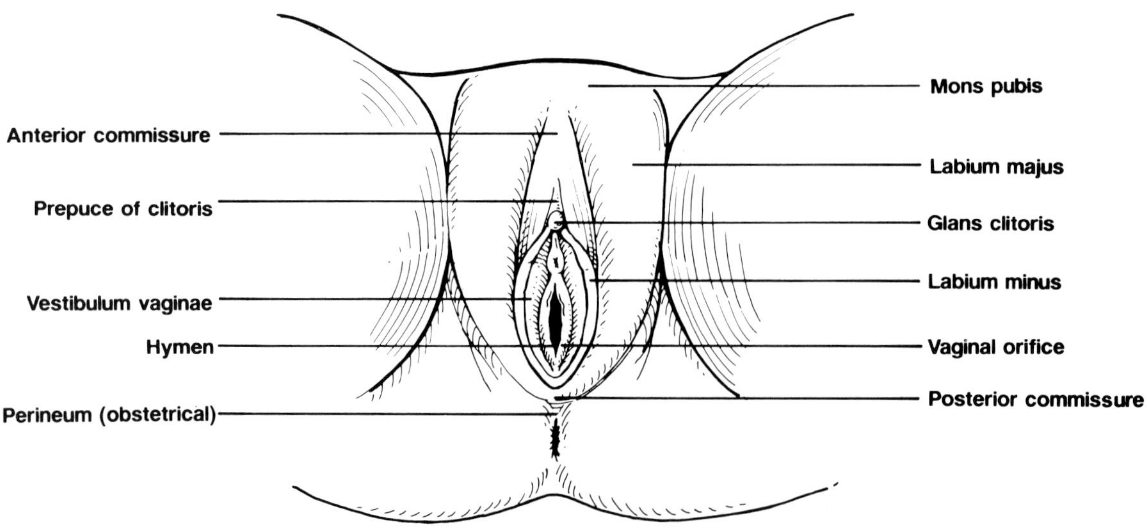

FIGURE 12–2. Surface anatomy of the vulva and perineum.

agnosis, but its eradication may prove problematic. Also, some authors have related it to verrucous carcinoma.[19] When the lesions are large (the size of a fingertip or larger), they require careful histological examination of the growth to exclude a carcinoma, and should ordinarily be excised because of poor response to other modalities.[2]

Malignant and premalignant lesions of the genitals are more common than the benign variety and are the main concern of this chapter.

PREMALIGNANT LESIONS AND CARCINOMAS IN SITU

Erythroplasia of Queyrat

Erythroplasia of Queyrat (EQ) is a squamous cell carcinoma in situ that affects the genital mucosae. In the male, it occurs almost exclusively on the inner surface of the prepuce and on the glans penis. The age range is 20 to 80 years.[3] Although the etiology of EQ remains unclear, the condition appears to be related to irritation from retention of smegma inside the preputial sack. In support of this is the fact that it is not seen in persons that have been circumsized during infancy. In the female, the lesion occurs predominantly on the labia minora.

In our experience, EQ is the most common malignant lesion of the genitalia. The lesions present as red, velvety, shiny plaques, which may be asymptomatic but are usually pruritic. Many cases have been diagnosed by clinicians as inflammatory conditions, notably eczema, contact dermatitis, and candidiasis (Fig. 12–3A). The development of ulceration usually signifies transformation into invasive epidermoid (squamous cell) carcinoma.[3] About 10% of EQ cases have evidence of squamous cell carcinoma, and 2% have lymph node metastasis by the time the patient presents for treatment.[4]

Generally, the histopathology of EQ is similar to that of Bowen's disease (Fig. 12–3B). However, it differs from it in several aspects that have certain prognostic and therapeutic implications. Unlike Bowen's disease, EQ is not associated with an increased incidence of internal malignancies nor related to the ingestion of arsenic, but is has a greater tendency toward invasiveness and metastasis.[3–5] In our series of 36 patients with EQ, invasive carcinoma had developed in 12 instances (33%) by the time they presented. One cannot overstress the importance of obtaining biopsy material from any recalcitrant lesion of the glans penis or prepuce. Also, it is advisable and proper to consult with a urologist before embarking on the treatment of a penile malignancy. This is particularly important when the lesion extends proximally along the urethra.

Topical chemotherapy with 5-fluorouracil

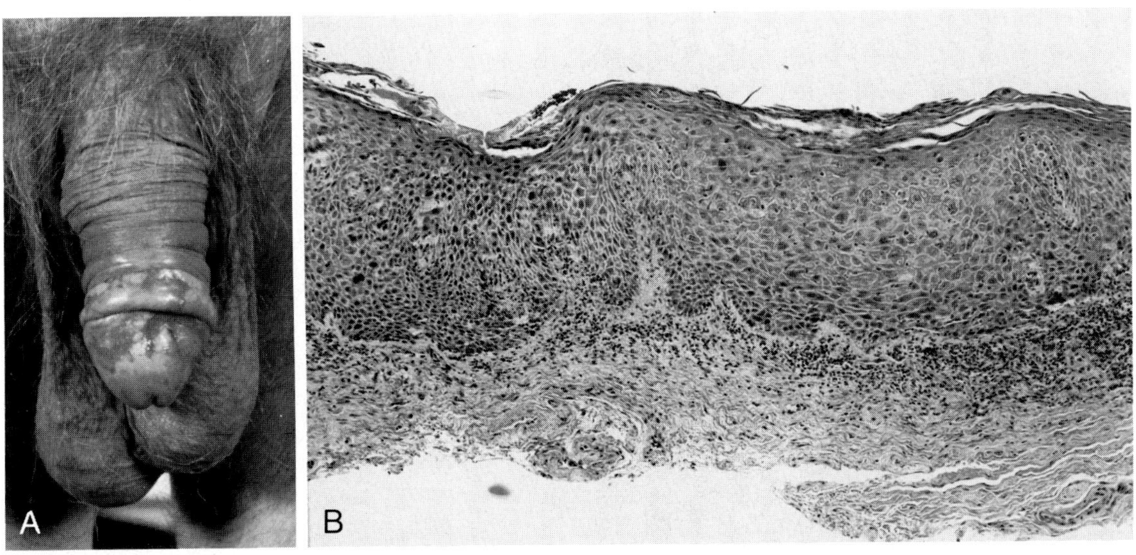

FIGURE 12–3. *A*, Erythroplasia of Queyrat of the glans penis and inner surface of the prepuce; a velvety, erythematous plaque. *B*, Section shows features of carcinoma in situ: atypical keratinocyte proliferation, malignant dyskeratosis and abnormal mitotic figures. The submucosa contains a dense infiltrate of plasma cells and lymphocytes.

(5-FU) for EQ in the male has been used with success by some authors.[6–8] We feel that this modality may be given a trial only in small nonulcerated lesions when the patient declines surgery. A 5% cream preparation is applied twice a day for at least 3 or 4 weeks. The inflammatory reaction that results takes 1 to 5 months to subside. The treatment is effective in some cases, but several courses may be necessary to achieve a cure. In our hands, as well as others, the modality has definitely proved to be of limited value.[1,9] The cases we have attempted to treat with 5-FU suffered severe disabling reactions caused by the inevitable contact of the penile and scrotal skin with the chemical. Wearing a rubber condom has been recommended to avoid such a complication. In a series of 24 cases without concomitant carcinoma, satisfactory results were obtained in only two of the four small lesions treated with 5-FU. The two other patients developed violent reactions that precluded the continuation of the therapy. The morbidity after surgery is much shorter than it is with 5-FU.

Because EQ is resistant to radiotherapy, ablation is the treatment of choice.[3] The type of

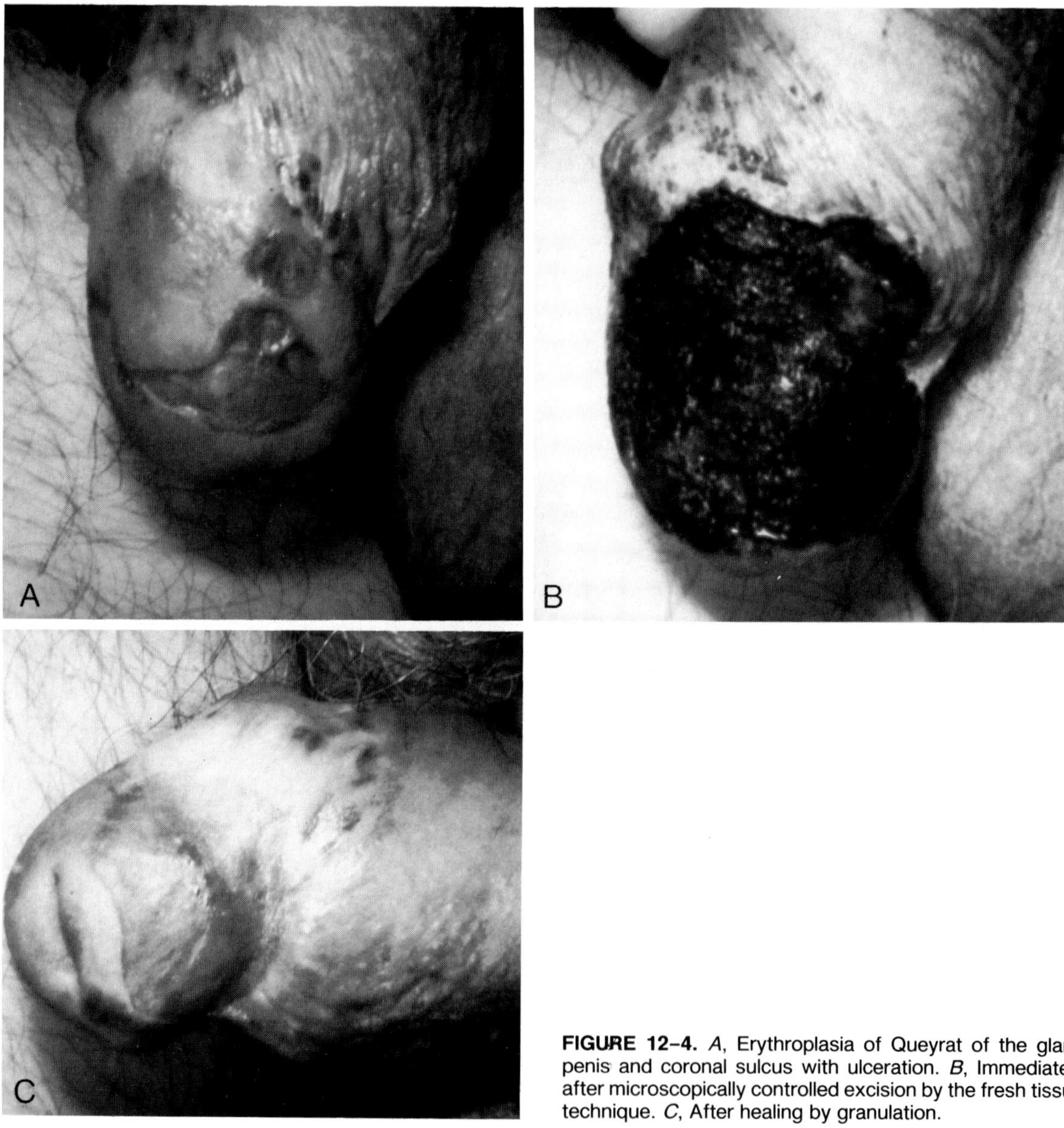

FIGURE 12–4. *A*, Erythroplasia of Queyrat of the glans penis and coronal sulcus with ulceration. *B*, Immediately after microscopically controlled excision by the fresh tissue technique. *C*, After healing by granulation.

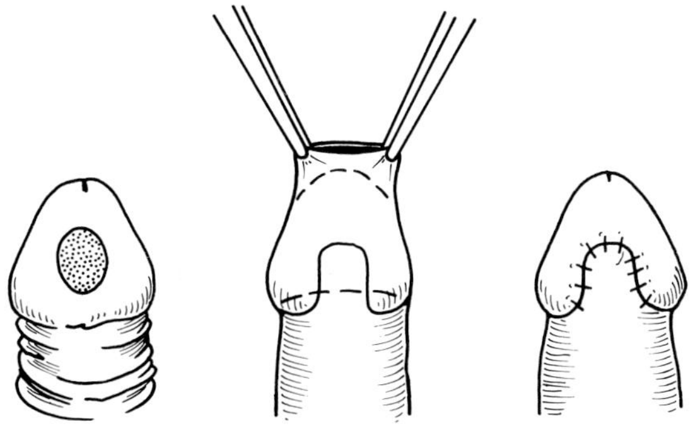

FIGURE 12–5. The Happle technique: Part of the preputial skin is used as a graft to cover the postexcision defect.

surgery depends upon the site of the lesion and its extent. Circumcision is curative only when the prepuce is involved. Lesions on the glans penis and labia minora can be adequately excised by using the fresh tissue technique of Mohs surgery. The base of the wound is usually electrocoagulated to control the bleeding and is left to heal by granulation. Healing is excellent even when the wounds are large (Fig. 12–4). When the foreskin is available, the defect on the glans may be covered by using the preputial skin as a pedicle graft.[10] We have used this technique in an elderly gentleman who could not take care of the open wound (Fig. 12–5 and 12–6). When the lesion is near the coronal sulcus, the wound can be closed by the simple approximation of its margins (Fig. 12–7).

In a series of 24 cases of EQ of the penis that were not associated with carcinoma, the treatment was as follows: 10 by the Mohs fresh tissue technique, eight by destruction with fulguration or vaporization with the carbon dioxide laser, four by the Mohs fixed tissue technique, and two with 5-FU.

Originally, it was our practice to treat EQ with the Mohs fixed tissue technique (four cases). Since 1975, we have exclusively used the fresh tissue technique (seven cases). Recently, we have treated lesions with fulgurating current or carbon dioxide laser. The rationale for using this last modality is that the mucosa, unlike the skin, does not contain pilosebaceous follicles along which the anaplastic cells may extend into deeper tissue, as is the case in Bowen's disease.[3–5] We have treated eight cases of EQ on the glans and the coronal sulcus with this modality with good results. Even large areas of fulgurated, denuded mucosa healed well in a comparatively short time (Fig. 12–8 and 12–9). An EQ that involved the mucosa of the prepuce and the glans was successfully treated by circumcision followed by fulguration of the area on the glans (Fig. 12–10). The carbon dioxide laser did not prove superior to the fulgurating current. Always remember that Mohs micrographic surgery becomes mandatory if the lesion is indurated, nodular, or ulcerated because these findings indicate an invasive carcinoma.

Follow-up observation in the above series of patients has been 5 to 10 years. The results were favorable in all cases except for a recur-

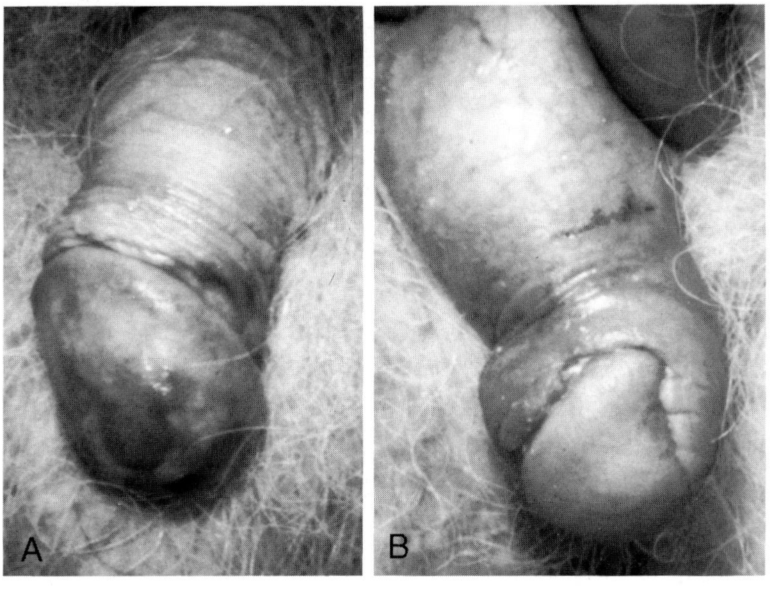

FIGURE 12–6. *A*, Erythroplasia of Queyrat of the glans penis and inner surface of prepuce. *B*, Lesion was excised by Mohs fresh tissue technique; circumcision was then undertaken, saving part of the skin of the prepuce for use as a pedicle graft to cover the defect on the glans (Happle technique).

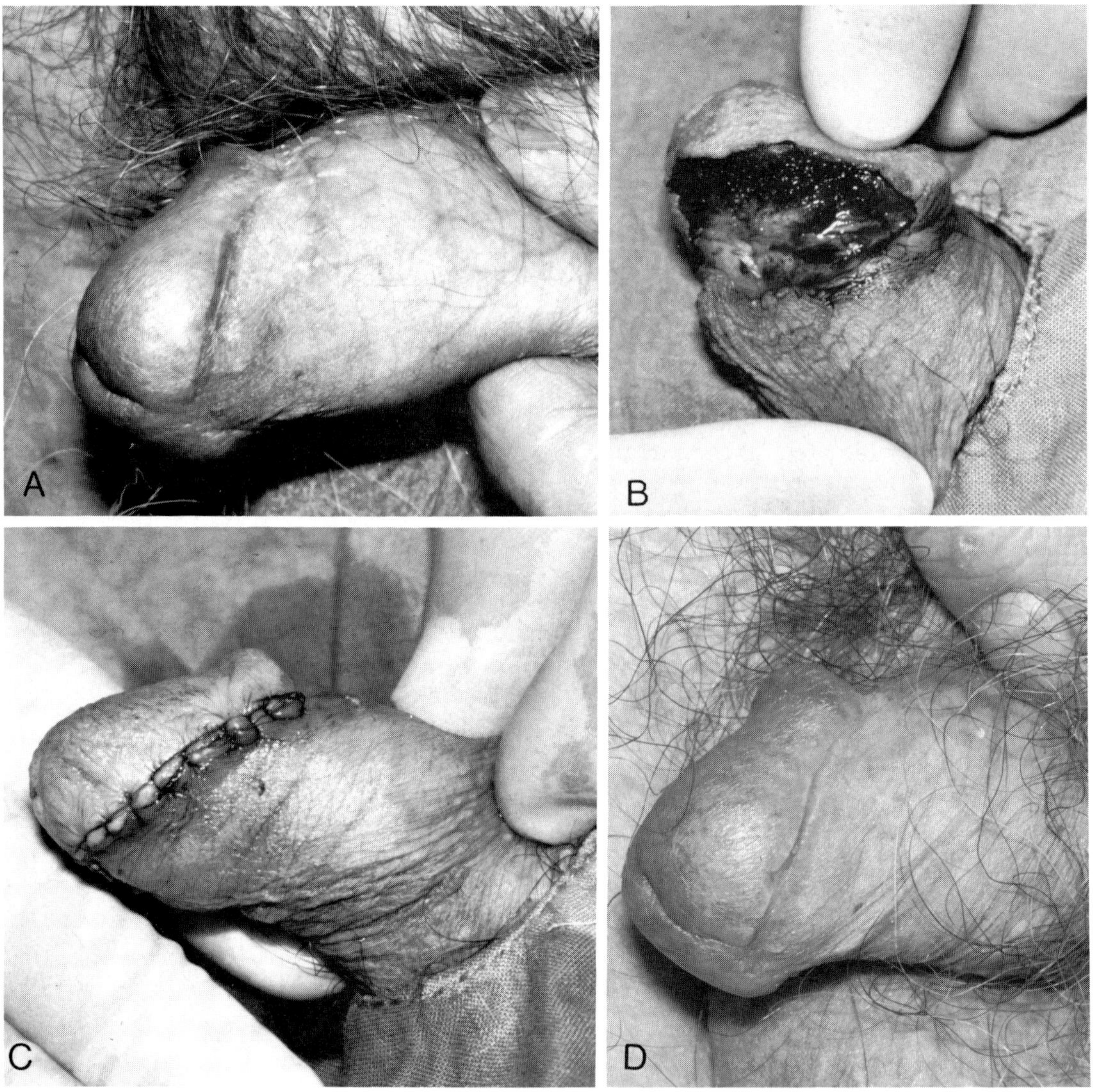

FIGURE 12–7. *A*, Wound after Mohs excision of erythroplasia of Queyrat of the glans and coronal sulcus. *B*, Sutured wound. *C*, Healed state 4 weeks later.

rence in one treated by Mohs fresh tissue technique, which was successfully retreated. There were no metastases in this series.

Five lesions of EQ on the labia minora have been treated by the Mohs fresh tissue technique followed by primary closure of the defect (Fig. 12–11). Two recurred but were retreated with a favorable outcome. None metastasized after more than 5 years follow-up.

It is important to bear in mind that patients with EQ have to be followed indefinitely. As long as mucosa exits, there is always the possibility of recurrence in previously uninvolved areas. Because of this, J. Mato and A. Vilalta of Barcelona, Spain, devised a procedure they call decortication of the glans in order to prevent recurrence. They presented it at the I International Congress of Dermatologic Surgery in Lisbon, Portugal, October 7–10, 1979. This technique removes the entire mucosal surface of the prepuce and glans penis, and the cutaneous part of the prepuce is used as a flap to cover the glans up to the urethral meatus. The operation is complicated and has a long morbidity but may be indicated when the involvement of the glans is unusually extensive. We have not found it applicable in any of our cases.

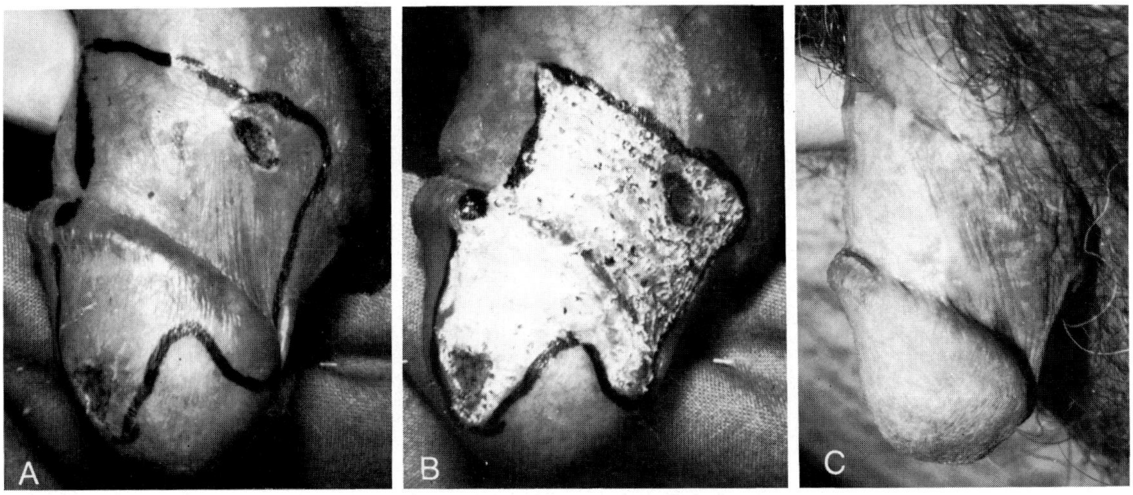

FIGURE 12–8. *A*, Extensive erythroplasia of Queyrat outlined; two biopsy sites are visible. *B*, Lesion fulgurated. *C*, Healed in 6 weeks.

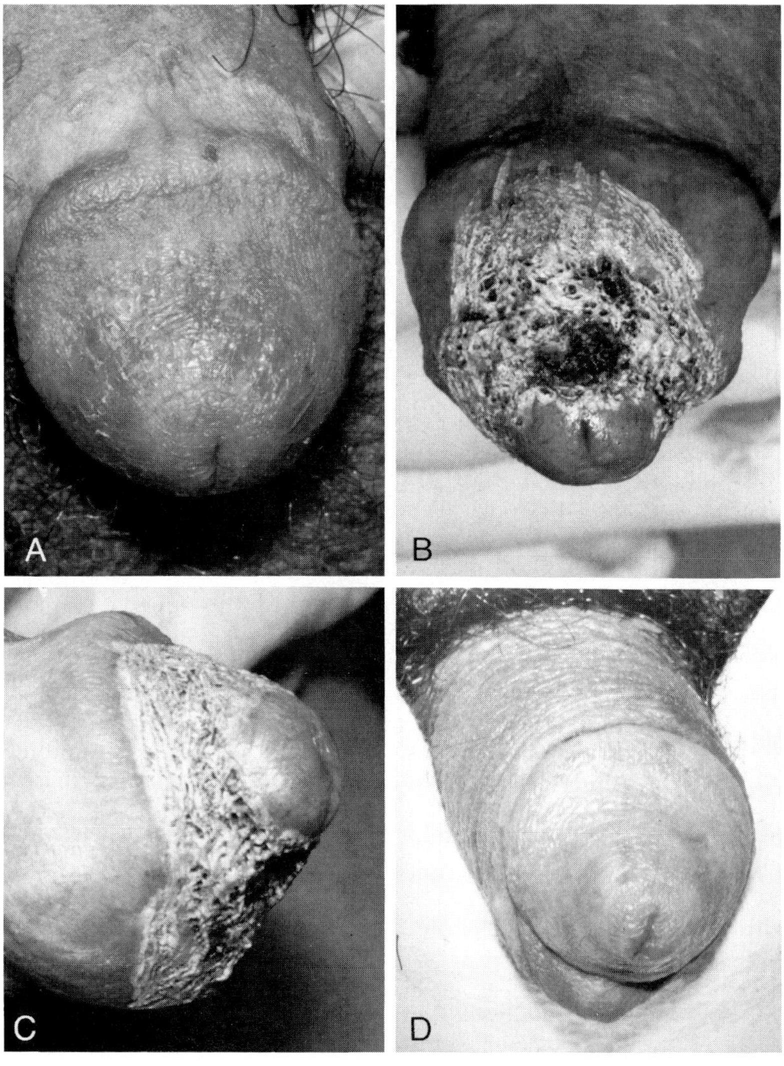

FIGURE 12–9. *A*, Erythroplasia of Queyrat of the glans. *B* and *C*, Appearance immediately after fulguration. *D*, Result 6 weeks later.

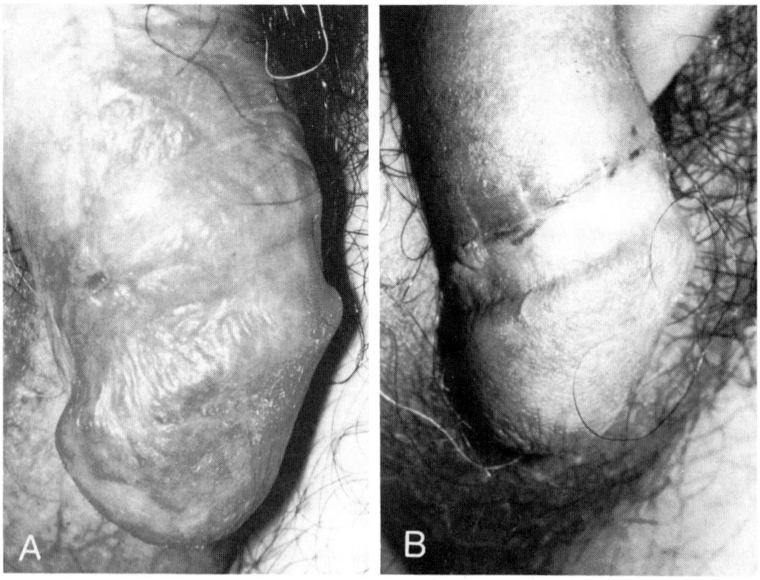

FIGURE 12–10. *A*, Erythroplasia of the mucosal surface of the prepuce and the glans penis. *B*, Final result after circumcision, followed by fulguration of the lesion on the glans.

Bowen's Disease

Bowen's disease is a squamous cell carcinoma in situ of the skin of middle-aged or elderly patients. In men, it may occur on the shaft of the penis, in the hairy skin of the inguinal and suprapubic areas, on the scrotum, and in the perineum. The labia majora is the commonest site in women. The lesion usually presents as a solitary, crusted, dull-red plaque that may simulate psoriasis, dermatophytosis, or other inflammatory conditions of the skin. As in erythroplasia of Queyrat, histologic examination is necessary to establish the diagnosis. Unlike EQ which involves the mucosae, Bowen's disease affects the epithelium of the skin and that of the pilosebaceous follicles and sweat ducts (Fig. 12–12). This feature renders topical chemotherapy with 5-FU inadequate because of the lack of deep penetration of the drug. This is especially important because invasive squamous cell carcinoma is likely to develop in 50% of the cases.[3–5] The standard recommended treatment is excision with a surgical margin of 0.5 cm, and the excised tissue should include subcutaneous fat in order to assure removal of any underlying carcinoma. As the histologic features are easily discernible to the trained eye in frozen tissue sections, the Mohs fresh tissue technique is well adapted for this condition.[11] We have practiced the technique in seven cases with excellent results. When the lesion is limited to the prepuce, circumcision is curative (Fig. 12–13).

Some authors have stressed that Bowen's disease, especially when it occurs on covered areas of the body, may be associated with internal malignancies.[3–5] In our experience, this has been a rare occurrence without a cause-and-effect relationship, aside from concomitant incidence in a certain old age group. The view that Bowen's disease is not a skin marker for internal malignancy is supported by other workers.[12–14]

Bowenoid Papulosis

Bowenoid papulosis of the genitalia is a comparatively recently reported lesion that occurs in young men and women,[15] in contrast to Bowen's disease, which occurs in people over age 50. The lesions of bowenoid papulosis are multiple and appear as small, hyperpigmented papules that resemble condylomata acuminata. The diagnosis is usually made by histologic examination and is to be suspected in sexually active, young people. It is without doubt, a sexually transmitted disease. In a series of 12 men, the condition was present in nine of their sex partners. Six of these women also had squamous cell carcinoma in situ of the cervix uteri. Therefore, all sexual contacts should be carefully examined. Subclinical penile human pap-

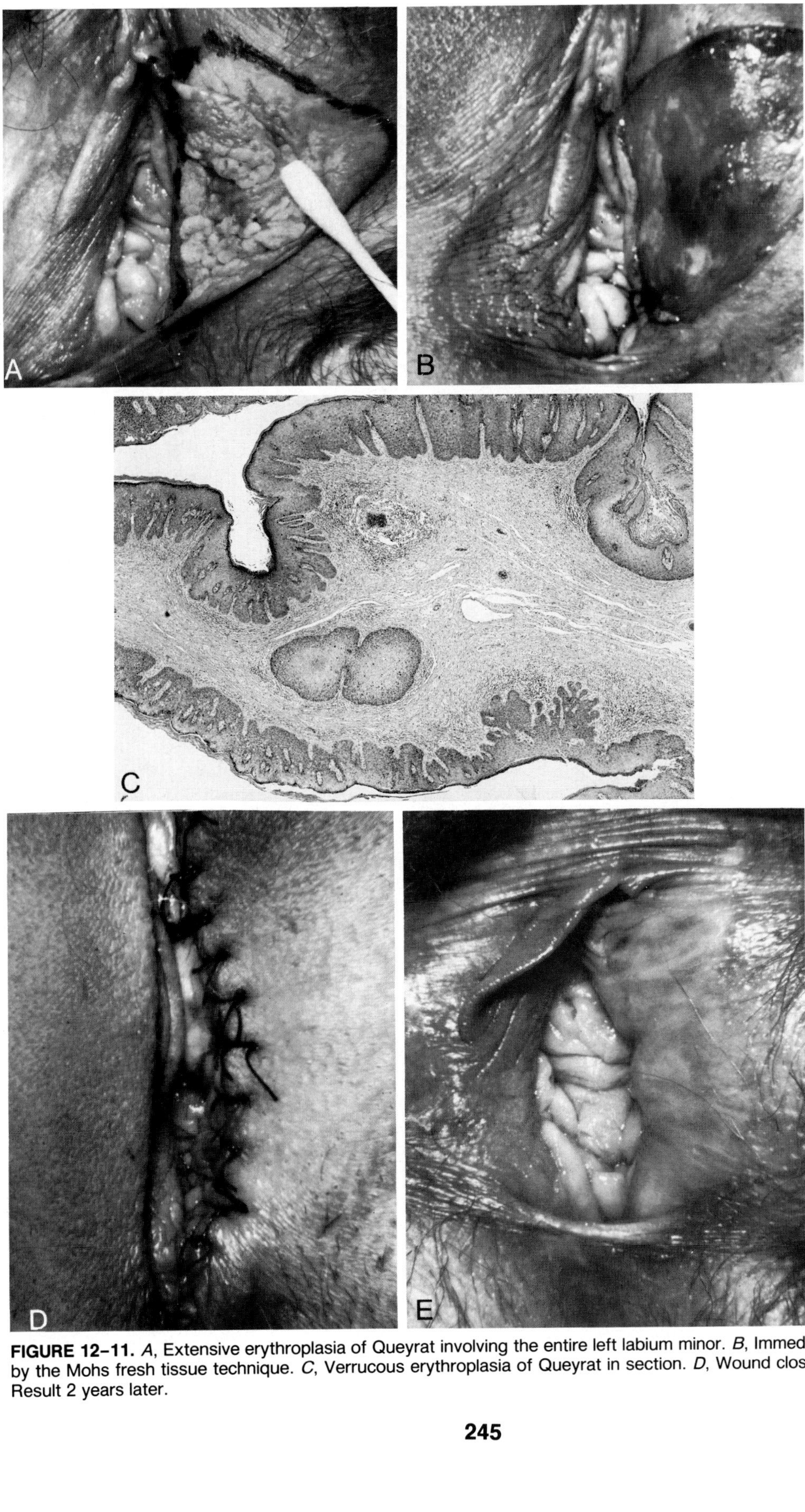

FIGURE 12–11. *A*, Extensive erythroplasia of Queyrat involving the entire left labium minor. *B*, Immediately after excision by the Mohs fresh tissue technique. *C*, Verrucous erythroplasia of Queyrat in section. *D*, Wound closed with sutures. *E*, Result 2 years later.

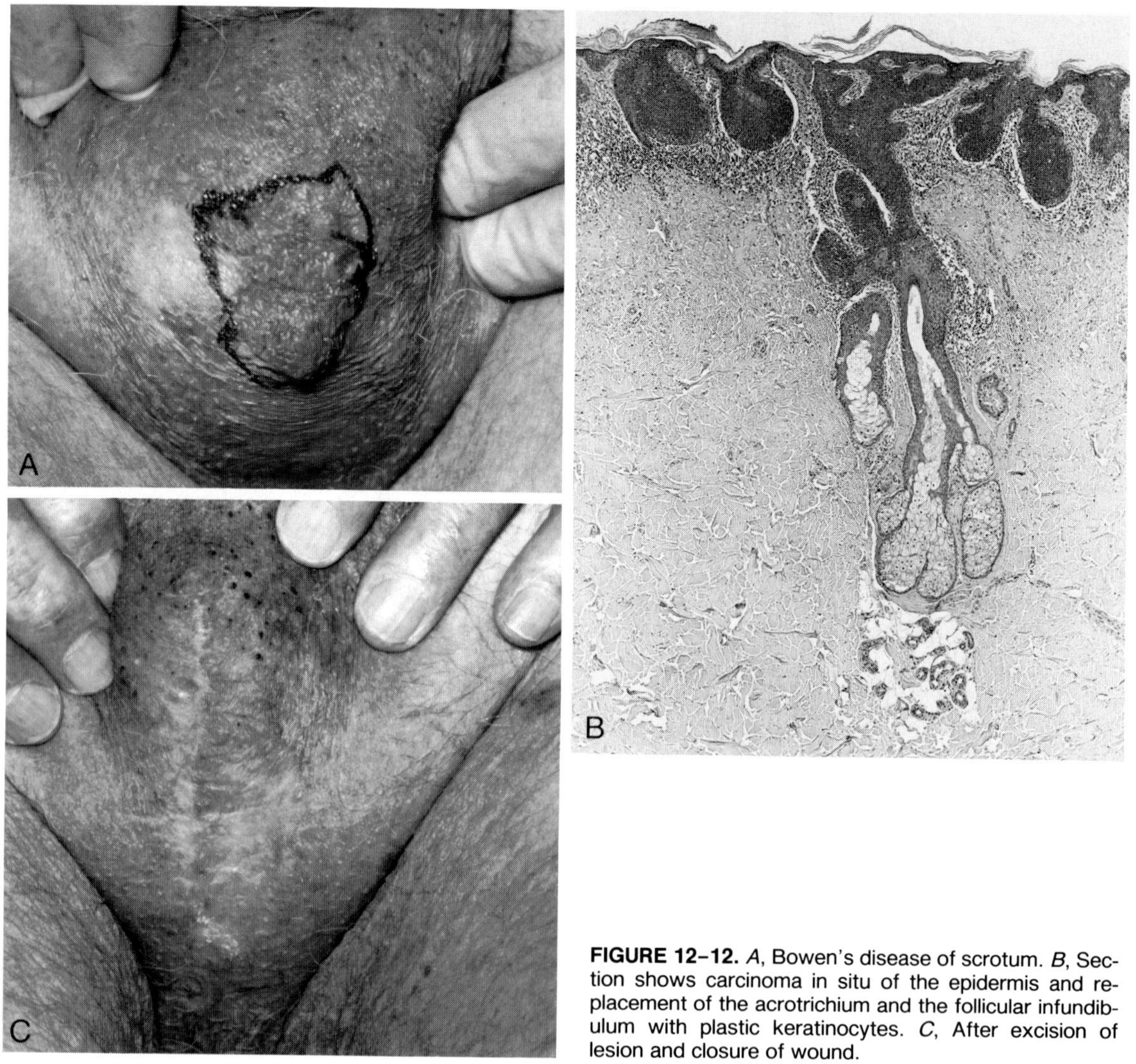

FIGURE 12–12. *A*, Bowen's disease of scrotum. *B*, Section shows carcinoma in situ of the epidermis and replacement of the acrotrichium and the follicular infundibulum with plastic keratinocytes. *C*, After excision of lesion and closure of wound.

illoma virus infection and dysplasia in consorts of women with cervical neoplasia have also been reported.[16]

The pathology is identical to that of Bowen's disease, but the lesions are usually smaller (Fig. 12–14). Viral particles have been demonstrated in many cases, and the condition has been shown to be caused by infection with the human papilloma virus, predominantly types 16 and 18.[15,17] Although spontaneous regression has occurred in some lesions,[18] they should be extirpated. This may be achieved by simple excision or by destruction with the fulgurating current. However, we have encountered large lesions that required microscopically controlled surgery (Fig. 12–15).

Leukoplakia

Leukoplakia of the mucosal surface of the glans penis or vulva is rare and appears to occur with greater frequency in diabetic patients. The condition is precancerous and considered by some pathologists to be an epidermoid carcinoma in situ.[19]

The lesion presents as a scaly, grayish-white patch, usually with a surrounding inflammatory component. The urethral meatus is commonly involved, which may lead to constriction of the urethra. The condition is often diagnosed as lichen sclerosus et atrophicus or kraurosis vulvae—the real diagnosis being recognized in retrospect after the development of

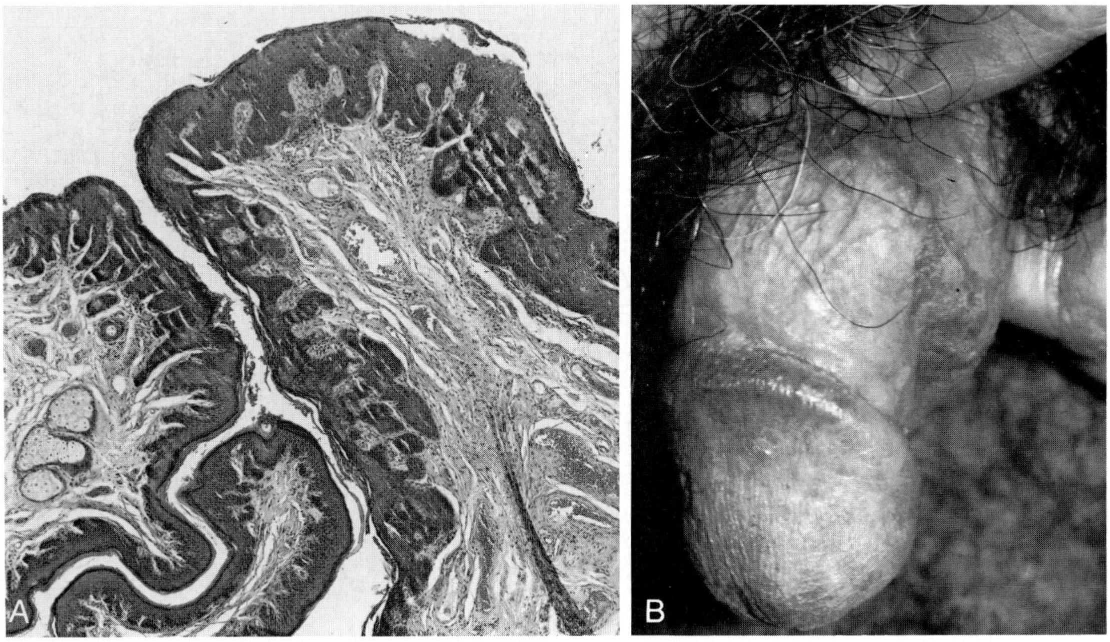

FIGURE 12–13. *A*, Bowen's disease in preputial skin. *B*, Condition after circumcision.

a frank carcinoma. The histology is identical to that of leukoplakia of the oral mucosa (Fig. 12–16). It is, therefore, advisable that biopsy material should be obtained from white lesions of the glans or the labia minora especially if they are recalcitrant to treatment or show a tendency to ulcerate (Fig. 12–17). These lesions are successfully removed by Mohs micrographic surgery.

Verrucous Carcinoma

Verrucous carcinoma, also called giant condyloma acuminatum and Buschke-Löwenstein tumor, is believed by some to be a variant of condyloma acuminatum which is caused by human papilloma virus. Others consider the lesion a low-grade malignancy which is slowly and locally aggressive but does not have the

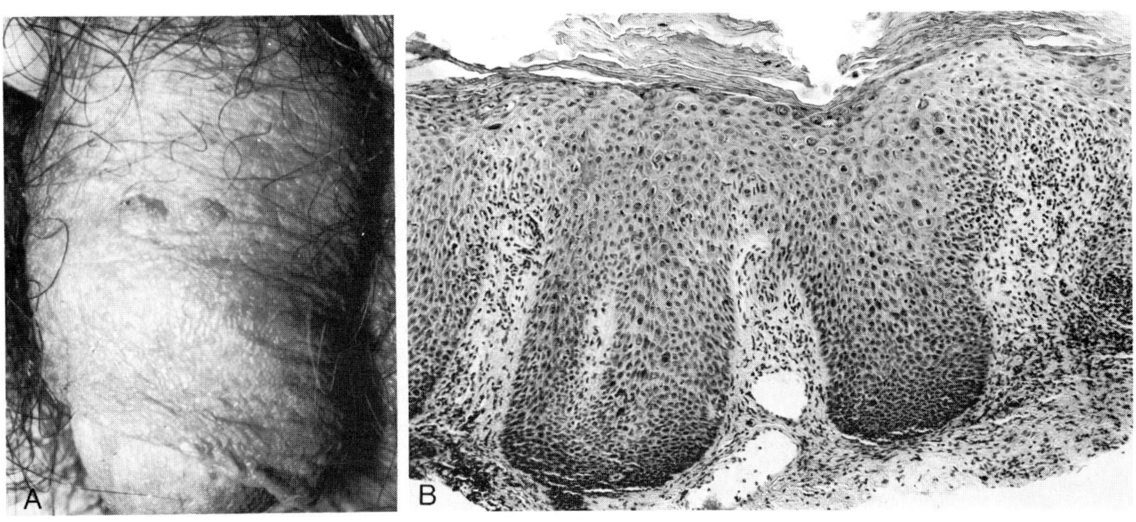

FIGURE 12–14. *A*, Bowenoid papulosis of the penis in a 25-year-old. *B*, The histopathology is similar to that of Bowen's disease; note the atypical mitoses and the dyskeratotic keratinocytes.

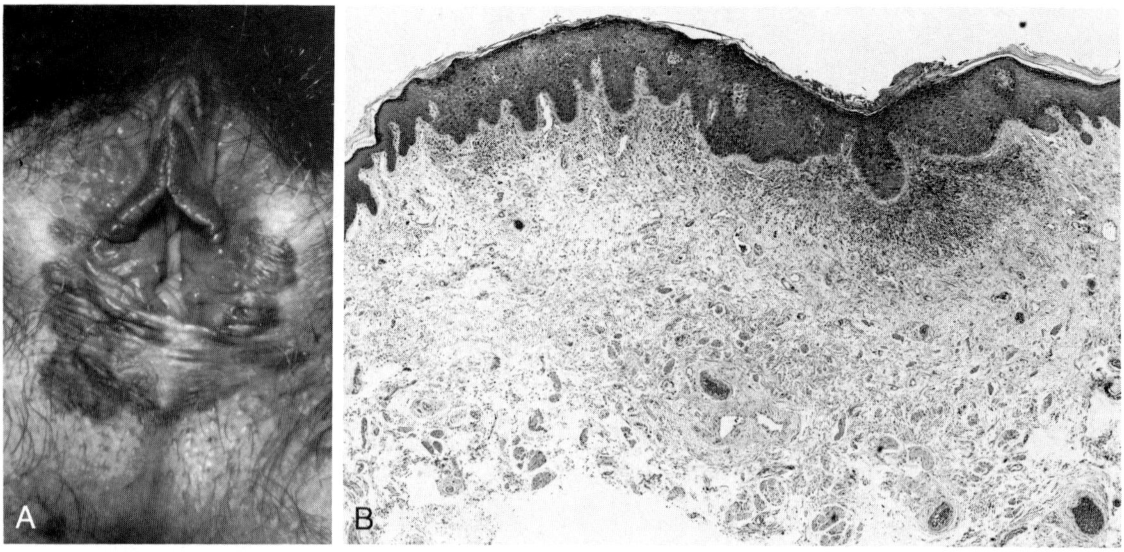

FIGURE 12–15. *A*, Bowenoid papulosis of the vulva and perineum in a woman age 28. Some of the lesions were in the form of large plaques, while the majority were small and papular. They were all excised by the Mohs fresh tissue technique. *B*, Note limited dysplastic epidermis; normal epidermis at margins of field.

tendency to metastasize.[19,20] The neoplasm develops as an exophytic and fungating mass that tends to occur on the glans and prepuce of uncircumcised men and usually grows to a large size. When the meatus is involved, there is a tendency of proximal extension of the tumor along the urethra. The histopathology is similar to that of condyloma acuminatum. The only satisfactory treatment is surgical ablation, and excellent functional results can be obtained by the Mohs technique.[11] The majority of cases can be ablated by the fresh tissue technique, which is described in detail later. We have treated four cases of this type with successful outcome after follow-up for 5 or more years (Fig. 12–18).

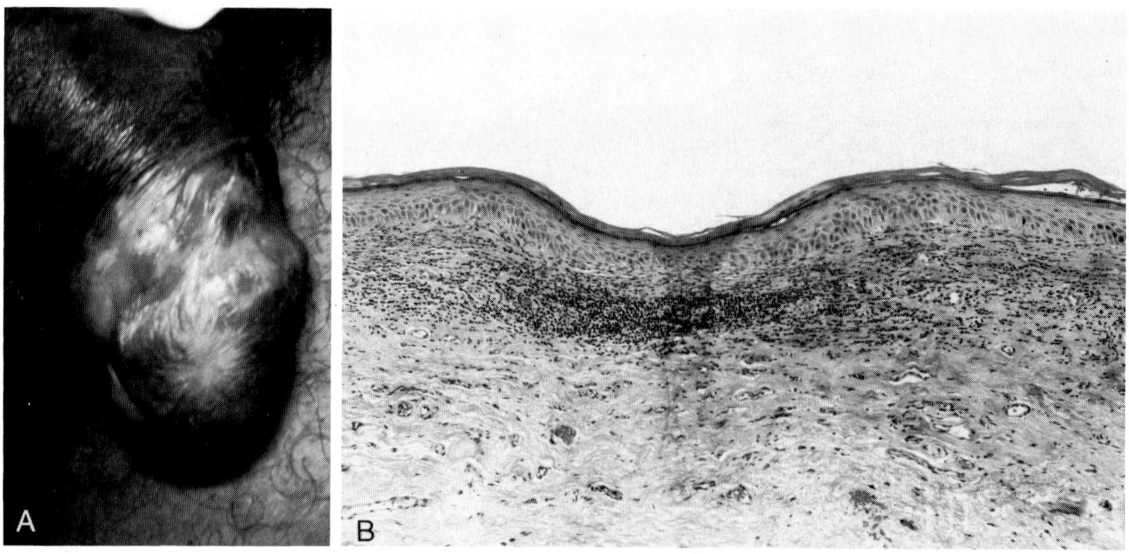

FIGURE 12–16. *A*, Advanced leukoplakia of the glans and coronal sulcus in a 60-year-old black man. *B*, Histology shows atrophic epidermis, dyskeratosis, disorderly arrangement of the keratinocytes, and inflammatory infiltrate in dermis.

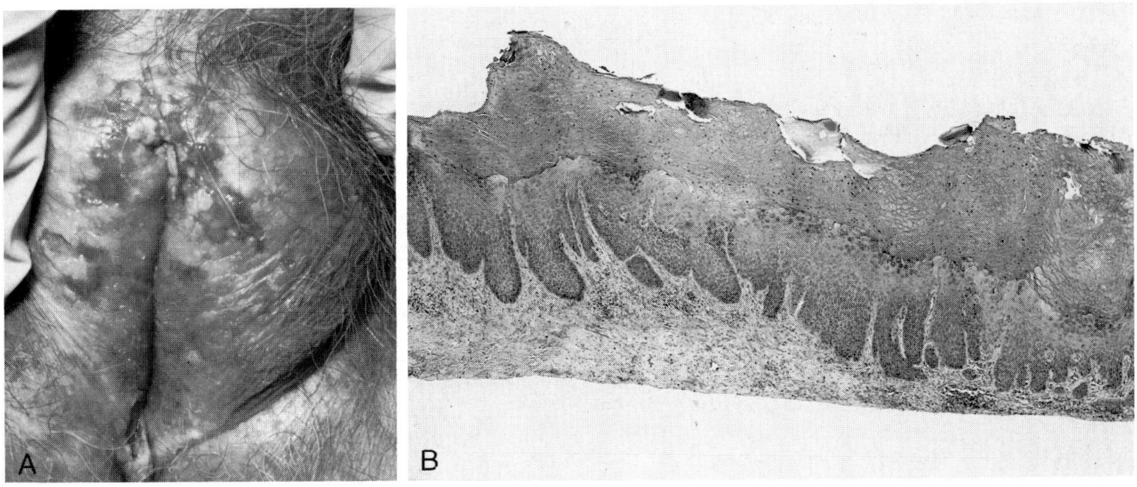

FIGURE 12–17. *A*, Leukoplakia of the vulva in a 72-year-old woman. The presence of ulceration is an ominous sign indicative of the development of carcinoma. *B*, Hyperkeratosis, dyskeratosis, and disorderly arrangement of keratinocytes are evident.

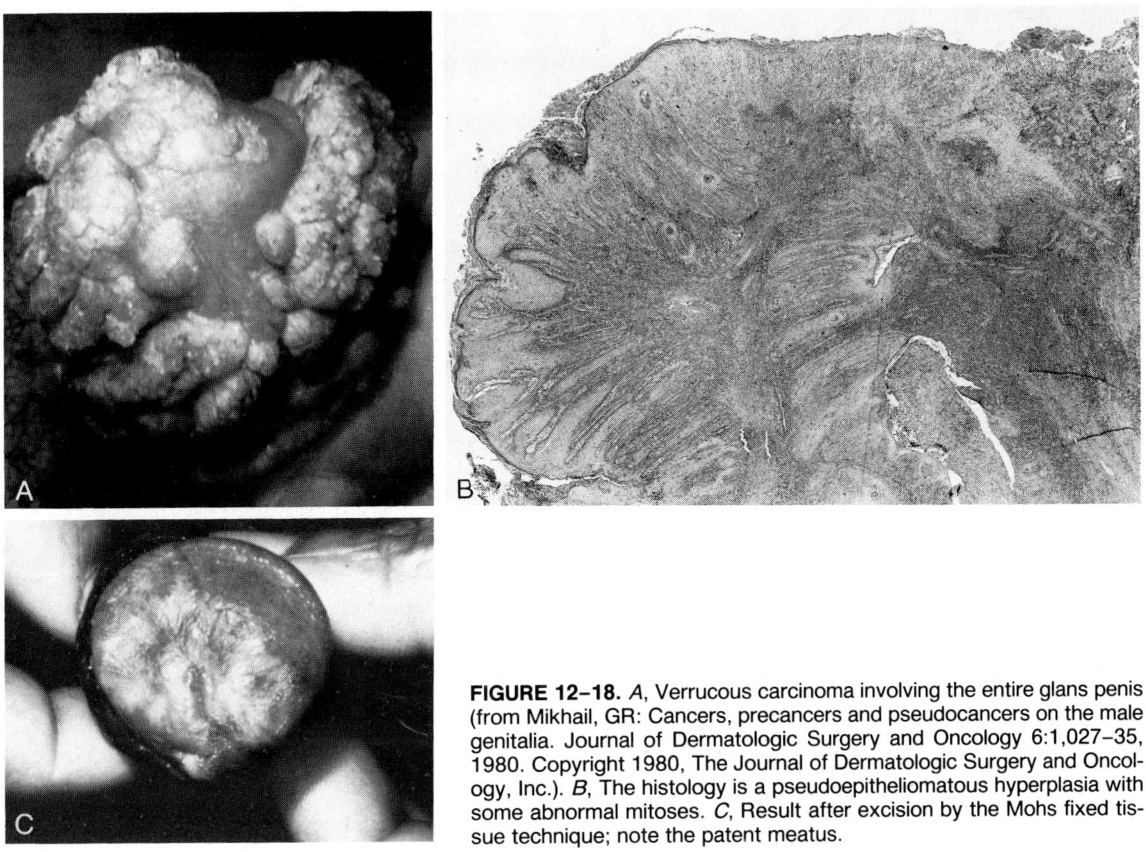

FIGURE 12–18. *A*, Verrucous carcinoma involving the entire glans penis (from Mikhail, GR: Cancers, precancers and pseudocancers on the male genitalia. Journal of Dermatologic Surgery and Oncology 6:1,027–35, 1980. Copyright 1980, The Journal of Dermatologic Surgery and Oncology, Inc.). *B*, The histology is a pseudoepitheliomatous hyperplasia with some abnormal mitoses. *C*, Result after excision by the Mohs fixed tissue technique; note the patent meatus.

Squamous Cell Carcinoma of the Penis

Although relatively rare, squamous cell carcinoma is the most common form of penile cancer, second only to squamous cell carcinoma in situ (erythroplasia of Queyrat and Bowen's disease). Many patients have advanced disease by the time they seek treatment, either because of fear of phallectomy or because of failure to recognize an early lesion beneath a phimotic foreskin.[18] As previously mentioned, the presence of malignancy should be suspected in recalcitrant penile lesions, which need a biopsy diag-

TABLE 12–1. Jackson Staging System for Carcinoma of the Penis

STAGE I	Tumor limited to glans penis and/or prepuce.
STAGE II	Invasion into the shaft or corpora cavernosa, but without lymph node or distant metastases.
STAGE III	Tumor confined to the shaft, with biopsy-proven regional node metastases
STAGE IV	Inoperable regional node involvement or distant metastases.

Adapted from Jackson SM: The treatment of carcinoma of the penis, British Journal of Surgery 53:33–35, 1966.

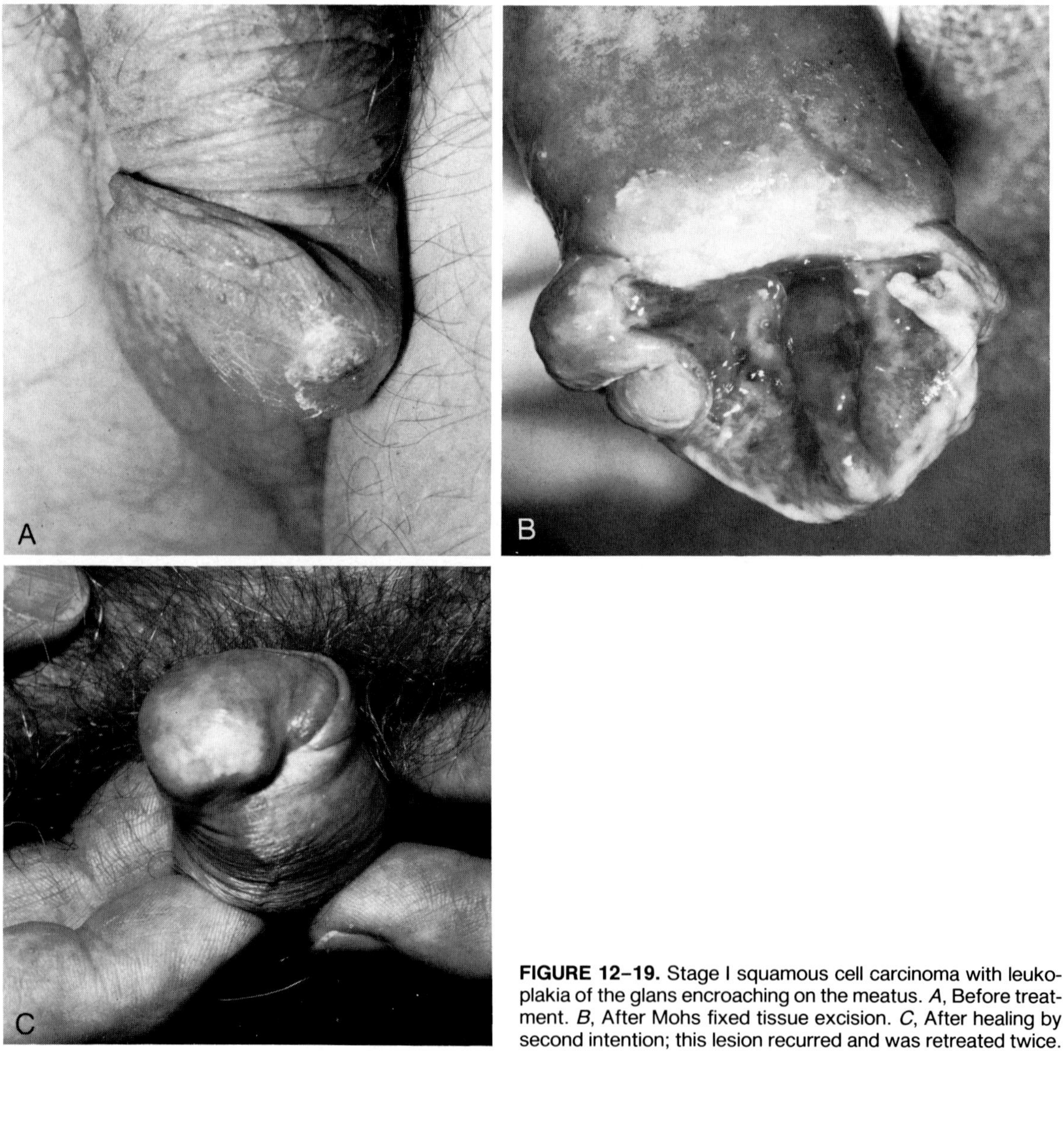

FIGURE 12–19. Stage I squamous cell carcinoma with leukoplakia of the glans encroaching on the meatus. *A*, Before treatment. *B*, After Mohs fixed tissue excision. *C*, After healing by second intention; this lesion recurred and was retreated twice.

nosis so that treatment may be instituted at an early stage.

The staging system devised by Jackson is universally recognized (Table 12–1), and prognosis has been found to correlate well with the stage of the tumor.[19,21] The standard surgical practice among urologists is along the following lines: (1) circumcision when the tumor is limited to the prepuce, (2) amputation at 2.0 to 2.5 cm beyond visible or palpable neoplasm when it occurs on the glans penis or coronal sulcus, or (3) radical phallectomy when the tumor occurs higher on the penile shaft. Since the majority of lesions occur on the glans penis, amputation 2.5 cm proximal to the clinical tumor is rather mutilating. Conservative therapy by the Mohs fixed or fresh tissue technique maximally saves unaffected tissue and is strongly advocated.[11] Mohs surgery has been most rewarding in the 19 cases of squamous

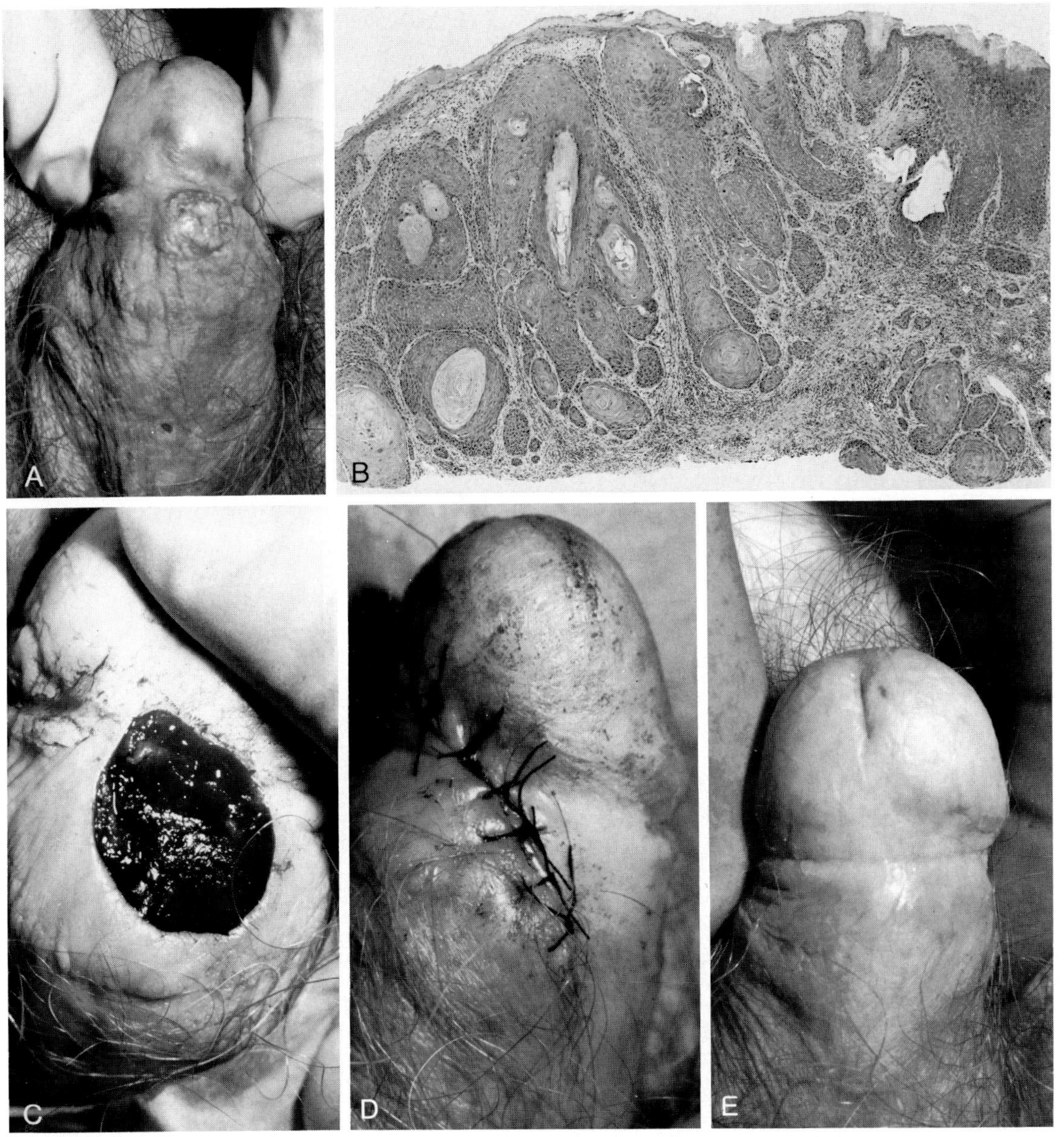

FIGURE 12–20. *A*, Stage I squamous cell carcinoma of the ventral surface of the penis. *B*, Section shows a deeply invasive carcinoma. *C*, Wound after Mohs fresh tissue excision. *D*, Sutured wound. *E*, Healed state.

cell carcinoma we have treated: 15 were Stage I, three were Stage II, and one was Stage III. There were two recurrences in a Stage I carcinoma that were successfully retreated. One Stage II patient had two recurrences, which can be ascribed to reactivation of underlying erythroplasia of Queyrat or leukoplakia (Fig. 12–19). Another patient, who clinicaly belonged to Stage II but was later classified Stage III (with biopsy-proved regional node metastasis), had prophylactic dissection of the inguinal and iliac nodes. Only the former contained tumor. He has remained free of disease for 7 years. Another Stage III case eventually needed penectomy.

Patients in Stages I and II can be adequately managed by the Mohs fresh tissue technique. Bleeding can be controlled with the fulgurating current and the application of oxidized cellulose (Oxycel) or absorbable gelatin sponges (Gelfoam) or by using the hot cautery. When the cancer is localized to the skin or mucosa of the coronal sulcus or frenulum, the wounds may be sutured (Fig. 12–20) or allowed to heal by granulation (Fig. 12–21).

In deeply invasive carcinomas, Stages II and III, the Mohs fixed tissue excision is, in our opinion, indicated. When this method is used on the penis, it is similar to that used elsewhere but with a few modifications. If the lesion is adjacent to or involves the urinary meatus, an indwelling catheter has to be placed and left in until the procedure is terminated. Regional block anesthesia of the penis has to be administered before the initial application of the zinc chloride paste. A plasticized hydrocarbon gel (Orbase) applied to the meatus is useful in protecting the zinc chloride fixative paste from becoming diluted by urine trickling down around the catheter. We have not encountered any bleeding from the corpora cavernosa after separation of the final fixed layer, nor have any of our cases developed stricture of the urethra (Fig. 12–22 and 12–23). This is because the reepithelization of wounds on mucosal surfaces is about three times as fast as that on skin.

Neither physical examination nor lymphangiography reliably and absolutely determines the presence or absence of metastasis in the inguinal nodes (which are the first to be involved). In patients with Stage I lesions, the probability of node metastasis, which may be either unilateral or bilateral, is less than 20%, and if metastases develop, they usually do so within 3 years. The question often arises whether prophylactic node dissection should be undertaken at the time when the carcinoma is excised. The consensus among urologists fa-

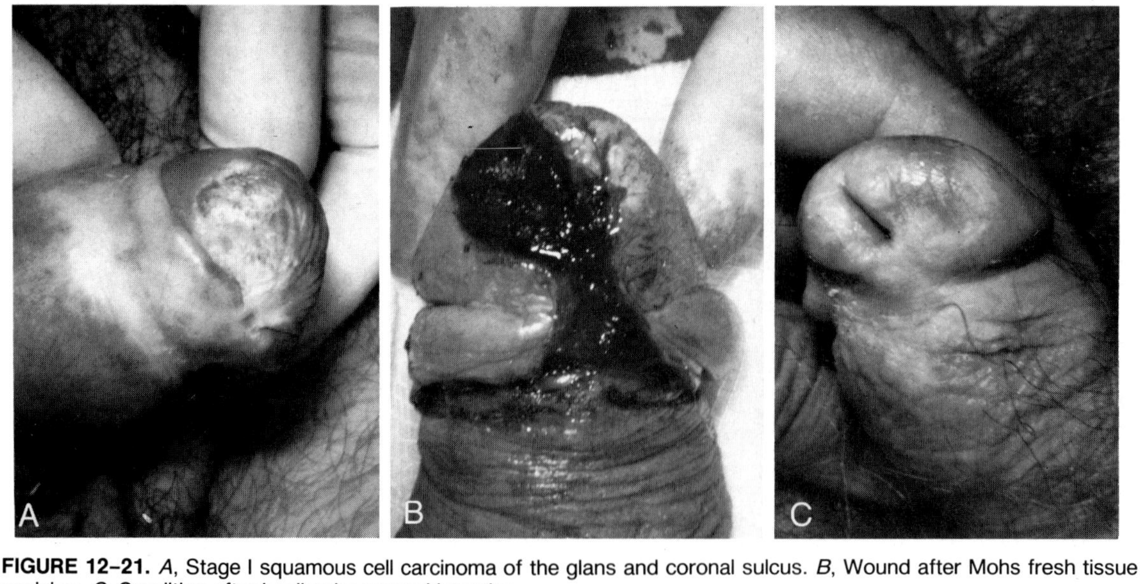

FIGURE 12–21. *A*, Stage I squamous cell carcinoma of the glans and coronal sulcus. *B*, Wound after Mohs fresh tissue excision. *C*, Condition after healing by second intention.

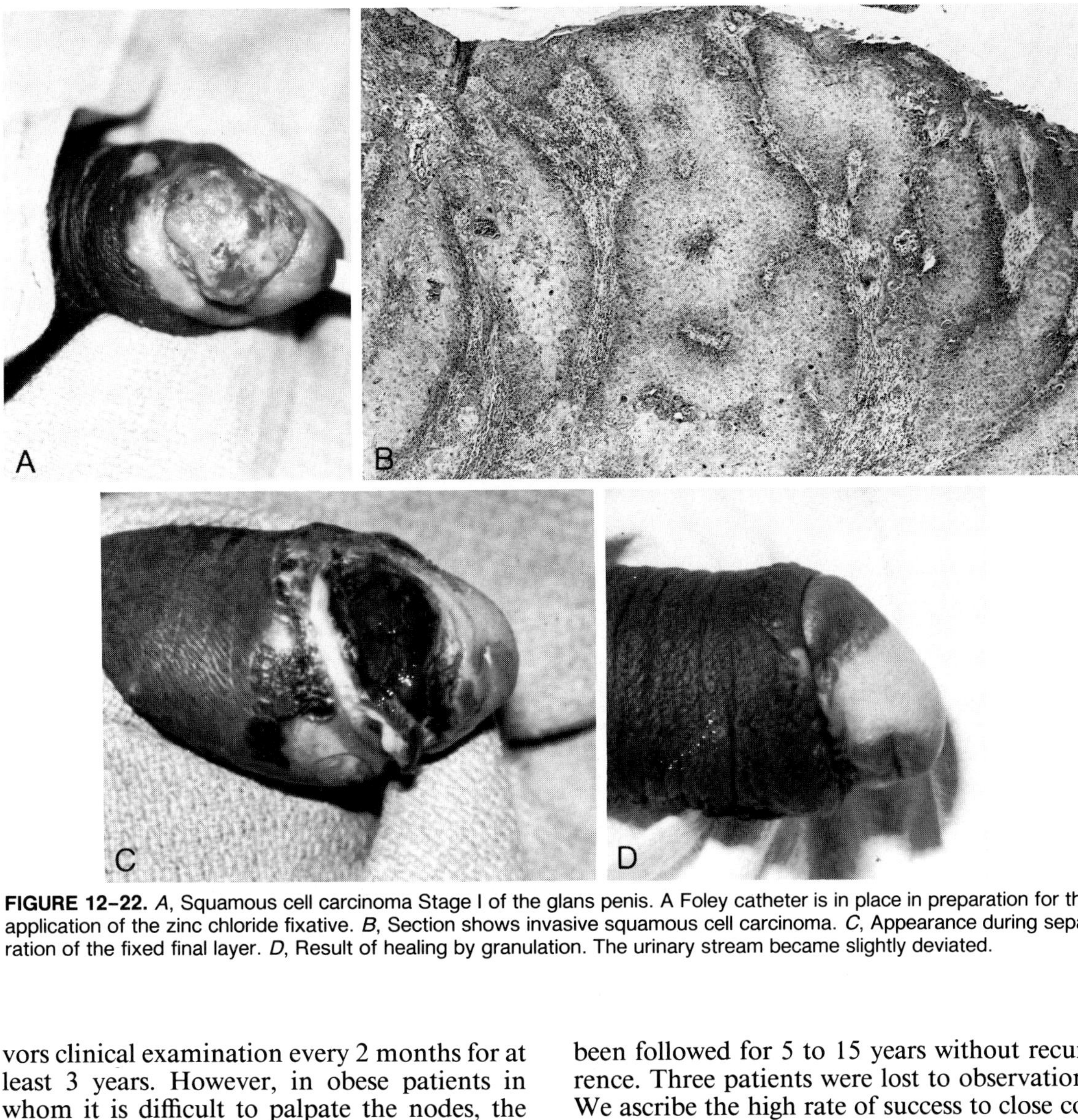

FIGURE 12–22. *A*, Squamous cell carcinoma Stage I of the glans penis. A Foley catheter is in place in preparation for the application of the zinc chloride fixative. *B*, Section shows invasive squamous cell carcinoma. *C*, Appearance during separation of the fixed final layer. *D*, Result of healing by granulation. The urinary stream became slightly deviated.

vors clinical examination every 2 months for at least 3 years. However, in obese patients in whom it is difficult to palpate the nodes, the nodes may be dissected to verify their condition.[19] We have experienced the value of this plan in an obese patient (see Fig. 12–23) with a clinical Stage II carcinoma who was mentioned earlier and who proved to be Stage III after node dissection. While no nodes could be palpated preoperatively in this case, one out of 20 nodes showed metastatic carcinoma.

Two of the 19 patients with squamous cell carcinomas treated by Mohs surgery had local recurrence within 6 months and 1 year. The case shown in Figure 12–18 recurred three times owing to extensive leukoplakia. The other recurred once (see Fig. 12–20). Both have been retreated and followed up for 2 and 4 years, respectively. Fourteen patients have been followed for 5 to 15 years without recurrence. Three patients were lost to observation. We ascribe the high rate of success to close cooperation with the urologists in our hospital, to early diagnosis, and to the proper selection of cases.

Squamous Cell Carcinoma of the Vulva

The four cases of squamous cell carcinoma of the vulva that we have treated were all associated with either leukoplakia (see Fig. 12–17) or EQ (Fig. 12–24). Most gynecologists tend to perform vulvectomy on these cases. We have found that Mohs surgery is adequate, of low morbidity, and the method least associated with anatomic complications.

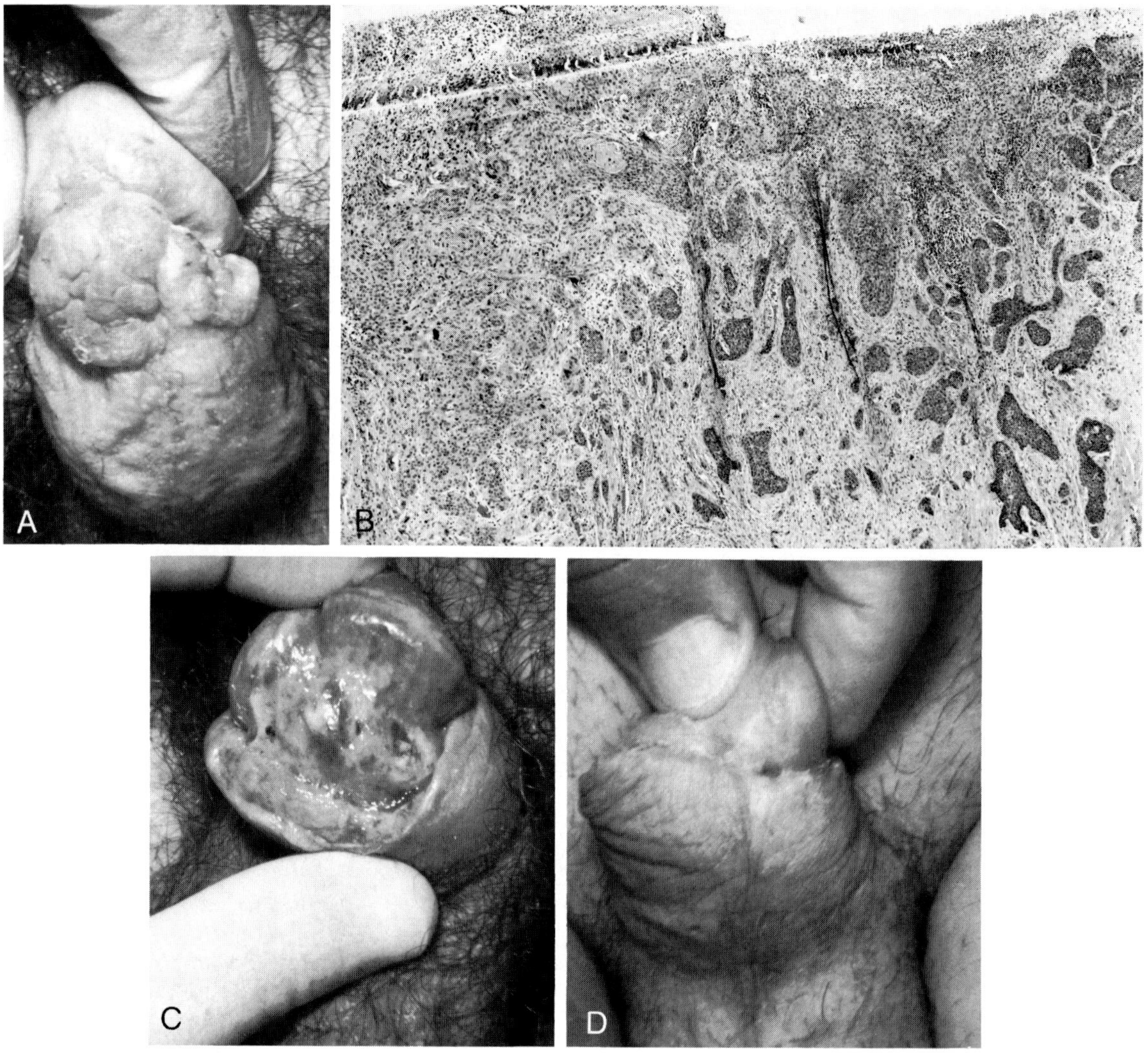

FIGURE 12–23. *A*, Stage III squamous cell carcinoma of the coronal sulcus, the ventral part of the glans, and the ventral shaft of the penis. *B*, The section shows a deeply invasive squamous cell carcinoma. *C*, Defect after fixed tissue excision. *D*, Result after healing by granulation. Note small urethral fistula to left of median raphe. This patient had inguinal node metastases (see text) and was well at seven years after surgery.

Extramammary Paget's Disease

Extramammary Paget's disease (EMPD) is a rare intraepidermal apocrine gland carcinoma mainly seen in postmenopausal women and elderly men. In the anogenital area, the disease presents clinically as one or more inflammatory, erythematous plaques on the genital, perigenital, or perianal skin. The lesions superficially resemble psoriasis, intertrigo, dermatophytosis, and candidiasis (Fig. 12–25). More than 50% of the patients complain of pruritus, and some experience pain or bleeding. The diagnosis of EMPD can only be established by histopathology, which is characteristic (Fig. 12–26). The epidermis contains distinctive clear cells which are large and have a pale cytoplasm replete with neutral and sulfonated mucopolysaccharides. Paget's cells can be traced from the epidermis downward along the epidermal appendages. The corium may be invaded, leading to lymph node metastasis. The EMPD cells are metastatic from apocrine gland carcinoma when the lesions occur in the genital and axillary regions or from cloacogenic carcinoma, arising in goblet cells located either on the surface epithelium or in the glands of the anal crypts at the anorectal junction.[22–24]

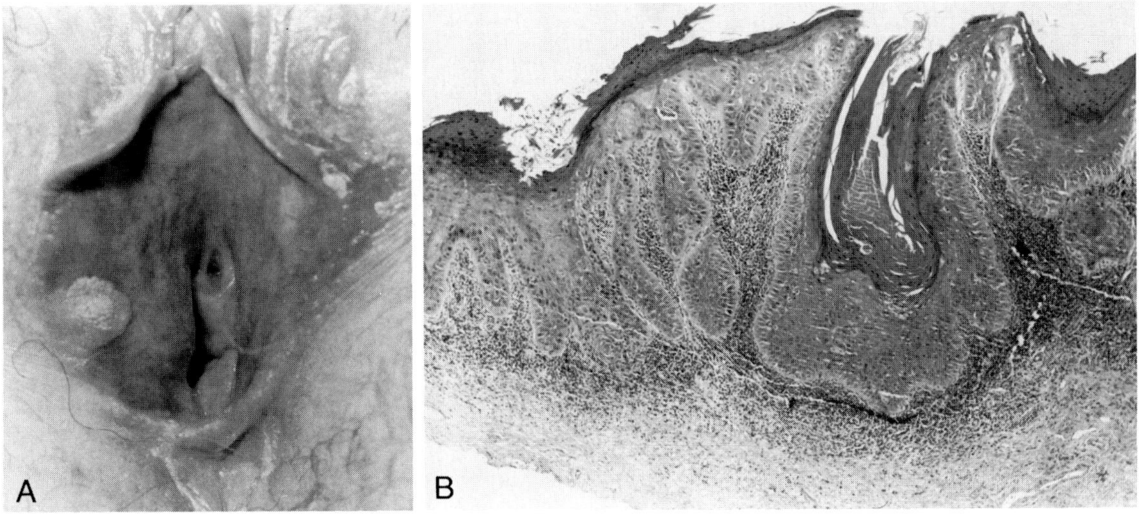

FIGURE 12–24. *A*, Squamous cell carcinoma of right labium minor; note erythroplasia of Queyrat in other areas. *B*, Section of nodule.

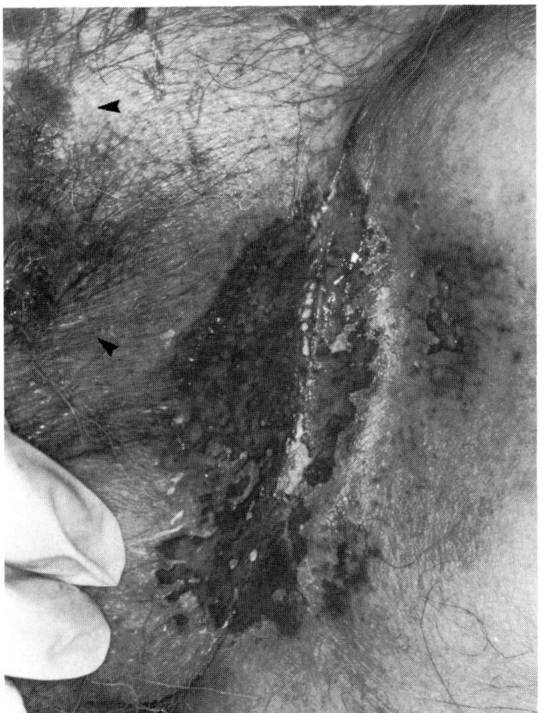

FIGURE 12–25. Extensive, inoperable, extramammary Paget's disease in the inguinal fold; lesion was mistaken for candidiasis. Also note lesions in suprapubic area (arrows). There was no response to topical bleomycin and 5-fluorouracil.

Examination for concomitant rectal or colonic carcinoma is mandatory when the lesion occurs in the anal region (Fig. 12–27).

Like Bowen's disease, EMPD can involve the epithelium of hair follicles and sweat ducts. Therefore, topical chemotherapy with 5-fluorouracil or bleomycin[25] is not effective. Also, the disease is resistant to radiotherapy.[3,5,8] The only effective treatment is an excision that is radically complete with careful microscopic examination of the margins of the excised tissue. Because the histologic picture is characteristic and easily discernible in frozen sections, the microscopically controlled surgery (Mohs) is well suited for the treatment of EMPD. It offers the most reliable means of removing all neoplastic cells.

Mohs and Blanchard[26] have reported five cases of EMPD treated successfully by microscopically controlled surgery. Their patients remained free of recurrence for periods ranging from 4 months to 9 years. The overall recurrence rate is about 44% after conventional surgical ablation.[4,27] Remember that in this condition recurrences may appear beyond 10 years.[28]

We have treated two patients with EMPD of the vulva by the Mohs technique (one by the fresh tissue method and one by the fixed tissue method). The patient treated on three occasions 15 years ago with the Mohs fixed tissue technique was a failure. The patient was initially treated by vulvectomy and radiotherapy, and by the time she was seen, the disease had

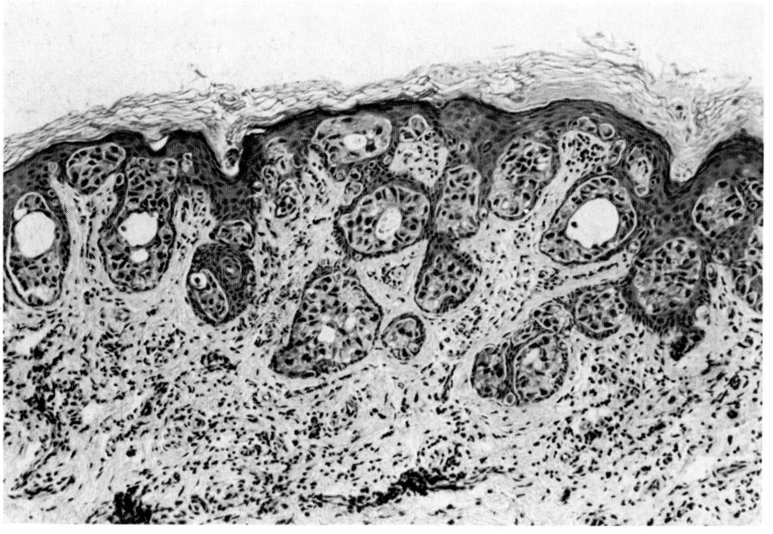

FIGURE 12–26. The histopathology of extramammary Paget's disease shows invasion of the epidermis by Paget's cells. The neoplastic cells, which are replete with mucin, are also present in the outer hair root epithelium and sweat ducts.

involved the entire vulva, pubic region, urethra, and vagina. The lesion then extended proximally into the urinary bladder, and deviation of the urinary flow to relieve pain had to be undertaken. She later succumbed from metastases. A third patient, an 80-year-old man with extensive EMPD that involved the suprapubic area, both inguinal folds, the scrotum, and almost the entire penis was considered inoperable (see Fig. 12–25). Topical chemotherapy with 5-fluorouracil and bleomycin over many months did not improve the condition. The patient finally expired with metastatic adenocarcinoma of the colon. The last two cases demonstrate the multicentricity characteristic of this disease.[28] At least 23% of the patients show multiple lesions.[3]

Squamous Cell Carcinoma of the Anal Region

Although rare, cancer of the anal region is often mistaken for benign or inflammatory conditions, causing delayed diagnosis and treatment. Pathologically, the great majority of

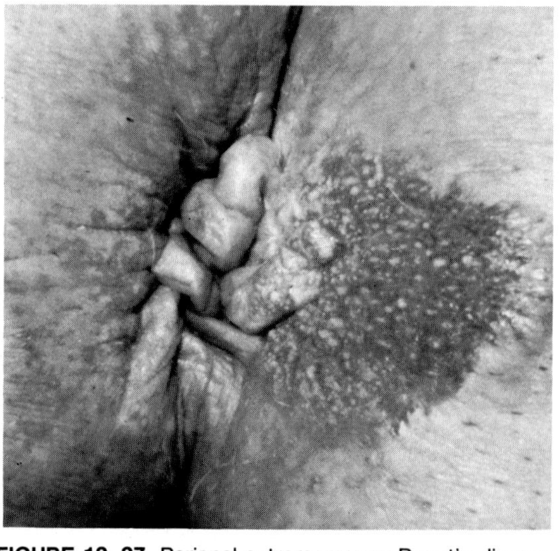

FIGURE 12–27. Perianal extramammary Paget's disease; The patient also had an adenocarcinoma of the rectum.

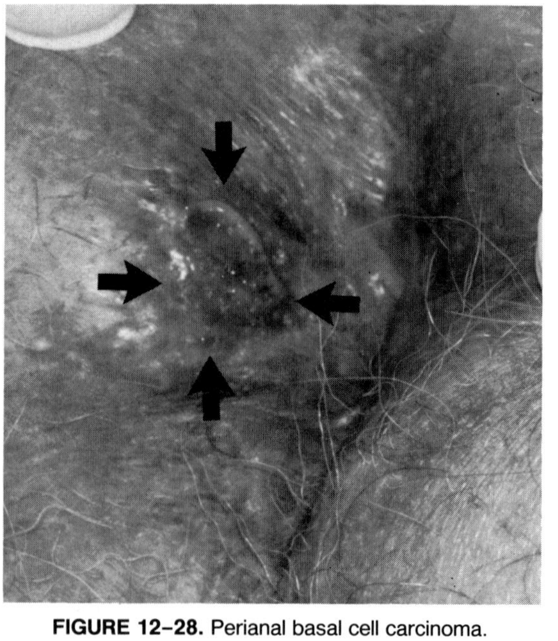

FIGURE 12–28. Perianal basal cell carcinoma.

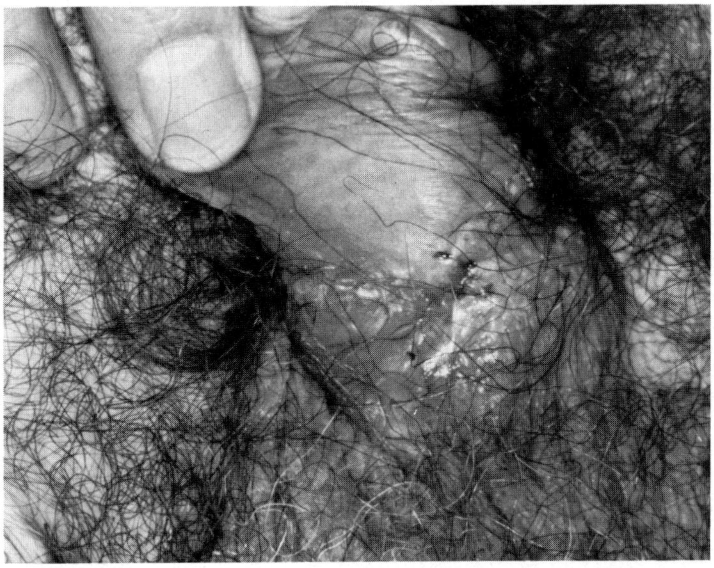

FIGURE 12–29. Basal cell carcinoma of the root of the penis and scrotum.

anal cancers are of the epidermoid type and arise in the cloacogenic zone (anorectal junction), which is lined with transitional epithelium, or the anal canal, which is lined with squamous epithelium. The peak frequency is at ages 55 to 60. The most common presenting symptom is bleeding and the sensation of an obstructing mass, which is often ulcerated and draining. Anal fistulae may be present.[28]

The extent of the tumor in the perineum is often underestimated, which accounts for the high recurrence rate. Extension into the prostate, vagina, and pelvis is frequent. These complications render the prognosis ominous.[29,30] Mohs has excised only a few carcinomas of the anal region by chemosurgery for palliative and exploratory reasons.[30] Radical surgery and/or radiotherapy are the prevailing modalities.

Basal Cell Carcinoma of the Anal Region and Genitals

Basal cell carcinomas are rare on the genitals. The cases we have encountered were nearly all of the pigmented nodular type (Fig. 12–28 to

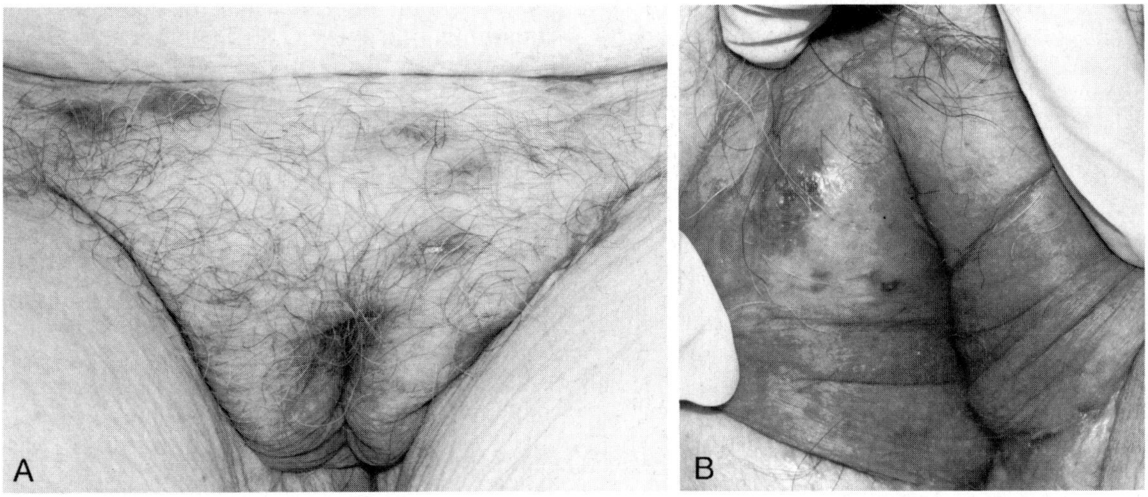

FIGURE 12–30. Multiple basal cell carcinomas in a nevoid basal cell carcinoma syndrome patient. *A*, Suprapubic lesions. *B*, Vulvar lesions.

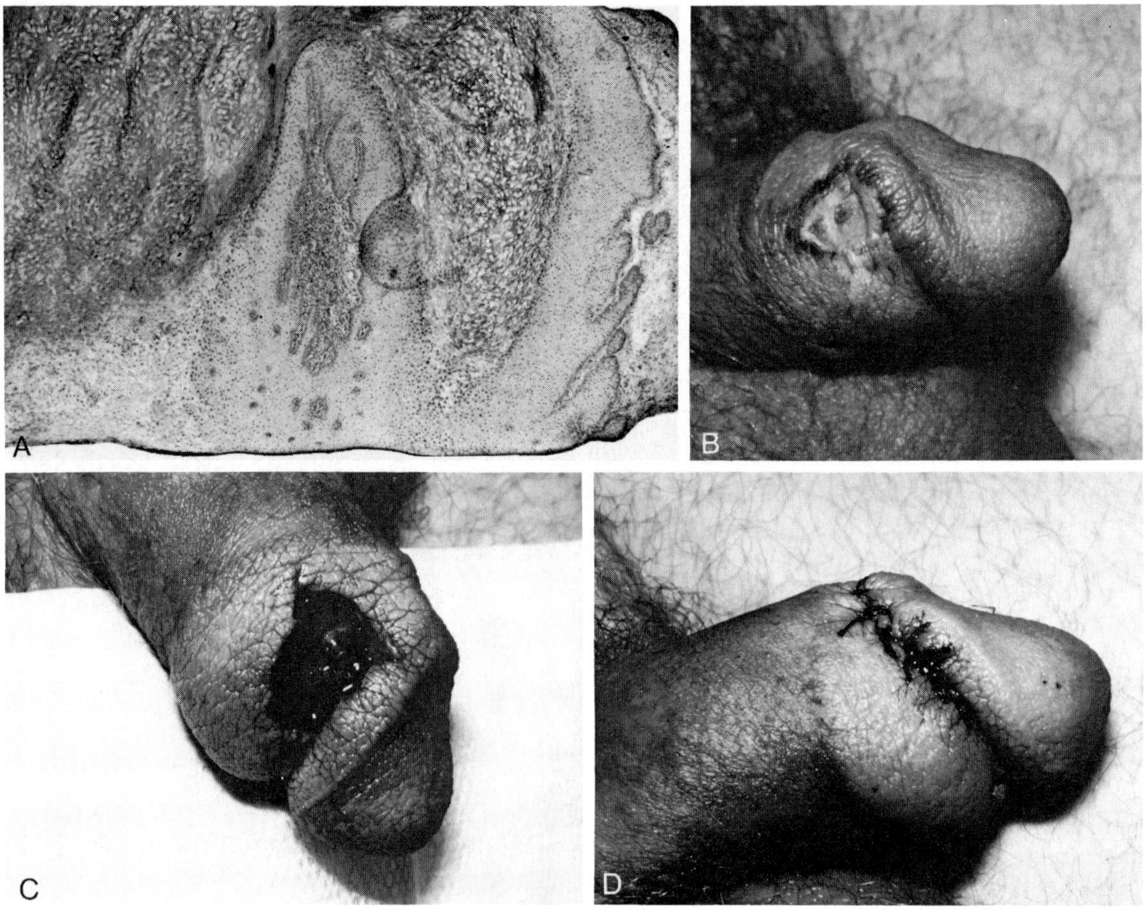

FIGURE 12–31. Keratoacanthoma in coronal sulcus: *A*, Section of half of the nodule removed by a biopsy; note the heavily keratinized mass on left (center of lesion) and the epithelial buttress on right. *B*, Crater-like lesion with raised margins after biopsy. *C*, After excision by Mohs surgery. *D*, Wound closed by approximation of margins.

12–30). The treatment modalities applicable to other parts of the body also apply here.

Malignant Melanoma

Malignant melanoma of the genitalia is rare. It accounts for less than 1% of all primary carcinomas of the penis.[25] The prognosis is poor even with radical surgery owing to the high frequency of early metastases.

Keratoacanthoma

Keratoacanthoma (KA) occurs most commonly on exposed skin surfaces. Ghadially's work led him to hypothesize that KA lesions start with hyperplasia of the infundibulum of one or several adjoining hair follicles and with squamous metaplasia of the attached sebaceous gland.[31] However, this cannot be universally valid because KA has been encountered on mucosal surfaces, e.g., conjunctiva[32] and oral mucosae,[33,34] in the nail bed,[35] on the mucosal surface of the prepuce,[36] and on the glans penis.[37]

It is our belief that keratoacanthomas should be considered a well-differentiated squamous cell carcinoma and should be handled accordingly. The reasons for this are detailed in Chapter 4.

We have encountered two cases of the so-called keratoacanthoma of the penis. One was in the coronal sulcus in a man age 40. It was excised and the wound sutured (Fig. 12–31). The other patient, age 55, presented with a large keratotic lesion of the tip of the glans

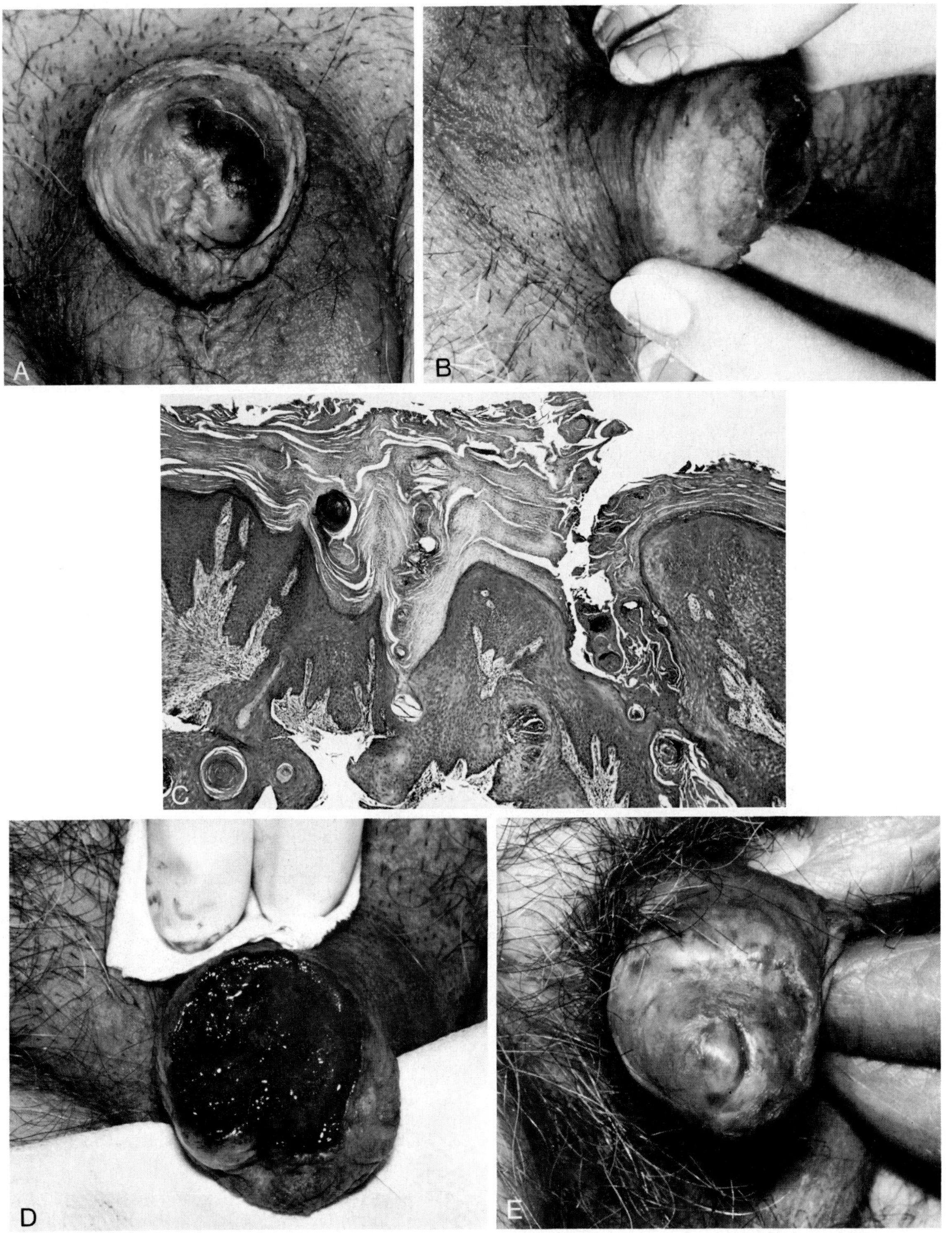

FIGURE 12–32. Keratoacanthoma on glans penis: *A*, Heavily keratinized tumor of glans, uniformly circular. *B*, Side view shows a central crater and the sloping wall of the lesion. *C*, Part of a section shows the buttress on the right and the keratinzed center on the left; the epidermal hyperplasia contains micro-abscesses, but hardly any cellular atypia. *D*, After excision by Mohs micrographic surgery. *E*, After healing by second intention.

penis. It was excised by Mohs surgery, and the wound was left to heal by second intention with a good result (Fig. 12–32).

REFERENCES

1. Kopf AW, Bart RS: Skin tumor conference No. 5: Erythematous plaque of the penis, J Dermatol Surg 2:14, 1976.
2. Boxer RJ, Skinner DG: Condylomata acuminata and squamous cell carcinoma, Urology 9:72–81, 1977.
3. Graham JH: Selected precancerous lesions. In Malkinson FD, Pearson RW (eds): Neoplasms of the Skin and Malignant Melanoma. Chicago: Year Book Medical Publishers, 1976.
4. Graham JH, Helwig EB: Erythroplasia of Queyrat: A clinicopathological and histochemical study, Cancer 32:1396–1414, 1973.
5. Graham JH, Helwig EB: Premalignant cutaneous and mucocutaneous disease. In Graham JH; Johnson WC, Helwig EB (eds): Dermal Pathology, Hagerstown, MD: Harper & Row, 1972, pp 581–597.
6. Goette DK, Carson TE: Erythroplasia of Queyrat, Cancer 38:1498–1502, 1976.
7. Honeycut WM, Jansen GT, Dillaha CJ: Topical antimetabolites and cytotoxic agents, Cutis 6:63–72, 1970.
8. Goette DK, Elgart M, De Villez RL: Erythroplasia of Queyrat. Treatment with topically applied fluorouracil, JAMA 232:934–937, 1975.
9. Lifshitz S, Roberts JA: Treatment of carcinoma in situ of the vulva with topical 5-fluorouracil, Obstet Gynecol 56:242–244, 1980.
10. Happle R: Surgical treatment of erythroplasia of Queyrat, Plast Reconst Surg 59:642–645, 1977.
11. Mohs FE: Chemosurgery: Microscopically Controlled Surgery for Skin Cancer, 2nd ed. Springfield, Ill.: Charles C. Thomas, 1978, pp 210–214.
12. Reymen F, Ravnborg L, Schou G, et al.: Bowen's disease and internal malignant diseases: A study of 581 patients, Arch Dermatol 124:677–679, 1988.
13. Chuang TY, Reizner GT: Bowen's disease and internal malignancy: A matched case-control study, J Am Acad Dermatol 19:47–51, 1988.
14. Marfing TE, Abel ME, Gallagher DM: Perianal Bowen's disease and associated malignancies, Dis Colon Rectum 30:782–785, 1987.
15. Turner MLC: Human papilloma virus infection of the genital tract, Prog Dermatol 23(2):1–12, 1989.
16. Campion MJ, McCane DJ, Mitchell HS, et al.: Subclinical penile human papillomavirus infection and dysplasia in consorts of women with cervical neoplasia, Genitourin Med 64:90–99, 1988.
17. Lupulescu A, Mehregan A: Bowen's disease of genital areas, J Cutan Pathol 4:266–274, 1977.
18. Berger BW, Hori Y: Multicentric Bowen's disease of the genitalia. Spontaneous regression of lesions, Arch Dermatol 114:1698–1699, 1978.
19. Schellhamer PE, Grabstald H: Tumors of the penis. In Campbell's Urology, 4th ed. Philadelphia: W. B. Saunders, 1979, pp. 1175–1188.
20. Hotchkiss RS: Cancer of the skin of the male genitalia. In Andrade R, Gumport SL, Popkin GL, et al. (eds): Cancer of the Skin. Philadelphia: W. B. Saunders, 1976, pp 1409–1432.
21. Jackson SM: The treatment of carcinoma of the penis, Brit J Surg 53:33–35, 1966.
22. Helwig EB, Graham JH: Anogenital (extramammary) Paget's disease, Cancer 16:387–395, 1963.
23. Janovski NA, Douglas CP: Diseases of the Vulva, New York: Harper & Row, 1972.
24. Klingmuller G, Ishibashi Y: Extramammary Paget's disease. In Andrade R, Gumport SL, Popkin GL, et al. (eds): Cancer of the Skin. Philadelphia: W. B. Saunders, 1976, pp 662–678.
25. Wade TR, Kopf AW, Ackerman AB: Bowenoid papulosis of the penis, Arch Dermatol 115:306–308, 1979.
26. Mohs FE, Blanchard L: Microscopically controlled surgery for extramammary Paget's disease, Arch Dermatol 115:706–708, 1979.
27. Boehm F, Morris JM: Paget's disease and apocrine carcinoma of the vulva, Obstet Gynecol 28:185–192, 1971.
28. Taylor PT, Stenwig JT, Clausen H: Paget's disease of the vulva, Gynecol Oncol 3:46–50, 1975.
29. Bradley B: Cancer of the anal and peri-anal areas. In Andrade R, Gumport SL, Popkin GL, et al. (eds): Cancer of the Skin. Philadelphia: W. B. Saunders, 1976, pp 1394–1407.
30. Mohs FE: Chemosurgical method for the microscopically controlled excision of cancer. Am J Proctol 8:273–277, 1957.
31. Ghadially FN: The role of the hair follicle in the origin and evolution of some cutaneous neoplasms of man and experimental animals, Cancer 14:801–816, 1961.
32. Roth AM: Solitary keratoacanthoma of the conjunctiva, Am J Ophthalmol 85:647–650, 1978.
33. Hume WJ, Quayle AA: An unusual epithelial neoplasm of gingiva resembling keratoacanthoma, Br J Oral Maxillofac Surg 23:366–370, 1985.
34. Eversole LF, Leider AS, Alexander G: Intraoral and labial keratoacanthoma, J Oral Surg Oral Med Oral Pathol 54:663–667, 1982.
35. Stoll DM, Ackerman AB: Subungual keratoacanthoma, Am J Dermatopathol 2:265–271, 1980.
36. Lejman K, Starzycki Z: Giant keratoacanthoma on the inner surface of the prepuce, Br J Vener Dis 53:65–67, 1977.
37. Thach JR, Thorne EG: Keratoacanthoma of the glans penis, Cutis 24:615–616, 1979.

Additional Readings

1. Adriani J: Labat's Regional Anesthesia, 4th ed. St. Louis: Warren H. Green, 1985, pp 580–582.
2. Johnson DE, Ayala AG: Primary melanoma of the penis, Urology 2:174–177, 1973.
3. Langman J, Woerdeman MW: Atlas of Medical Anatomy. Philadelphia: W. B. Saunders, 1982.
4. Mikhail GR: Squamous cell carcinoma of the penis, J Dermatol Surg 2:406–408, 1976.
5. Mikhail GR: Cancers, precancers and pseudocancers on the male genitalia, J Dermatol Surg Oncol 6:1027–1035, 1980.
6. Mikhail GR, Farah RN: Surgery of the skin of the male genitalia. In Epstein E, Epstein E Jr (eds): Skin Surgery, 6th ed. Philadephia: W. B. Saunders, 1987, pp 518–533.
7. Watring WG, Roberts JA, Lagasse LD, et al.: Treatment of recurrent Paget's disease of the vulva with topical bleomycin, Cancer 41:10–11, 1978.

CHAPTER 13

Treatment of Rare Malignancies

William C. Hanke, M.D.
Melissa W. Lee, B.S.

The most commonly accepted indications for Mohs micrographic surgery (MMS) are recurrent basal cell carcinoma and recurrent squamous cell carcinoma. Other problematic types of basal cell carcinoma and squamous cell carcinoma are also often treated. A number of additional unusual malignancies have been treated with MMS including verrucous carcinoma, keratoacanthomas (aggressive or mutilating), hemangioendothelioma, dermatofibrosarcoma protuberans, malignant fibrohistiocytoma, leiomyosarcoma, adenocystic carcinoma of the skin, malignant melanoma, sebaceous carcinoma of the eyelid, extramammary Paget's disease, penile erythroplasia of Queyrat, oral and central facial paranasal sinus neoplasms, Merkel cell carcinoma, microcytic adnexal carcinoma, neurosarcoma, fibromyosarcoma, endothelioma, angiosarcoma, fibrosarcoma, and Bowen's disease.

In this chapter, we will discuss the advantages of MMS in the treatment of six types of unusual malignancies: dermatofibrosarcoma protuberans, verrucous carcinoma, leiomyosarcoma, microcytic adnexal carcinoma, Merkel cell carcinoma, and Bowen's disease of the scalp. Each malignancy is illustrated with a case report, followed by a discussion of the entity.

DERMATOFIBROSARCOMA PROTUBERANS

A woman age 34 first noticed a pea-sized growth at the left frontal hairline in 1985. The patient was referred for MMS in 1987. Examination at that time revealed a 30×25 mm erythematous nodule adjacent to the left frontal hairline (Fig. 13–1). Biopsy findings were typical of dermatofibrosarcoma protuberans (Fig. 13–2), and the lesion was treated with MMS. Eleven stages and 46 horizontal frozen sections were required to achieve a tumor-free plane. The final surgical defect measured 70×50 mm and extended to the cranium (Fig. 13–3). The wound healed by second intention in 20 weeks (Fig. 13–4). There has been no evidence of recurrence during follow-up.

Dermatofibrosarcoma protuberans (DFSP) is an uncommon, locally invasive malignant tumor.[1] It arises in the dermis and rarely metastasizes, but it is notorious for recurrence after wide excision.[1–3] DFSP most commonly occurs on the trunk and proximal extremities. It grows slowly, and a history of antecedent trauma is present in 10% of the patients.

Clinically, DFSP often appears as a dusky indurated plaque. After a period of time, the tumor may become nodular or multinodular and ulcerate.

The tumor infiltrates laterally between the collagen bundles of the reticular dermis and merges into the normal dermis. The fibroblasts in the dermis may extend into the subcutaneous fat or even deeper into striated muscles.[1] The spread of tumor by finger-like extensions makes complete removal by standard surgical excision difficult. High rates of recurrence following standard surgical excision have been reported.[1,2] Published series of patients with DFSP have reported recurrence rates as high as

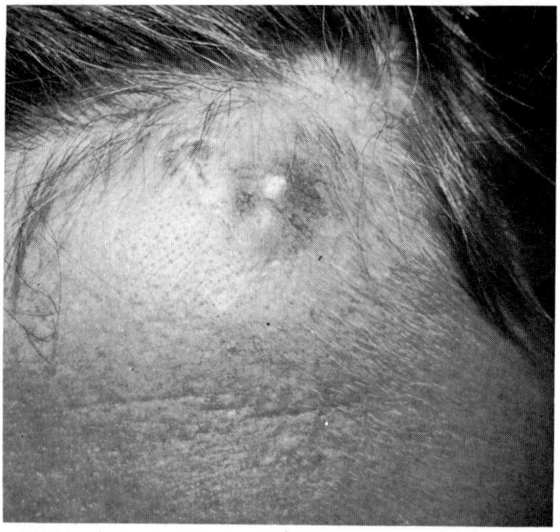

FIGURE 13–1. Dermatofibrosarcoma protuberans in a woman age 34 at the left frontal hairline of 2 years' duration.

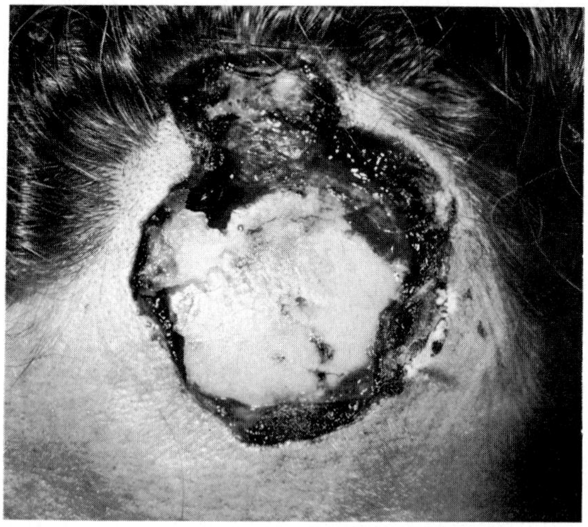

FIGURE 13–3. Dermatofibrosarcoma protuberans: The surgical defect measured 70×50 mm following Mohs micrographic surgery and extended to the periosteum.

54%, and rates of 10% to 20% have been reported even with excisional margins of greater than 3 cm including the underlying fascia.[3]

Because of the tendency of DFSP to extend and spread beneath normal-appearing skin, some physicians have practiced MMS rather than wide excision.[1] This allows microscopic examination of all excised tissue margins for any remaining tumor. Microscopically controlled margins are invaluable in treating DFSP. In addition to complete removal of the tumor, MMS allows preservation of as much normal tissue as possible.

Peters and colleagues[4] used MMS to treat a patient with DFSP on the face that had recurred four times following standard surgical excision. There was no evidence of recurrence after 5 years. The histologic determination between tumor and normal tissue in frozen sections did not pose a problem during the MMS procedure.

Mikhail and Lynn have reported on the successful treatment of two cases of DFSP by the

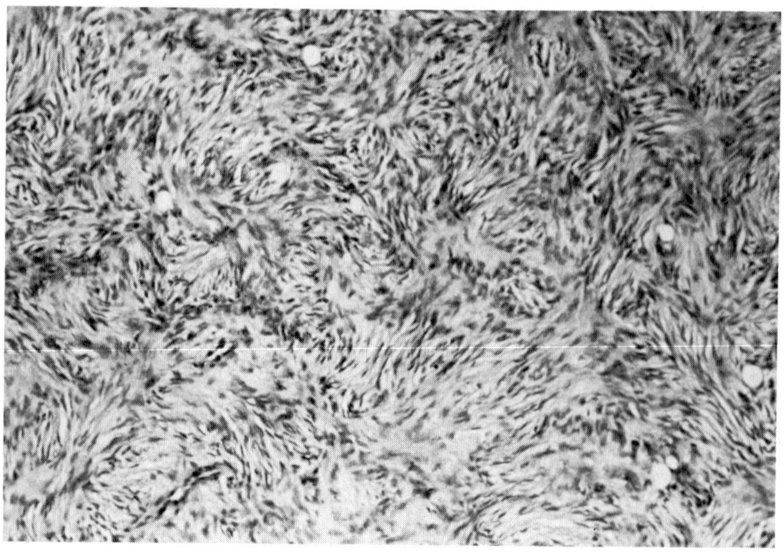

FIGURE 13–2. Biopsy of the lesion shown in Figure 13–1 is typical of dermatofibrosarcoma protuberans.

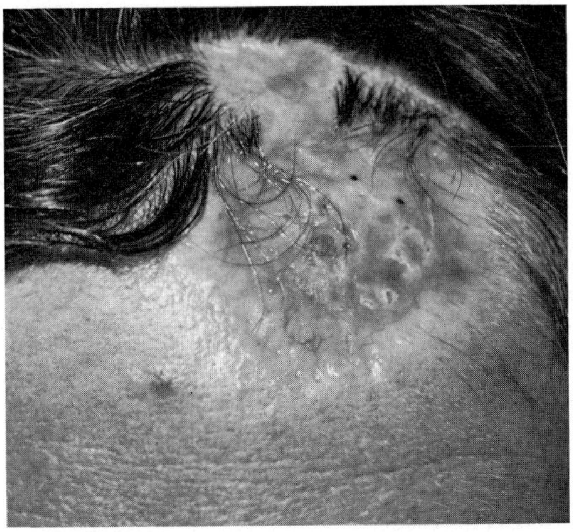

FIGURE 13-4. The wound shown in Figure 13-3 healed by second intention in 20 weeks.

Mohs technique in 1978. Both lesions were on the chest of young women. One of the lesions had recurred twice.[5] Both women were followed for 10 years without evidence of recurrence.

Hess and coworkers[2] treated a patient with DFSP on the chest wall with MMS. There was no recurrence after 18 months. The authors reported no difficulty in differentiating DFSP from normal tissue in frozen sections. It is recommended, especially with the myxoid variety of DFSP, that the Mohs micrographic surgeon perform several preoperative biopsies in order to become familiar with the histologic pattern in frozen section.[2,5]

Robinson treated four patients with DFSP by MMS. All patients were examined at 4-month intervals for lymphadenopathy or recurrence. There were no recurrences at 5 years.[1]

Hobbs and coworkers[3] treated 10 patients with DFSP by MMS. All 10 patients had been treated previously by unsuccessful conventional excisional surgery. The average follow-up was 43 months, and no recurrence developed. It was also pointed out that there was no difficulty in distinguishing tumor from normal tissue in frozen sections.

No recurrences of DFSP following MMS have been reported. MMS allows complete removal of tumor with maximum preservation of normal tissue. In view of the tendency of DFSP to recur locally and metastasize rarely, several authors have recommended MMS as the treatment of choice for this lesion.[2,3]

VERRUCOUS CARCINOMA OF THE FOOT

A man age 54 noticed a growth on the ball of the left foot in 1975. The lesion continued to enlarge, and was treated with excision and a skin graft in 1977. The tumor recurred and the patient was referred for MMS in October 1979. Examination revealed a 25×57 mm, exophytic tumor that involved the plantar aspect of the left sole overlying the third, fourth, and fifth metatarsal heads (Fig. 13-5).

A biopsy of the lesion showed features of verrucous carcinoma. The sections demonstrated a neoplasm arising from the epidermis and infiltrating the underlying tissues. The individual cells contained abundant quantities of eosinophilic cytoplasm. Central areas of keratinous pearls were present throughout. The nuclei were oval and exhibited little pleomorphism. Most of the nuclei had a single prominent nucleolus. Mitoses were present, but not abundant. Prominent parakeratotic epithelial tracts were present in the dermis. The overlying epidermis showed marked hyperkeratosis and parakeratosis. A prominent inflammatory infiltrate, composed of lymphocytes, plasma cells, and a few eosinophils, was present adjacent to the margins of the lesion. The epidermis was acanthotic adjacent to the foci of downward proliferation. X-rays of the foot and a three-phase bone scan showed no evidence of bony involvement by the tumor.

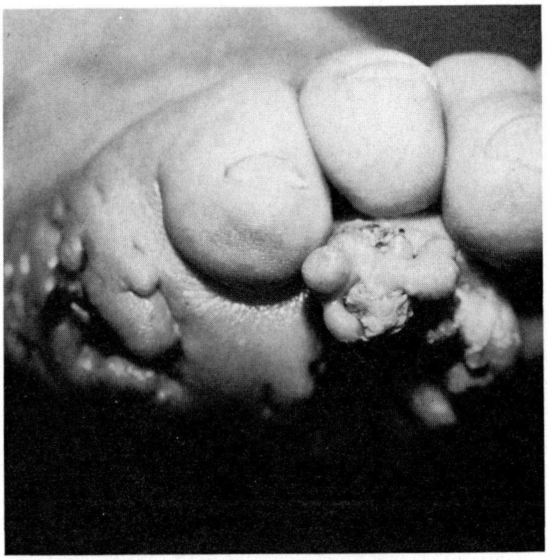

FIGURE 13-5. A man age 54 developed this verrucous carcinoma on the sole in 1977.

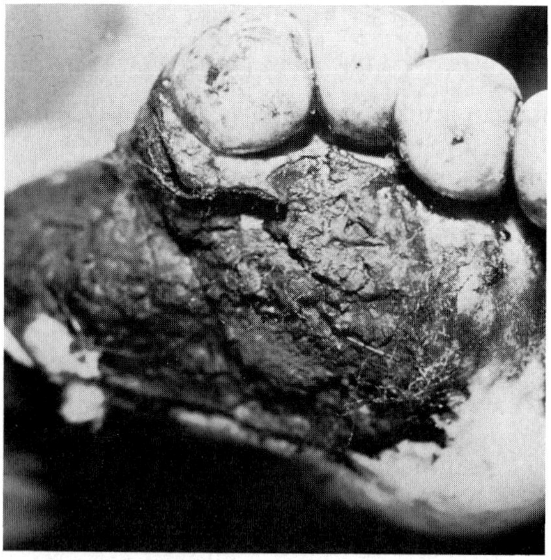

FIGURE 13-6. The tumor in Figure 13-5 was treated with the Mohs fixed tissue micrographic surgery in 1979. The zinc chloride fixative paste is shown in place before excision of a layer of tissue.

On December 11, 1979, treatment was initiated with the fixed tissue method of MMS. The zinc chloride fixative paste was applied to the tumor on each of 4 consecutive days (Fig. 13-6). After each application of the fixative paste, the surgical site was bandaged, and the patient was sent home overnight. A total of 134 horizontal frozen sections were prepared over the 4 days of MMS. The fifth toe was heavily involved with tumor and was amputated during the final stage. The final defect measured 80×75 mm, and extended entirely through the fat pad and the periosteum of the metatarsal bones. The residual fixed tissue separated 2 weeks later revealing healthy granulation tissue. The wound healed by second intention in 12 weeks (Fig. 13-7).

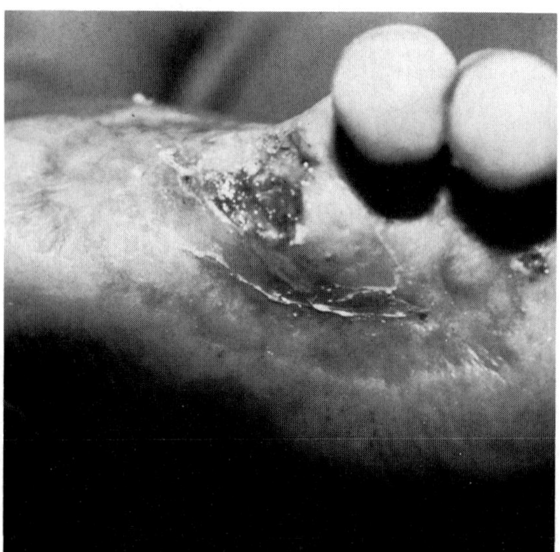

FIGURE 13-7. The surgical site in Figure 13-6 shows healing at 8 weeks after termination of Mohs micrographic surgery. The fifth toe was removed during the procedure.

A tender ulceration developed adjacent to the surgical scar in October 1981, and a biopsy again showed verrucous carcinoma. In view of the extensiveness of the original MMS procedure, it was felt that another attempt at local eradication of the tumor would not be indicated. Therefore, the patient was referred to an orthopedic surgeon for a below-knee amputation. This was performed, and the surgical margins showed no evidence of residual verrucous carcinoma. The patient did well following the amputation and was fitted with a prosthesis. There has been no evidence of recurrence during follow-up.

Verrucous carcinoma of the foot was first described in the English literature by Aird and colleagues[6] as "epithelioma cuniculatum." The tumor has since been classified as verrucous carcinoma by Brownstein and Shapiro,[7] and more specifically as "plantar verrucous carcinoma" by Mohs and Sahl.[8] Approximately 50 cases of verrucous carcinoma of the foot have been reported to date.

Verrucous carcinoma of the foot occurs predominantly on the moist macerated epithelium of the sole and heel.[8,9] Extrapedal sites of occurrence have been reported including the knee, lower leg, wrist, and finger.[7,9–11]

Verrucous carcinoma of the foot consists of large, fungating masses of moist squamous epithelium containing numerous interconnecting crypts and sinuses.[8,9] The crypts and sinuses resemble rabbit burrows, hence the name *cuniculatum.*[6] A foul-smelling greasy material containing keratin and cellular debris can be extruded from the sinus openings by the application of gentle pressure.

Verrucous carcinoma of the foot is characterized histopathologically by acanthosis, papillomatosis, moderate hyperkeratosis, and focal areas of parakeratosis. The tumor has a dense fibrous stroma and a moderate inflammatory infiltrate composed chiefly of lymphocytes in the dermis and polymorphonuclear leukocytes in the crypts.[8] The abnormal epithelial growth infiltrates the underlying dermis as broad columns or as thin trabeculae.[9] Tumors that invade deeply tend to grow around bones and tendons. However, invasion of these structures has only occasionally been reported.[9,12,13] In general, verrucous carcinoma of the foot does not exhibit the classic histologic features of malignancy but resembles carcinoma only by virtue of its aggressive behavior.[8]

The etiology of verrucous carcinoma remains unclear. Several possibilities have been suggested, including: (1) development of a de novo squamous cell carcinoma, (2) the result of chronic trauma to the plantar surface, (3) the result of low-dose radiation therapy, and (4) the result of viral infection.[6,12,14]

Almost all of the reports of verrucous carcinoma of the foot describe clinical and histopathologic difficulties in reaching a specific diagnosis because of the protracted growth and subtle microscopic features of the neoplasm.[14] Mohs and Sahl[8] feel that the diagnosis of verrucous carcinoma of the foot should be based on both the clinical and the histologic features of the lesion as well as its biological behavior. The tumors are frequently misdiagnosed because biopsies are usually either too small or too superficial for proper evaluation or because the pathologist is unaware of the size, site, and duration of the lesion.[9,13] The differential diagnosis includes plantar wart, pseudoepitheliomatous hyperplasia, giant keratoacanthoma, deep fungal infection, amelanotic malignant melanoma, basal cell carcinoma, and squamous cell carcinoma.[11,15]

Several therapeutic modalities have been used in the treatment of verrucous carcinoma of the foot including curettage and electrodesiccation, intralesional injection of 5-fluorouracil, and wide surgical excision followed by skin grafting. Amputation may be indicated when extensive growth of tumor results in severe deformity of the foot or when there is evidence of bone involvement or regional metastases.[11] Anaplastic transformation of verrucous carcinoma of the oral cavity, i.e., oral florid papillomatosis, following radiation treatment has been reported, suggesting that radiation therapy may not be a good alternative.[16]

In view of the low metastatic potential of verrucous carcinoma of the foot, an ideal therapeutic modality would be one that would destroy or ablate all of the neoplastic growth while preserving the normal uninvolved tissues. MMS has been employed successfully in the treatment of these tumors.[8,11] The maximal conservation of normal tissue provided by MMS offers the greatest chance of preserving a functional leg and foot. We recommend MMS rather than conventional wide surgical excision or surgical amputation as the treatment of choice for the majority of verrucous carcinomas of the foot. The patients must be followed closely postoperatively for recurrence.

LEIOMYOSARCOMA

A man age 48 had an enlarging mass on the chest for 1 year. Examination in May 1986, revealed a 1-cm firm nodule over the inferior part of the sternum. There were no lymphadenopathies. A biopsy of the lesion showed elongated bundles of spindle cells, with blunted ends, infiltrating the reticular dermis (Fig. 13–8 and 13–9). The tumor did not involve the subcutaneous fat. Atypical nuclei and mitotic figures were occasionally observed. The deep and lateral margins of the biopsy specimen were involved with tumor. A Masson trichrome stain confirmed the smooth-muscle origin of the cells. Staining for S-100 protein was negative.

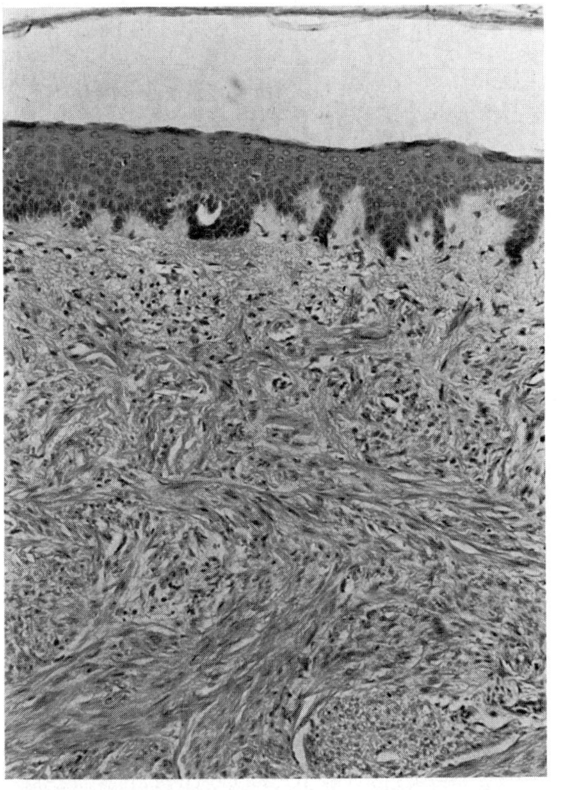

FIGURE 13–8. Biopsy from a chest lesion shows spindle cells of leiomyosarcoma that invaded the reticular dermis.

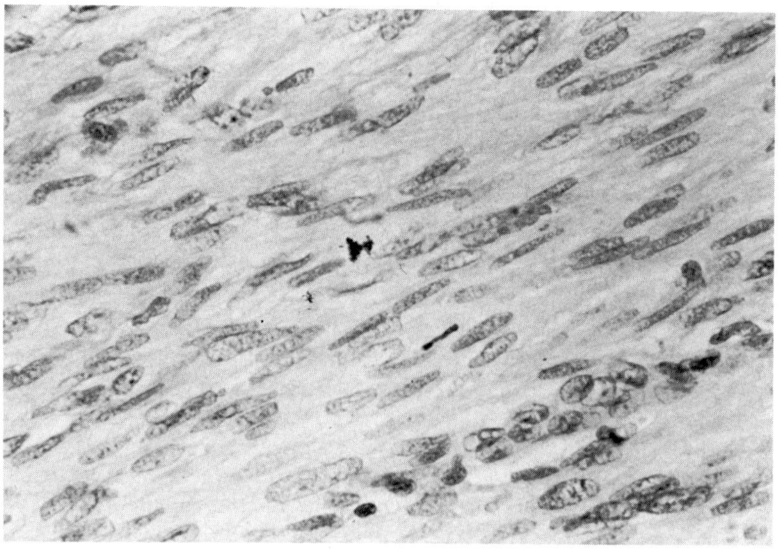

FIGURE 13–9. A high-power photomicrograph of section shown in Figure 13–8 shows the blunt-ended nuclei of leiomyosarcoma.

The lesion was treated with MMS. Two stages, utilizing 16 horizontal frozen sections, were required in order to achieve a microscopic tumor-free plane. The final surgical defect measured 45×30 mm (Fig. 13–10), and the surgical site was allowed to heal by second intention (Fig. 13–11). Follow-up examination at 30 months revealed no evidence of recurrence.

Leiomyosarcoma is a rare tumor that arises in the cutaneous or subcutaneous tissue, generally between the ages of 50 and 70. Cutaneous leiomyosarcoma arises from the smooth muscle surrounding the sweat glands or in the arrector muscle of the hair follicle. Consequently, cutaneous leiomyosarcoma appears mostly on the hair-bearing extensor surfaces. Cutaneous leiomyosarcoma is less aggressive than subcutaneous leiomyosarcoma and has a tendency to recur locally rather than metastasize. Cutaneous leiomyosarcoma is usually smaller clinically than the subcutaneous variety when first detected. It usually appears as a

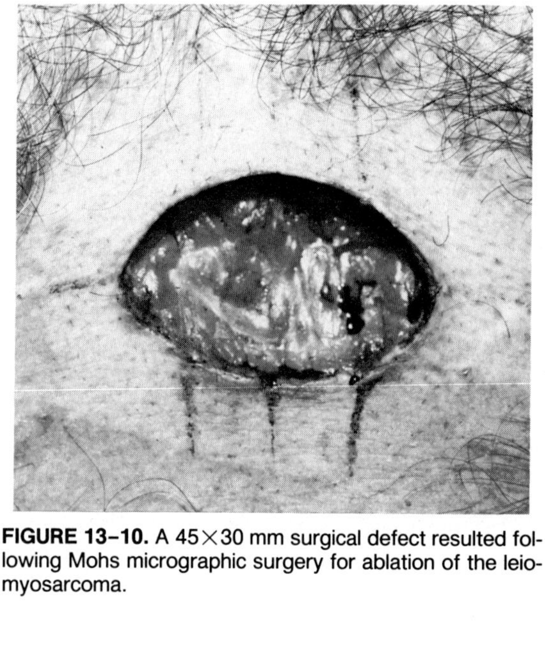

FIGURE 13–10. A 45×30 mm surgical defect resulted following Mohs micrographic surgery for ablation of the leiomyosarcoma.

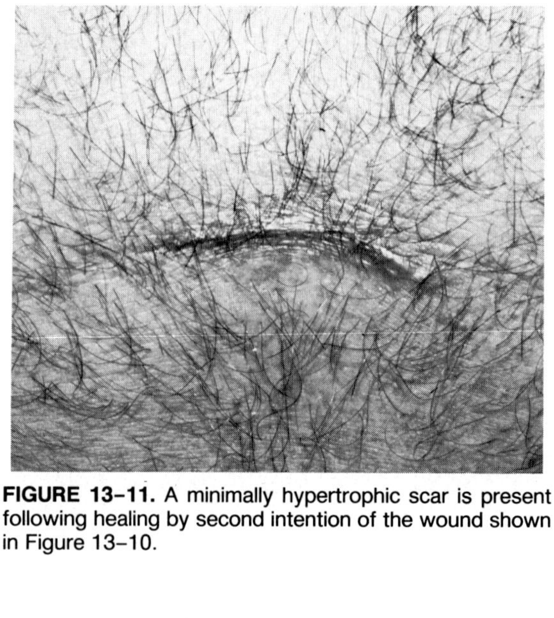

FIGURE 13–11. A minimally hypertrophic scar is present following healing by second intention of the wound shown in Figure 13–10.

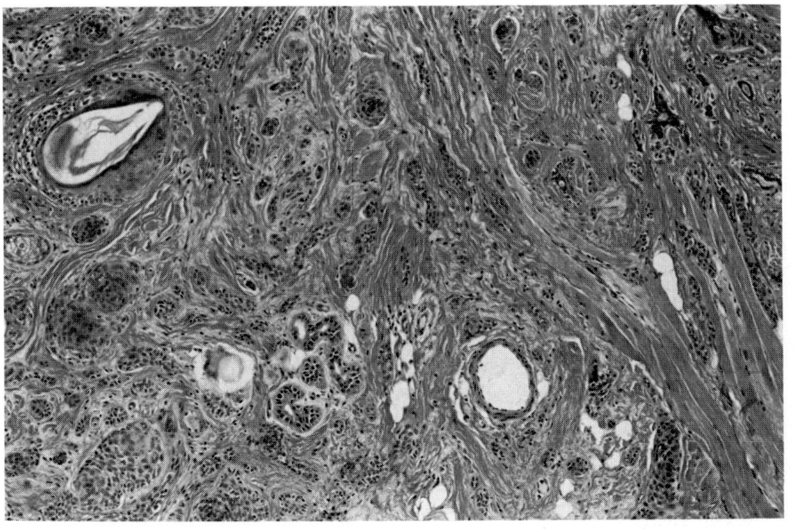

FIGURE 13–12. The histopathology of microcystic adnexal carcinoma shows squamous microcysts and anastomosing epithelial strands and cords with ductal differentiation.

firm solitary nodule and may develop discoloration, umbilication, or ulceration.[5]

Subcutaneous leiomyosarcoma is distinctive in that it arises from the muscular media of blood vessels. These lesions have a rapid rate of growth and tend to metastasize.[17] Therefore, the prognosis for these tumors is poor.

A review of 80 patients with cutaneous leiomyosarcoma by Fields and Helwig[18] revealed that local recurrence developed in 32% of the tumors that were confined to the dermis and 47% of the tumors that arose in the subcutaneous fat. Subcutaneous leiomyosarcoma has a 33% incidence of metastases, while cutaneous leiomyosarcoma rarely metastasizes.[17]

Treatment of leiomyosarcoma has traditionally consisted of wide excision, amputation, fulguration, or radiotherapy; wide excision being the treatment of choice.[17] Our patient with primary cutaneous leiomyosarcoma was treated with MMS without substantial normal tissue loss and with no recurrence after 30 months. Since most recurrences develop within 5 years of the initial surgery, the results with MMS are promising.

MICROCYTIC ADNEXAL CARCINOMA

A woman age 77 was treated with curettage and electrosurgery for a "basal cell carcinoma" on the right alar rim in 1985. The tumor recurred and a biopsy in April 1987 was interpreted as microcytic adnexal carcinoma (Fig. 13–12). Examination revealed a 10×12 mm crusted plaque at the mucocutaneous junction of the right alar rim (Fig. 13–13). The lesion was treated with MMS, and five stages utilizing 18 horizontal frozen sections were required in order to achieve a microscopic tumor-free plane. The final surgical defect was 31×26 mm in size (Fig. 13–14). During the procedure, the tumor was observed to extend along the perichondrium and also within the perineural sheath. The wound was allowed to heal by second intention. The patient was fitted with a

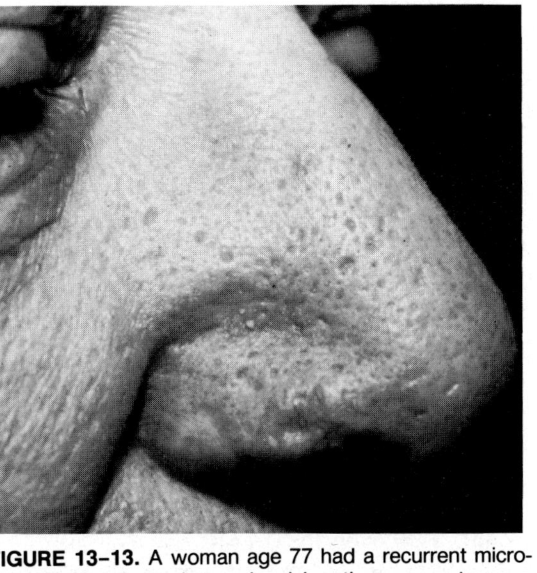

FIGURE 13–13. A woman age 77 had a recurrent microcystic adnexal carcinoma involving the mucocutaneous junction of the right alar rim. Note the small clinical size.

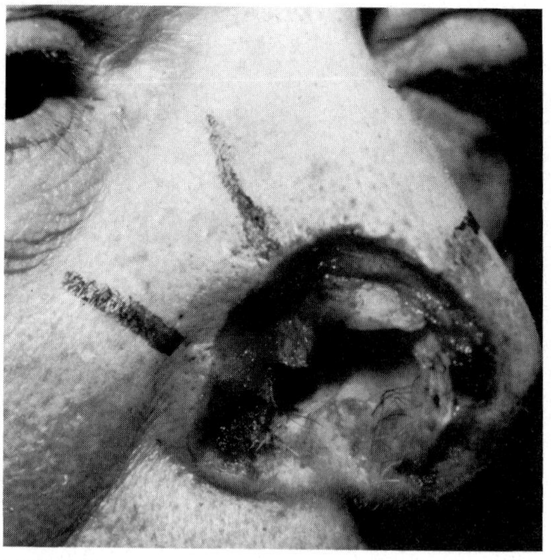

FIGURE 13–14. The extent of the microcystic adnexal carcinoma is disclosed following five Mohs micrographic surgical stages.

partial nasal prosthesis, and there has been no evidence of recurrence of tumor during follow-up.

Microcytic adnexal carcinoma (MAC), a rare, locally aggressive neoplasm, is a recently described clinicopathologic entity that demonstrates both pilar and eccrine differentiation.[19–22] In 1982, six patients with a tumor that showed unusual histologic features were given the designation "microcytic adnexal carcinoma" by Goldstein and coworkers.[23] Twenty-two cases of MAC have been reported in the literature,[19] and of these, 21 have occurred on the face, most commonly on the lip. Twelve of the patients were women, and the mean age was 47 years.

Clinically, MAC often presents as a papular, flesh-colored tumor in the middle-aged. It usually involves the mucocutaneous junction of the upper lip or alar rim. The lesion appears clinically and histologically benign.[21] However, it is locally invasive and may spread extensively into the adjacent subcutaneous tissues, nerves, muscles, cartilage, and bone. Perineural involvement has been also reported.[19,21] Pathologically, the bidirectional extension of this carcinoma may make diagnosis difficult. Microscopically, MAC may be confused with various benign tumors, including desmoplastic trichoepithelioma, syringoma, and trichoadenoma. However, the deeply invasive nature of the tumor and prominent perineural involvement should rule out benign conditions.[19]

Treatment of MAC includes conventional surgery, radiation therapy or a combination of both. In 21 cases in which follow-up information was available, 10 (48%) recurred.[19] Therefore, conventional surgery and radiation therapy are not particularly effective. MMS, on the other hand, is advantageous in that it provides precise microscopic control of the margins and insures complete removal. Another advantage is the preservation of as much normal tissue as possible.[21]

Birkby and colleagues treated a man age 51 with MAC on the left lower lip. The patient had been previously treated unsuccessfully with standard surgical excision. The authors found evidence of direct invasion of bone, and a partial hemimandibulectomy was performed, followed by radiation therapy. There was no evidence of recurrence 18 months later.

Hamm and coworkers[21] treated three patients with MAC using MMS. The first patient was a woman age 68 with MAC on the right side of the nose which extended onto the upper lip. There was no evidence of recurrence or metastasis 2 years following MMS. The second patient was a woman age 72 with MAC in the right nasolabial angle. There was no evidence of recurrence 18 months following MMS. The third patient was a man age 75 with MAC on the left cheek. Seven months following treatment with MMS, the patient was free of tumor.[20] Nickoloff and colleagues[22] also reported a woman age 45 with MAC on the left upper lip which extended into the nasolabial fold and onto the nasal ala. There was no evidence of recurrence 13 months following MMS.

MMS is an ideal treatment for MAC because of the tumor's low rate of metastasis and its tendency to recur following conventional surgery. In our opinion, this technique will become the standard treatment for this unusual tumor.

MERKEL CELL CARCINOMA

A man age 71 noticed a rapidly enlarging tumor on the left forehead in December 1987. Examination revealed an 11×9 mm crusted nodule on the central left forehead (Fig. 13–15). A biopsy showed Merkel cell carcinoma (Fig. 13–16 and 13–17). A work-up for systemic malignancy was negative. The past history was significant in that the patient had received x-ray treatments to the face for acne

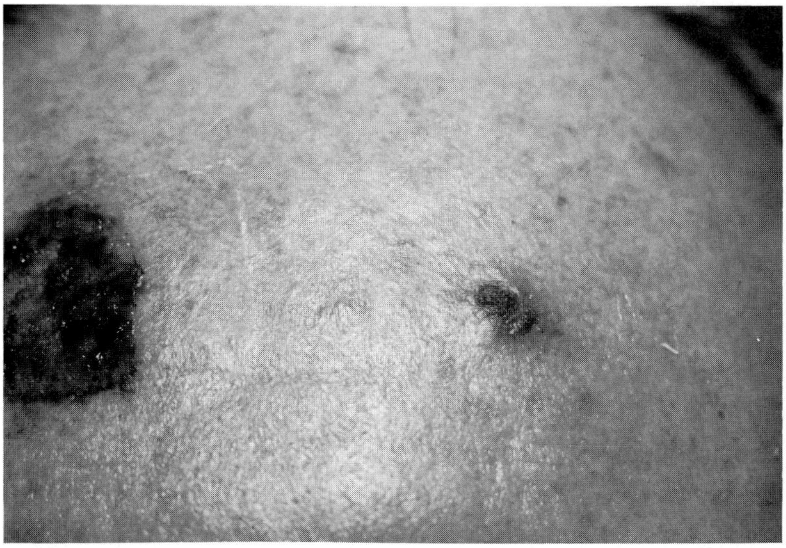

FIGURE 13–15. Merkel cell carcinoma: A man age 71 developed a rapidly enlarging growth on the left forehead in December of 1987; the tumor enlarged to this size 4 months later. The larger superficial wound on the right forehead was created by electrosurgery for a basal cell carcinoma.

during his teens. The lesion was treated with MMS in March 1988. Four stages and 11 horizontal frozen sections were required in order to achieve a microscopic tumor-free plane. The surgical defect measured 32×38 mm at the completion of the procedure and extended to the periosteum (Fig. 13–18). The wound was left to heal by second intention.

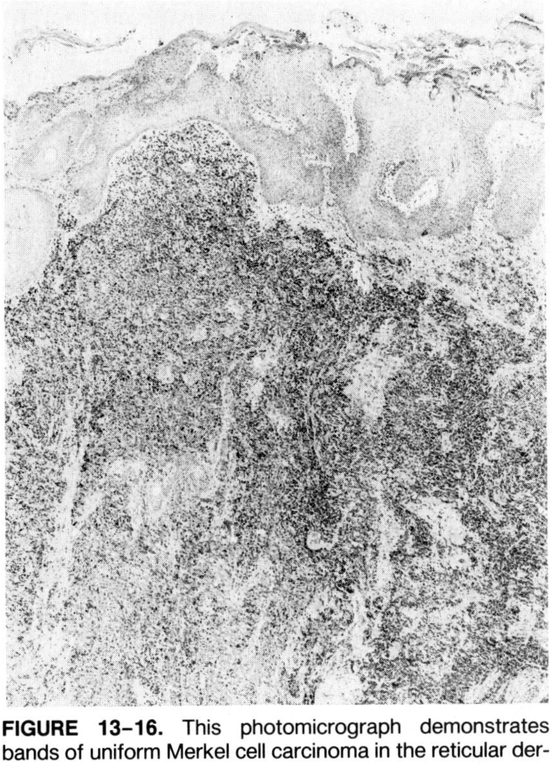

FIGURE 13–16. This photomicrograph demonstrates bands of uniform Merkel cell carcinoma in the reticular dermis.

In May 1988, a nodule appeared inferior and to the left forehead scar. A needle aspiration biopsy from an enlarged left infra-auricular lymph node demonstrated Merkel cell carcinoma. A reexcision of the left forehead surgical site and scar, including the outer table of the bone was undertaken. A modified neck dissection was also done. Twenty-seven of 45 lymph nodes harvested during the neck dissection were positive for Merkel cell carcinoma. The surgical defect was allowed to heal by second intention (Fig. 13–19 and 13–20).

Multiple erythematous papules developed adjacent to the forehead scar in July 1988. A biopsy from a 4 mm nodule in the left eyebrow area contained Merkel cell carcinoma. Chemotherapy was begun with cyclophosphamide, doxorubicin hydrochloride, and vincristine sulfate. The patient was later given two courses of cisplatin (20 mg m^2 daily for 4 days). The clinically evident cutaneous metastases resolved.

The patient expired in August 1989. A postmortem showed metastatic Merkel cell carcinoma in the liver, vertebral bodies, adrenal glands, and peripancreatic lymph nodes.

Merkel cell carcinoma (MCC), also called trabecular carcinoma or neuroendocrine carcinoma, is an unusual primary neoplasm, and approximately 400 cases have been reported in the literature. MCC occurs most commonly on sun-exposed areas of the skin in elderly patients. The tumor is aggressive and appears

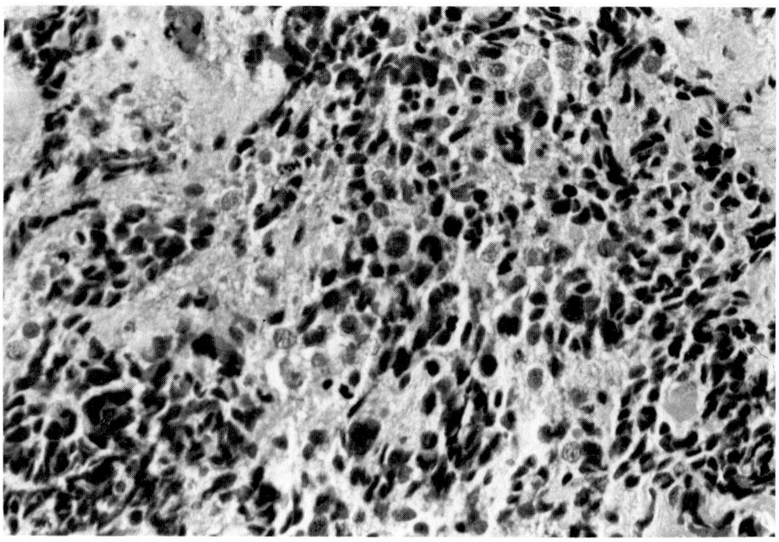

FIGURE 13–17. This high-power photomicrograph shows a dense infiltrate of Merkel cell carcinoma in the subcutaneous fat.

clinically as a rapidly growing nodule. The tumor infiltrates subcutaneous fat and muscles, and then the lymphatics and blood vessels. Considering the aggressive nature of this neoplasm, it is not surprising that 40% of the 400 documented cases of MCC have experienced local recurrence following surgical treatment. Twelve months following surgery, distant metastases occurred in 49.3% of the patients.[24]

The medical literature indicates that the survival rate for patients with MCC is 55% at 3 years. Because of the potentially lethal nature of the tumor, early diagnosis and treatment are essential. Diagnosis should be early and accurate and should be based upon clinical evaluation and pathologic examination with light and electron microscopy.[24]

The treatment methods that have been reported include MMS, traditional surgical excision, chemotherapy, and radiation therapy. The results of treatment have been variable. Wide local excision is the most common method for managing Merkel cell carcinoma. The use of MMS is also beneficial because of the specific identification of microscopic tumor-free planes. Radiation may also be given to the primary tumor site in order to maximize the cure rate.

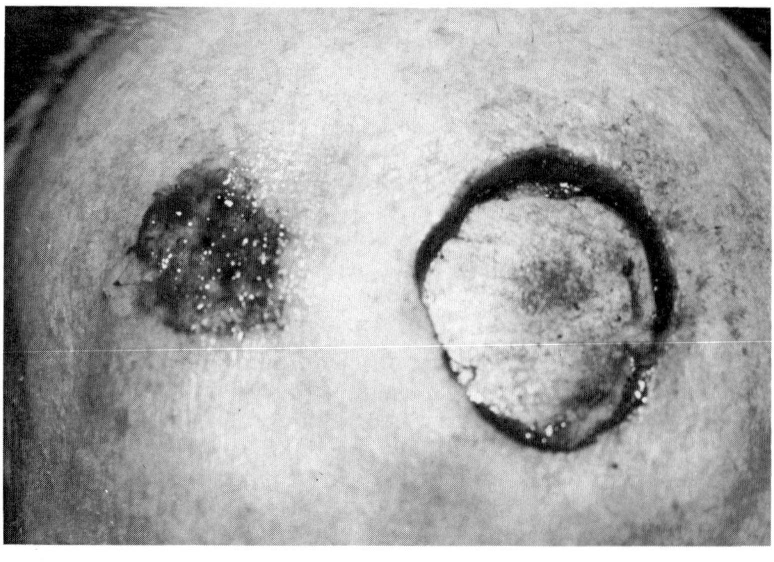

FIGURE 13–18. The surgical defect for the lesion in Figure 13–15 measured 38×32 mm following Mohs micrographic surgery. The right forehead wound is healing following electrosurgery for a basal cell carcinoma.

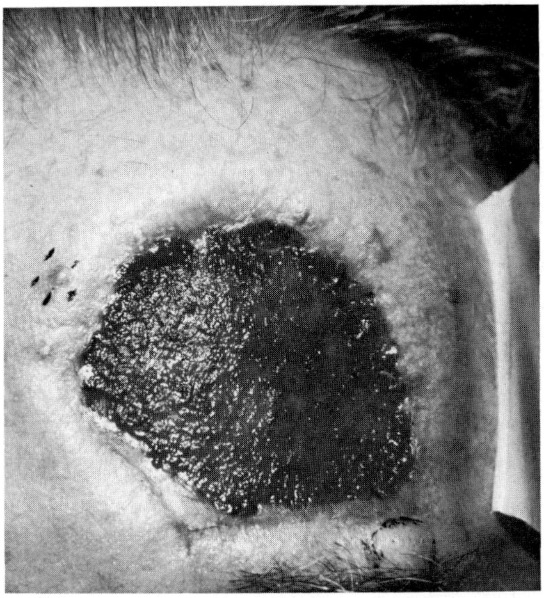

FIGURE 13–19. The Mohs micrographic surgery wound is granulating well following removal of the outer table of bone.

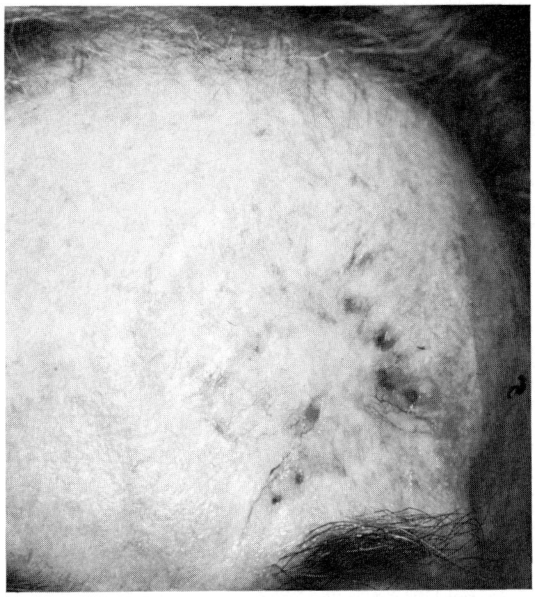

FIGURE 13–20. The surgical site demonstrates a scar after healing by second intention.

Hanke and coworkers[24] treated four patients with MCC who were between 68 and 76 years of age. Three patients experienced local recurrences and regional and distant metastases and died after 11, 19, and 39 months following treatment. The fourth patient was without evidence of recurrence at 41 months.

After treatment, patients should be followed closely with frequent and complete examinations. If the primary lesion is extensive, recurrent, or associated with regional or distant metastases, systemic chemotherapy should be considered.[24]

BOWEN'S DISEASE OF THE SCALP

A woman age 56 first noticed a crusted area on the scalp in March 1986. Examination revealed a 55×45 mm scaling, erythematous plaque on the right parietal scalp. A punch biopsy showed

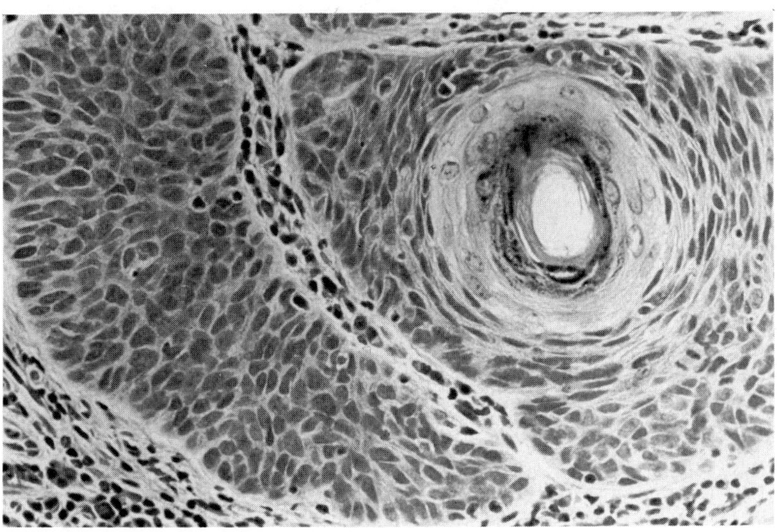

FIGURE 13–21. Photomicrograph of squamous cell carcinoma in situ (Bowen's disease) with extension into the follicular epithelium in the subcutaneous tissue of the scalp.

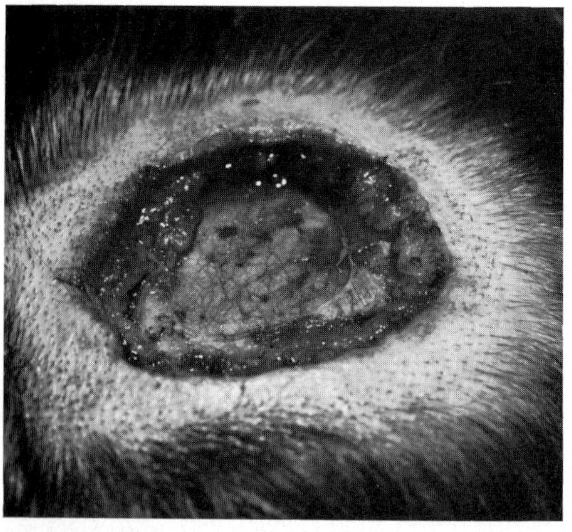

FIGURE 13–22. A woman age 56 underwent Mohs micrographic surgery for Bowen's disease of the right parietal scalp. This 60×55 mm surgical defect resulted following ablation of the lesion by three Mohs micrographic surgery stages and 33 horizontal frozen sections.

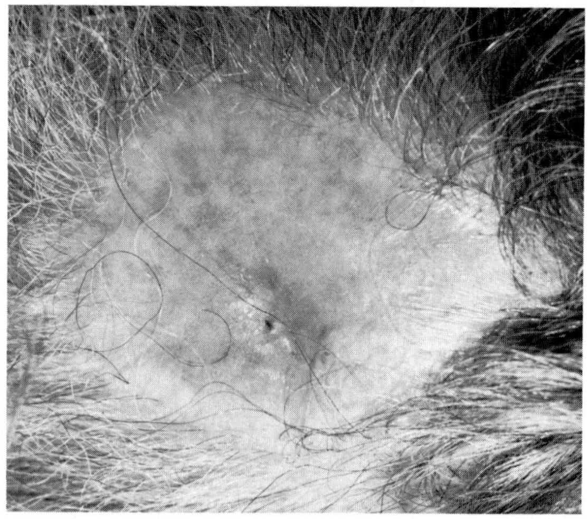

FIGURE 13–24. The wound shown in Figure 13–23 healed completely by second intention and resulted in a 50 mm area of alopecia.

Bowen's disease. Atypical dyskeratotic cells involved the full-thickness of the epidermis and the hair follicle epithelium. The lesion was treated with MMS. Three extensive stages requiring 33 horizontal frozen sections were required in order to achieve a microscopic tumor-free plane. During the procedure Bowen's disease was observed in hair follicle epithelium deep in the subcutaneous tissue (Fig. 13–21). The final surgical defect measured 60×55 mm and extended to the periosteum (Fig. 13–22). The wound was given a trial for healing by second intention, but a 12×12 mm area of bone remained exposed after 5 months. Portions of the outer table of bone were then removed with a chisel, and the area subsequently healed completely in 8 more weeks (Fig. 13–23 and 13–24), but the patient then complained of the inability to cover the 50 mm area of alopecia with the remaining hair. The scar was serially excised on 2 occasions, 6 months apart,

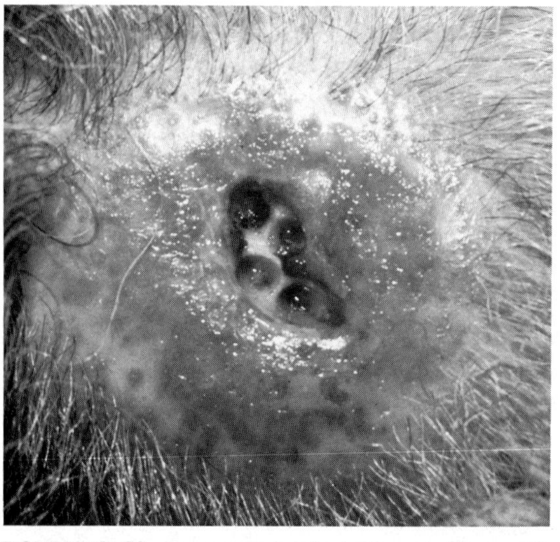

FIGURE 13–23. The surgical defect shown in Figure 13–22 healed by second intention except for a 10 mm area of exposed cranium. This photograph shows the surgical site following removal of areas of the outer table of bone with an osteotome.

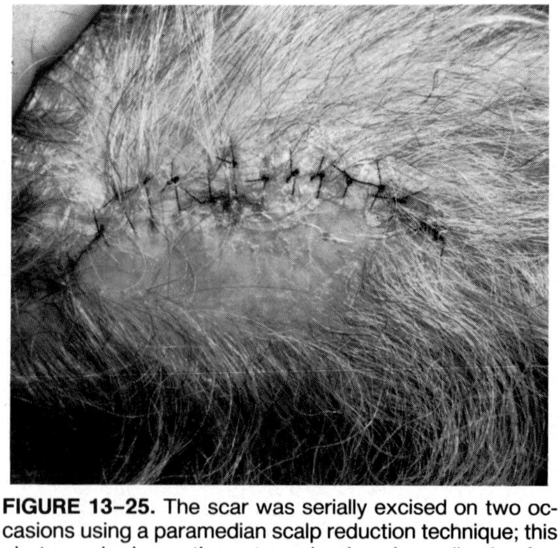

FIGURE 13–25. The scar was serially excised on two occasions using a paramedian scalp reduction technique; this photograph shows the sutures in place immediately after the first scalp reduction.

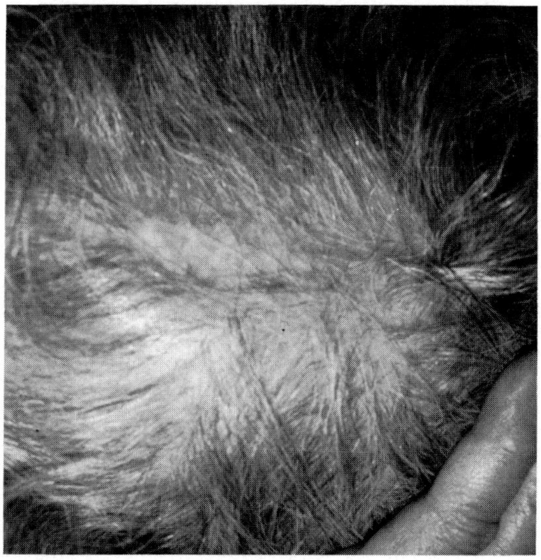

FIGURE 13–26. Following the second scalp reduction, the scar measured 5×50 mm and could be easily covered with the surrounding hairs.

using a paramedian scalp reduction technique (Fig. 13–25). This resulted in a 4×50 mm scar that the patient could easily camouflage with the remaining hair (Fig. 13–26). There has been no evidence of recurrence of Bowen's disease during follow-up.

Bowen's disease (squamous cell carcinoma in situ) occurs on sun-exposed areas in fair-skinned individuals as a result of ultraviolet radiation. It may also occur on unexposed skin as a result of inorganic arsenic ingestion.

The skin lesions of Bowen's disease are typically slowly enlarging, hairless, annular, and scaling erythematous patches or plaques. It is often difficult clinically to differentiate between Bowen's disease and bowenoid actinic keratosis, which may be similar clinically and histopathologically. Lesions of bowenoid actinic keratosis, however, are usually smaller clinically than the lesions of Bowen's disease.

Bowen's disease is a precancerous condition that progresses to invasive squamous cell carcinoma in up to 11% of cases.[25] Regional and visceral metastases may occur once invasive squamous cell carcinoma develops. The association between Bowen's disease and internal malignancy continues to be a matter of debate.

The histopathology of Bowen's disease shows acanthosis with large dyskeratotic cells involving the full-thickness of the epidermis. The stratum corneum is thickened with parakeratotic cells that have hyperchromatic nuclei. The atypical cells may involve the follicular epithelium and the sebaceous glands.[26] This deep follicular involvement probably accounts for the recurrences of Bowen's disease that are seen following superficial x-ray, curettage, cryosurgery, and topical 5-fluorouracil treatment.[27] When recurrence develops following previous treatment, a more aggressive approach utilizing MMS or standard wide surgical excision is indicated.

Mohs achieved a 97.9% 5-year cure rate in treating Bowen's disease with MMS.[28] In the patient illustrated in this report, MMS was recommended after a biopsy showed follicular involvement. The final surgical defect and subsequent reconstructions were minimized because MMS allows the maximum conservation of normal tissue.

REFERENCES

1. Robinson JK: Dermatofibrosarcoma protuberans resected by Mohs' surgery (chemosurgery). J Am Acad Dermatol 12:1093–1098, 1985.
2. Hess KA, Hanke CW, Estes NC, et al.: Chemosurgical reports: Myxoid dermatofibrosarcoma protuberans. 11:268–271, 1985.
3. Hobbs ER, Wheeland RG, Bailin PL, et al.: Treatment of dermatofibrosarcoma protuberans with Mohs micrographic surgery. Ann Surg 207:102–107, 1988.
4. Peters CW, Hanke CW, Pasarell HA, et al.: Chemosurgical reports: Dermatofibrosarcoma protuberans of the face. J Dermatol Surg Oncol 8:823–826, 1982.
5. Mikhail GR, Lynn BH: Dermatofibrosarcoma protuberans. J Dermatol Surg Oncol 4:81–84, 1978.
6. Aird I, Johnson HD, Lennon B, et al.: Epithelioma cuniculatum: A variety of squamous cell carcinoma peculiar to the foot. Br J Surg 42:245–250, 1954.
7. Brownstein MH, Shapiro L: Verrucous carcinoma of the skin: Epithelioma cuniculatum plantare. Cancer 38:1710–1716, 1976.
8. Mohs FE, Sahl WJ: Chemosurgery for verrucous carcinoma. J Dermatol Surg Oncol 5:302–306, 1979.
9. McKee PH, Wilkinson JR, Black MM, et al.: Carcinoma (epithelioma) cuniculatum: A clinico-pathological study of nineteen cases and a review of the literature. Histopathology 5:425–436, 1981.
10. Klima M, Kurtis B, Jordan PH: Verrucous carcinoma of the skin. J Cut Pathol 7:88–95, 1980.
11. Mora RG: Microscopically controlled surgery (Mohs chemosurgery) for treatment of verrucous squamous cell carcinoma of the foot. J Am Acad Dermatol 8:354–362, 1983.
12. Owen WR, Wolfe ID, Burnet JW, et al.: Epithelioma cuniculatum. South Med J 71:477–479, 1978.
13. Reingold IM, Smith BR, Graham JH: Epithelioma cuniculatum pedis a variant of squamous cell carcinoma. Am J Clin Pathol 69:561–565, 1978.
14. Kao GF, Graham JH, Helwig EB: Epithelioma cuniculatum: A preliminary clinico-pathological study. J Assoc Milit Dermatol 6:14–16, 1980.
15. Seehafer JR, Rahman D, Soderstrom CW: Epithelioma cuniculatum: Verrucous carcinoma of the foot. Cutis 23:287–290, 1979.

16. Perez CA, Kraus FT, Evans JC, et al.: Anaplastic transformation in verrucous carcinoma of the oral cavity after radiation therapy. Radiology 86:108–115, 1966.
17. Davidson LL, Frost ML, Hanke CW, et al.: Primary leiomyosarcoma of the skin. J Am Acad Dermatol 21:1156–1160, 1989.
18. Fields JP, Helwig EB: Leiomyosarcoma of the skin and subcutaneous tissue. Cancer 47:156–169, 1981.
19. Birkby CS, Argenyi ZB, Whitaker DC: Microcystic adnexal carcinoma with mandibular invasion and bone marrow replacement. J Dermatol Surg Oncol 15:308–312, 1989.
20. Fleischmann HE, Roth RJ, Wood C, et al.: Microcystic adnexal carcinoma treated by microscopically controlled excision. J Dermatol Surg Oncol 10:873–875, 1984.
21. Hamm JC, Argenta LC, Swanson NA: Microcystic adnexal carcinoma: An unpredictable aggressive neoplasm. Ann Plastic Surg 19:172–180, 1987.
22. Nickoloff BJ, Fleischmann HE, Carmel J, et al.: Microcystic adnexal carcinoma. Arch Dermatol 122:290–294, 1986.
23. Goldstein DJ, Barr RJ, Santa Cruz DJ: Microcystic adnexal carcinoma: A distinct clinicopathologic entity. Cancer 50:566–572, 1982.
24. Hanke CW, Conner AC, Temofeew RK, et al.: Merkel cell carcinoma. Arch Dermatol 125:1096–1100. 1989.
25. Graham JH, Helwig EB: Bowen's disease and its relationship to systemic cancer. Arch Dermatol 80:133–159, 1959.
26. Brownstein MH, Rabinowitz AD: The precursors of cutaneous squamous cell carcinoma. Int J Dermatol 18:1–16, 1979.
27. Mohs FE: Chemosurgery: Microscopically Controlled Surgery For Skin Cancer. Springfield, Ill.: Charles C. Thomas, 1978, p 278.
28. Mohs FE: Chemosurgery: Microscopically Controlled Surgery For Skin Cancer. Springfield, Ill.: Charles C. Thomas, 1978, p 150.

CHAPTER 14

Mohs Surgery for Melanoma

John A. Zitelli, M.D.

The treatment of melanoma is an emotional issue that often precludes rational scientific thinking, a problem that is perpetuated for many reasons. Melanoma affects people during their most productive years. A small and innocent lesion may result in metastases and eventual death. While earlier diagnosis and treatment are now possible, the incidence of melanoma is increasing, as is the death rate, fear of the disease, and increased public awareness. The literature is filled with unanswered questions and controversy over its best treatment. While some physicians stand staunch in their beliefs of the need for wide margins or elective node dissections, others are reluctant to get caught in the controversy for reasons including medicolegal fears. The treatment of melanoma has changed slowly in the past century and has lagged behind the scientific evidence that supports the better results obtained by the recent trends in management. Mohs micrographic surgery is still a "new" treatment for melanoma despite its use for decades. Based on sound scientific evidence, it offers a conservative, less disfiguring, and safe alternative to the current practice of wide excision.

HISTORY OF TREATMENT FOR MELANOMA

In order to understand the biological behavior of the tumor and rationale for treatment, it is important to review the history of melanoma. Until the last 100 years, little was known about melanoma other than the appearance of a black, enlarging, and friable nodule was an ominous sign that usually meant impending death.

The Age of Dogma

The early treatments of melanoma were not based on data, only theories supported for decades by surgical dogma. In 1820, William Norris reported the first case of melanoma in the English literature.[2] His patient had a nodular melanoma that was treated by simple excision, but the tumor soon recurred in the surgical scar. He later reported a patient whose melanoma was treated by wide excision and was alive 8 years later. Norris attributed this prolonged survival to wide excision and was the first to advocate wide excision of normal tissue in the treatment of melanoma.

It is W. Sampson Handley,[3] however, who is generally given credit for establishing the rationale for wide excision. In 1907, he published his observations of the route of spread of tumor deposits around a metastatic nodule overlying the inguinal lymph nodes in a patient with a primary melanoma on the ankle. He saw visible nodules in the subcutaneous tissue and muscle that extended widely around the metastatic nodule of the skin (Fig. 14–1). He then suggested that it was necessary to "cut a circular incision . . . through the skin about an inch from the edge of the tumor to expose the subcutaneous fat. The skin (should now be) separated from the deep fascia to be dissected from

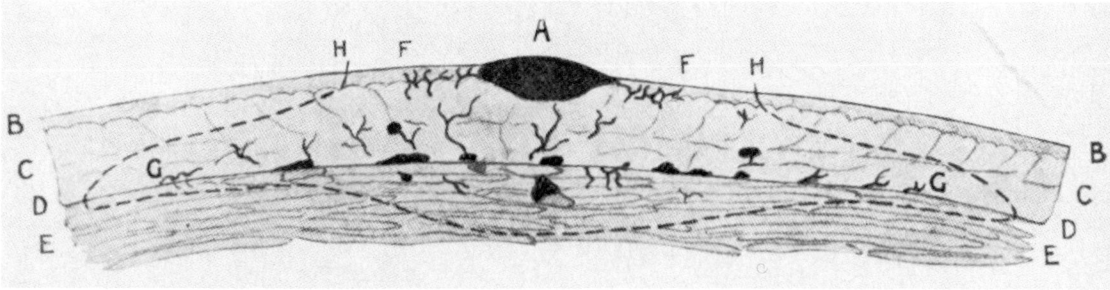

FIGURE 14–1. Distribution of tumor deposits around a cutaneous metastasis. From this, Handley deduced that wide excision should be necessary to treat melanoma, an idea refuted decades later. From Handley WS: The pathology of melanocytic growths in relation to their operative treatment. *Lancet* 1:927–933 and 996–1003, 1907. Copyright 1907, Little Brown and Company.

the muscles. Finally, the whole mass with the growth at its center is removed."

Although Handley's recommendation for wide excision was based on a faulty extrapolation of data from a metastatic lesion, it became surgical dogma for decades to come. This may be in part because it was published at a time when surgical thinking was fertile for the recommendation of wide excision. William Halsted's radial mastectomy was becoming popular, Miles had proposed the abdominal-perineal resection for rectal carcinoma, and Basset was using radial vulvectomy for vulvar carcinoma, all with apparent success. So the idea of wide excision was readily adopted.

Over the next three decades, it was recognized that some patients survived whose melanomas were excised with very wide margins, apparently further supporting radical excision. However, others continued to succumb to metastatic disease after excision, and the drive for super-radical surgery continued. George Pack popularized super-radical procedures such as hemipelvectomy and interscapular thoracic amputation. Still, patients died from melanoma despite these heroic and mutilating procedures. By 1963, Haagenson expressed the feelings of many other surgeons when he said, "we have reached the limits of the radical attack on cancer, and we are beginning to restrict its use."[4]

During this time of radical surgery, there was little scientific evidence to support its use. Most support came from studies showing an improved survival compared to historical controls, but there was no recognition that thin tumors had a better prognosis, so that fair comparisons as we know them were impossible. In 1965, Mundth reported that melanomas excised with narrow margins often left residual tumor behind.[5] In 55 patients whose melanomas were initially excised with narrow margins, 20 patients (36%) showed residual tumor in the re-excision specimen. Unfortunately, neither the size or depth of the lesion nor the stage of disease was reported.

Other apparent support for wide excision came from independent studies by Wong[6] and Cochran,[7] who found atypical melanocytes in the epidermis surrounding melanomas at a distance up to 5 cm from the tumor's visible margin. Some of these melanocytes were cytologically bizarre, and they felt these cells should be excised with the melanoma. However, Cochran and later others also showed an increase in the number of atypical melanocytes in benign nevi, other epidermal tumors, and dermatitis, refuting the importance of Wong's and Cochran's initial conclusions.

The most compelling support for wide excision was the observation of local satellites, or in-transit metastases around the melanoma excision sites. The desire that wider excision could include these local tumor deposits and therefore prevent recurrence was overwhelming. This rationale assumes that, as melanoma invades, there is a point in time when the tumor disseminates locally before systemic involvement occurs.[3,8] This assumption is false, as pointed out later by others.

The Age of Reason

Only in the last 25 years have we begun to critically evaluate the biological behavior, prognostic features, and rationale for the treatment of melanoma. The work of Clark,[9–11] Breslow[12] and others[13–15] has allowed us to make earlier and more accurate diagnoses and to compare patient groups with similar prognoses in order to test theories on biological behavior and treatment.

A surprising finding that led to a better understanding of the biological behavior of melanoma was reported in 1966 by Grete Olsen,[16] who found that surgical margins did not affect the survival of patients with melanoma. In a study of 456 patients with Stage I melanoma, there was no significant difference between the survival or recurrence rate in the group excised with margins less than 5 mm and the group with margins greater than 5 cm. Likewise, she found that lymph node metastases were no more common in patients with narrow margins than wide-margin excisions.

Her findings were important for they refuted the theory that there exists a time when melanoma spreads locally, a few centimeters from the main tumor, before it spreads to more distant sites or systemically. Instead, her findings confirm that once tumor cells break away from the main tumor mass, wider margins to include these local deposits are not successful.

Olsen's findings were not easy to accept, but every study since that time has similarly concluded that survival is unrelated to the surgical margin. Breslow and Macht[17] studied 62 thin melanomas (less than 0.76 mm) excised with margins that varied from 1 mm to 5 cm. All patients were alive and none had recurrence at 5 years. Well-known leaders in melanoma research and surgery such as Bagley,[18] Balch,[19] Cascinelli,[20] Day,[21,22] Elder,[23] Schmoeckel,[24] and Veronesi[25] as well as the World Health Organization multicenter studies[25] have examined the same question and have come to the same conclusion that survival is unrelated to surgical margins.

An important corollary to this concept, however, is that very narrow margins (less than 1.5 cm) may result in a higher local recurrence rate due to melanoma in the radial growth phase that was not visible to the surgeon's eye.[20,22,24-28] Recurrence of radial growth phase melanoma, if noted early, may not have competence for metastasis. While recurrence may not affect survival if re-excised promptly, it supports the concept that tumor may extend beyond the clinical margins in the radial growth phase and emphasizes the need to include some margin of normal-appearing skin during standard melanoma surgery. Thus, the goal of surgery for melanoma is to remove the main mass of tumor including the contiguous subclinical extensions. There is no benefit to undertake more extensive surgery hoping to remove invisible satellite lesions.

MOHS MICROGRAPHIC SURGERY FOR MELANOMA

Rationale

For Mohs micrographic surgery to be effective in the treatment of melanoma, two criteria must be fulfilled. First, the treatable components of the tumor must be in continuity. Second, the tumor cells must be distinguishable by the light microscopy (usually frozen sections) from those of normal tissue.

The first criterion—that surgically curable melanoma grows in a contiguous fashion—is supported by the finding that surgical margins do not influence survival. This means that any tumor outside the main mass of tumor is not amenable to surgical excision, since wide excision that would include noncontiguous satellites does not improve survival. On the other hand, narrow margins may result in local recurrences in radial growth phase melanoma when neoplastic cells are contiguous with the main tumor mass. Although Mohs surgery may not offer better survival than standard surgical excision, it does allow excision with narrower margins without increasing total recurrences.

The second criterion that melanoma cells must be visible by light microscopy is supported both by research and clinical experience. Multiple studies have established the accuracy for diagnosis of melanoma by frozen sections at the 95% to 99% level[29-32] and that the identification at the surgical margins of a previously undiagnosed unkown tumor is more difficult than the detection of a histologically known tumor. In a study of frozen sections for the evaluation of surgical margins, frozen section specimens from melanoma treated by Mohs surgery were compared to paraffin sections of the same specimens.[33] It was demonstrated that frozen sections were 100% sensitive for detecting melanomas. In this study, 221 specimens from 59 patients were examined by routine Mohs micrographic frozen section techniques. The same specimens were then blindly interpreted after paraffin sections by another investigator. The results of comparing the interpretations showed that when melanoma was present at the margin, it was always detected in the frozen sections (100% sensitivity). Frozen sections, on the other hand, over-read melanoma in 10% of the specimens (90% specificity), although this never influenced the final cosmetic or functional result. Furthermore, frozen sections were reliable in finding both intraepidermal as well as deep dermal deposits of tumor. Of the specimens positive for melanoma at the margin, 80% were present in the epidermis. Only 20% of the positive margins were found in the deep margin, and these were almost exclusively in recurrent melanomas or neurotropic, desmoplastic melanomas. As previously emphasized, the evaluation of frozen sections for tumor margins of a known melanoma is a simpler task than performing frozen sections for diagnosis of an unknown disease.

Further support for the ability to see melanoma by frozen sections are the reports of Mohs surgery that document a success rate at least as good as wide excision as well as a low local recurrence rate, thus demonstrating the efficacy of the technique.[33–41]

Techniques

Both fresh and fixed tissue techniques have been used for melanoma with success. Mohs prefers the fixed tissue technique for thicker melanomas because of the presumed security in the event the tumor is transected. Zitelli prefers the fresh-tissue technique because of the superior quality of frozen sections and the ability for immediate reconstruction. With either method, there are some important differences between treating melanoma and treating other neoplasms. First, any sign of regression of melanoma must be excised in order to assure complete removal of all contiguous elements of the tumor. This requires excision of areas with dermal melanophages, dermal fibrosis, and any lymphohistiocytic infiltrate as if they contain melanoma. Fortunately, regression at the surgical margin is a rare event.

The second difference is less emphasis on extreme conservation of tissue. While the surgical margins for basal cell carcinoma are 1 to 2 mm or less, they are usually wider for melanoma. For fresh tissue surgery, the tumor is debulked with a 3-mm margin of normal tissue before taking the first layer for delineation of margins. Thus, the minimum margin is usually 6 mm. Similarly, for the fixed tissue technique, wider margins are excised initially, then after a tumor-free plane is reached, a final thin layer of fixative is applied to sterilize the field from tumor cells and to remove an additional margin for safety. Both alterations still provide a more conservative excision than the standard wide surgical margin (Figs. 14–2 and 14–3).

The detection of melanoma by frozen sections of either fresh tissue or fixed tissue is not as difficult as some physicians imagine (Fig. 14–4). The fresh tissue sections minimize the contrast between melanocytes and keratinocytes, while the zinc chloride–fixed tissue produces artifacts. In either fresh or fixed tissue method, one looks for nests or groups of atypical melanocytes, or areas of marked melanocytic hyperplasia. An isolated atypical melanocyte does not require re-excision. A lymphocytic infiltrate beneath the epidermis is often a clue to the presence of melanoma within the epidermis.

Difficulties may be encountered in identifying melanoma in severely sun-damaged skin because atypical keratinocytes and loss of normal epidermal architecture may simulate in situ melanoma.[42] In this case, review of multiple serial frozen sections usually results in correct interpretation. If difficulties persist, an additional tissue layer may be excised and examined, or the tissue in question may be submitted for paraffin sections.

Difficulties are also encountered interpreting frozen sections of melanoma in the mucous membranes of the conjunctiva and the nose. Again, the use of formalin-fixed paraffin-embedded techniques may be helpful if frozen sections are difficult to interpret.

In any case, the detection of melanoma by frozen sections is reliable and no more difficult than the interpretation of tumors where Mohs surgery is useful, such as Bowen's disease,[43] extramammary Paget's disease,[44] or dermatofibrosarcoma protuberans.[45]

Results

Although many studies support the theory that Mohs surgery would be useful for melanoma, the long-term results of Mohs surgery prove its efficacy and value. The majority of published data have been authored by Mohs,[34–41] although the initial published data by Zitelli concur with those findings.[33] Mohs reported his first results of treating melanoma in a study of 20 patients,[37] 10 of whom had metastatic disease at the time of treatment and 12 of whom had previous treatment. After 5 years, seven (35%) were still alive without disease. Although

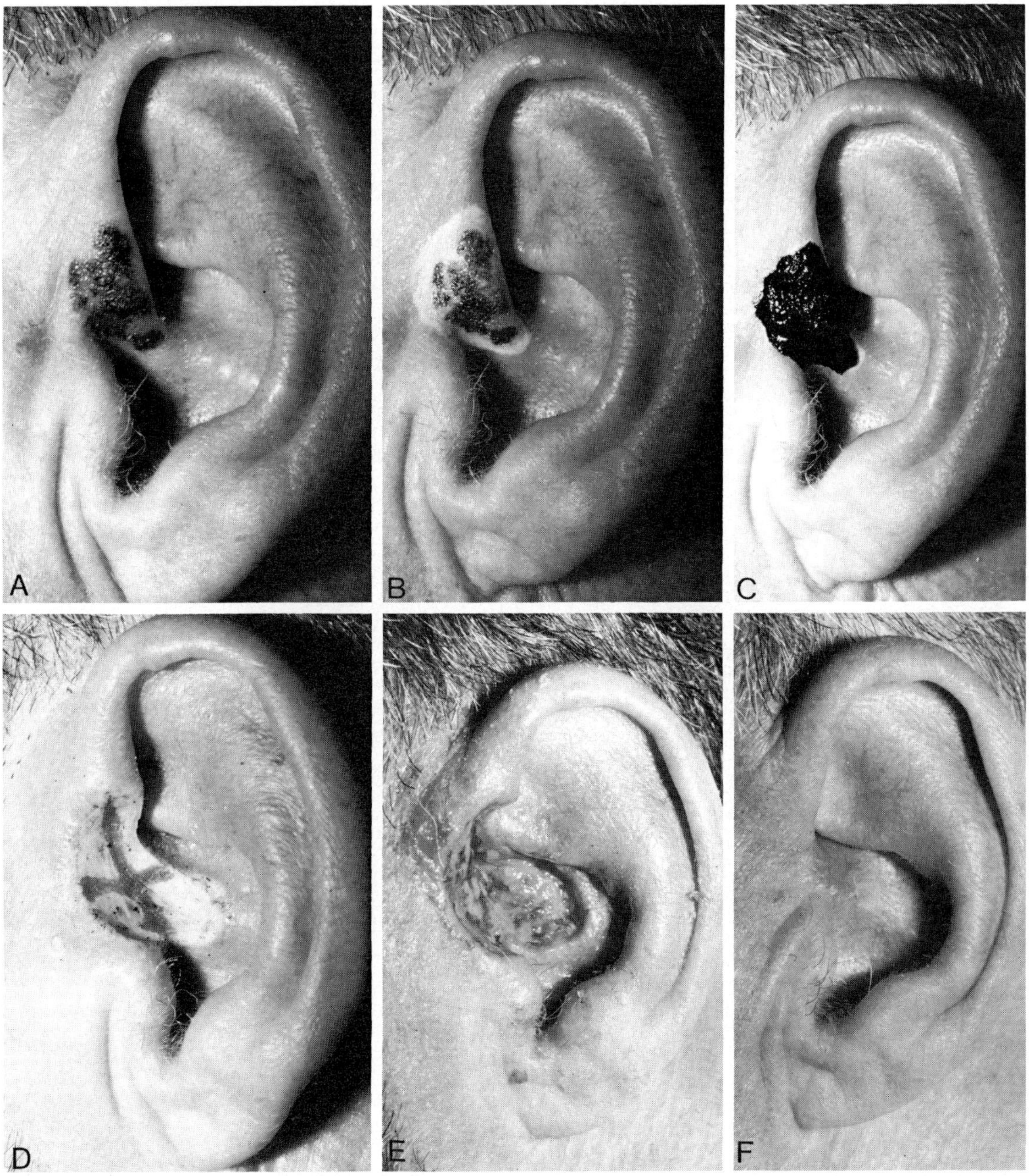

FIGURE 14–2. Fixed tissue technique for melanoma: *A*, Preoperative appearance of melanoma on the ear. *B*, Application of dichloracetic acid to enhance penetration of fixative. *C*, Application of zinc chloride paste to melanoma and narrow margin of normal skin. *D*, Excision of specimens through fixed tissue. *E*, Wound after separation of fixed tissue. *F*, Result about 1 year later; no evidence of disease 5 years later. (Courtesy of Frederic E. Mohs, M.D.)

Clark's level and Breslow's thickness had not yet been described to estimate prognosis, Mohs' report was encouraging because many of his patients had thick or recurrent lesions. Furthermore other published cure rates for melanoma at that time ranged from 2% to 38%.

In his report, Mohs mentioned the modification of the usual fixed tissue technique of other tumors that he used for the treatment of melanomas. This included the excision of an additional margin of tissue up to 2 cm wide after the melanoma was excised. He began this practice after his first patient developed satel-

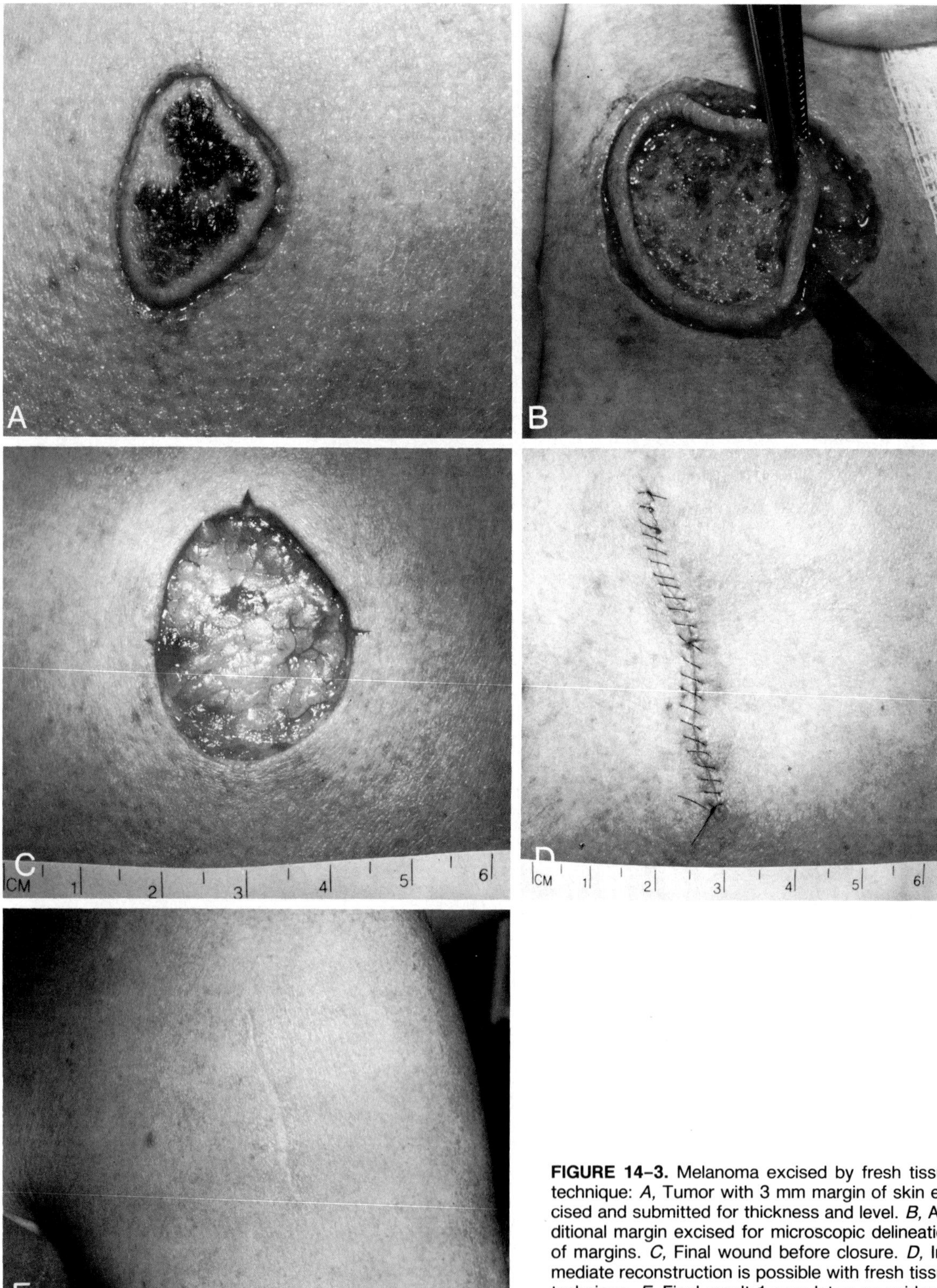

FIGURE 14–3. Melanoma excised by fresh tissue technique: *A,* Tumor with 3 mm margin of skin excised and submitted for thickness and level. *B,* Additional margin excised for microscopic delineation of margins. *C,* Final wound before closure. *D,* Immediate reconstruction is possible with fresh tissue technique. *E,* Final result 1 year later; no evidence of disease 5 years later.

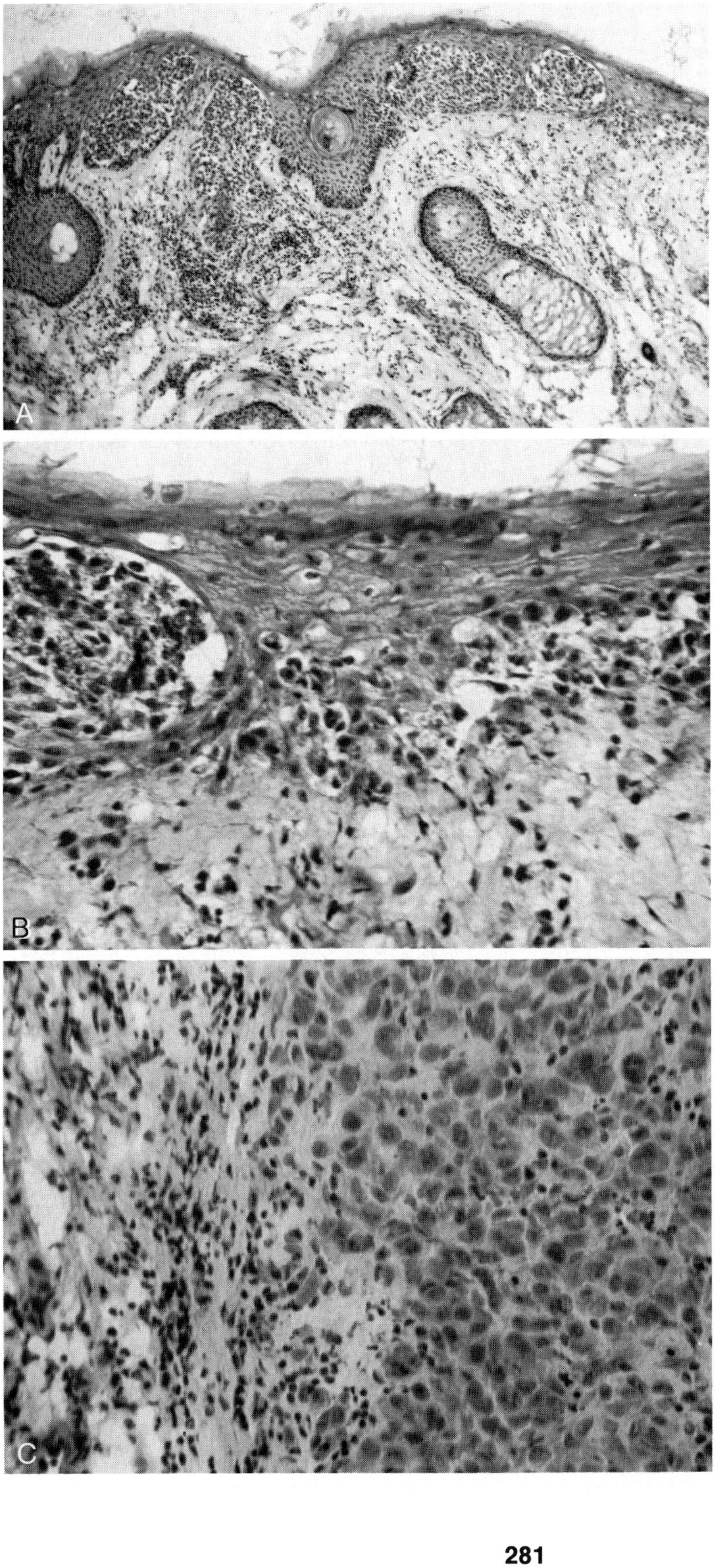

FIGURE 14–4. Melanoma histology by frozen section. *A,* Low-power view of melanoma in situ with nests and aggregates of tumor within the epidermis. *B,* High-power view. *C,* Tumor nest detected in a deep margin of a recurrent melanoma. (From Zitelli JA, Mohs FE, Larson P, Snow S: Mohs micrographic surgery for melanomas. *Dermatology Clinics* 7:833–843, 1989. Copyright 1989, W.B. Saunders, with permission.)

lites within 2 cm of the wound, shortly after treatment. Mohs excised the satellites by micrographic surgery and thereafter recommended taking an additional margin after the tumor was excised in order to include any possible invisible satellites. Later reports by others documented the futility of wider margins to remove "visible" satellites in the hope of achieving better results,[16–25] and Mohs has gradually reduced the margin of the additional normal tissue especially in areas where vital structures sit close to the wound.

In 1956, Mohs updated his statistics, reporting 31 patients with a 50% 5-year cure rate, including the same single local recurrence of his original report.[35] By 1977, Clark had defined levels of invasion, and Mohs reported 103 patients stratified according to Clark's levels.[38] He compared his results with historical controls treated by wide excision for each level. He showed that Mohs surgery (fixed tissue technique) surpassed the results of standard surgery for each Clark's level (50% 5-year cure rate, and 3% local recurrence rate for Mohs surgery). Mohs' most recent updated statistics include 200 consecutive patients with a minimum 5-year follow-up and a 65.2% cure rate for all Clark's levels combined (Table 14–1).[33]

In other reports, Mohs emphasized the tissue-sparing advantage of Mohs surgery for melanoma and treating tumors of the periorbital area[40] and ear[36] and for melanomas in patients with dysplastic nevus syndrome.[39] Each report documents that Mohs surgery conserves tissue and minimizes the disfigurement of wide excision while still offering the highest survival rate and a low local recurrence rate.

The fresh tissue technique for melanoma was adopted after confirmation that fixed tissue surgery was both safe and effective. The concern about cutting through viable melanoma and spreading tumor cells through the wound and into the circulation was minimized by the findings of several investigators that incisional biopsies of melanoma did not increase the chance of metastases.[46] Further support followed the documentation that standard surgical excisions with narrow margins did not decrease survival, which has dispelled the fear that disturbing invisible satellites might increase the risk of metastasis.

Mohs first reported the use of fresh tissue surgery for certain periorbital melanomas in 1985[40] and later in 1988 for thin melanomas in other areas.[36] Zitelli presented his 6 years of data on fresh tissue surgery for melanoma at the American College of Chemosurgery annual meeting in 1986. He emphasized that the difference between treating melanoma and basal cell carcinoma was less conservation of tissue in the former, usually taking a 6 mm minimum margin. The most recent data on 200 consecutive patients treated from 1980 to 1988 are shown in Table 14–2. The patients are stratified according to Breslow's thicknesses and compared to historical controls from the same time period and similar geographic areas.[33]

Zitelli also documented the tissue-sparing advantage of Mohs surgery. In a study of 200 patients with melanoma, the subclinical microscopic extension of melanoma was measured from the visible margin. Microscopic evidence of melanoma was found to extend in the epidermis up to 1.5 cm from the visible margin (in tumors less than 4 cm in diameter). However, most tumors (80%) had microscopic extensions of 6 mm or less.[33] Thus, if standard surgical excision is to include visible as well as invisible

TABLE 14–1. Effect of Level of Invasion on 5-Year Results of Melanoma Treated by Fixed Tissue Micrographic Surgery

Level *(Clark)*	Total Number*	Indeterminate Cases†	Total	Cure Rate	
				Successful Cases	*Percent*
II	45	9	36	32	89
III	45	11	34	30	88
IV	42	15	27	17	63
V	68‡	10	58	22	38
ALL	200	45	155	101	65.2

*Series of consecutive patients with Stage I melanomas.
†Patients without evidence of melanoma when they died or lost to follow-up before 5 years.
‡Note the unusually high proportion of deep melanomas.
From Zitelli JA, Mohs FE, Larson P, Snow S: Mohs micrographic surgery for melanoma, *Dermatology Clinics* 7:833–843, 1989. Copyright 1989, W. B. Saunders Co., with permission.

TABLE 14–2. Effect of Tumor Thickness on Survival of Patients with Melanoma Treated by the Fresh Tissue Technique

	2½-Year Follow-up			5-Year Follow-up		
Tumor Thickness	*No. of Patients*	*Expected Deaths**	*Actual Deaths*	*No. of Patients*	*Expected Deaths**	*Actual Deaths*
In situ	12	–	–	6	–	0
<0.85	38	0.38	0	10	0.10	0
0.86–1.6	11	0.33	1	4	0.24	1
1.70–3.64	12	1.44	0	4	0.96	0
>3.64	4	1.72	0	2	1.08	0
	77†	3.87	1	26‡	2.38	1

*Determined by life-table analysis of 98 clinical stage I patients from the Massachusetts General Hospital and New York University Medical Center[57]

†Out of 95 patients, 77 were determinate.

‡Out of 36 patients, 26 were determinate.

From Zitelli JA, Mohs FE, Larson P, Snow S: Mohs micrographic surgery for melanoma, *Dermatology Clinics* 7:833–843, 1989. Copyright 1989, W. B. Saunders Co., with permission.

contiguous tumor in all cases, a margin of 1.5 cm is necessary. On the other hand, since Mohs surgery conserves normal skin, 80% of melanomas can be excised with a margin of 6 mm of normal skin, preserving 1.8 cm (9 mm on each side).

Furthermore, this study showed that deeply invasive melanomas do not extend more widely beyond the margins than thin melanomas, thus refuting the common practice of excising wider margins for thicker melanomas. This study also showed that the subclinical extension was not different for melanomas in any location or for melanomas of different sizes (less than 4 cm in diameter).

The results of fresh tissue surgery, like those of fixed tissue surgery, confirm that Mohs surgery offers a survival and recurrence rate as good as wide excision but conserves significantly more skin.

Indications

Because of the microscopic control and tissue-sparing advantages of Mohs surgery, the technique is useful in managing many routine and difficult melanomas. The microscopic control offers particular advantage in treating melanomas with poorly defined clinical margins, such as lentigo maligna, lentigo maligna melanoma, and amelanotic melanoma. The clinical margins of subungual and mucosal melanomas are often indistinct, and microscopic control is useful for detecting the true margins of the tumor. In addition, desmoplastic melanomas often have wide subclinical microscopic extensions with perineural invasion that can be traced and excised with Mohs surgery (Fig. 14–5).

The tissue-sparing ability of Mohs surgery results in significantly less disfigurement than the excision of wider margins required by standard surgical procedures intended to minimize recurrences. This conservation of tissue is important on the head and neck, particularly around the eyes, nose, and lips as well as for melanomas on the hands, feet and genitalia. In these areas, Mohs surgery can often safely remove the melanoma without the need for amputation, loss of function or disfigurement (Fig. 14–6).

MANAGEMENT OF THE PATIENT WITH MELANOMA

The Mohs surgeon who treats patients with melanoma must also understand the broader picture of patient management. The patient referred for evaluation of an undiagnosed melanoma or who has had a biopsy first requires a complete evaluation and a significant amount of time to discuss the diagnosis and the treatment. A diagnosis is best made by an excisional biopsy if possible, although an incisional biopsy will not increase the risk of metastases if it must be done.[46] A deep saucerization excision biopsy can provide a good specimen since the experienced surgeon can accurately estimate the tumor thickness well enough to excise below the deepest portion of the tumor. The

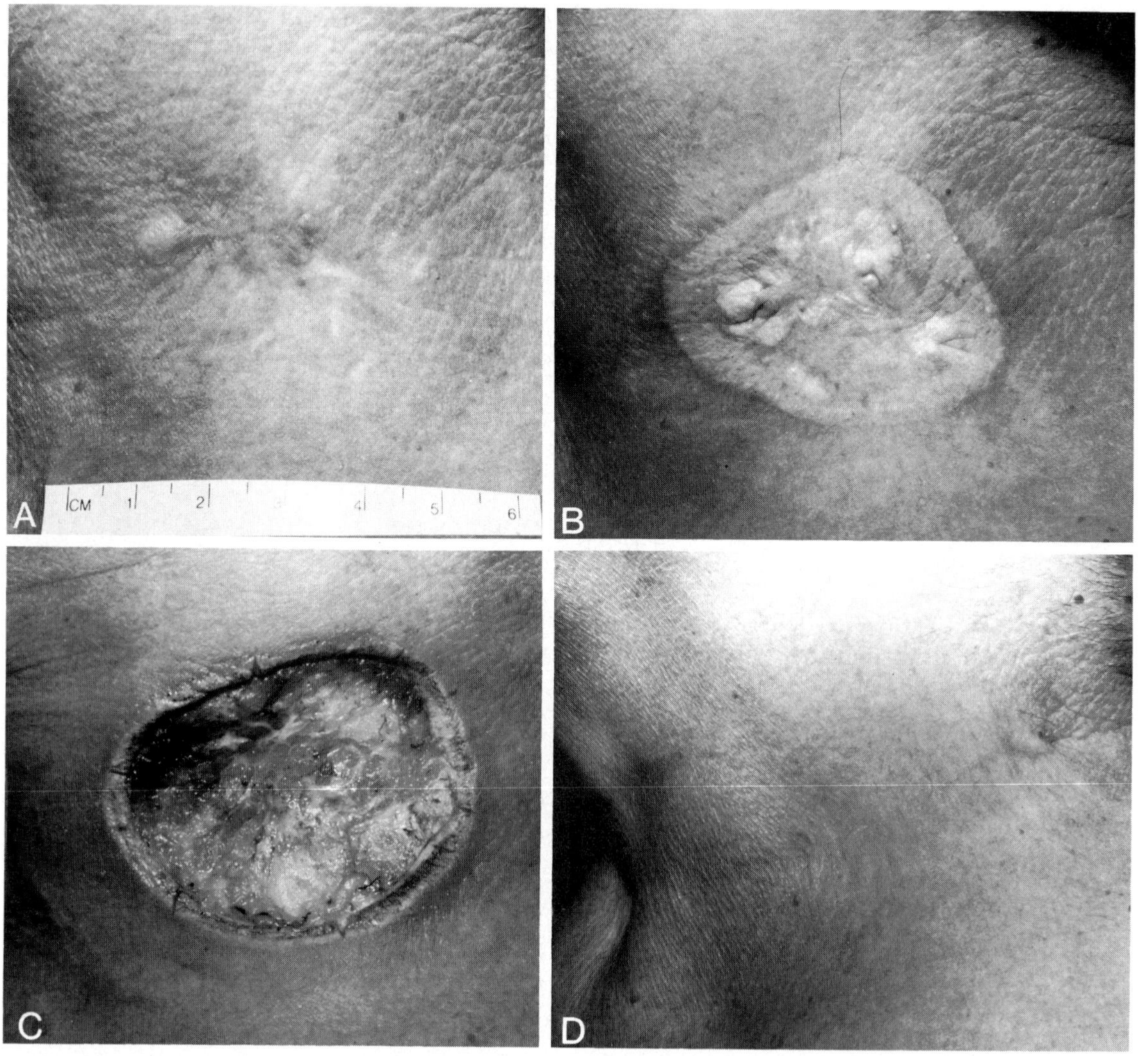

FIGURE 14–5. Mohs surgery for poorly defined melanoma: *A,* Recurrent amelanotic, desmoplastic melanoma. *B,* Application of dichloracetic acid. *C,* Tumor-free wound after fixed tissue Mohs surgery. *D,* Appearance of scar 1 year after healing by second degree intention; no evidence of disease 6 years later.

specimen is then sent for diagnosis and determination of Breslow's thickness and Clark's levels.

Once a diagnosis is made, a thorough history and physical exam is performed. The history should include both the patient's and family's history of melanoma, dysplastic nevi, or congenital nevi, and the physical exam should include a careful evaluation of lymph nodes and other skin lesions. Any signs or symptoms suggestive of metastatic disease should be further evaluated. The necessary work-up is dictated by the unfortunate fact that there is no effective treatment for most asymptomatic metastatic disease. For the asymptomatic patient, one looks only for surgically correctable disease, i.e., metastases to the lymph nodes, lung, or liver. A chest x-ray is most effective in serching for isolated, surgically correctable lung metastases.[47] A lactate dehydrogenase (LDH) level is helpful in the search for liver metastases.[48] On the initial visit, patients are also instructed in self-examination and palpation for enlarged lymph nodes.

After the initial visit, follow-up visits are scheduled to identify symptomatic or surgically correctable disease. The frequency of follow-up visits usually depends on the prognostic factors, particularly tumor thickness. Thin melanomas (less than 0.76 mm) are unlikely to

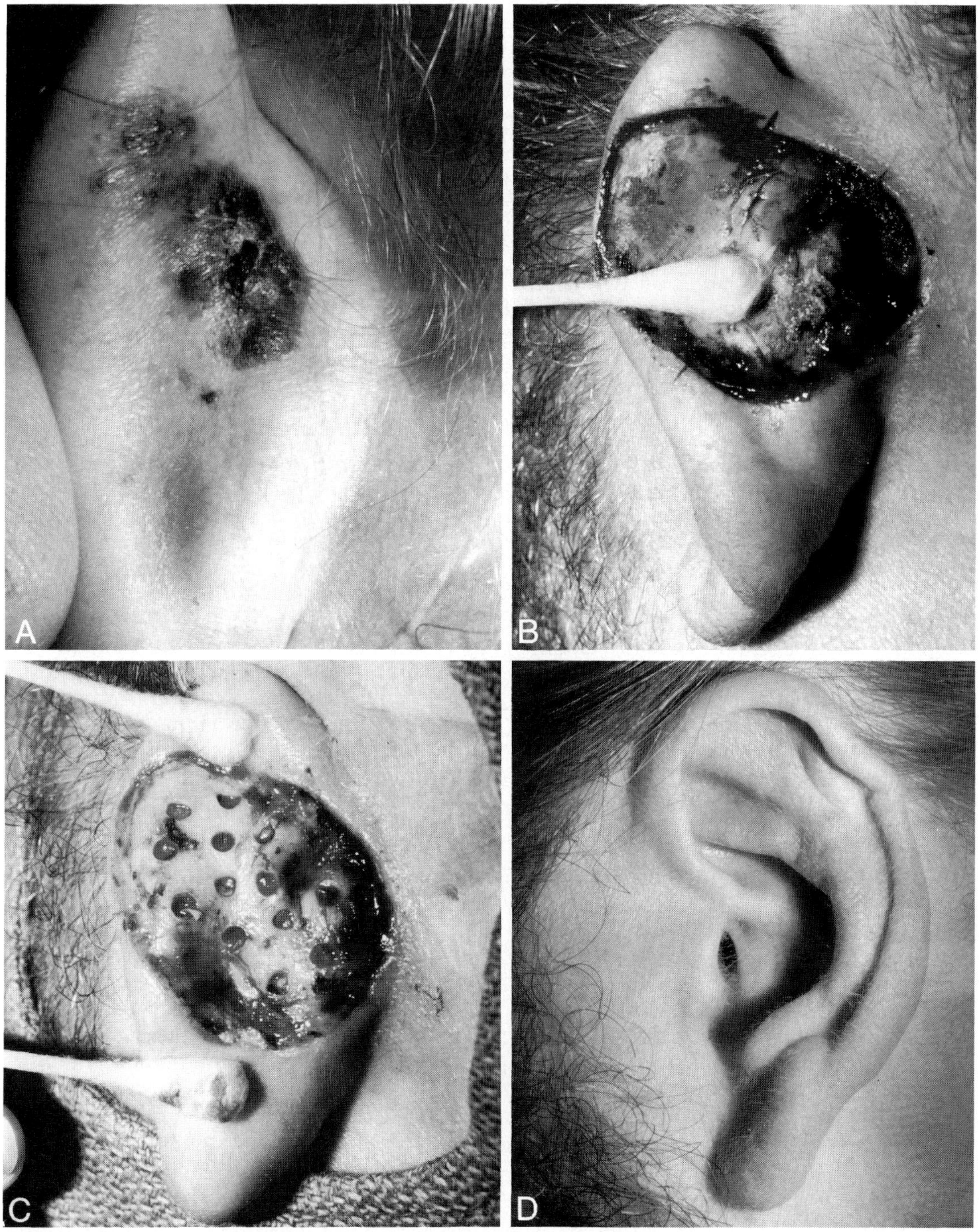

FIGURE 14–6. Mohs surgery to conserve tissue: *A,* Melanoma on posterior surface of the ear with satellites. *B,* Wound appearance after excision by the fresh tissue technique. *C,* Fenestration of the cartilage to enhance healing by second intention. *D,* Appearance of the ear 1 year after surgery; no evidence of disease after 5 years of follow-up.

metastasize, and follow-up visits are scheduled every 6 months. Patients with thick melanomas (greater than 3.5 mm) which are more likely to metastasize are seen every 2 to 3 months. Patients with intermediate thickness melanomas are seen every 3 to 4 months.

The duration of follow-up is indefinite but should be for at least 10 years. Data from New York University show that deaths from thin melanomas occur later than for thicker melanomas.[49] The time of peak incidence of death for thin melanomas (less than 0.76 mm) is 6 years and trails off to low values by 10 years. The peak incidence of death for thicker melanomas (greater than 3.0 mm), however, is between 3 and 4 years after diagnosis but also trails off at 10 years. Thus, patients with melanoma cannot be labeled as a cure by 5 years of follow-up. During the follow-up period, the office visit consists of a complete exam looking especially for signs of local recurrence, in-transit metastic nodules, and palpation of lymph nodes. Once each year, a chest x-ray and LDH level are repeated and further investigated if abnormal.

The controversy over elective versus therapeutic lymph node dissection remains unanswered. Most surgeons agree that there is no benefit of elective node dissection for patients with thin melanomas, or very thick melanomas. Two prospective studies addressing the issue have shown no benefit for any patient.[50,51] However, less well-controlled studies have shown some benefit for patients with intermediate thickness melanomas with well-defined lymph node drainage patterns.[52] There is no standard of care for clinically negative nodes, and the answer to the controversy will only come after the larger prospective studies already begun are completed.

The treatment of metastatic disease is discouraging. The treatment of local and regional recurrences is worthwhile and associated with a slightly improved survival than without treatment.[53] Satellite lesions and in-transit metastases can be excised successfully with Mohs surgery, as reported by Mohs using the fixed tissue technique.[54] Therapeutic dissection of clinically involved nodes is the standard of care in the absence of more widespread disease. Local perfusion chemotherapy to limbs with regional disease has shown promising results.[55] It consists of surgical isolation of the limb and perfusion with heated chemotherapeutic drugs. Treatment of asymptomatic patients with widespread or surgically incorrectable disease is not necessary unless the patients are entered into a protocol to gather information about the efficacy of new treatments. Symptomatic patients, however, may benefit from radiation therapy and some forms of chemotherapy.

CONCLUSION

Mohs micrographic surgery has significant advantages in the management of patients with melanoma. It has been shown to be safe and effective and allows conservation of tissue compared with the standard surgical practice of wide excision which requires at least a 1.5 cm margin. This conservation of tissue is especially important for melanomas on the head and neck, hands, feet, and genitalia. Mohs surgery is also useful for treating melanomas with poorly defined margins, such as amelanotic melanomas, lentigo maligna, subungual melanoma, and desmoplastic melanoma.

The technical aspects of treating melanoma differ slightly from treating other tumors. Less emphasis is placed on extreme conservation of tissue in melanoma, but technical preparation of slides is more critical. Slides must be thin (4 to 6 microns) and stained with hematoxylin and eosin rather than toluidine blue. With experience, the ability to identify melanoma is no more difficult than identifying other tumors treated by Mohs surgery, such as Bowen's disease, extramammary Paget's disease, or dermatofibrosarcoma protuberans.

As surgical margins for melanoma decrease with standard surgery, the importance of margin examination increases in order to insure complete removal. The most reliable method for examining margins is Mohs surgery because it examines 100% of the margins as compared with the less than 1% usually examined by standard histologic techniques.[56] Since frozen sections are reliable for margin exam, it is certainly better to look at the entire margin, rather than a small sample, and Mohs surgery achieves that goal.

We now have long-term results from large numbers of patients, confirmed by multiple investigators to support the concept that Mohs surgery plays an important role in the treatment of melanoma.

REFERENCES

1. Lee JAH: Melanoma. In Schottenfeld D, Fraumeni JF Jr (eds): Cancer Epidemiology and Prevention. Philadelphia: WB Saunders, 1982, pp 984–995.

2. Davis NC: William Norris, a pioneer of melanomas, Med J Aust 1:52–54, 1980.
3. Handley WS: The pathology of melanocytic growths in relation to their operative treatment, Lancet, Lecture 1 1:927–933, 1907.
4. Haagenson CD: Advances in the treatment of cancer, Practitioner 191:437–481, 1963.
5. Mundth ED, Guralnick EA, Raker JW: Malignant melanoma—a clinical study of 427 cases, Ann Surg 162:15–28, 1965.
6. Wong CK: A study of melanocytes in the normal skin surrounding malignant melanomata, Dermatologica 141:215–225, 1970.
7. Cochran AA: Studies of the melanocytes of the epidermis adjacent to tumors, J Invest Dermatol 57:38–43, 1971.
8. Scanlon EF: The process of metastasis, Cancer 55:1163–1166, 1985.
9. Clark WH:A classification of malignant melanoma in man correlated with histogenesis and biologic behavior. In Montagna W, Hu F (eds): Advances in the Biology of Skin. New York: Pergamon Press, 1966, pp 621–647.
10. Clark WH, From L, Bernardino EA, Mihm ML: The histogenesis and biologic behavior of primary human malignant melanomas of the skin, Cancer Research 29:705–726, 1969.
11. Clark WH, Ainsworth AM, Bernardino EA, et al.: The developmental biology of primary human malignant melanomas, Semin Oncol 2:83–103, 1975.
12. Breslow A: Thickness, cross-sectional area, and depth of invasion in the prognosis of cutaneous melanoma, Ann Surg 172:902–908, 1970.
13. Mihm MC, Clark WH, Reed RJ: The clinical diagnosis of malignant melanoma, Semin Oncol 2:105–118, 1975.
14. McGovern VJ: The classification of melanoma and its relationship with prognosis, Pathology 1:85–98, 1970.
15. Price NM, Rywlin AM, Ackerman AB: Histologic criteria for the diagnosis of superficial spreading malignant melanoma, Cancer 38:2434–2441, 1976.
16. Olsen G: The malignant melanoma of the skin—new theories based on a study of 500 cases, Acta Chir Scan (Suppl) 365:1–220, 1966.
17. Breslow A, Macht SD: Optimal size of resection margin for thin cutaneous melanoma, Surg Gynecol Obstet 145:691–692, 1977.
18. Bagley FH, Caddy B, Lee A, Legg MA: Changes in clinical presentation and management of malignant melanoma, Cancer 47:2126–2134, 1981.
19. Balch CM, Murad TM, Soong SJ, et al.: Tumor thickness as a guide to surgical management of clinical stage I melanoma patients, Cancer 43:883–888, 1979.
20. Cascinelli N, Vander Esch EP, Breslow A, et al.: Stage I melanoma of the skin: The problem of resection margins, Europ J Cancer 16:1079–1085, 1980.
21. Day CL, Mihm ML, Suber AJ, et al.: Narrower margins for clinical stage I malignant melanoma, N Engl J Med 306:479–481, 1982.
22. Day CL, Lew RA: Malignant melanoma prognostic factors 3: Surgical margins, J Dermatol Surg Oncol 9:797–801, 1983.
23. Elder DE, Gverry D, Heiberger RM, et al.: Optimal resection margin for cutaneous malignant melanoma, Plast Reconstr Surg 71:66–72, 1983.
24. Schmoeckel C, Bockelbrink A, Bockelbrink H, et al.: Low and high risk malignant melanoma—III, prognostic significance of the resection margin, Eur J Cancer Clin Oncol 19:245–249, 1983.
25. Veronesi V, Cascinelli N, Adamus J, et al.: Thin stage I primary cutaneous malignant melanoma, N Engl J Med 318:1159–1162, 1988.
26. Zeitels J, LaRossa D, Hamilton R, et al.: A comparison of local recurrence and resection margins for stage I primary cutaneous malignant melanomas, Plast Reconstr Surg 81:688–693, 1988.
27. Rampen F: Melanoma: The problem with resection margins, Eur J Cancer 17:589, 1981.
28. Kelly JW, Sagebiel RW, Calderon W, et al.: The frequency of local recurrence and microsatellites as a guide to re-excision margins for cutaneous malignant melanoma, Ann Surg 200:759–763, 1984.
29. Davis N: Melanoma, Curr Probl Surg 13:1–63, 1976.
30. Milton GW, Jelihuvsky, T: Frozen section examination in the diagnosis of cutaneous malignant melanoma (melanoblastoma), Med J Austral 2:503–504, 1962.
31. Shafir, R, Hiss J, Tsur H, Bubis JJ: Pitfalls in frozen section diagnosis of malignant melanoma, Cancer 51:1168–1170, 1983.
32. Little JH, Davis NC: Frozen section diagnosis of suspected malignant melanomas of the skin, Cancer 34:1163–1172, 1974.
33. Zitelli JA, Mohs FE, Larson P, Snow S: Mohs micrographic surgery for melanoma. Dermatol Clin 7:833–843, 1989.
34. Mohs FE: Chemosurgery: Microscopically Controlled Surgery for Skin Cancer. Springfield, Ill.: Charles C. Thomas, 1978, pp 225–248.
35. Mohs FE: Chemosurgery in Cancer, Gangrene and Infections. Springfield, Ill.: Charles C. Thomas, 1956, pp 168–178.
36. Mohs FE: Fixed-tissue micrographic surgery for melanoma of the ear, Arch Otolaryngol Head Neck Surg 114:625–631, 1988.
37. Mohs FE: Chemosurgical treatment of melanoma: A microscopically controlled method of excision, Arch Dermatol 62:269–279, 1950.
38. Mohs FE: Chemosurgery for melanoma, Arch Dermatol 113:285–291, 1977.
39. Mohs FE, Bloom RF, Sahl WL: Chemosurgery for familial malignant melanomas, J Dermatol Surg Oncol 5:127–131, 1979.
40. Mohs FE: Microscopically controlled surgery for periorbital melanoma: Fixed-tissue and fresh-tissue techniques. J Dermatol Surg Oncol 11:284–291, 1985.
41. Fewkes J, Mohs FE: Microscopically controlled surgical excision (the Mohs technique). In Fitzpatrick TB, Eisen AZ, Wolff K, et al. (eds): Dermatology in General Medicine. New York: McGraw-Hill, 1987, pp 2557–2563.
42. Montagna W, Kirchner S, Carlisle K: Histology of sun-damaged human skin, J Amer Acad Dermatol 21:907–918, 1989.
43. Mikhail GR: Chemosurgery in the treatment of skin cancer, Int J Dermatol 14:33–38, 1975.
44. Mohs FE, Blanchard L: Microscopically controlled surgery for extramammary Paget's disease, Arch Dermatol 115:706–708, 1979.
45. Peters CW, Hanke CW, Pasarell HA, Bennett JE: Chemosurgical reports: Dermatofibrosarcoma protuberans of the face, J Dermatol Surg Oncol 8:823–828, 1982.
46. Epstein E: Thoughts on melanoma. In Epstein E, Epstein E Jr (eds): Skin Surgery, 6th ed. Philadelphia: W. B. Saunders, 1987, p 554.
47. Iscoe N, Kersey P, Gapski J, et al.: Predictive value of staging investigation in patients with clinical stage I

malignant melanoma, Plast Reconstr Surg 80:233–237, 1987.
48. Garg R, McPherson A, Lentle, et al.: Usefulness of an elevated serum lactate dehydrogenase value as a marker of hepatic metastasis, Can Med Assoc J 120:1114–1117, 1977.
49. Rogers GS, Kopf AW, Rigel DS, et al.: Hazard-rate analysis in stage I malignant melanoma, Arch Dermatol 122:999–1006, 1986.
50. Veronesi U, Adamus J, Bandiera DC, et al.: Inefficacy of immediate node dissection in stage I melanoma of the limbs, N Engl J Med 297:627–630, 1977.
51. Sim FH, Taylor WF, Pritchard DJ, Soule EH: A prospective randomized study of the efficacy of routine elective lymphadenectomy in the management of malignant melanoma, Cancer 41:948–956, 1978.
52. Balch CM: The role of elective lymph node dissection in melanoma: Rationale, results and controversies, J Clin Oncol 6:163–172, 1988.
53. Cascinelli N, Vaglini M, Nava M, et al.: Prognosis of skin melanoma with regional node metastases (stage II), J Surg Oncol 25:240–247, 1984.
54. Mohs FE: Micrographic surgery for satellites and in-transit metastases of malignant melanoma, J Dermatol Surg Oncol 12:471–476, 1986.
55. Rege VB, Leone LA, Soderberg CH, et al.: Hyperthermic adjuvant perfusion chemotherapy for stage I malignant melanoma of the extremity with literature review, Cancer 52:2033–2039, 1983.
56. Abide JM, Nahai F, Bennett RG: The meaning of surgical margins, Plast Reconstr Surg 73:492–496, 1984.
57. Sober AJ, Day CL, Koh HK, et al.: Melanoma in the Northeastern United States: Experience of Melanoma Clinical Cooperative Group. In Balch CM, Milton GW (eds): Cutaneous Melanoma. Philadelphia: J. B. Lippincott, 1985, p 441.

CHAPTER 15

The Use of the Zinc Chloride Fixative

George R. Mikhail, M.D., M.S.

Mohs micrographic surgery was originally called *chemosurgery* by its originator, Frederic E. Mohs, in the late 1930s. It was carried out by employing chemical fixations in situ prior to excision by means of a zinc chloride paste. The preparation consists of stibnite (40 gm), *Sanguinaria canadensis* (10 gm), and a saturated solution of zinc chloride (35 ml). The interested reader should read Mohs' book[1] for details of its application, but he or she is strongly urged not to use this very potent preparation without receiving first-hand instructions from someone proficient in its use.

The Mohs fresh tissue technique was first used by the originator in the late 1950s for treatment of eyelid lesions.[2] By the 1970s the method had become routine. At the present time it is the prevalent method and used exclusively by many Mohs surgeons. It has certain distinct advantages over the fixed tissue method, namely, it causes less discomfort to the patient, allows the excision of as many layers as are needed on the same day, and permits the repair of defects immediately after the ablation of tumors. Furthermore, the success rates for both techniques are comparable.[3] However, there are certain situations, now rather uncommon, in which the use of fixative paste can have a distinct advantage in achieving a favorable outcome. Examples include bone involvement, especially the paranasal sinuses, and invasion of deep fascial planes and the brain. Even then, some surgeons may debate the need for its use.

MALIGNANT MELANOMAS

Opinions about the preferred method for managing malignant melanomas also remain divided. Frederic E. Mohs is a strong proponent of the treatment of these lesions with the fixed tissue technique.[4,5]

Although our experience in the treatment of melanomas is rather limited, there are some conclusions that may be deduced. We have treated 10 superficial spreading melanomas, Clark's levels II and III, and 21 lentigo maligna melanomas, levels II and III, with the fresh tissue technique. All were 2.5 mm or less (Breslow[6]) in thickness. None of them recurred locally, but lymph node metastasis occurred in one of the level III superficial spreading type. Six lesions of nodular lentigo maligna melanomas, 4.0 to 8.0 mm thick, were treated. One, on the nose, was ablated by the fixed tissue technique, and almost the entire nose had to be removed. Despite this, the tumor recurred and metastasized. Another nodular lentigo maligna melanoma on the cheek had metastasized to the parotid nodes by the time the patient presented for treatment. The lesion was ablated by the fresh tissue method. Metastases to the lung were later detected, but all metastases spontaneously resolved at 7 months after excision of the skin lesion.[6] The other four cases were successfully treated, two by the fixed and two by the fresh tissue method.

It is difficult to draw conclusions from this meager and limited series, but our experience tends to favor the use of fixed tissue surgery in melanomas that are greater than 2.5 mm in thickness.

As an illustration, the case of a man age 65 with a large nodular lentigo maligna melanoma, 8 mm thick, in the left parotid area is presented. The lesion was ablated with the fixed tissue method, and the wound was left to heal by second intention. The cosmesis was reasonably good, and the patient was well and without metastasis for more than 5 years (Fig. 15–1).

DEEPLY INVASIVE BASAL CELL CARCINOMA

In our hands, the zinc chloride fixative has undoubtedly proved itself of immense value in the management of certain cases of basal cell carcinoma (BCC).

A man age 56 had a deeply seated, recurrent basal cell carcinoma of the chin that had been treated with deep cryosurgery. He presented with a large indurated, subcutaneous mass that impinged on the buccal mucosa. The fixed tissue method was applied, and fistula resulted after separation of the final fixed layer. However, it gradually became obliterated, and eventually the site became inconspicuous (Fig. 15–2). It appears that zinc chloride contributed toward this favorable result. It is contended that rapid healing, healthy granulation tissue, and scar contraction after the use of the fixative are inherent effects of the zinc chloride.

A man age 60 presented with a large sclerotic BCC of the right zygomatic area and the outer portions of the eyelids. It was excised by

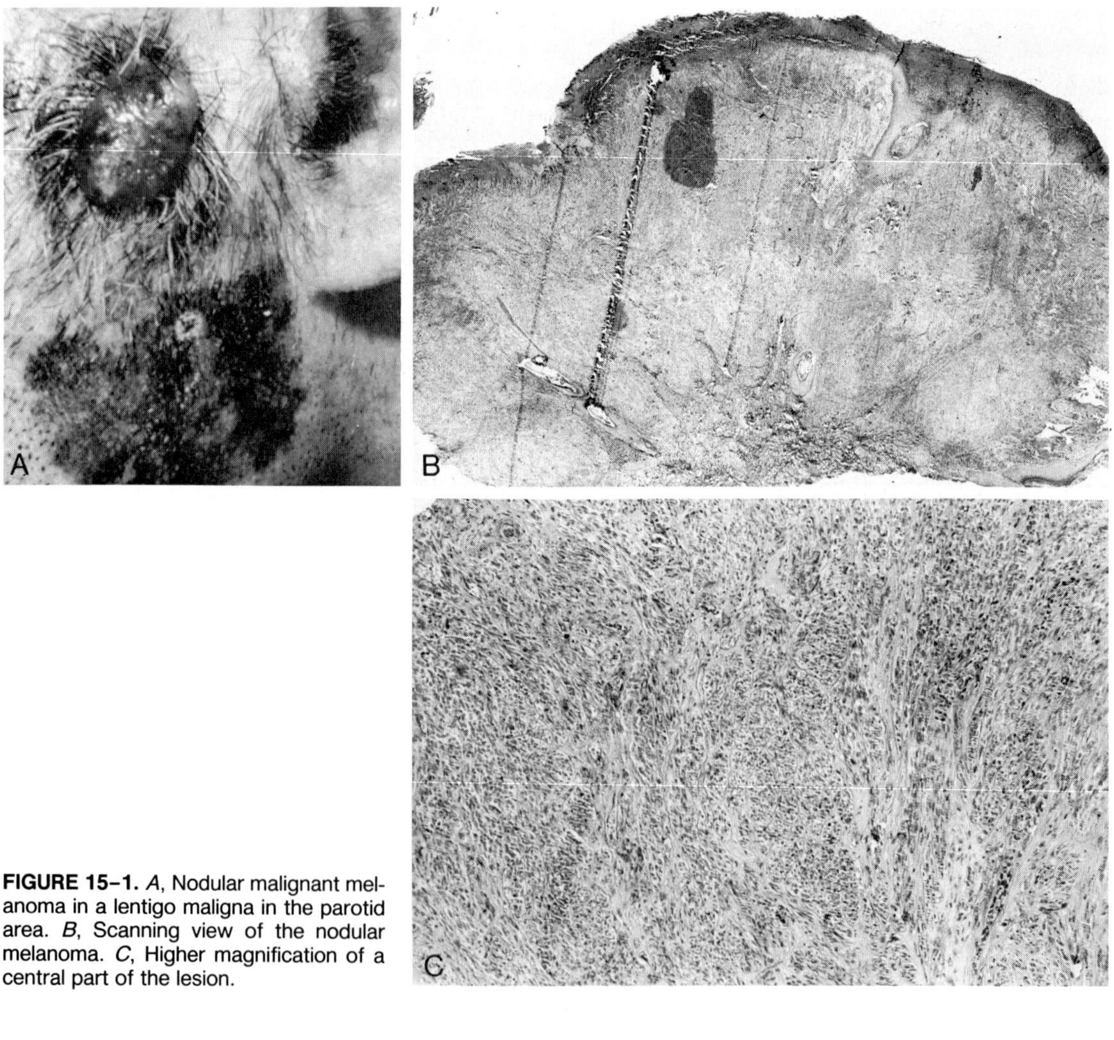

FIGURE 15–1. *A*, Nodular malignant melanoma in a lentigo maligna in the parotid area. *B*, Scanning view of the nodular melanoma. *C*, Higher magnification of a central part of the lesion.

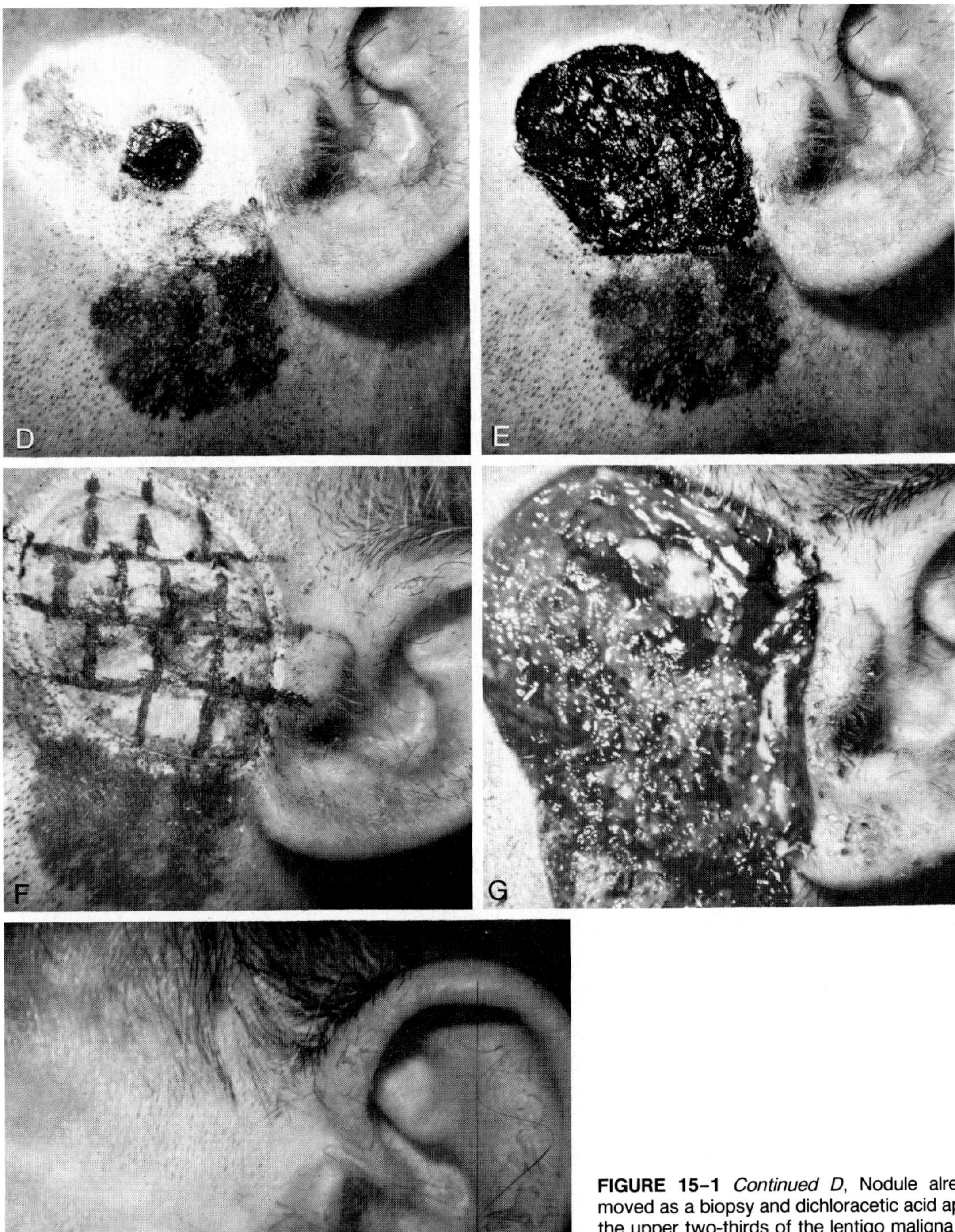

FIGURE 15–1 *Continued D*, Nodule already removed as a biopsy and dichloracetic acid applied to the upper two-thirds of the lentigo maligna and the melanoma component as a keratolytic. *E*, The zinc chloride fixative applied. *F*, First layer excised; note sites of sections. *G*, Wound after separation of final fixed layer. *H*, Result after healing by second intention; there was no local recurrence or metastasis after five years.

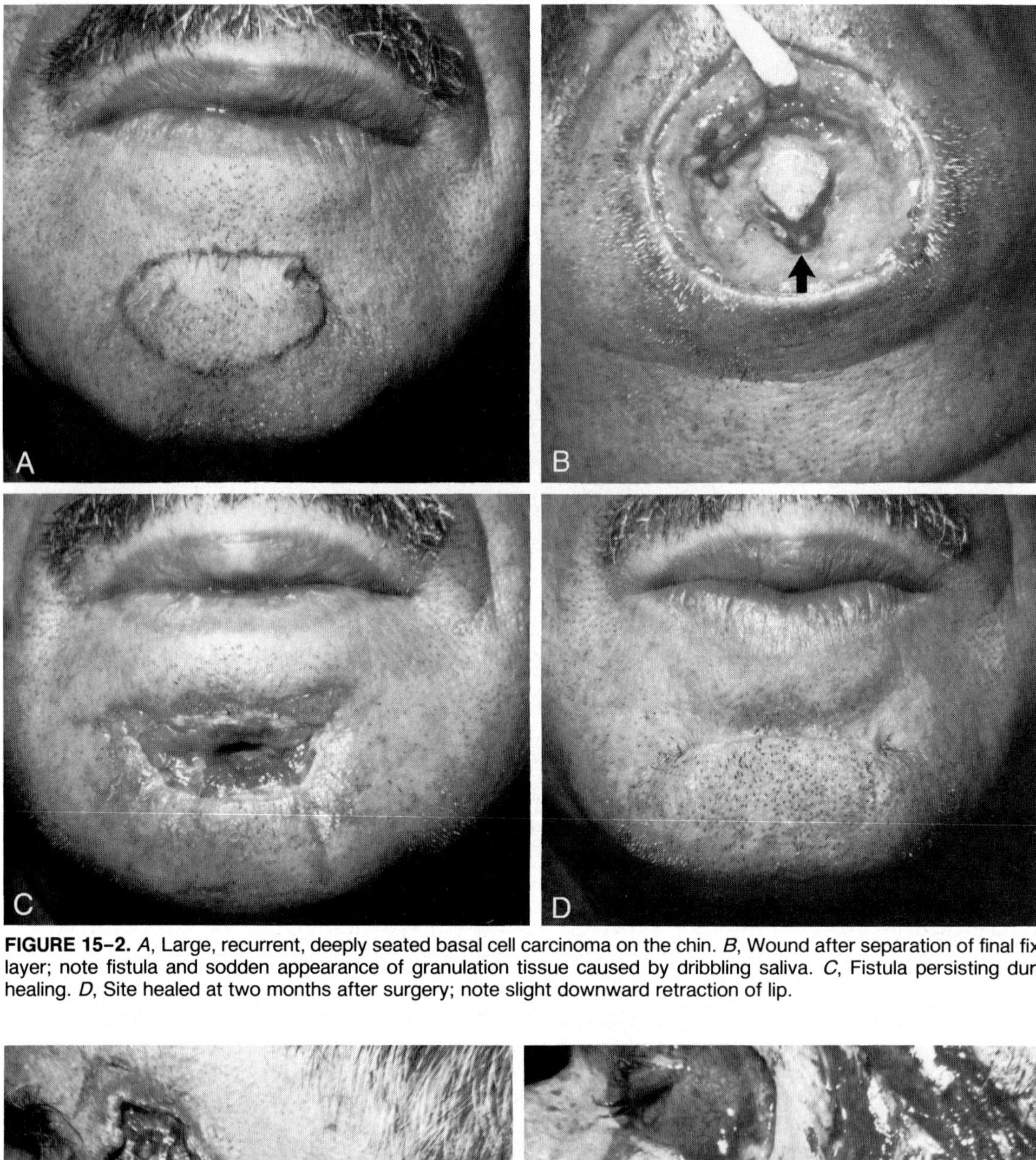

FIGURE 15–2. *A*, Large, recurrent, deeply seated basal cell carcinoma on the chin. *B*, Wound after separation of final fixed layer; note fistula and sodden appearance of granulation tissue caused by dribbling saliva. *C*, Fistula persisting during healing. *D*, Site healed at two months after surgery; note slight downward retraction of lip.

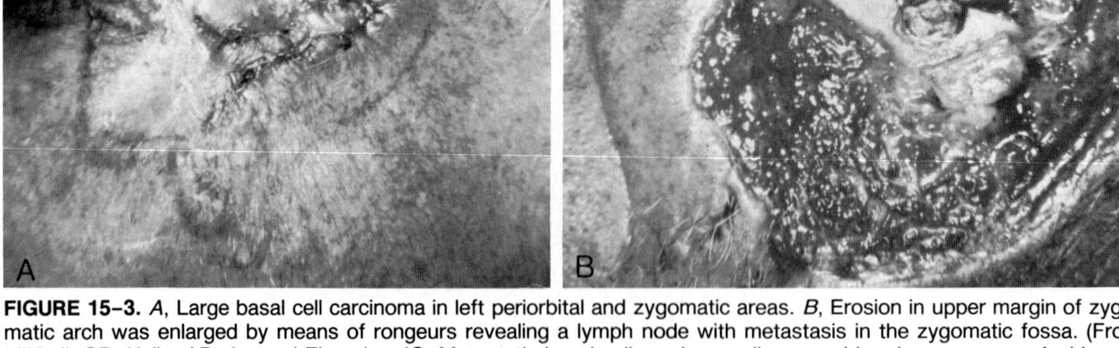

FIGURE 15–3. *A*, Large basal cell carcinoma in left periorbital and zygomatic areas. *B*, Erosion in upper margin of zygomatic arch was enlarged by means of rongeurs revealing a lymph node with metastasis in the zygomatic fossa. (From Mikhail, GR; Kelly, AP, Jr.; and Elmquist, JG: Metastatic basal cell carcinoma discovered by chemosurgery. *Archives of Dermatology* 105:103–104, 1972. Copyright 1972, American Medical Association.)

the fixed tissue method. During surgery, when an erosion in the upper margin of the zygomatic arch was removed with rongeurs, metastatic BCC in a deeply-seated zygomatic lymph node was discovered (Fig. 15–3). It might be argued that this discovery was fortuitous. However, it is doubtful that the metastasis could have been found and eradicated by any other modality.

CARCINOMA IN BONE

The zinc chloride fixative paste is one, if not the best, means of extirpating a carcinoma that invades bone. Such a condition can be recognized either by the presence of pits or honeycombing of the exposed bone or by the microscopic presence of carcinoma in the periosteum, even when the surface of the bone appears smooth to the naked eye. A case in point, illustrated in Figure 15–4, is of a patient with a recurrent BCC underneath a graft in the right supraorbital area. When lesion was ablated with Mohs fixed tissue technique, the tumor was found to extend to the frontal bone. The fixed outer table of the bone separated and was lifted off 7 weeks later as a wafer disclosing a healthy granulating base. The wound healed uneventfully by second intention.

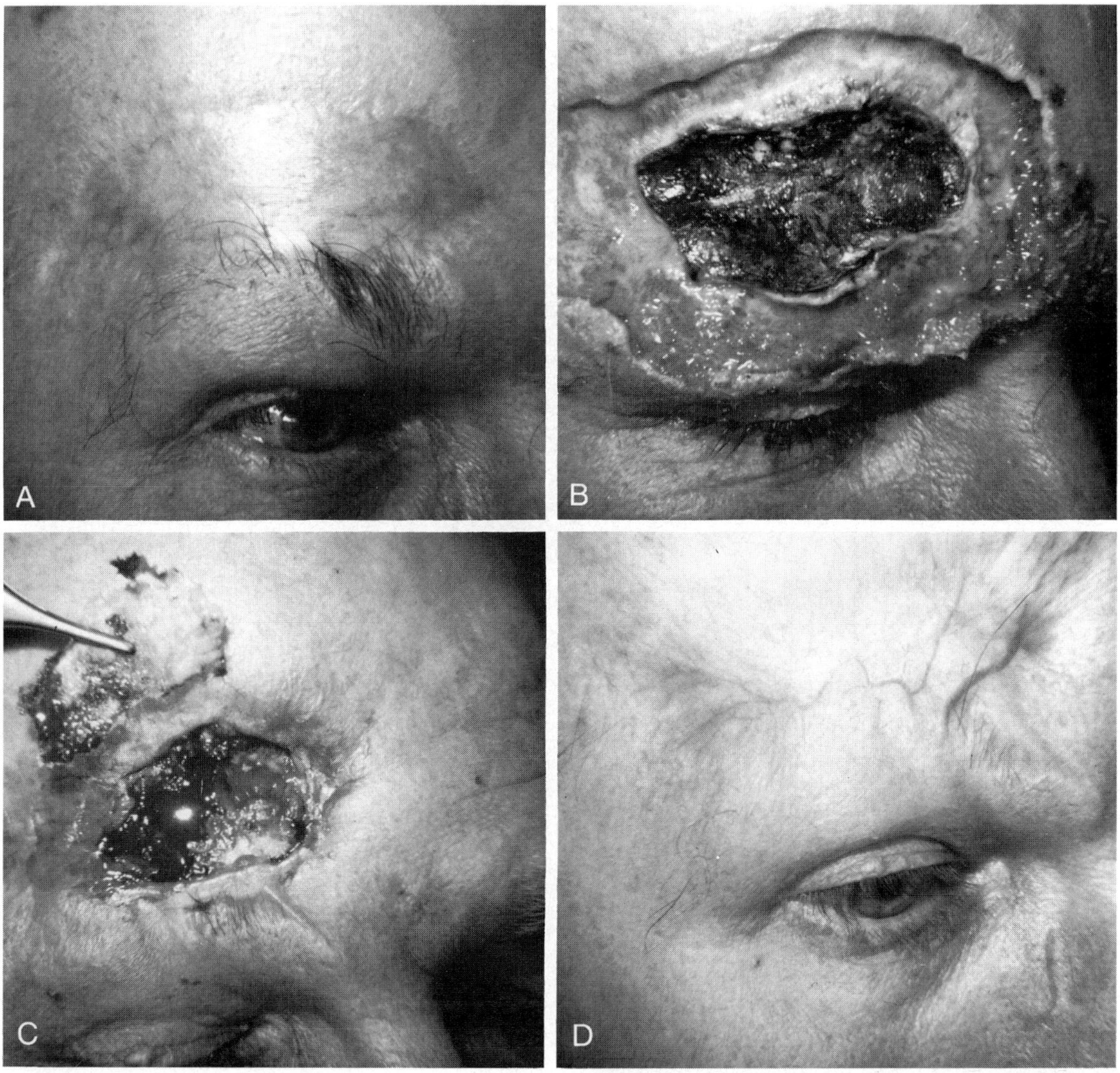

FIGURE 15–4. *A*, Recurrent basal cell carcinoma in right supraorbital graft. *B*, At termination of Mohs fixed tissue excision; bone fixed in center of wound. *C*, Outer table of frontal bone removed in one piece; note granulating base. *D*, Result after healing by second intention.

DEEPLY INVASIVE SQUAMOUS CELL CARCINOMA

The Mohs fixed tissue technique can be of great value in deeply invasive squamous cell carcinomas. A man age 60 was referred by a plastic surgeon for excision of a large squamous cell carcinoma on the right cheek that had invaded the parotid glands. Stenson's duct was severed during the fixed tissue procedure and a parotid fistula resulted. The plastic surgeon was naturally perturbed. However, the wound healed nicely, the contracting granulation tissue having obliterated the fistula (Fig. 15–5). Again, this favorable outcome could be ascribed to zinc.

CARCINOMAS IN VASCULAR TISSUE

The fixed tissue technique is particularly indicated in squamous cell carcinomas of the penis when the corpora cavernosa (noncontractile vascular channels) are involved. Examples are included in Chapter 12. Analogous to this situation is the case of a man age 55 with a recurrent squamous cell carcinoma in a cavern-

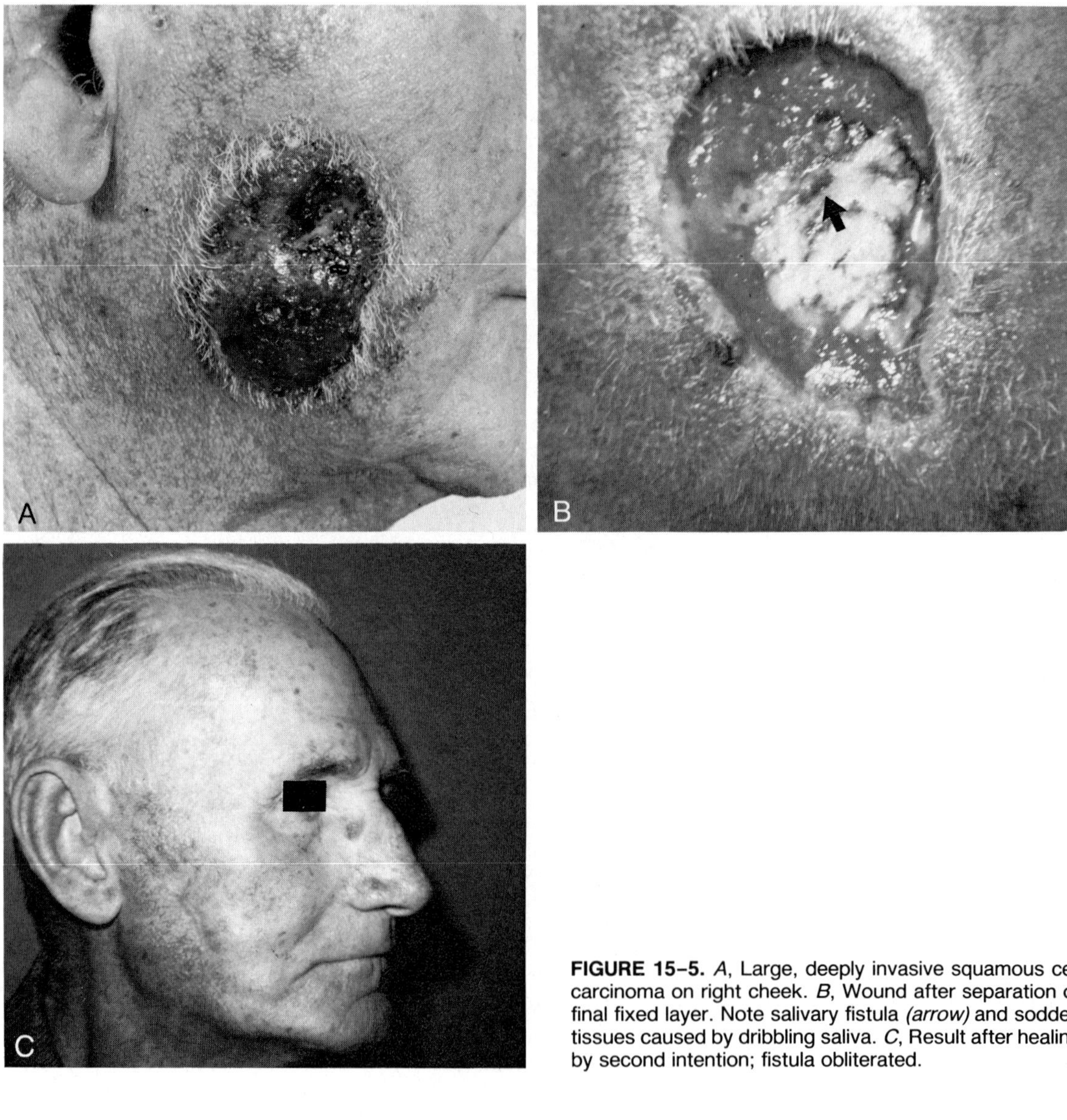

FIGURE 15–5. *A*, Large, deeply invasive squamous cell carcinoma on right cheek. *B*, Wound after separation of final fixed layer. Note salivary fistula *(arrow)* and sodden tissues caused by dribbling saliva. *C*, Result after healing by second intention; fistula obliterated.

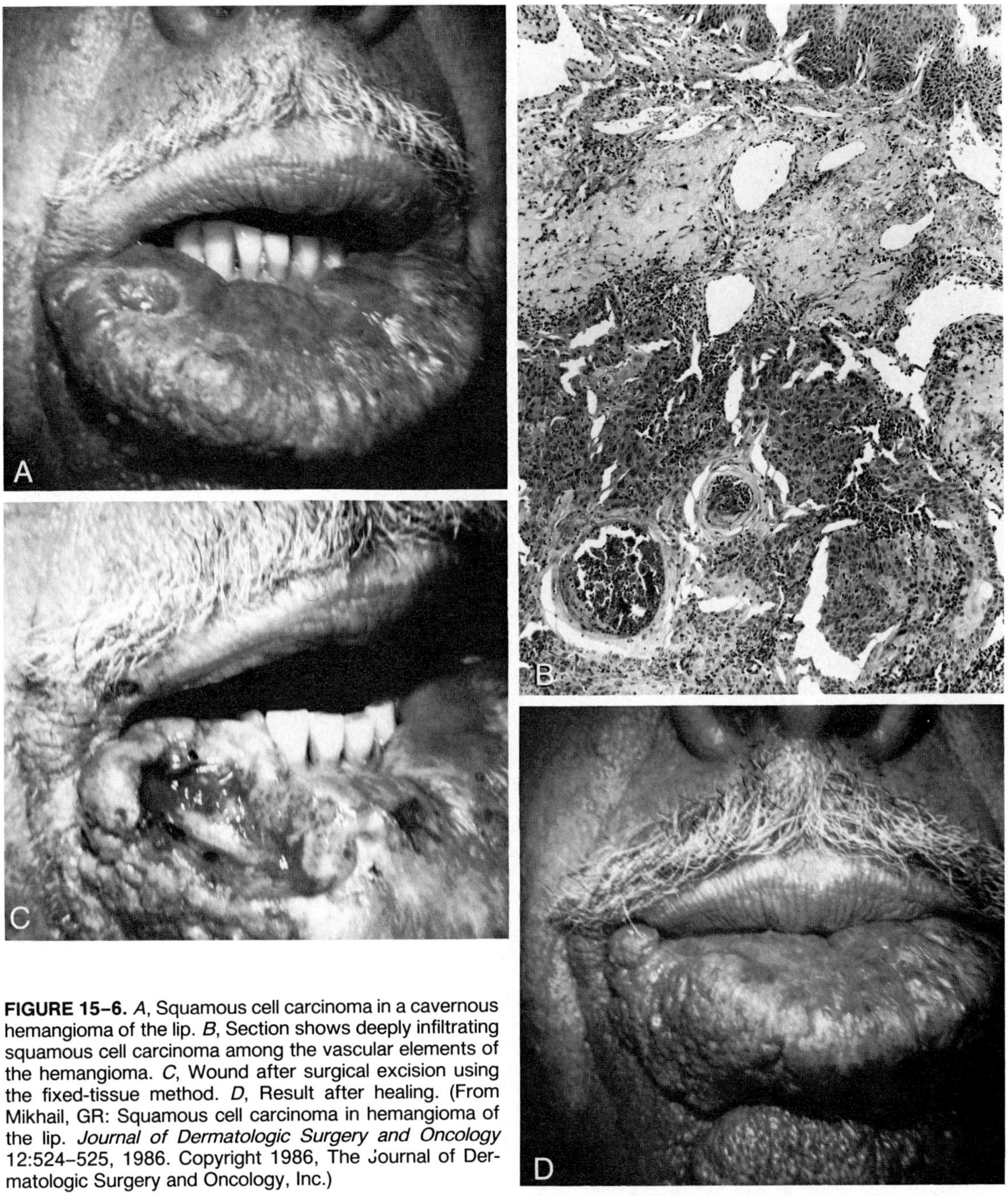

FIGURE 15–6. *A*, Squamous cell carcinoma in a cavernous hemangioma of the lip. *B*, Section shows deeply infiltrating squamous cell carcinoma among the vascular elements of the hemangioma. *C*, Wound after surgical excision using the fixed-tissue method. *D*, Result after healing. (From Mikhail, GR: Squamous cell carcinoma in hemangioma of the lip. *Journal of Dermatologic Surgery and Oncology* 12:524–525, 1986. Copyright 1986, The Journal of Dermatologic Surgery and Oncology, Inc.)

ous hemangioma of the lip. Treatment by radiotherapy had failed. The tumor was ulcerated and deeply infiltrating by palpation. It was excised using the fixed tissue method without bleeding, either during surgery or after separation of the final fixed tissue layer, and prompt healing took place (Fig. 15–6). This case could not have been managed so easily by any other means.

OTHER APPLICATIONS OF MOHS FIXED TISSUE SURGERY

During the era when the fixed tissue technique was the rule, the plastic surgeons who grafted the wounds remarked that grafts took exceptionally readily and well. They did not even have to suture the grafts in place, a simple dressing was sufficient. At the present time,

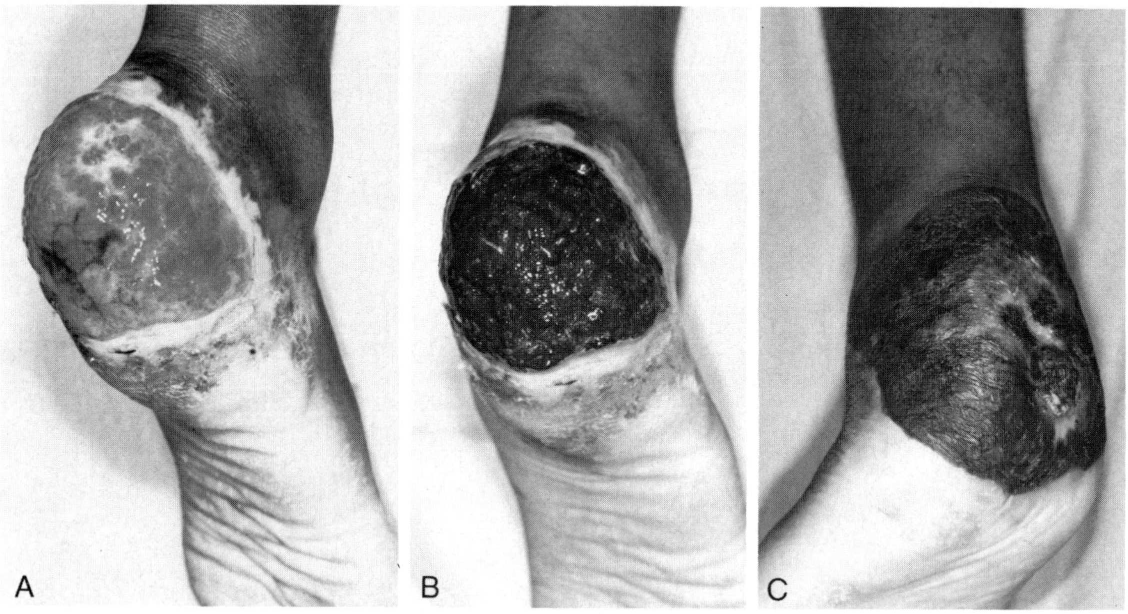

FIGURE 15–7. *A*, Third-degree burn on heel; repeated grafting failed. *B*, Zinc chloride fixative applied. *C*, Result was 100% take of graft.

they find grafting wounds after fresh tissue excisions is not as easy as it used to be. These observations led to three situations where the zinc chloride fixative was used to stimulate the production of healthy granulation tissue readily receptive of grafts. The first patient is a boy age 15 who had third-degree burns on both heels. Repeated attempts at grafting the burn wounds failed. A thin layer of zinc chloride fixative was applied for 20 minutes and then wiped off with a wet sponge. Five days later, a thin layer of fixed tissue separated. The area was then grafted with a prompt 100% take (Fig. 15–7).

The second patient had an arteriosclerotic ulcer on the instep of the foot that failed to heal after systemic and topical therapy and repeated split-thickness grafts. Amputation was being considered, but the plastic surgeon, familiar with the Mohs fixed tissue method, suggested a referral consultation. The zinc fixative was applied to the residual ulcer in a thin film. A layer of tissue was excised the following day. No ma-

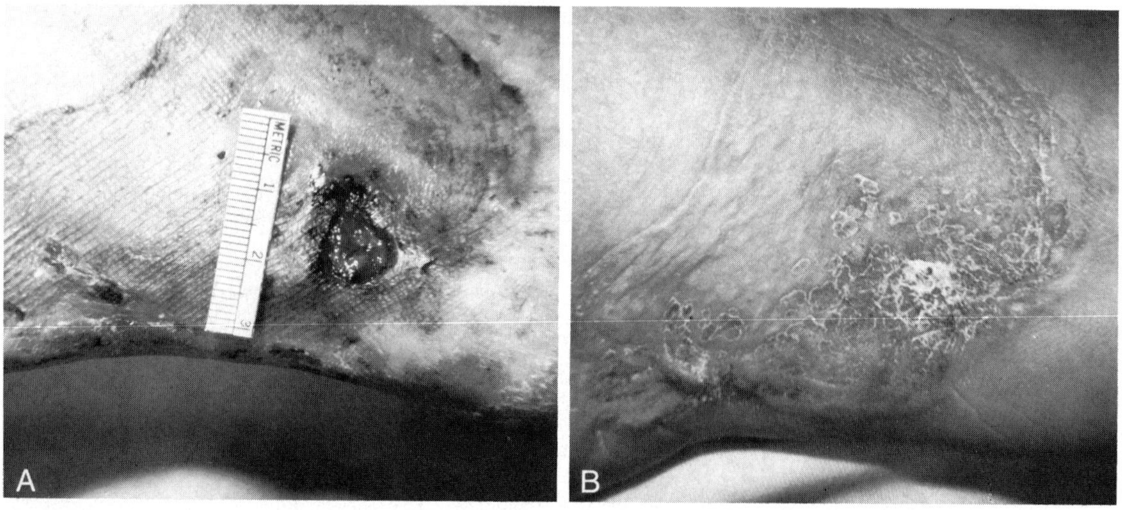

FIGURE 15–8. *A*, Arteriosclerotic ulcer of the foot; note grafted area. *B*, Ulcer healed after excision of ulcer by the fixed-tissue method.

lignancy was detected. Following separation of the final layer, the wound healed uneventfully within 3 weeks by second intention (Fig. 15–8).

The third patient presented with an ulcer of the glans penis with a granulomatous base of many months duration. Tests for granulomatous disease including syphilis, tuberculosis, leprosy, deep fungal infection, and atypical mycobacterial infection were all negative. The histology was that of a nonspecific granuloma. Several therapies were used to no avail. In order to exclude an underlying malignancy, the lesion was excised using the zinc chloride fixative. No carcinoma could be detected. Prompt healing took place after separation of the final fixed layer (Fig. 15–9).

These cases demonstrate that the Mohs fixed tissue method has merits that cannot be denied. It was certainly valuable in the case of melanoma and in the carcinoma in a hemangioma. The other three cases were the outcome of observation and serendipity.

The advent and continuing spread of the acquired immunodeficiency syndrome (AIDS) is having its impact on the practice of Mohs surgery. The cutting of fresh tissue frozen sections imposes a real danger to the histotechnologist handling the tissues. The use of gloves is inadequate in the face of a sharp knife, and we all know that a cut hand is always possible in this occupation. As long as the technicians cannot be immunized against this deadly disease, other measures have to be adopted in treating patients with AIDS. If small, the lesion may be excised, the margins marked, and routine par-

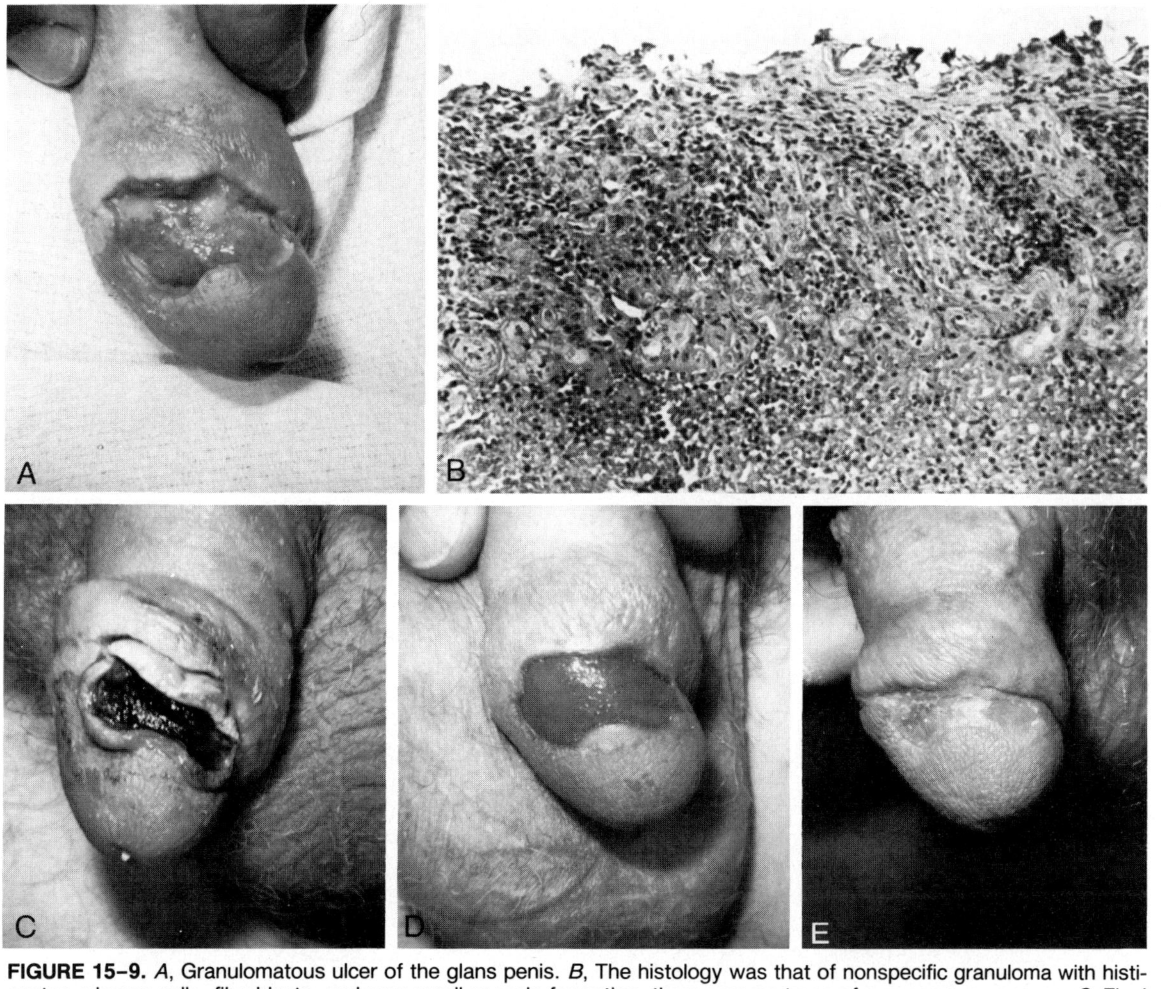

FIGURE 15–9. *A*, Granulomatous ulcer of the glans penis. *B*, The histology was that of nonspecific granuloma with histiocytes, plasma cells, fibroblasts, and new small vessels formation; there was no trace of a cancerous process. *C*, Final fixed layer separating. *D*, Smooth granulation tissue after separation of final layer. *E*, Result after healing.

affin sections examined. In the case of large tumors, the Mohs fixed tissue method would be indicated. For other situations, see Chapter 2.

REFERENCES

1. Mohs FE: Chemosurgery. Microscopically Controlled Surgery for Skin Cancer. Springfield, Ill.: Charles C. Thomas, 1978, pp 3–29.
2. Ibid., p 106.
3. Ibid., pp 123–130.
4. Ibid., pp 246–248.
5. Mohs FE: Chemosurgery for melanoma, Arch Dermatol 113:285–291, 1977.
6. Breslow A: Thickness, cross-sectional areas and depth of invasion in the prognosis of cutaneous melanoma, Ann Surg 172:902–908, 1970.
7. Mikhail GR, Gorsulowsky DC: Spontaneous regression of metastatic malignant melanoma, J Dermatol Surg Oncol 12:497–500, 1986.

CHAPTER 16

The Mohs Laboratory

Linda S. Selak, H.T.(A.S.C.P.)

The laboratory is an integral part of Mohs micrographic surgery. Because of the important role it plays, the surgeon and histotechnologist need to communicate and develop a close relationship so that optimal performance is achieved. There are various techniques that give the same result when preparing microsections from a piece of tissue. In this chapter we describe how a Mohs lab is set up, and the materials and methods we use in processing the tissues from the time they are excised until they are examined microscopically.

SETTING UP THE LABORATORY

The Environment

When setting up a Mohs laboratory, the first concern should be the environment. The room should be conveniently located near the surgery rooms to minimize transport time and to avoid the disturbance of tissues. Good ventilation as well as air conditioning is important to maintain the equipment in proper working order. The cryostat, like any refrigeration unit, generates heat into the outside air. Without adequate ventilation and air conditioning, the optimal temperature for cutting is difficult to maintain.

There should be a water supply for staining purposes. Plumbing may require modification to accommodate an automatic stainer if one is used.

Equipment and Supplies

There are important decisions to be made when choosing the equipment and supplies for a Mohs laboratory. The basic set up shown in Table 16–1 has worked well for us. Various equipment suppliers are listed in Table 16–2. The microtome inside the cryostat should be easy to adjust for the angles of difference between the tissue block and blade edge. It should also have an anti-roll device, which helps shorten the cutting time, although this can be a matter of personal preference for the technologist. It is helpful to have a quick-freeze area in the cryostat where the temperature is lower than the rest of the chamber in order to expedite the freezing process. This is particularly helpful when cutting fatty tissues.

The choice between the standard microtome knife and a disposable blade system can also be a matter of personal preference. In our experience disposable blades are perfectly suited for Mohs surgery. The blades are of much higher quality at present as compared to when they were first introduced. If surgery necessitates the cutting of suture material, hair, cartilage, or bone, using a disposable blade eliminates the apprehension of damaging a standard knife. A damaged standard knife needs repeated honing and sharpening, which can be expensive and time-consuming, with the eventual loss of the proper cutting edge, but when the disposable blade is damaged, another is readily available.

An automatic stainer is an optional piece of equipment. When first setting up a lab one can

TABLE 16–1. Equipment and Supplies

Cryostat with Anti-roll Quick freeze area Extra specimen holders	**Hydrochloric acid,** concentrated
Microscope with objectives (3.5×, 10×, and 40×)	**10% Formalin or OmniFix** for postfixation of tissue sections
Microtome knives and knife sharpener or disposable blade system	**Liquid nitrogen** for rapid freezing
Knife guard	**100% Ethyl or reagent alcohol** (also used to make up 70% and 95% alcohol)
Automatic slide stainer (optional)	**Xylene** or another clearing agent
Trays for drying slides and file system	**Solutions** Concentrated blue dye and mercurochrome (40% aqueous solution for marking tissue) Gill's triple-strength hematoxylin or Harris formula hematoxylin Scott's tap water (bluing reagent)
Fume exhaust hood or fume extractor with activated charcoal	**Embedding medium** (used for orientation and freezing of tissue)
Safety cans for the flammable liquids	**Decalcifying solution** (a chelating agent in dilute HCl)
Glassware Erlenmeyer flask, 500 ml Graduated cylinder, 500 ml Graduated transfer pipettes, 5 ml Funnel, 150 mm Staining dishes and lids Staining racks (10-slide capacity)	**Mounting medium** for cover slipping
Tissue forceps without teeth	**Spray freeze** for cooling tissue
Small curved scissors	**Miscellaneous** Latex gloves nonsterile Microscopic slides Microscopic slide labels Square petri dishes, 100 mm × 100 mm disposable Qualitative filter paper 4 × 4 inch gauze, nonsterile
Camel hair brush, No. 5	
Heat extractor (used for flattening tissue)	

use glass or plastic staining dishes and racks. This manual method gives satisfactory results, but when the case load increases, one may want to consider an automatic stainer, which gives the technologist more time for the orientation and cutting of tissues or to assist in the operating room. The automatic stainer used in our lab allows for one or many slides to be stained in a continuous flow pattern (Fig. 16–1). It contains a slide dryer which, although not normally used for regular frozen sections, is helpful for preparing sections that tend to fall off during staining, e.g., decalcified bone and zinc chloride–fixed tissues. The automatic stainer provides consistent and reliable results using any staining technique. It also permits efficient use of the staining reagents by reducing contamination from one solution to the next.

Safety is another important factor when establishing a laboratory. Items necessary to maintain safety in a Mohs laboratory are: a permanent fume hood or fume extractor, safety cans for storage of flammable liquids, knife guard, latex gloves, and pipette pump.

Whether one chooses xylene or a substitute, such as a clearing agent, one must have adequate ventilation for the toxic fumes and strong odors. In our laboratory we use activated charcoal fume extractors in the cover slipping area, and there is also another built into the automatic stainer. The fume extractor is a good choice where a permanent fume hood

TABLE 16–2. Sources for Laboratory Equipment and Supplies for Mohs Surgery

An-Con Genetics, Inc.*
1 Huntington Quadrangle
Melville, NY 11747
1-800-888-4999

Baxter Healthcare Corporation
Scientific Products Division
1430 Waukegan Road
McGaw Park, IL 60085-6786
(312) 689-8410

Columbia Diagnostics, Inc.
8001 Research Way
Springfield, VA 22153
(703) 569-7511

Dermatologic Lab and Supply, Inc.
205 Ridge #205
Council Bluffs, IA 51503
(800) 831-6273

Fisher Scientific International
50 Fadem Road
Springfield, NJ 07081
(201) 467-6400

Hacker Instruments, Inc.
Box 657
Fairfield, NJ 07007
(201) 226-8450

International Equipment Company
300 Second Ave.
Needham Heights, MA 02194
(617) 449-0800

Luther Ford and Company†
100 North Seventh Street
Minneapolis, MN 55403
(612) 332-2441

Thomas Scientific
99 High Hill Road
P. O. Box 99
Swedesboro, NJ 08085-0099
(609) 467-2000

*For OmniFix tissue fixative.
†For super-concentrated bluing for marking tissue sections.

cannot be installed (Fig. 16–1). Although xylene substitutes are nontoxic and less flammable, there is still need for good ventilation because of the strong odors.[1]

For the technologist's safety, gloves should be worn while cutting. Latex gloves are preferred over the plastic type because they conform better to the hand, which reduces the chance of injury from the glove catching on the microtome or blade.

The purchase of a slide file system is something that should not be overlooked. It is our medicolegal responsibility to store this material.[2] It is not only important for keeping the surgery cases, but also for filing frozen section biopsies performed on site and for slides sent in from referring physicians. For the Mohs surgery cases we assign a number, which begins with an *M* to represent Mohs, followed by the year and case number, e.g., M-90-001 (Fig. 16–2). The biopsy slides from referring physicians are filed alphabetically by patient's name. The period of retention recommended by the College of American Pathologists is 20 years.[3] The original diagrams should also be kept on file even if they are duplicated in the patients' charts. One should also check for local, state, and federal requirements.

TISSUE PROCESSING

The layer removal, dissection, and marking of the tissue sections is covered in detail in Chapter 2. This chapter explains the important steps in the Mohs method for achieving good quality frozen sections with minimal trimming.

When removing a layer of tissue in Mohs surgery, it is important that the layer be beveled at the periphery at approximately a 45-degree angle from the epidermis to the deep margin. This angle makes it possible for the technologist to make frozen sections of the entire cut surface. With such sections the surgeon can assess the presence of tumor at the lateral and deep margins of the tissue.[4] If the cut is made at a 90-degree angle at the epidermal surface, it would be difficult to obtain a plane of tissue showing all the epidermis and the deep margins without having to trim too deeply into the block. This could give a false-positive result, after trimming away an excess of normal tissues in attempting to achieve a complete section. No amount of flattening of the sections, which is used by some technologists during embedding, can rectify an improperly cut layer.

When dividing the layer of tissue, several points should be kept in mind. The sections should be of such size so that the technologist can embed them on the cryostat holder or disk with enough room for the supporting medium to be placed all around it. The usual size is 0.5 to 1.0 cm. This helps to maintain a level surface for cutting. Square pieces of tissue are not appropriate in peripheral sections. It is ex-

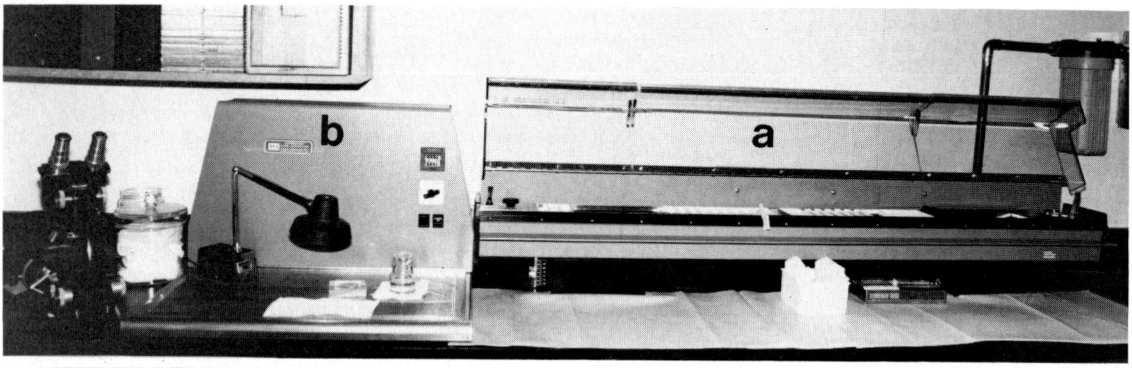

FIGURE 16–1. The Baxter GLX linear stainer (*a*) and Hacker Instrument's downdraft fume extraction (*b*).

tremely difficult to embed square tissue pieces if two sides of epidermis are to be obtained without too much trimming into the block. Optimally, the section should have a short, relatively straight edge of epidermis. A large section with a long curved edge of epidermis is difficult to embed and cut. Appropriate and inappropriate examples of dissecting techniques are shown in Figure 16–3.

The marking of the tissue is not only a guide for the surgeon when reading the slides, it also serves to direct the technologist in the process of orientation and embedding. When it is difficult to grossly recognize the epidermal edge, one has to examine the diagram for the orientation of the color dyes. The tissue edges must be thoroughly marked so that when the tissue is turned upside-down to begin sectioning from the cut surface, the dyes are clearly seen. Too much dye should be avoided because this can confuse the technologist and can be the cause for improper orientation.

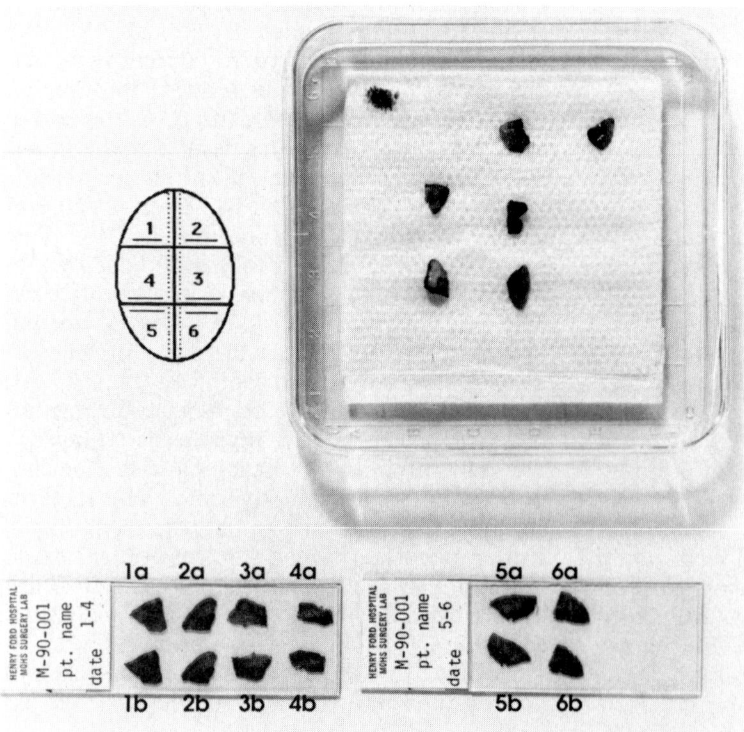

FIGURE 16–2. Slides show the serial numbering of cases and the sequence of sections. The square petri dish contains six sections. The reference for the sequence is the dot in the upper left-hand corner; the diagram shows the origin of each section.

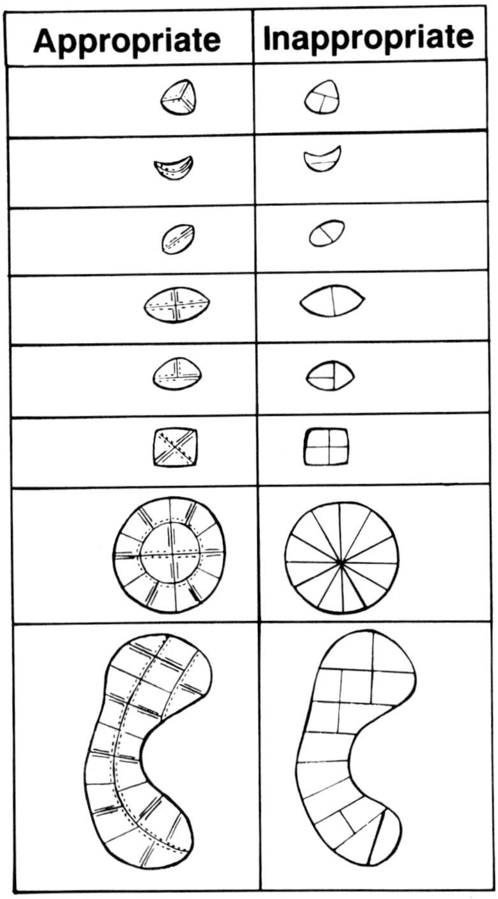

FIGURE 16–3. Appropriate and inappropriate methods of dividing tissue layers. (Reprinted by permission of publisher from "Technical procedures for Mohs fresh tissue surgery" by M. Picoto and A. Picoto, *Journal of Dermatologic Surgery and Oncology* 12(2):134–138. Copyright 1986, by Elsevier Science Publishing Company, Inc.)

ORIENTATION AND EMBEDDING OF THE TISSUE

The dissected and marked layer of tissue is delivered to the laboratory in a petri dish on a 4 × 4-inch gauze moistened with tap water (Fig. 16–2). The tissue sections are arranged in three vertical rows on the gauze. The first row has two tissue sections starting under one red dot placed in the upper left-hand corner. Then there are three sections in each of the next two rows, allowing for a maximum of eight sections per square of gauze. For additional tissue sections, the dot would change to blue for the next set of eight, then two red dots for the next series, alternating the colors and increasing the number of dots as necessary. The numbering of the sections begins with row one, section one below the dot, then numbering from the top of each row ending in the lower right-hand corner. The surgeon places the side to be examined, the undersurface of the section, facedown on the gauze. It is necessary to adhere to this routine in order to eliminate possible confusion.

Before embedding, the cryostat should be checked for the proper temperature. For skin with fat the recommended temperature is −16° to −25°C, for muscle −13° to −20°C.[5] A good mean temperature for the section we deal with in Mohs surgery would be −20°C. To begin embedding, we start with the first section of the layer and compare it to the corresponding area on the diagram to make sure the markings are correct. At this point one can detect if the tissue has been misplaced or incorrectly marked. On our diagrams a dotted line on the edge of the section represents the blue dye on the tissue and the solid line represents the red (Fig. 16–2).

After checking the tissue markings, one begins embedding by applying a small amount of the mounting medium to the cryostat object disk. When the medium begins to turn from clear to milky-white, the disk is ready for the tissue.

Several good media are commercially available. The qualities most suited for Mohs surgery are minimal water content (to reduce ice artifact), lack of a residue on the slide after staining, the ability to produce sections with minimal curling, and good adherence to the object disk. One begins embedding by removing the piece of tissue from the petri dish and turning it upside-down to examine the side to be cut. It is helpful to notice if the tissue contains cartilage, muscle, mucosa, or fat because recognizing these components after the tissue has been frozen is sometimes difficult and the orientation for cutting is different for each of these tissues. Also, one should make sure from the diagram whether the section should contain epidermis. A piece of tissue from the middle of a first layer may have epidermis on the top but it should not appear in the frozen section because we are only concerned with the undersurface of such a piece. Inadvertently getting epidermis on a section when it should not be seen can give a false result and is caused by undue compression during embedding and rolling over of the upper surface of the section.

The tissue should be handled carefully with forceps while it is embedded into the partially

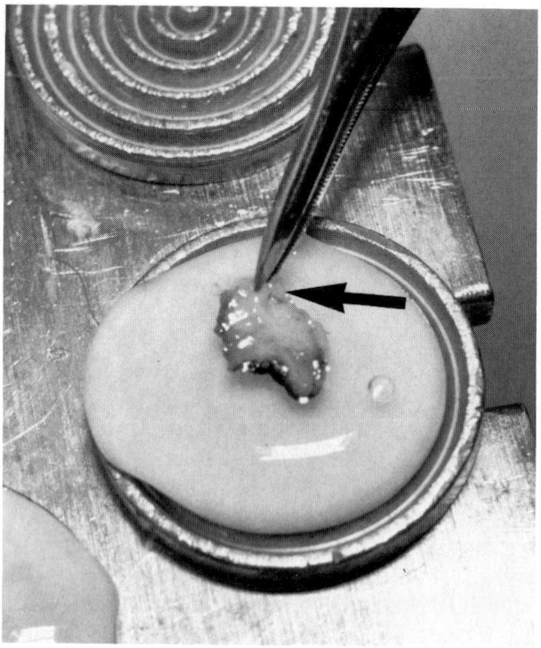

FIGURE 16–4. Tissue section being placed into the embedding medium on the tissue disk. Note that the epidermal margin is held by the forceps (*arrow*).

frozen medium. The medium should surround the tissue but not cover it. Because the embedding medium is viscid, it supports the tissue at any angle at which it is embedded while freezing. If the section is thick, additional medium may need to be added around it. If it has epidermis, one must pay careful attention while embedding to make sure that the epidermis is level with the surface of medium and can be viewed for cutting (Fig. 16–4). At this point, just before the tissue is completely frozen, a flattening device may be applied. The type we use is a heavy metal cylinder with a handle known as a heat extractor. One can use any flat metal object or even a glass slide for this purpose. The device should be kept in the cryostat at all times so that it is always cold and ready for use. In most sections that are properly beveled during surgery, we do not find it necessary to use a flattening device, but sections may require flattening if they are thick or not properly beveled, especially tissues obtained from the thick skin of the back, chest, and back of the neck. The flattening device is applied with slight pressure after the section begins to freeze. One must be careful not to distort the tissue when flattening by pressing the epidermis or any other part of the tissue too deeply into the medium because excessive trimming may be required to reach a full representative section.

For fatty sections, which are sometimes difficult to freeze, one may immerse the embedded tissue in liquid nitrogen for a few seconds. However, it should not be left in to the point where the tissue becomes brittle since this causes the tissue to chip into small pieces during cutting. Letting the tissue warm up slightly corrects the problem. For the experienced technologist the entire embedding process takes 2 to 3 minutes for each piece of tissue.

ORIENTATION AND CUTTING

To begin cutting, the tissue and the medium should be thoroughly frozen. Special consideration must be given to tissues that contain bone before embedding. It will be necessary to decalcify them first to permit proper cutting. We use a chelating agent in a weak solution of hydrochloric acid. The tissue is placed between layers of gauze to maintain orientation and is deposited in a small jar into which the decalcifying solution is poured slowly and the time is noted. The tissue is checked every hour until it has a rubbery consistency. When this is achieved, the decalcification process is complete. The tissue is then washed in water to produce good nuclear detail after staining. This is done by discarding the decalcifying solution and filling the jar with tap water while being careful to maintain the orientation. The tissue should wash in three changes of water for 5 minutes each.

We start the orientation for cutting by placing the disk into the microtome holder. Most specimen disks have an indentation in the stem which, when placed in the microtome holder, can be locked into place with a screw. The holder is usually adjustable in order to align the tissue with the knife edge by moving it from side to side or up and down. In our particular cryostat, the adjustment is made simply by loosening and tightening one part, the orientation handle (Fig. 16–5). By loosening it, one can swivel the tissue disk which is held in a ball-and-socket joint. In some cryostats this same procedure takes several steps, making the adjustment more difficult. Because of the differences in cryostat microtomes, one should refer to the manufacturer's manual for specific instructions on adjusting the tissue block. The

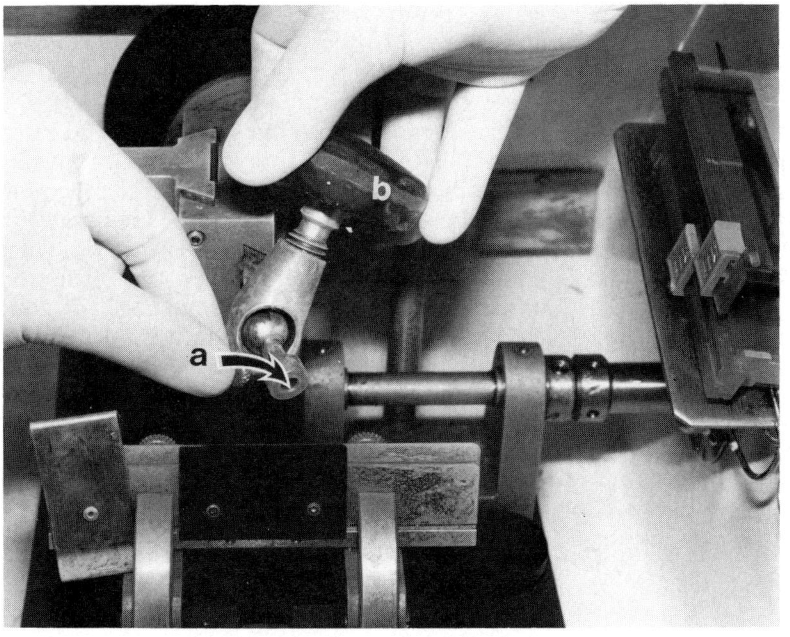

FIGURE 16–5. Positioning of the tissue disk holder (*a*) is demonstrated. The orientation handle (*b*) can be easily maneuvered.

microtome automatic feed mechanism should also be set to the desired thickness of the microsections. In our laboratory sections are cut at 4 to 6 microns.

Adjustment of the tissue block should be such that it is parallel to the angle of the microtome blade. This orientation minimizes the amount of trimming. If the tissue contains epidermis, one should rotate the tissue block so that the epidermis is perpendicular to the blade edge (Fig. 16–6). The same applies to the conjunctiva and other mucosa. This will eliminate

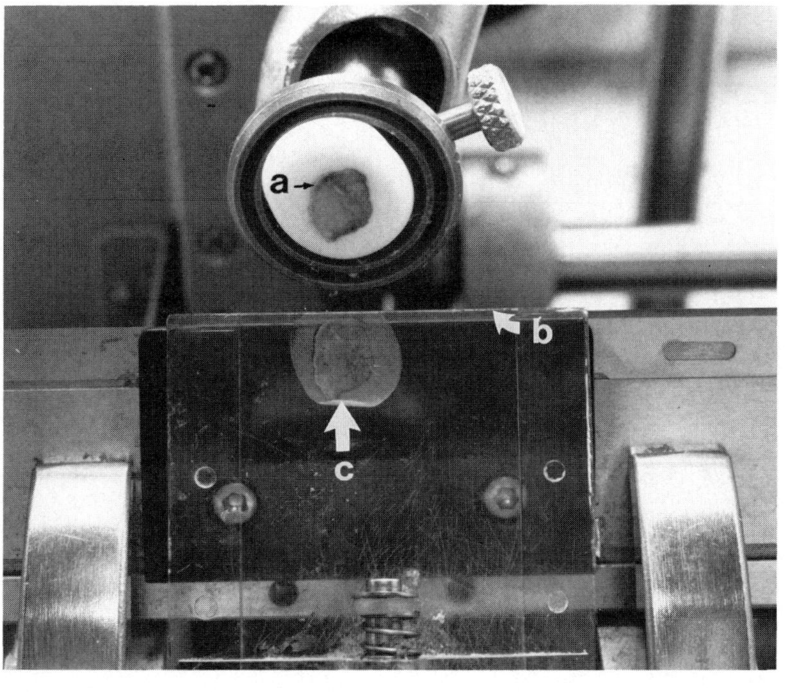

FIGURE 16–6. Tissue section mounted on the object holder with the epidermis (*a*) perpendicular to the edge of the blade. The anti-roll plate is in place during cutting (*b*). Note full section (*c*) on knife.

artifactual separations in the microsections. Muscle should also be oriented in a similar way, with the fiber direction perpendicular to the edge of the blade. If not properly oriented, the section will shatter. If this happens one should rotate the block 90 degrees.

After the tissue is properly aligned to the blade, one can begin trimming. The goal is to trim just enough to where one can obtain a complete section. This is achieved, in most cases, after 3 to 4 microlayers are removed. To obtain a section, first engage the automatic feed mechanism and the anti-roll plate. One pass over the blade should produce a full, flat section (Fig. 16–6). To insure that the section is a full one, compare it to the tissue block. It is vital that not even the smallest amount of tissue be missing from either the deep or superficial margins, otherwise one could possibly be leaving tumor behind.[6] Any difficulties in obtaining good frozen sections are usually caused by a warm temperature or by debris on the blade or the anti-roll plate. To maintain the proper temperature, one can use a freezing spray. There are new sprays that do not contain ozone-damaging chemicals. Remember to spray the anti-roll plate as well as the tissue and blade. To clear away debris, one should use cooled gauze and gently wipe the blade and anti-roll plate. When cleaning the blade, one should wipe away from its edge to avoid injury. To pick up a section, simply swing the anti-roll plate away and place a slide at room temperature above the section, bringing it carefully closer. The warm slide will attract the cold section, and the section will then thaw and adhere to the glass slide. In our lab we cut two sections from each piece of tissue in case one should fall

TABLE 16–3. Methods of Hematoxylin and Eosin Staining for Mohs Surgery

Manual Steps

1. Stain in **hematoxylin** (Harris formula) for 1 minute.
2. Wash in **lukewarm running tap water** until all of the embedding residue is removed.
3. Dip into **bluing reagent** until the color develops from a reddish purple to blue.
4. Rinse in tap water.
5. Stain in **1% alcoholic eosin Y** for 10 seconds.
6. Dehydrate in 2 changes of 95% alcohol, 15 dips each.
7. Dehydrate in 5 changes of 100% alcohol, 15 dips each.
8. Dip in clearing reagent **(xylene or xylene substitute)** until clear (when the solution flows smoothly over the slide).
9. Coverslip.

Automatic Method for the Baxter S/P* GLX Linear Stainer

Solution	No. of Changes†
Hematoxylin (Gill's triple-strength)	×2
Tap water (38°C)	×5
Bluing reagent	×1
95% Alcohol	×1
1% Eosin Y	×1
95% Alcohol	×2
100% Alcohol	×8
Xylene	until ready to coverslip

*Scientific Products Division of Baxter Healthcare Corporation.
†Each change is 15 seconds in solution.

off during staining. The sections are mounted, starting at the frosted end of the slide. The first of the two sections from each piece is mounted on the upper half of the slide (Fig. 16–2). This order is maintained so that false positives can be recognized. If section 1b, the second and deeper section into the block is positive and section 1a is not, the positive could be a false one because the deeper the section into the block the closer it is to the tumor.

The cutting is the most time-consuming part of tissue processing and depends on the type of tissue, the temperature, and how well the tissue was beveled. Under ideal conditions an average four-section case should take about 8 to 10 minutes.

FIXATION AND STAINING OF THE SECTIONS

The selection of the best stain for frozen sections is really a matter of personal choice. Many modifications to the standard hematoxylin and eosin (H&E) stain exist; they all serve the general purpose. Table 16–3 shows two methods we have used. The modifications in the technique were made to achieve optimal results with sections that are easy to read and that can be saved for a long time. Using warm water, as opposed to the usual cold water, removes any residue left from the embedding medium. This is especially helpful in the case of thicker, fatty sections. Using a bluing reagent like Scott's tap water substitute (2 gm of potassium bicarbonate and 20 gm of magnesium sulfate in 1 liter of distilled water) speeds up the bluing after staining in hematoxylin.[7] We also find that the stain does not fade with time when compared to sections treated with lithium carbonate. Choosing H&E over another type of stain is really a matter of personal preference. In our experience H&E retains its quality longer than other rapid stains, e.g., toluidine blue.

Recent studies have indicated that postfixation of frozen sections from Mohs surgery improves cellular preservation and stain intensity. The cut frozen sections are submersed for 1 minute in either 95% ethyl, 10% formalin, fixative cocktail (ethyl alcohol, formalin, and glacial acetic acid), or OmniFix (a commercially prepared alcohol-based fixative).[8] The best staining intensity was achieved after 10% formalin fixation, but OmniFix gave good staining intensity and better cellular preservation.

The staining method shown for the automatic stainer in Table 16–3 is slightly modified from the manual method to fit the mechanical flow. The slide travels in a constant linear motion, from solution to solution, at the rate of 15 seconds in each container. To control the timing for a stain, one adds or subtracts the number of containers for solutions. The hematoxylin solution was changed from the Harris formula to Gill's triple strength to shorten the staining time while balancing the increased intensity of eosin. The stainer was modified with a hot and cold water mixer to obtain a flowing warm water at a temperature of 38°C. A 95% alcohol container was added after the water rinse to aid dehydration and fixation before the eosin. Additional absolute alcohol (Table 16–3, step 7) was also added for adequate dehydration before the clearing agent.

The automatic stainer provides the technologist with valuable time for other responsibilities. It allows one to view the surgeries as they are being performed and to observe how the surgeon is dividing and marking the tissues. In difficult cases this helps to better understand the proper orientation for embedding.

If the staining procedure fails, the sections can be decolorized in a solution of 1% hydrochloric acid in 70% alcohol after rehydration. After decolorization, the sections are carefully washed in water so they do not float off. For tissues that have a tendency to float off during staining, e.g., decalcified bone and zinc chloride–fixed tissue or cartilage, one can mount the sections on slides smeared with albumin, then heat them over a burner or in a slide dryer before staining.

After the sections are stained they are preserved by covering them with a mounting medium and glass coverslip.

The entire staining process should take about 5 minutes. For the automatic stainer, an additional 5 minutes are required for travel time between solutions.

REFERENCES

1. Grande DJ, Phillips FW: Histo-Clear to replace xylene in dermatopathology laboratory, J Dermatol Surg Oncol 11(2):102–105, 1985.
2. Scott WL: Legal aspects of laboratory records, Medical Laboratory Observer 11:119–131, 1979.
3. Guidelines for Retention of Laboratory Records and Materials. College of American Pathologists. Northfield, Ill: Commission on Laboratory Accreditation, 1988 edition.

4. Abide JM, Nahai F, Bennett RG: The meaning of surgical margins, Plast Reconstr Surg 73(3):492–496, 1984.
5. The IEC Cryotomy Handbook, 1st ed. Needham, Mass.: International Equipment Co., 1975, p 10.
6. Dzubow LM: Chemosurgical report: Recurrence (persistence) of tumor following excision by Mohs surgery, J Dermatol Surg Oncol 13(1):27–30, 1987.
7. Culling CFA, Allison RT, Barr WT: Cellular Pathology Technique, 4th ed. London: Butterworth, 1985, p 137.
8. Rustad OH, Kaye V, Cerio R, Zachary CB: Post-fixation of cryostat sections improves tumor definition in Mohs surgery, J Dermatol Surg Oncol 15(12):1262–1267, 1989.

CHAPTER 17

Data Collection and Analysis

Daniel W. Collison, M.D.
George R. Mikhail, M.D., M.S.
Gary B. Rosen, M.D.

Mohs micrographic surgery (MMS) is relatively novel and not widely practiced when compared to other therapeutic methods for cutaneous cancers. This renders information regarding cure rates obtained by this method both desirable and significant. Previous chapters have discussed the techniques of MMS, including the advantages of microscopic verification of margins of excised cancers. As with any therapy, the results of these techniques should be evaluated and compared with other modalities.

Two reviews by Rowe and colleagues summarized the recurrence rates of primary and recurrent basal cell carcinomas (BCC) treated by various modalities.[1,2] There were wide variations in the follow-up periods and in the definition of cure or recurrence. In addition, some authors grouped primary and recurrent lesions together and did not differentiate the cure rates according to category, demonstrating the need for standarized methods of data collection and analysis. However, certain conclusions can be drawn from the above reviews. The data indicate that the cure rates after Mohs surgery were superior to the more commonly practiced modalities, which included curettage and electrodesiccation, radiation therapy, cryotherapy, and traditional excision (see Table 1–2).

The recordings and analyses of Mohs surgery data hitherto have varied in method. In this chapter we will present a system of prospective and retrospective record-keeping for MMS cases developed by one of us (D.W.C.). This system is especially adaptable to a computerized database, and the results of the retrospective application of this system to cases treated and followed by one of us (G.R.M.) for 5 or more years will be presented.

METHODS

Starting in the late 1960s, case data of patients referred to one of us (G.R.M.) for treatment by MMS were recorded in a logbook. In the early 1970s, the previously collected data and data from subsequent cases were stored on preprinted 3″ × 5″ rotary file index cards; the most recent card design is shown in Figure 17–1. Basic data regarding patient, tumor, and treatment were collected for each treated lesion (Table 17–1). Dates of follow-up as well as pertinent clinical information, such as dates of recurrence and dates of death, were recorded on the back of the cards. In cases where the patient was not seen in follow-up, additional data were obtained by letter questionnaire or telephone from the patient, relatives, or referring physician.

A coding system for tumor sites (Tables 17–2 and 17–3) and accompanying body diagrams (Figs. 17–2 and 17–3) were designed. The system of site codes using three-digit numbers was suggested by a tentative system currently used by the Tumor Registry of the American College of Mohs Micrographic Surgery and Cutaneous Oncology. In retrospect, a system devel-

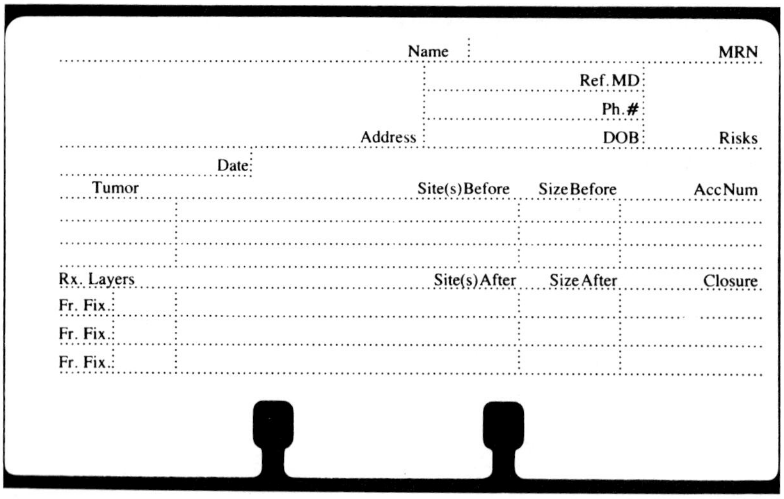

FIGURE 17–1. Rotary file index card, 3″ × 5″, showing basic case data.

oped by Kopf predates both systems.[3] Our system of coding has the advantages of a more consistent structure and the inclusion of codes for both prospective and retrospective analyses. For example, both specific codes ("columella") and general codes ("nose, site not otherwise specified," abbreviated "nose NOS") are included. Specific codes are more desirable, but nonspecific codes may be needed for retrospective studies in which medical records may be incomplete or nonspecific.

In order to provide a consistency that makes the codes easier to use, the codes are grouped to represent certain body areas and certain conventions are used. For example, whenever possible, code endings 0, 2, or 4 are used for the left side of the body; endings 1, 3, and 5 are used for the right side; the ending 8 is used for the midline, and the ending 9 is used for non-

Text continued on page 315

TABLE 17–1. Data Collected for Each Lesion

- Patient name
- Patient address
- Patient phone number
- Medical record number of patient
- Date of birth
- Date treated
- Tumor type
- Site(s) before treatment
- Size before treatment
- Size after treatment
- Treatment type
- Layers required for excision
- Date of last follow-up
- Date of recurrence (if any)
- Date of death (if any)
- Referring physician

TABLE 17–2. Overview of Site Codes

Head and Neck	100–599
Scalp, temple, forehead, and eyebrows	100–199
Scalp	100–139
Temple	150–159
Forehead and eyebrows	160–179
Eyelids and ears	200–299
Eyelids and ocular mucosa	200–229
Ears	240–299
Nose and nasal mucosa	300–399
Lips and oral mucosa	400–499
Cheeks, jaw, chin, and neck	500–599
Cheeks and jaw	500–539
Chin	540–549
Neck	550–589
Trunk and Extremities	600–899
Trunk	600–699
Anterior thorax	600–622
Abdominal, inguinal, and crural areas	624–649
Shoulders, back, and buttocks	650–699
Extremities	700–899
Upper extremities	700–799
Lower extremities	800–899
Anogenital Areas	900–999
Genitalia	900–959
Female genitalia	900–919
Male genitalia	930–959
Perineum and perianal areas	970–989
Mucosal Areas	
Ocular	220–229
Nasal	350–369
Vermilion lip	440–449
Intraoral	450–499
Female genitalia	900–919
Male genitalia	930–959
Anal	980–989

TABLE 17–3. Site Codes and Body Sites

Scalp: 100–139

Code	Site
100	left frontal scalp
101	right frontal scalp
102	left anterior scalp NOS*
103	right anterior scalp NOS
104	mid anterior scalp NOS
105	anterior scalp NOS
108	mid frontal scalp
109	frontal scalp NOS
110	left parietal scalp
111	right parietal scalp
118	mid parietal scalp
119	parietal scalp NOS
120	left occipital scalp
121	right occipital scalp
122	left posterior scalp NOS
123	right posterior scalp NOS
124	mid posterior scalp NOS
125	anterior scalp NOS
128	mid occipital scalp
129	occipital scalp NOS
130	left scalp NOS
131	right scalp NOS
138	mid scalp NOS
139	scalp NOS

Temple: 150–159

Code	Site
150	left temple
151	right temple
159	temple NOS

Forehead and Eyebrows: 160–179

Code	Site
160	left forehead
161	right forehead
168	mid forehead
169	forehead NOS
170	left eyebrow
171	right eyebrow
172	left supraorbital NOS
173	right supraorbital NOS
178	glabella
179	eyebrow(s) NOS

Eyelids: 200–219

Code	Site
200	left upper eyelid
201	right upper eyelid
202	upper eyelid NOS
203	lower eyelid NOS
204	left lower eyelid
205	right lower eyelid
206	left eyelid NOS
207	right eyelid NOS
209	eyelids NOS
210	left lateral canthus
211	right lateral canthus
212	left medial canthus
213	right medial canthus
214	left eye canthus NOS
215	right eye canthus NOS
216	left eye NOS
217	right eye NOS
218	canthus NOS
219	eye NOS

Ocular Mucosae: 220–229

Code	Site
220	left upper conjunctiva
221	right upper conjunctiva
222	upper conjunctiva NOS
223	lower conjunctiva NOS
224	left lower conjunctiva
225	right lower conjunctiva
226	left ocular mucosa NOS
227	right ocular mucosa NOS
228	conjunctiva NOS
229	ocular mucosa NOS

Ears: 240–299

Code	Site
240	left preauricular
241	right preauricular
242	preauricular NOS
244	left tragus of ear
245	right tragus of ear
246	tragus NOS
250	left superior helix
251	right superior helix
252	superior helix NOS
253	inferior helix NOS
254	left inferior helix
255	right inferior helix
256	left helix NOS
257	right helix NOS
259	helix NOS
260	left earlobe
261	right earlobe
262	earlobe NOS
263	fossa of helix, superior antihelix, or fossa of antihelix NOS
264	left fossa of helix, superior antihelix, or fossa of antihelix
265	right fossa of helix, superior antihelix, or fossa of antihelix
266	left inferior antihelix or antitragus
267	right inferior antihelix or antitragus
269	inferior antihelix or antitragus NOS
270	left conchal bowl or crus of helix
271	right conchal bowl or crus of helix
272	conchal bowl or crus of helix NOS
274	left ear canal
275	right ear canal
279	ear canal NOS
280	left nonhelix posterior ear
281	right nonhelix posterior ear
282	left posterior ear NOS
283	right posterior ear NOS
284	posterior ear NOS
286	left ear NOS
287	right ear NOS
289	ear NOS
290	left retroauricular sulcus
291	right retroauricular sulcus
292	retroauricular sulcus NOS
294	left postauricular (left mastoid)
295	right postauricular (right mastoid)
299	postauricular NOS

Nose: 300–349

Code	Site
300	left root of nose
301	right root of nose
302	mid root of nose
303	root of nose NOS
304	left paranasal
305	right paranasal
309	paranasal NOS
310	left dorsum (bridge) of nose
311	right dorsum (bridge) of nose
312	left nose NOS
313	right nose NOS
314	dorsum (bridge) of nose NOS
318	mid dorsum (bridge) of nose
319	nose NOS
320	left alar crease
321	right alar crease
322	alar crease NOS
324	left nasal ala
325	right nasal ala
329	nasal ala NOS
330	left tip of nose
331	right tip of nose
338	mid tip of nose
339	tip of nose NOS
348	columella of nose

Nasal Mucosae: 350–369

Code	Site
350	left nasal septum
351	right nasal septum
352	nasal septum NOS
354	left nasal vestibule
355	right nasal vestibule
356	nasal vestibule NOS
360	left nasal mucosa NOS
361	right nasal mucosa NOS
362	nasal mucosa NOS

Cutaneous Lips: 400–439

Code	Site
400	left nasolabial fold
401	right nasolabial fold
409	nasolabial fold NOS
410	left upper cutaneous lip
411	right upper cutaneous lip
412	philtrum or mid upper cutaneous lip
413	upper cutaneous lip NOS
414	left upper lip NOS
415	right upper lip NOS
416	mid upper lip NOS
419	upper lip NOS
420	left angle of mouth
421	right angle of mouth
429	angle of mouth NOS
430	left lower cutaneous lip
431	right lower cutaneous lip
432	mid lower cutaneous lip
433	lower cutaneous lip NOS
434	left lower lip NOS
435	right lower lip NOS
436	mid lower lip NOS
437	lower lip NOS
438	cutaneous lips NOS
439	lips NOS

Vermilion Lips: 440–449

Code	Site
440	left upper vermilion lip
441	right upper vermilion lip
442	mid upper vermilion lip
443	upper vermilion lip NOS
444	left lower vermilion lip
445	right lower vermilion lip

Table continued on following page

TABLE 17–3. Site Codes and Body Sites *Continued*

Vermillion Lips *Continued*
446 mid lower vermilion lip
447 lower vermilion lip NOS
449 vermilion lip NOS

Intraoral Mucosa: 450–499
450 left upper lip intraoral (vestibular) mucosa
451 right upper lip intraoral (vestibular) mucosa
452 mid upper lip intraoral (vestibular) mucosa
453 upper lip intraoral (vestibular) mucosa NOS
454 left lower lip intraoral (vestibular) mucosa
455 right lower lip intraoral (vestibular) mucosa
456 mid lower lip intraoral (vestibular) mucosa
457 lower lip intraoral (vestibular) mucosa NOS
459 lip intraoral (vestibular) mucosa NOS
460 left lower gingival mucosa
461 right lower gingival mucosa
462 mid lower gingival mucosa
463 lower gingival mucosa NOS
464 left upper gingival mucosa
465 right upper gingival mucosa
466 mid upper gingival mucosa
467 upper gingival mucosa NOS
469 gingival mucosa NOS
470 left floor of mouth
471 right floor of mouth
472 mid floor of mouth
473 floor of mouth NOS
474 left undersurface of tongue
475 right undersurface of tongue
476 mid undersurface of tongue
479 undersurface of tongue NOS
480 left dorsum of tongue
481 right dorsum of tongue
482 mid dorsum of tongue
483 dorsum of tongue NOS
484 tongue NOS
486 left hard palate
487 right hard palate
488 mid hard palate
489 hard palate NOS
490 left upper buccal mucosa
491 right upper buccal mucosa
492 upper buccal mucosa NOS
493 lower buccal mucosa NOS
494 left lower buccal mucosa
495 right lower buccal mucosa
496 left buccal mucosa NOS
497 right buccal mucosa NOS
499 buccal mucosa NOS

Cheeks: 500–529
500 left zygomatic area
501 right zygomatic area
502 zygomatic NOS
504 left parotideomasseteric area
505 right parotideomasseteric area
506 left parotid NOS
507 right parotid NOS
508 parotid NOS
509 parotideomasseteric area NOS
510 left malar (infraorbital) area
511 right malar (infraorbital) area
512 malar (infraorbital) area NOS
513 buccal area NOS
514 left buccal area
515 right buccal area
516 left cheek or maxilla NOS
517 right cheek or maxilla NOS
519 cheek(s) or maxilla NOS
526 left face NOS
527 right face NOS
528 mid face NOS
529 face NOS

Jaw: 530–539
530 left posterior mandible (angle of jaw)
531 right posterior mandible (angle of jaw)
532 posterior mandible (angle of jaw) NOS
533 anterior mandible NOS
534 left anterior mandible
535 right anterior mandible
536 left jaw or mandible NOS
537 right jaw or mandible NOS
539 jaw or mandible NOS

Chin: 540–549
540 left chin
541 right chin
548 mid chin
549 chin NOS

Neck: 550–589
550 left submandibular
551 right submandibular
552 submandibular NOS
554 left submental
555 right submental
558 mid submental
559 submental NOS
560 left anterior neck
561 right anterior neck
562 throat or mid anterior neck
569 anterior neck NOS
570 left supraclavicular
571 right supraclavicular
572 suprasternal
574 left lateral neck
575 right lateral neck
576 lateral neck NOS
579 supraclavicular NOS
580 left posterior neck
581 right posterior neck
582 posterior neck NOS
584 left neck NOS
585 right neck NOS
588 mid posterior neck or nape
589 neck NOS

Anterior Thorax: 600–622
600 left upper anterior thorax
601 right upper anterior thorax
602 mid upper anterior thorax (sternum)
603 upper anterior thorax NOS
604 left lower anterior thorax
605 right lower anterior thorax
606 left chest NOS
607 right chest NOS
608 chest NOS
609 lower anterior thorax NOS
610 left axilla
611 right axilla
612 axilla NOS
613 breast NOS
614 left breast
615 right breast
616 left areola
617 right areola
618 left nipple
619 right nipple
620 left lateral thorax
621 right lateral thorax
622 lateral thorax NOS

Abdominal, Inguinal, and Crural Areas: 624–649
624 upper abdomen NOS
625 lower abdomen NOS
626 left abdomen NOS
627 right abdomen NOS
628 mid abdomen NOS
629 abdomen NOS
630 left upper abdomen
631 right upper abdomen
632 left lower abdomen
633 right lower abdomen
634 umbilicus
636 left flank
637 right flank
639 flank NOS
640 left inguinal
641 right inguinal
642 inguinal NOS
643 suprapubic NOS
644 left suprapubic
645 right suprapubic
646 left crural fold
647 right crural fold
649 crural fold NOS

Shoulders, Back, and Buttocks: 650–699
650 left anterior shoulder
651 right anterior shoulder
652 left posterior shoulder
653 right posterior shoulder
654 left shoulder NOS
655 right shoulder NOS
659 shoulder NOS
660 left upper back
661 right upper back
668 mid upper back
669 upper back NOS
670 left lower back
671 right lower back
673 lower back NOS
676 left back NOS
677 right back NOS
678 mid lower back
679 back NOS
680 left anterior hip
681 right anterior hip

TABLE 17–3. Site Codes and Body Sites *Continued*

Code	Site
682	left posterior hip
683	right posterior hip
684	left hip NOS
685	right hip NOS
689	hip NOS
690	left buttock
691	right buttock
692	buttocks NOS
694	left intergluteal cleft
695	right intergluteal cleft
699	intergluteal cleft NOS
Upper Extremities: 700–799	
700	left extensor arm
701	right extensor arm
702	left flexor arm
703	right flexor arm
704	left lateral arm
705	right lateral arm
706	left medial arm
707	right medial arm
708	left arm NOS
709	right arm NOS
710	arm NOS
711	elbow NOS
712	left elbow
713	right elbow
714	left antecubital area
715	right antecubital area
716	left lateral elbow
717	right lateral elbow
718	left medial elbow
719	right medial elbow
720	left extensor forearm
721	right extensor forearm
722	left flexor forearm
723	right flexor forearm
724	left radial forearm
725	right radial forearm
726	left ulnar forearm
727	right ulnar forearm
728	left forearm NOS
729	right forearm NOS
730	forearm NOS
731	wrist NOS
732	left dorsal (extensor) wrist
733	right dorsal (extensor) wrist
734	left ventral (flexor) wrist
735	right ventral (flexor) wrist
736	left radial wrist
737	right radial wrist
738	left ulnar wrist
739	right ulnar wrist
740	left wrist NOS
741	right wrist NOS
742	left hand dorsum
743	right hand dorsum
744	left palm
745	right palm
746	left hand NOS
747	right hand NOS
748	hand NOS
749	finger NOS
750	left extensor first finger
751	right extensor first finger
752	left palmar first finger
753	right palmar first finger
754	left radial or ulnar first finger
755	right radial or ulnar first finger
756	left first finger nail unit
757	right first finger nail unit
758	left first finger NOS
759	right first finger NOS
760	left extensor second finger
761	right extensor second finger
762	left palmar second finger
763	right palmar second finger
764	left radial or ulnar second finger
765	right radial or ulnar second finger
766	left second finger nail unit
767	right second finger nail unit
768	left second finger NOS
769	right second finger NOS
770	left extensor third finger
771	right extensor third finger
772	left palmar third finger
773	right palmar third finger
774	left radial or ulnar third finger
775	right radial or ulnar third finger
776	left third finger nail unit
777	right third finger nail unit
778	left third finger NOS
779	right third finger NOS
780	left extensor fourth finger
781	right extensor fourth finger
782	left palmar fourth finger
783	right palmar fourth finger
784	left radial or ulnar fourth finger
785	right radial or ulnar fourth finger
786	left fourth finger nail unit
787	right fourth finger nail unit
788	left fourth finger NOS
789	right fourth finger NOS
790	left extensor fifth finger
791	right extensor fifth finger
792	left palmar fifth finger
793	right palmar fifth finger
794	left radial or ulnar fifth finger
795	right radial or ulnar fifth finger
796	left fifth finger nail unit
797	right fifth finger nail unit
798	left fifth finger NOS
799	right fifth finger NOS
Lower Extremities: 800–899	
800	left anterior thigh
801	right anterior thigh
802	left posterior thigh
803	right posterior thigh
804	left lateral thigh
805	right lateral thigh
806	left medial thigh
807	right medial thigh
808	left thigh NOS
809	right thigh NOS
810	thigh NOS
811	knee NOS
812	left knee
813	right knee
814	left popliteal area
815	right popliteal area
816	left lateral knee
817	right lateral knee
818	left medial knee
819	right medial knee
820	left anterior leg
821	right anterior leg
822	left posterior leg
823	right posterior leg
824	left lateral leg
825	right lateral leg
826	left medial leg
827	right medial leg
828	left leg NOS
829	right leg NOS
830	leg NOS
831	ankle NOS
832	left anterior ankle
833	right anterior ankle
834	left posterior ankle
835	right posterior ankle
836	left lateral ankle
837	right lateral ankle
838	left medial ankle
839	right medial ankle
840	left ankle NOS
841	right ankle NOS
842	left foot dorsum
843	right foot dorsum
844	left sole
845	right sole
846	left foot NOS
847	right foot NOS
848	foot NOS
849	toe NOS
850	left extensor first toe
851	right extensor first toe
852	left plantar first toe
853	right plantar first toe
854	left lateral or medial first toe
855	right lateral or medial first toe
856	left first toe nail unit
857	right first toe nail unit
858	left first toe NOS
859	right first toe NOS
860	left extensor second toe
861	right extensor second toe
862	left plantar second toe
863	right plantar second toe
864	left lateral or medial second toe
865	right lateral or medial second toe
866	left second toe nail unit
867	right second toe nail unit
868	left second toe NOS
869	right second toe NOS
870	left extensor third toe
871	right extensor third toe
872	left plantar third toe
873	right plantar third toe
874	left lateral or medial third toe
875	right lateral or medial third toe
876	left third toe nail unit
877	right third toe nail unit
878	left third toe NOS
879	right third toe NOS
880	left extensor fourth toe
881	right extensor fourth toe
882	left plantar fourth toe
883	right plantar fourth toe

Table continued on following page

TABLE 17–3. Site Codes and Body Sites *Continued*

Code	Body Site
Lower Extremities *Continued*	
884	left lateral or medial fourth toe
885	right lateral or medial fourth toe
886	left fourth toe nail unit
887	right fourth toe nail unit
888	left fourth toe NOS
889	right fourth toe NOS
890	left extensor fifth toe
891	right extensor fifth toe
892	left plantar fifth toe
893	right plantar fifth toe
894	left lateral or medial fifth toe
895	right lateral or medial fifth toe
896	left fifth toe nail unit
897	right fifth toe nail unit
898	left fifth toe NOS
899	right fifth toe NOS
Female Genitalia: 900–919	
900	left labia majora
901	right labia majora
902	labia majora NOS
904	left labia minora
905	right labia minora
906	labia minora NOS
910	clitoris
912	vagina
915	female urinary meatus
916	left vulva or female genitalia NOS
917	right vulva or female genitalia NOS
919	vulva or female genitalia NOS
Male Genitalia: 930–959	
930	left scrotum
931	right scrotum
932	scrotum NOS
934	left shaft of penis
935	right shaft of penis
936	dorsal shaft of penis
937	ventral shaft of penis
939	shaft of penis NOS
940	left foreskin
941	right foreskin
942	dorsal foreskin
943	ventral foreskin
944	foreskin NOS
945	left coronal sulcus
946	right coronal sulcus
947	dorsal coronal sulcus
948	ventral coronal sulcus
949	coronal sulcus NOS
950	left glans penis
951	right glans penis
952	dorsal glans penis
953	ventral glans penis
954	glans penis NOS
955	male urinary meatus
958	penis NOS
959	male genitalia NOS
Perineum and Perianal Areas: 970–989	
970	left perineum
971	right perineum
972	mid perineum
979	perineum NOS
980	left perianal area
981	right perianal area
982	anterior perianal area
983	posterior perianal area
984	perianal area NOS
989	anus

*NOS = not otherwise specified.

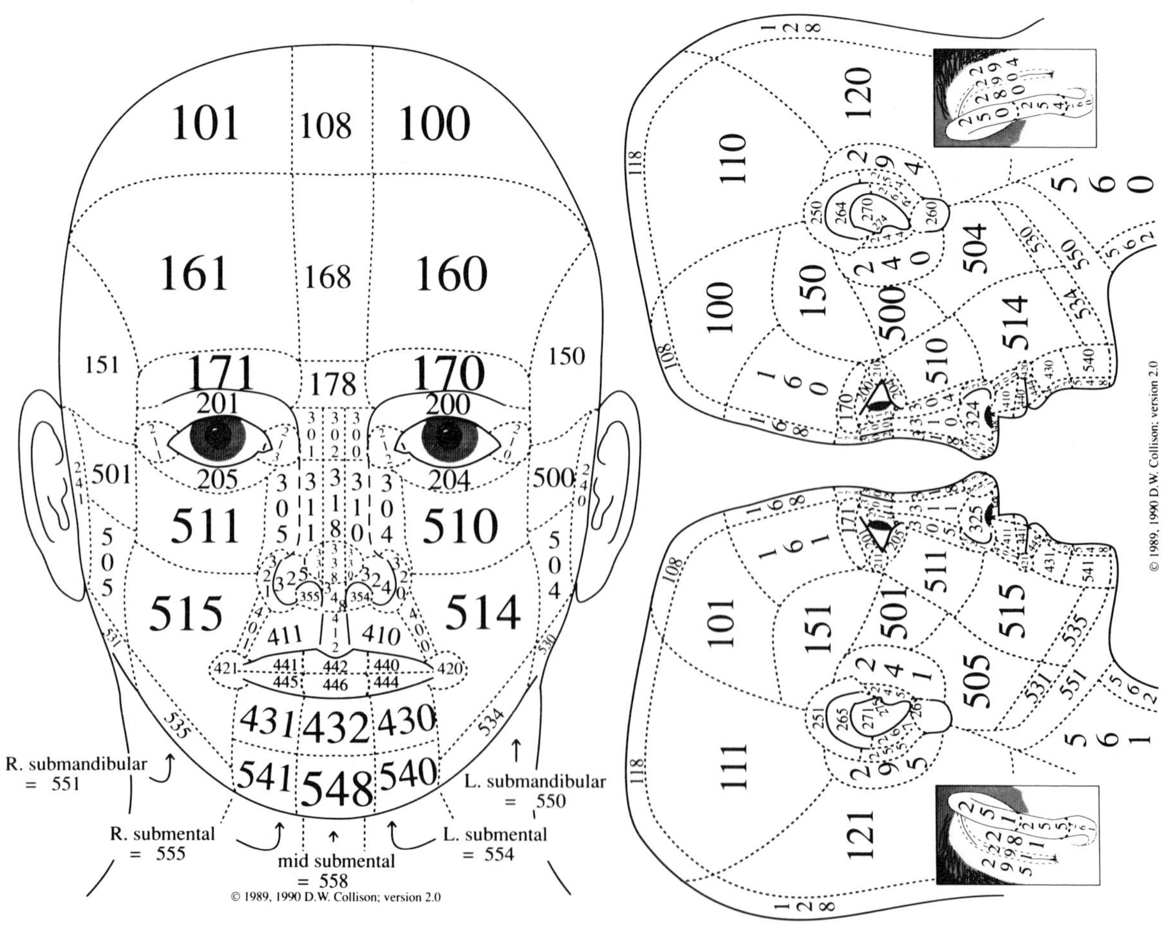

FIGURE 17–2. Head and neck diagrams with specific site codes. Copyright © Daniel W. Collison, M.D.

specific codes. Exceptions to these guidelines are made in order to preserve consistency of grouping of numbers.

In our study, all body sites affected by tumors were coded. This meant that large lesions or lesions that overlapped anatomic boundaries were assigned more than one code. For example, a lesion involving the left malar area, the left paranasal area, and the left dorsum of the nose was given all three site codes.

The types of skin tumors or conditions treated by MMS were also coded and grouped for ease of data entry and retrieval (Table 17–4). Whether the lesion had been previously treated was an important criterion; thus, categories for primary and recurrent tumors were delineated.

Lesions treated from 1968 through 1984 were identified in order to allow for at least a 5-year period of follow-up prior to the time of data evaluation (1990). Each treated lesion was given its own accession number so that the natural history of each individual lesion could be followed. Lesions that recurred were identified by a new accession number as well as by the accession number of the preceding lesion.

Each treated lesion was coded according to site, tumor type, and treatment outcome. The most specific codes for a given tumor type or tumor site were recorded. In many cases, however, data items were incomplete or missing. Site information was frequently nonspecific. The extensive use of nonspecific site codes in our coding system allowed the maximum amount of information to be preserved without assigning the data too much specificity. For example, a frequent problem was the use of the term "upper lip" or "lower lip," which did not indicate whether the cutaneous or vermilion lip was involved. These sites were denoted using a nonspecific code. This assured the integrity of the data; a study of lip lesions known to involve the mucous membranes would not be influenced by data representing nonmucosal tumors. Correspondingly, nonspecific tumor codes were also used. If a BCC was not specified as being primary or recurrent, it was coded as "BCC, type not otherwise specified," abbre-

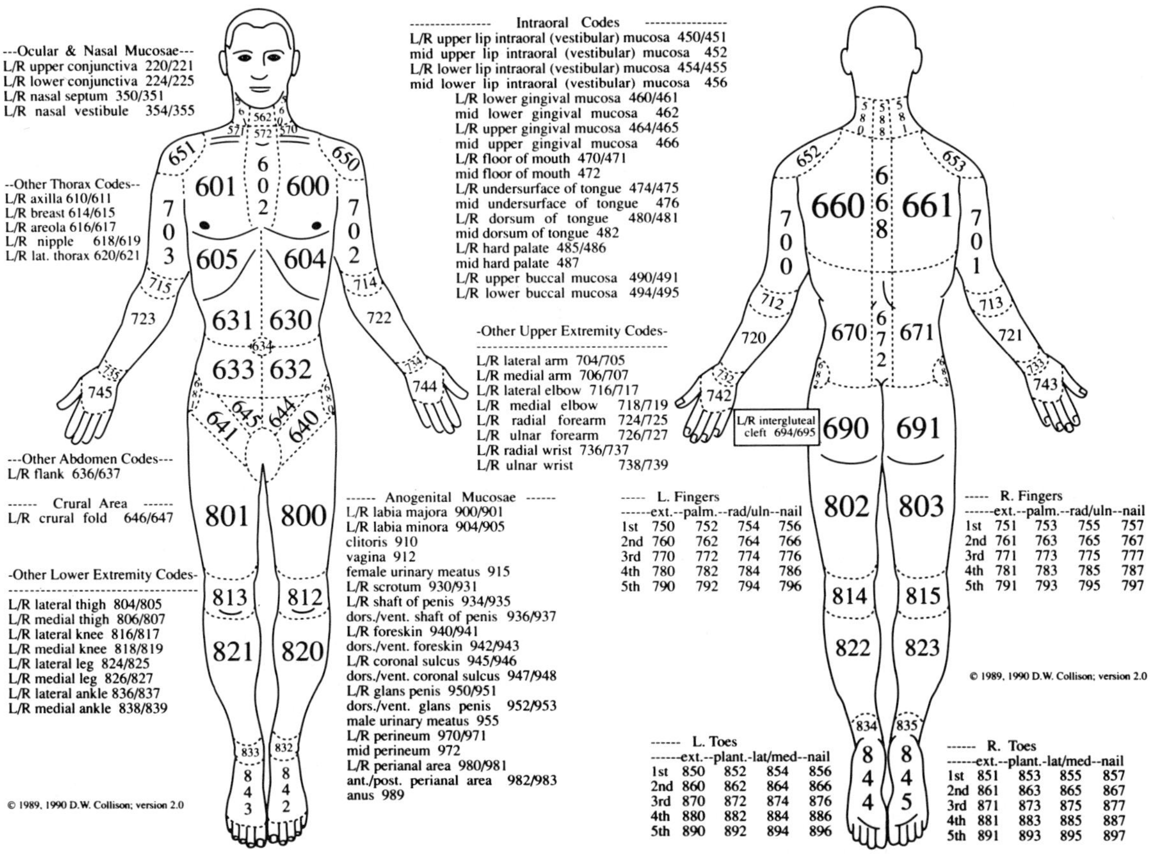

FIGURE 17–3. Diagrams of the trunk and extremities with specific site codes. Copyright © Daniel W. Collison, M.D.

TABLE 17–4. Tumor Codes and Types

N.	Not specified*	21.	Primary dermatofibrosarcoma protuberans
0.	See comments†	22.	Secondary dermatofibrosarcoma protuberans
1.	Primary basal cell carcinoma (BCC)	23.	Dermatofibrosarcoma protuberans NOS
2.	Recurrent BCC	24.	Lentigo maligna
3.	BCC NOS‡	25.	Lentigo maligna melanoma
4.	Sclerotic BCC	26.	Primary superficial spreading malignant melanoma
5.	Recurrent sclerotic BCC	27.	Recurrent superficial spreading malignant melanoma
6.	Metatypical ("basosquamous") BCC	28.	Primary nodular malignant melanoma
7.	Trichoepithelioma	29.	Seconary nodular malignant melanoma
8.	Recurrent trichoepithelioma	30.	Primary acral lentiginous malignant melanoma
9.	Desmoplastic trichoepithelioma	31.	Secondary acral lentiginous malignant melanoma
10.	Recurrent desmoplastic trichoepithelioma	32.	Primary malignant melanoma NOS
11.	Primary squamous cell carcinoma (SCC)	33.	Secondary malignant melanoma NOS
12.	Recurrent SCC	34.	Lymphangiosarcoma
13.	SCC NOS	35.	Nevus sebaceus
14.	Primary Bowen's disease	36.	Meningioma
15.	Recurrent Bowen's disease	37.	Metastatic carcinoma NOS
16.	Bowen's disease NOS	38.	Chronic ulcer
17.	Solitary keratoacanthoma	39.	Sebaceous carcinoma
18.	Recurrent solitary keratoacanthoma	40.	Eccrine carcinoma
19.	Primary verrucous carcinoma	41.	Apocrine carcinoma
20.	Recurrent verrucous carcinoma	42.	Paget's disease

*N is to be used if no data are available.
†O is to be used in cases in which the listed codes are not appropriate. An explanatory comment may be made in the "Comments" category.
‡NOS = Not otherwise specified.

viated "BCC NOS." It is obvious that more precise data could have been entered had our system been in place all along.

A microcomputer database was written to assist in the analysis of data. Coded data as shown in Table 17–1 were transferred from the index cards to the microcomputer by secretaries. Computer programs were used to detect errors both during and following data entry. Lesions were analyzed according to the following parameters:

1. Follow-up period
2. Tumor type
3. Tumor site (before treatment)
4. Tumor size (largest dimension of defect following excision)
5. Patient's sex
6. Treatment result (recurrence, cure, or indeterminate).

With regard to treatment results, lesions followed for more than 5 years without recurrence were considered cured. However, if the lesion recurred at the treated site after the 5-year cutoff, it was considered a recurrence. Patients with whom contact was lost or who died without tumor before the 5-year cutoff were considered indeterminate cases. Lesions that recurred after MMS were identified, and those that were cured by retreatment using MMS were separately tabulated.

RESULTS

Of the 4,484 patients referred by 413 physicians in the Great Lakes states and Ontario, 3,959 patients had BCC, and 427 patients had squamous cell carcinoma (SCC). Ninety-eight patients were treated for a variety of condi-

TABLE 17–5. Results of Treatment of Primary Basal Cell Carcinomas by Lesion Size

Sizes	Men	Women	Total Patients*	Total Lesions*	Lesions Lost from Follow-up	Lesions Lost Through Patient Death
<1 cm	30	62	92	109 (5.3%)	43	8
1–1.9 cm	326	345	671	777 (37.9%)	293	35
2–2.9 cm	221	154	375	423 (20.6%)	150	15
>2.9 cm	369	274	643	743 (36.2%)	252	46
Total	946	835	1,781	2,052 (100%)	738	104

*Lesions outnumber patients because some patients had more than one lesion.
†MMS = Mohs micrographic surgery.

tions, including solitary keratoacanthoma, malignant melanoma, and dermatofibrosarcoma protuberans. Of the BCC cases, 62% were followed for at least 5 years after treatment, and 32% were lost to follow-up because patients moved, returned to their local physician, or did not see any physician. Only 6% of the cases were lost to follow-up by the patient's death.

The results obtained by this study are shown in Tables 17–5 to 17–18 and are self-explanatory. They include patients with BCC and SCC (invasive and in situ) according to size and site of lesions as well as the sex distribution.

DISCUSSION

Previous large series of cases treated with MMS have resulted in cure rates approaching 99% for primary BCC and 94.4% for recurrent BCC. Our results for primary BCC indicate cure rates of 94.6% using one treatment, and 97.5% after retreatment of recurrent lesions. Cure rates for recurrent BCC are 90.0% using one treatment, and 96.2% after retreatment. Differences between our cure rates and previously published rates for BCC could arise through differences in study populations, surgical technique, or histologic interpretation.

Regarding our study population, our lower rate of cure may be due to the large size of lesions in our series: 36% of primary BCC and 47% of recurrent BCC were 3.0 cm or larger. Additionally, some cured patients may not have been included in the determinate category because a large percentage (38%) were lost to follow-up. We suspect that patients with recurrences were more likely to seek physician attention than those who were cured. This was supported by information obtained through periodic letter questionnaires and telephone calls made to obtain follow-up data about patients who did not return to us for continuing care. This task was complicated by the fact that over 400 physicians had referred patients for treatment.

In our series, the rate of failure for treatment of BCC was 2.5% for primary lesions (Table 17–5) and 3.8% for recurrent lesions (Table 17–6). Failure rates in summary data from previous MMS series have been 1% and 5.6%, respectively (see Table 1–2). This difference might well have arisen from the fact that our staff failed to designate the status of the tumor and simply recorded it as "BCC." These nonspecified lesions have been apportioned to each category using the ratio of the designations in other cases. However, it is significant that the ultimate failure rate in our series for all cases, primary and recurrent, was 3.2% (Table 17–7), a figure comparable to the average of the combined figures cited by Mohs in Table 1–2.

It is evident that the use of computers will increase and enhance the number of studies involving cutaneous oncology. Many of the problems of data collection, storage, and analysis have been partially solved through the use of computers. Kopf was a pioneer in this area. He designed a punch card system with a mainframe computer program that analyzed the characteristics of over 9,000 cutaneous tumors seen at New York University from 1954 through 1978.[4] In a similar fashion, Robins used a mainframe computer to analyze nearly 7,597 lesions in 6,954 patients who were treated by Mohs surgery at the same institutions.[5] In the 10 years since these computer studies were completed, the power and ease of use of computers have increased tremendously. Desktop microcomputers now can perform the functions of mainframe computers that took up an entire room when Kopf first designed his system. Individual researchers, with the aid of clerical help, can now perform computerized studies that formerly required the assistance of computer scientists.

Another advantage of using computer records is the ease of updating information on individual patients and individual lesions. Similarly, the disadvantage of computer records is that data may be electronically lost or cor-

Text continued on page 326

Total Indeterminate Lesions	Total Recurrent Lesions	Total Determinate Lesions	Cure Rate after One Treatment	Recurrences after MMS† Cured after Retreatment	Treatment Failures	Ultimate Cure Rate
51	2	58	96.55%			
328	19	449	95.77%			
165	13	258	94.96%			
298	31	445	93.03%			
842	65	1,210	94.63%	35	30	97.52%

TABLE 17–6. Results of Treatment of Recurrent Basal Cell Carcinomas by Lesion Size

Sizes	Men	Women	Total Patients*	Total Lesions*	Lesions Lost from Follow-up	Lesions Lost Through Patient Death
<1 cm	21	38	59	89 (3.4%)	27	6
1–1.9 cm	297	323	620	742 (28.2%)	224	31
2–2.9 cm	266	211	477	561 (21.3%)	165	27
>2.9 cm	588	434	1,022	1,236 (47.1%)	364	79
Total	1,172	1,006	2,178	2,628 (100%)	780	143

*Lesions outnumber patients because some patients had more than one lesion.
†MMS = Mohs micrographic surgery.

TABLE 17–7. Results of Treatment of All Basal Cell Carcinomas (Primary and Recurrent) by Lesion Size

Sizes	Men	Women	Total Patients*	Total Lesions*	Lesions Lost from Follow-up	Lesions Lost Through Patient Death
<1 cm	51	100	151	198 (4.2%)	70	14
1–1.9 cm	623	668	1,291	1,519 (32.5%)	517	66
2–2.9 cm	487	365	852	984 (21.0%)	315	42
>2.9 cm	957	708	1,665	1,979 (42.3%)	616	125
Total	2,118	1,841	3,959	4,680 (100%)	1,518	247

*Lesions outnumber patients because some patients had more than one lesion.
†MMS = Mohs micrographic surgery.

TABLE 17–8. Results of Treatment of Primary Basal Cell Carcinomas by Body Site

Sites	Men	Women	Total Patients*	Total Lesions*	Lesions Lost from Follow-up	Lesions Lost Through Patient Death
Nose	331	339	670	714	275	38
Ears	172	37	209	223	82	12
Eyelids	102	88	190	196	73	12
Cheeks	119	108	227	233	85	11
Chin	16	24	40	44	14	2
Forehead and temples	134	122	256	274	85	14
Lips	93	130	223	227	83	11
Scalp	24	25	49	53	21	3
Neck	25	10	35	34	16	1
Trunk and extremities	43	29	72	79	24	5
Anogenital area	1	1	2	2	1	0
Total‡	1,060	913	1,973	2,079	759	109

*Lesions outnumber patients because some patients had more than one lesion.
†MMS = Mohs micrographic surgery.
‡Totals add up to more than those in Table 17–5 because some lesions involved more than one coded site.

Total Indeterminate Lesions	Total Recurrent Lesions	Total Determinate Lesions	Cure Rate after One Treatment	Recurrences after MMS† Cured after Retreatment	Treatment Failures	Ultimate Cure Rate
33	5	56	91.07			
255	30	487	93.84			
192	27	369	92.68			
443	108	793	86.38			
923	170	1,705	90.03	106	64	96.25

Total Indeterminate Lesions	Total Recurrent Lesions	Total Determinate Lesions	Cure Rate after One Treatment	Recurrences after MMS† Cured after Retreatment	Treatment Failures	Ultimate Cure Rate
84	7	114	93.86			
583	49	936	94.76			
357	40	627	93.62			
741	139	1,238	88.77			
1,765	235	2,915	91.94	141	94	96.78

Total Indeterminate Lesions	Total Recurrent Lesions	Total Determinate Lesions	Cure Rate after One Treatment	Recurrences after MMS† Cured after Retreatment	Treatment Failures	Ultimate Cure Rate
313	17	401	95.76	9	8	98.00
94	10	129	92.25	7	3	97.67
85	9	111	91.89	2	7	93.69
96	8	137	94.16	3	5	96.35
16	1	28	96.43	1	0	100
99	13	175	92.57	8	5	97.14
94	10	133	92.48	4	6	95.49
24	2	29	93.10	2	0	100
17	1	17	94.12	1	0	100
29	2	50	96.00	1	1	98.00
1	0	1	100	0	0	100
868	73	1,211	93.97	38	35	97.11

TABLE 17–9. Results of Treatment of Recurrent Basal Cell Carcinomas by Body Site

Sites	Men	Women	Total Patients*	Total Lesions*	Lesions Lost from Follow-up	Lesions Lost Through Patient Death
Nose	381	406	787	865	272	55
Ears	185	41	226	259	72	17
Eyelids	102	68	170	195	51	13
Cheeks	142	131	273	294	90	12
Chin	17	26	43	45	11	2
Forehead and temples	219	192	411	461	127	17
Lips	105	155	260	285	86	13
Scalp	27	23	50	56	17	5
Neck	33	13	46	50	13	2
Trunk and extremities	64	34	98	111	29	5
Anogenital area	1	0	1	1	1	0
Total‡	1,276	1,089	2,365	2,622	769	141

*Lesions outnumber patients because some patients had more than one lesion.
†MMS = Mohs micrographic surgery.
‡Totals add up to more than those in Table 17–6 because some lesions involved more than one coded site.
**NA = Not applicable.

TABLE 17–10. Results of Treatment of All Basal Cell Carcinomas (Primary and Recurrent) by Body Site

Sites	Men	Women	Total Patients*	Total Lesions*	Lesions Lost from Follow-up	Lesions Lost Through Patient Death
Nose	712	745	1,457	1,579	547	93
Ears	357	78	435	482	154	29
Eyelids	204	156	360	391	124	25
Cheeks	261	239	500	527	175	23
Chin	33	50	83	89	25	4
Forehead and temples	353	314	667	735	212	31
Lips	198	285	483	512	169	24
Scalp	51	48	99	109	38	8
Neck	58	23	81	84	29	3
Trunk and extremities	107	63	170	190	53	10
Anogenital area	2	1	3	3	2	0
Total‡	2,336	2,002	4,338	4,701	1,528	250

*Lesions outnumber patients because some patients had more than one lesion.
†MMS = Mohs micrographic surgery.
‡Totals add up to more than those in Table 17–7 because some lesions involved more than one coded site.

TABLE 17–11. Results of Treatment of Primary Invasive Squamous Cell Carcinomas by Lesion Size

Sizes	Men	Women	Total Patients*	Total Lesions*	Lesions Lost from Follow-up	Lesions Lost Through Patient Death
<1 cm	4	2	6	6 (3.0%)	2	0
1–1.9 cm	26	20	46	53 (26.8%)	18	4
2–2.9 cm	28	11	39	45 (22.7%)	18	9
>2.9 cm	65	22	87	94 (47.4%)	39	7
Total	123	55	178	198 (100%)	77	20

*Lesions outnumber patients because some patients had more than one lesion.
†MMS = Mohs micrographic surgery.

Total Indeterminate Lesions	Total Recurrent Lesions	Total Determinate Lesions	Cure Rate after One Treatment	Recurrences after MMS† Cured after Retreatment	Treatment Failures	Ultimate Cure Rate
327	37	538	93.12	26	11	97.96
89	27	170	84.12	21	6	96.47
64	21	131	83.97	15	6	95.42
102	15	192	92.19	6	9	95.31
13	1	32	96.88	1	0	100
144	31	317	90.22	14	17	94.64
99	21	186	88.71	13	8	95.70
22	3	34	91.18	1	2	94.12
15	1	35	97.14	1	0	100
34	9	77	88.31	5	4	94.81
1	0	0	NA**	0	0	NA
910	166	1,712	90.30	103	63	96.32

Total Indeterminate Lesions	Total Recurrent Lesions	Total Determinate Lesions	Cure Rate after One Treatment	Recurrences after MMS† Cured after Retreatment	Treatment Failures	Ultimate Cure Rate
640	54	939	94.25	35	19	97.98
183	37	299	87.63	28	9	96.99
149	30	242	87.60	17	13	94.63
198	23	329	93.01	9	14	95.74
29	2	60	96.67	2	0	100
243	44	492	91.06	22	22	95.53
193	31	319	90.28	17	14	95.61
46	5	63	92.06	3	2	96.83
32	2	52	96.15	2	0	100
63	11	127	91.34	6	5	96.06
2	0	1	100	0	0	100
1,778	239	2,923	91.82	141	98	96.65

Total Indeterminate Lesions	Total Recurrent Lesions	Total Determinate Lesions	Cure Rate after One Treatment	Recurrences after MMS† Cured after Retreatment	Treatment Failures	Ultimate Cure Rate
2	0	4	100			
22	3	31	90.32			
27	2	18	88.89			
46	8	48	83.33			
97	13	101	87.13	3	10	90.10

TABLE 17–12. Results of Treatment of Recurrent Invasive Squamous Cell Carcinomas by Lesion Size

Sizes	Men	Women	Total Patients*	Total Lesions*	Lesions Lost from Follow-up	Lesions Lost Through Patient Death
<1 cm	4	0	4	4 (2%)	2	0
1–1.9 cm	16	12	28	34 (17%)	10	3
2–2.9 cm	26	10	36	42 (21%)	14	5
>2.9 cm	80	23	103	120 (60%)	43	10
Total	126	45	171	200 (100%)	69	18

*Lesions outnumber patients because some patients had more than one lesion.
†MMS = Mohs micrographic surgery.

TABLE 17–13. Results of Treatment of All Invasive Squamous Cell Carcinomas (Primary and Recurrent) by Lesion Size

Sizes	Men	Women	Total Patients*	Total Lesions*	Lesions Lost from Follow-up	Lesions Lost Through Patient Death
<1 cm	8	2	10	10 (2.5%)	4	0
1–1.9 cm	42	32	74	87 (21.9%)	28	7
2–2.9 cm	54	21	75	87 (21.9%)	32	14
>2.9 cm	145	45	190	214 (53.7%)	82	17
Total	249	100	349	398 (100%)	146	38

*Lesions outnumber patients because some patients had more than one lesion.
†MMS = Mohs micrographic surgery.

TABLE 17–14. Results of Treatment of Primary Invasive Squamous Cell Carcinomas by Body Site

Sites	Men	Women	Total Patients*	Total Lesions*	Lesions Lost from Follow-up	Lesions Lost Through Patient Death
Nose	22	14	36	35	13	3
Ears	33	1	34	35	13	8
Eyelids	6	3	9	9	2	2
Cheeks	15	10	25	26	10	1
Chin	0	1	1	1	1	0
Forehead and temples	16	10	26	27	13	4
Lips	14	8	22	24	10	5
Scalp	10	0	10	10	4	2
Neck	2	1	3	3	1	0
Trunk and extremities	13	11	24	25	12	2
Anogenital area	8	1	9	11	3	0
Oral	0	0	0	0	0	0
Total‡	139	60	199	206	82	27

*Lesions outnumber patients because some patients had more than one lesion.
†MMS = Mohs micrographic surgery.
‡Totals add up to more than those in Table 17–11 because some lesions involved more than one coded site.
**NA = Not applicable.

Total Indeterminate Lesions	Total Recurrent Lesions	Total Determinate Lesions	Cure Rate after One Treatment	Recurrences after MMS† Cured after Retreatment	Treatment Failures	Ultimate Cure Rate
2	0	2	100			
13	3	21	85.71			
19	2	23	91.30			
53	20	67	70.15			
87	25	113	77.88	14	11	90.27

Total Indeterminate Lesions	Total Recurrent Lesions	Total Determinate Lesions	Cure Rate after One Treatment	Recurrences after MMS† Cured after Retreatment	Treatment Failures	Ultimate Cure Rate
4	0	6	100			
35	6	52	88.46			
46	4	41	90.24			
99	28	115	75.65			
184	38	214	82.24	17	21	90.19

Total Indeterminate Lesions	Total Recurrent Lesions	Total Determinate Lesions	Cure Rate after One Treatment	Recurrences after MMS† Cured after Retreatment	Treatment Failures	Ultimate Cure Rate
16	3	19	84.21	0	3	84.21
19	3	16	81.25	1	2	87.50
4	0	5	100	0	0	100
11	2	15	86.67	0	2	86.67
1	0	0	NA**	0	0	NA
16	2	11	81.82	0	2	81.82
13	1	11	90.91	0	1	90.91
6	1	4	75.00	0	1	75.00
1	0	2	100	0	0	100
14	2	11	81.82	0	2	81.82
3	3	8	62.50	1	2	75.00
0	0	0	NA	0	0	NA
104	17	102	83.33	2	15	85.29

TABLE 17–15. Results of Treatment of Recurrent Invasive Squamous Cell Carcinomas by Body Site

Sites	Males	Females	Total Patients*	Total Lesions*	Lesions Lost from Follow-up	Lesions Lost Through Patient Death
Nose	26	12	38	41	13	3
Ears	24	1	25	31	6	3
Eyelids	6	1	7	8	1	0
Cheeks	17	4	21	28	8	3
Chin	0	0	0	0	0	0
Forehead and temples	12	6	18	23	10	2
Lips	12	5	17	18	9	0
Scalp	6	1	7	9	6	0
Neck	2	2	4	4	2	1
Trunk and extremities	14	10	24	24	8	0
Anogenital area	9	0	9	11	2	0
Oral	1	0	1	1	0	0
Total‡	129	42	171	198	65	12

*Lesions outnumber patients because some patients had more than one lesion.
†MMS = Mohs micrographic surgery.
‡Totals add up to more than those in Table 17–12 because some lesions involved more than one coded site.
**NA = Not applicable.

TABLE 17–16. Results of Treatment of All Invasive Squamous Cell Carcinomas (Primary and Recurrent) by Body Site

Sites	Men	Women	Total Patients*	Total Lesions*	Lesions Lost from Follow-up	Lesions Lost Through Patient Death
Nose	48	26	74	76	26	6
Ears	57	2	59	66	19	11
Eyelids	12	4	16	17	3	2
Cheeks	32	14	46	54	18	4
Chin	0	1	1	1	1	0
Forehead and temples	28	16	44	50	23	6
Lips	26	13	39	42	19	5
Scalp	16	1	17	19	10	2
Neck	4	3	7	7	3	1
Trunk and extremities	27	21	48	49	20	2
Anogenital area	17	1	18	22	5	0
Oral	1	0	1	1	0	0
Total‡	268	102	370	404	147	39

*Lesions outnumber patients because some patients had more than one lesion.
†MMS = Mohs micrographic surgery.
‡Totals add up to more than those in Table 17–13 because some lesions involved more than one coded site.
**NA = Not applicable.

TABLE 17–17. Results of Treatment of All In Situ Squamous Cell Carcinomas (Primary and Recurrent) by Lesion Size

Sizes	Men	Women	Total Patients*	Total Lesions*	Lesions Lost from Follow-up	Lesions Lost Through Patient Death
<1 cm	2	1	3	3 (3.5%)	1	0
1–1.9 cm	13	6	19	20 (23.5%)	7	2
2–2.9 cm	10	6	16	18 (21.2%)	2	2
>2.9 cm	25	15	40	44 (51.8%)	22	5
Total	50	28	78	85 (100%)	32	9

*Lesions outnumber patients because some patients had more than one lesion.
†MMS = Mohs micrographic surgery.

Total Indeterminate Lesions	Total Recurrent Lesions	Total Determinate Lesions	Cure Rate after One Treatment	Recurrences after MMS† Cured after Retreatment	Treatment Failures	Ultimate Cure Rate
16	3	25	88.00	0	3	88.00
11	5	20	75.00	5	0	100
1	2	7	71.43	1	1	85.71
11	4	17	76.47	1	3	82.35
0	0	0	NA**	0	0	NA
13	5	10	50.00	4	1	90.00
11	3	7	57.14	0	3	57.14
6	0	3	100	0	0	100
3	0	1	100	0	0	100
8	0	16	100	0	0	100
2	2	9	77.78	2	0	100
0	1	1	0	0	1	0
82	25	116	78.45	13	12	89.66

Total Indeterminate Lesions	Total Recurrent Lesions	Total Determinate Lesions	Cure Rate after One Treatment	Recurrences after MMS† Cured after Retreatment	Treatment Failures	Ultimate Cure Rate
32	6	44	86.36	0	6	86.36
30	8	36	77.78	6	2	94.44
5	2	12	83.33	1	1	91.67
22	6	32	81.25	1	5	84.38
1	0	0	NA**	0	0	NA
29	7	21	66.67	4	3	85.71
24	4	18	77.78	0	4	77.78
12	1	7	85.71	0	1	85.71
4	0	3	100	0	0	100
22	2	27	92.59	0	2	92.59
5	5	17	70.59	3	2	88.24
0	1	1	0	0	1	0
186	42	218	80.73	15	27	87.61

Total Indeterminate Lesions	Total Recurrent Lesions	Total Determinate Lesions	Cure Rate after One Treatment	Recurrences after MMS† Cured after Retreatment	Treatment Failures	Ultimate Cure Rate
1	1	2	50.00			
9	2	11	81.82			
4	1	14	92.86			
27	1	17	94.12			
41	5	44	88.64	1	4	90.91

TABLE 17–18. Results of Treatment of All In Situ Squamous Cell Carcinomas (Primary and Recurrent) by Body Site

Sites	Men	Women	Total Patients*	Total Lesions*	Lesions Lost from Follow-up	Lesions Lost Through Patient Death
Nose	0	2	2	2	1	0
Ears	4	2	6	6	1	3
Eyelids	0	0	0	0	0	0
Cheeks	3	1	4	4	3	0
Chin	0	0	0	0	0	0
Forehead and temples	3	3	6	6	2	1
Lips	0	0	0	0	0	0
Scalp	2	0	2	2	2	0
Neck	2	0	2	2	0	1
Trunk and extremities	23	12	35	42	14	2
Anogenital area	15	6	21	21	8	2
Oral	0	0	0	0	0	0
Total‡	52	26	78	85	31	9

*Lesions outnumber patients because some patients had more than one lesion.
†MMS = Mohs micrographic surgery.
‡Totals add up to more than those in Table 17–17 because some lesions involved more than one coded site.
**NA = Not applicable.

rupted. We recommend making backup copies of data in both electronic and paper form.

A microcomputer-based MMS database in a surgeon's office can also be coordinated to handle routine office paperwork, such as using the same data to prepare operative notes and letters to referring physicians. We plan to use our database to automate the next generation of follow-up questionnaires to referring physicians, a task done manually in the past. The microcomputer database will prepare lists of patients sent by each referring physician, giving the patient's name, date of birth, date of treatment, tumor type, and tumor site. Better fol-

TABLE 17–19. Suggested Mohs Micrographic Surgery Database Categories

1. Lesion accession number
2. Previous lesion accession number (if any)
3. Patient name
4. Patient medical record number
5. Sex of patient
6. Race of patient (see Table 17–20)
7. Date of birth of patient
8. Allergies
9. Risk factors (if any; see Table 17–21)
10. Previous treatment (if any; list each treatment type and number of times; see Table 17–22)
11. Resuscitation status (e.g., "CPR only, do not intubate.")
12. Date(s) of surgery
13. Surgeon number
14. Preoperative biopsy number
15. Tumor type (see Table 17–4)
16. Site(s) before treatment (see Table 17–3)
17. Tumor length before treatment
18. Tumor width before treatment
19. Tumor depth before treatment
20. Treatment (see Table 17–22)
21. Site(s) after treatment (see Table 17–3)
22. Defect length after treatment
23. Defect width after treatment
24. Defect depth after treatment
25. Debulking performed (if any)
26. Layers required
27. Sections required
28. Frozen-section biopsy number (if any)
29. Frozen-section slide number(s)
30. Permanent section biopsy number(s) (if any)
31. Intraoperative procedures used (if any)
32. Method of healing/closure (see Table 17–23)
33. Deep suture (if any)
34. Superficial suture
35. Dressings
36. Adjunct perioperative therapies (if any)
37. Adjunct postoperative therapies (if any)
38. Date of last follow-up
39. Complications (if any; see Table 17–24)
40. Date of recurrence (if any)
41. Date of death (if any)
42. Referring physician
43. Comments

Ancillary Data

44. Patient address
45. Patient phone number
46. Emergency contact
47. Emergency contact phone number
48. Kodachrome slide numbers
49. Date follow-up questionnaire sent
50. Date follow-up questionnaire received
51. Time interval for next follow-up

Total Indeterminate Lesions	Total Recurrent Lesions	Total Determinate Lesions	Cure Rate after One Treatment	Recurrences after MMS† Cured after Retreatment	Treatment Failures	Ultimate Cure Rate
1	0	1	100	0	0	100
4	0	2	100	0	0	100
0	0	0	NA**	0	0	NA
3	0	1	100	0	0	100
0	0	0	NA	0	0	NA
3	1	3	66.67	0	1	66.67
0	0	0	NA	0	0	NA
2	0	0	NA	0	0	NA
1	0	1	100	0	0	100
16	3	26	88.46	0	3	88.46
10	1	11	90.91	0	1	90.91
0	0	0	NA	0	0	NA
40	5	45	88.89	0	5	88.89

low-up data will certainly be obtained by using this method.

Whatever system is used to keep track of MMS cases, applying that system retrospectively is an effective way to test it before applying it to prospective studies. Our prospective cases will now be followed with a more detailed database according to the characteristics and variables listed in Tables 17–19 through 17–24.

In summary, as MMS is being more widely used, accurate data will be collected regarding its overall efficacy and the efficacy of changing individual variables in the technique. Comparison between the cure rates of individual surgeons may reveal the elements important in achieving cures. Also, valuable information can be made readily available about the results obtained with different types of tumors, new surgical techniques, and other therapeutic modalities. Carefully designed studies with meticulous data collection and analysis will help analyze these variables. The tables and figures in this chapter are provided to assist in data collection.

TABLE 17–20. Race Codes

N. Not specified*
0. See comments†
1. White
2. Black
3. Oriental
4. Native American

*N is to be used if no data are available.
†O is to be used in cases in which the listed codes are not appropriate. An explanataory comment may be made in the "Comments" category.

TABLE 17–21. Risk Factors

N. Not specified*
0. See comments†
1. Recreational actinic damage
2. Occupational actinic damage
3. Actinic damage not otherwise specified
4. History of (other) basal cell carcinoma
5. History of (other) squamous cell carcinoma
6. History of (other) malignant melanoma
7. History of actinic keratoses
8. Previous actinic keratosis at site
9. Other cutaneous malignancy
10. Phototherapy NOS or NEC‡
11. Psoralen and ultraviolet A (PUVA) therapy
12. Ultraviolet B therapy
13. Ionizing radiation (x-ray)
14. Radium implants
15. Immunosuppressive therapy
16. Arsenic exposure
17. Lymphoma
18. Leukemia
19. Other noncutaneous malignancy
20. Other immunosuppressed state
21. Basal cell nevus syndrome
22. Xeroderma pigmentosum
23. Dysplastic nevus syndrome
24. Other genodermatosis
25. Chronic scar
26. Chronic skin ulcer
27. Chronic inflammation
28. Coronary artery disease
29. Diabetes mellitus
30. Bleeding disorder
31. Pacemaker
32. Cardiac dysrhythmia
33. Epinephrine sensitivity
34. History of hypertrophic scarring or keloids
35. History of hepatitis (any type)
36. Positive for antibodies to Human Immunodeficiency Virus-1 (HIV-1)

*N is to be used if no data are available.
†O is to be used in cases in which the listed codes are not appropriate. An explanatory comment may be made in the "Comments" category.
‡NOS = not otherwise specified; NEC = not classified elsewhere.

TABLE 17–22. Treatment Codes

N. Not specified*
0. See comments†
1. Mohs fresh tissue technique
2. Mohs fixed tissue technique
3. Mohs fresh and fixed tissue techniques (both)
4. Mohs fresh tissue technique (intermittent)
5. Mohs fixed tissue technique (intermittent)
6. Mohs fresh and fixed tissue techniques (both, intermittent)
7. Mohs surgery not otherwise specified
8. Excision
9. Electrosurgery and curettage
10. Electrosurgery only
11. Curettage only
12. Cryotherapy
13. Cryotherapy with thermocouple
14. Ionizing radiation (x-ray)
15. Grenz ray
16. Topical 5-fluorouracil
17. Other topical chemotherapy
18. Systemic chemotherapy
19. Flap
20. Graft
21. Inpatient
22. No previous treatment

*N is to be used if no data are available.
†O is to be used in cases in which the listed codes are not appropriate. An explanatory comment may be made in the "Comments" category.

TABLE 17–23. Closure Codes

N. Not specified*
0. See comments†
1. Primary closure NOS‡
2. Second intention
3. Layered closure
4. Partial closure
5. Side-to-side
6. Burow's triangle
7. M-plasty
8. Z-plasty
9. Rhomboid flap
10. Bilobed flap
11. Island advancement flap
12. A-to-T plasty
13. O-to-T plasty
14. O-to-Z plasty
15. V-to-Y plasty
16. Y-to-V plasty
17. Advancement flap NEC§ or NOS
18. Rotation flap NEC or NOS
19. Transposition flap NEC or NOS
20. Flap NOS or NEC
21. Split-thickness skin graft
22. Full-thickness skin graft
23. Skin graft NOS
24. By plastic surgeon NOS
25. By oculoplastic surgeon NOS
26. By head and neck surgeon NOS
27. By dermatologic surgeon NOS

*N is to be used if no data are available
†O is to be used in cases in which the listed codes are not appropriate. An explanatory comment may be made in the "Comments" category.
‡NOS = Not otherwise specified.
§NEC = Not elsewhere classified.

TABLE 17–24. Complication Codes

N. Not specified*
0. See comments†
1. Wound infection
2. Necrosis involving flap
3. Necrosis NOS or NEC‡
4. Hematoma
5. Hemorrhage requiring hospitalization or transfusion
6. Hemorrhage NOS or NEC
7. Dehiscence before suture removal
8. Dehiscence after suture removal
9. Dehiscence NOS
10. Sloughing of graft
11. Subsequent ulceration of grafted site
12. Hypertrophic scar
13. Keloid
14. Stitch abscess
15. Suture splitting
16. Perforation of normal structure, e.g., pinna
17. Ectropion
18. Eclabium
19. Stenosis, e.g., of nares or ear canal
20. Other distortion of anatomy or poor cosmesis
21. Fistula
22. Paresthesia
23. Anesthesia
24. Motor palsy
25. Neurologic damage NOS or NEC
26. Local lymphadenopathy
27. Local lymphatic metastasis
28. Distant metastasis
29. Cardiac arrhythmia
30. Myocardial infarction
31. Stroke
32. Hepatitis (any type)
33. Death

*N is to be used if no data are available.
†O is to be used in cases in which the listed codes are not appropriate.
‡NOS = Not otherwise specified; NEC = Not elsewhere classified.

REFERENCES

1. Rowe DE, Carroll RJ, Day CL: Long-term recurrence rates in previously untreated (primary) basal cell carcinoma: Implications for patient follow-up, J Dermatol Surg Oncol 15:315–328, 1989.
2. Rowe DE, Carroll RJ, Day CL: Mohs surgery is the treatment of choice for recurrent (previously treated) basal cell carcinoma, J Dermatol Surg Oncol 15:424–431, 1989.
3. Kopf AW: Organization and function of an oncology service for skin tumors. In Andrade R, Gumport SL, Popkin GL, Rees TD (eds.): Cancer of the Skin. Philadelphia: W. B. Saunders, 1976, pp 6–15.
4. Kopf AW: Computer analysis of 3531 basal-cell carcinomas of the skin, J Dermatol (Tokyo) 6:267–281, 1979.
5. Robins P: Chemosurgery: My 15 years of experience, J Dermatol Surg Oncol 7(10):779–789, 1981.

CHAPTER 18

Maxillofacial Prosthetics

Robert A. Mohr, B.A.

Maxillofacial prosthetics are always a consideration in Mohs micrographic surgery because any degree of disfigurement is a major concern to patients and often becomes as psychologically damaging as the initial diagnosis of cancer. Therefore, to reduce the apprehension and anxiety associated with a potentially disfiguring procedure, corrective plastic surgical reconstruction and/or a temporary or permanent prosthesis should be thoroughly discussed. If available, good photographic examples of corrective postoperative reconstructive plastic surgery results as well as various prostheses are also recommended.

If the operative plan involves ablation of the ear or nose or extensive periorbital or maxillary excisions, it is advisable to obtain a preoperative mold of the anatomic area. For optimal results, the mold should have a 2 to 3 cm margin beyond the primary site, providing the affected area has not been too badly distorted. This procedure serves the dual purpose of producing a very close replica of the specimen to be removed and indicates the restoration of the surrounding area that may be involved. Good quality preoperative photographic color slides or prints are also recommended for the patient record and for the plastic surgeon's and prosthetist's reference.

Because this chapter primarily addresses the needs of patients with concomitant external facial defects from Mohs micrographic surgery and/or preexisting eroded cancerous lesions, intraoral, deep mandibular, and maxillary reconstruction techniques are not discussed.

Following surgery, it is very important that the healing process and contracture of the surrounding tissue is complete before an impression is made of the defect. If the patient is very anxious to have the area replaced, a temporary prosthesis can be fashioned, but this should be attached with great caution and never affixed to a fresh graft or granulating area.

REFERRALS

Neither the prosthetic practitioner's credentials nor the size of their affiliated institution should be the sole basis for patient referrals. There are many highly skilled prosthodontists, prosthetists, and medical illustrators who do excellent work. It is, therefore, incumbent upon the referring physicians to familiarize themselves with the work of the prosthetist before the referral. Many times, an optimal result will require a team effort involving the cooperation of the dermatologist, plastic surgeon, and prosthodontist or prosthetist.

ADVANTAGES AND DISADVANTAGES

When a prosthesis is recommended as an alternative to plastic surgery, the patient should be thoroughly versed in the positive and negative aspects of the appliance. The disadvantages are the adhesive applications and removal of adhesive from the prosthesis and the skin every

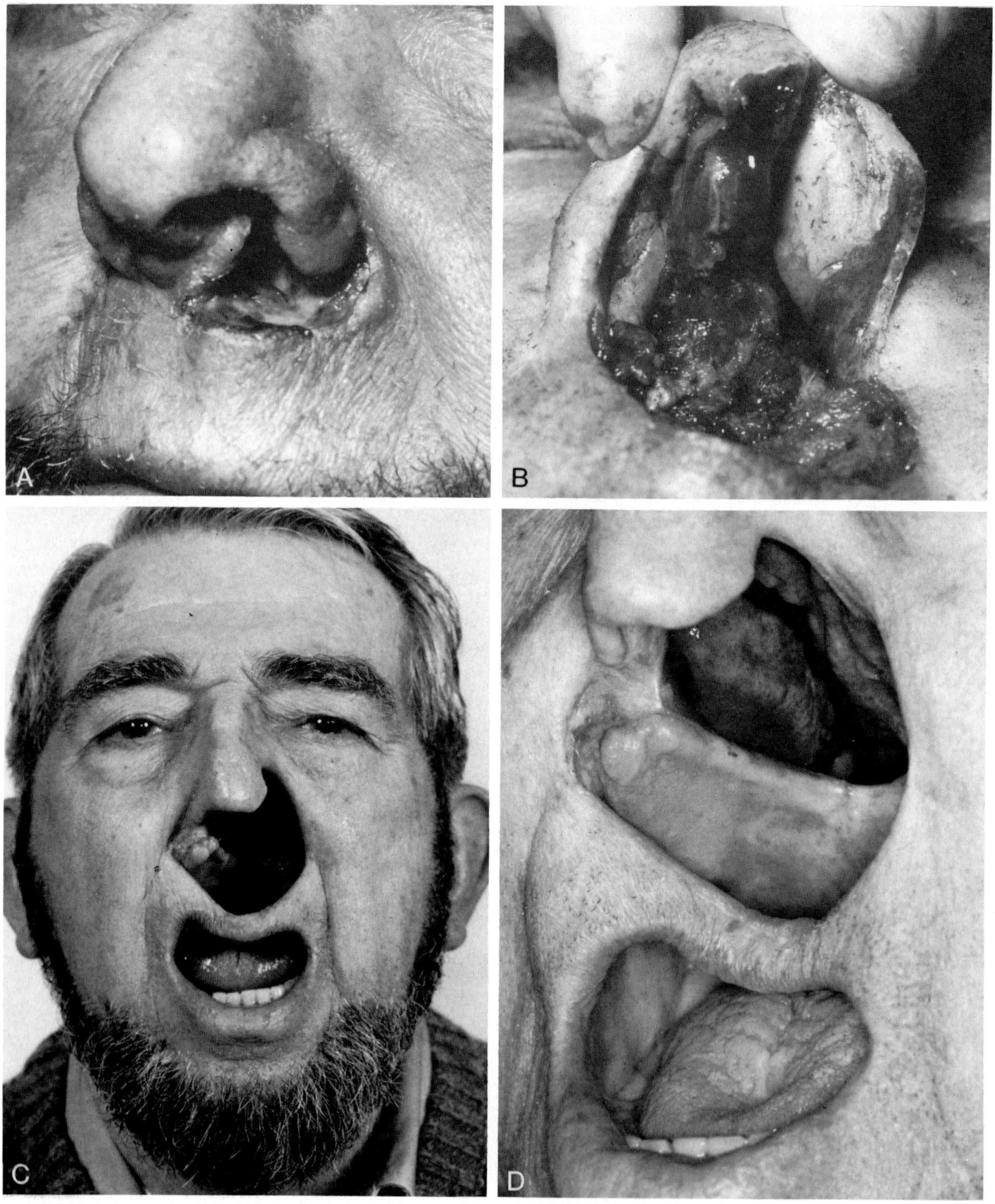

FIGURE 18–1. *A*, Squamous cell carcinoma of nose and left upper lip. *B*, Result after Mohs surgery; because the palate and maxilla were involved, they were partially resected by otolaryngologist, Dr. Jack L. Clark. *C*, Final result after surgery; note the defect in the nose, maxilla, and palate. *D*, Intraoral palate defect.

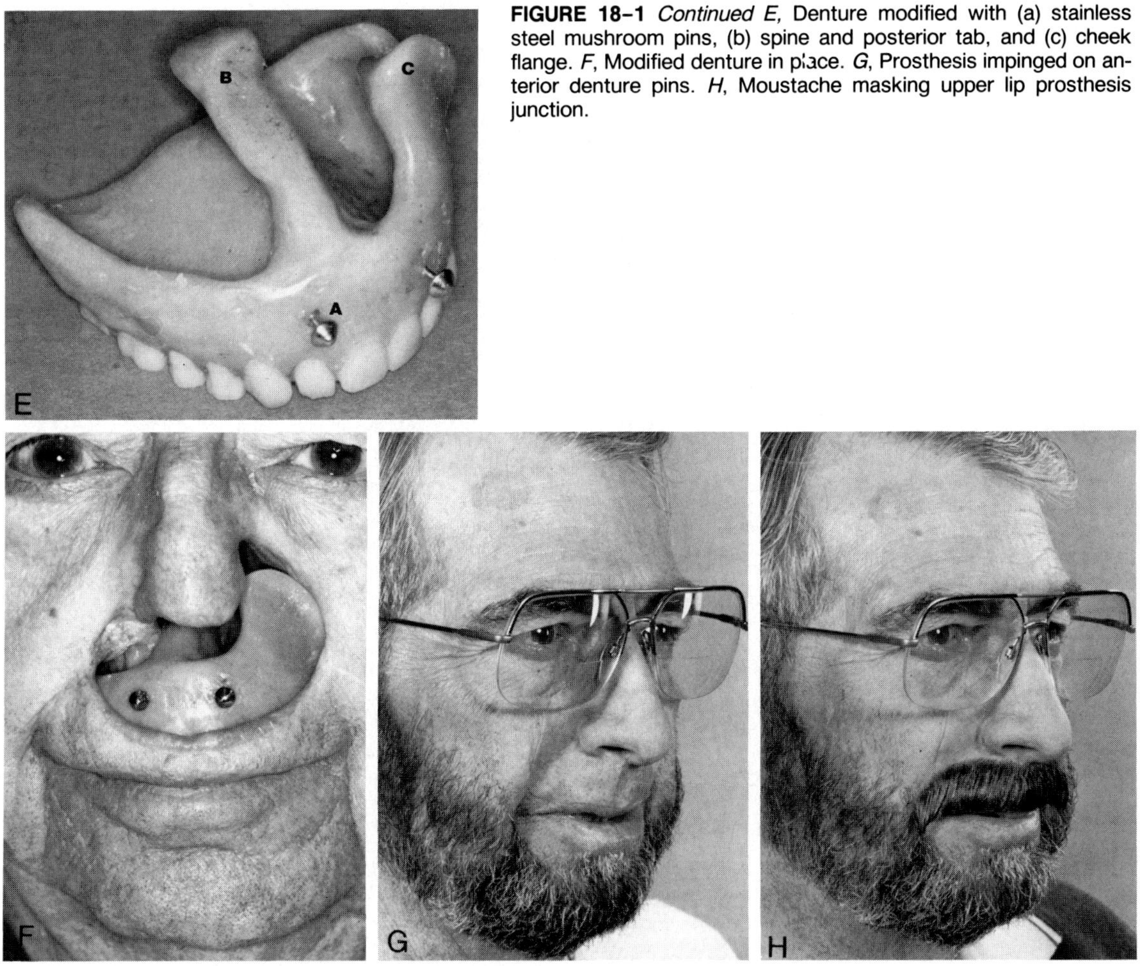

FIGURE 18–1 *Continued E,* Denture modified with (a) stainless steel mushroom pins, (b) spine and posterior tab, and (c) cheek flange. *F,* Modified denture in place. *G,* Prosthesis impinged on anterior denture pins. *H,* Moustache masking upper lip prosthesis junction.

other day, plus the periodic need for a new prosthesis. The advantage is that it does not usually require additional surgical procedures which may involve skin grafts with added patient recovery periods. When produced by a competent prosthetist, the results are usually much more natural looking than reconstructed surgical areas.

MATERIALS AND FABRICATION

There are many types of materials for fabricating prostheses, including methyl methacrylate, vinyl polymers, copolymers, urethane, latex, and silicones. The choice is dictated by the anatomic part to be replaced, its function (fixed or mobile), the size of the defect, and to some degree, the ability of the recipient to properly manage and care for the prosthesis.

In the fabrication process, the minor skin color variations are mixed into the base material and thickly deposited into the mold. This is followed by the larger deposit of base color material which is mixed with red and violet fibers to simulate arteries and veins, thus providing durable intrinsic coloring. The mold is packed with this material and clamped tightly during the curing process. When the prosthesis is removed from the mold and appropriately trimmed, it is placed on the patient. Additional tinting can be applied followed by a clear coat with a matte finish to complete the prosthesis.

The acceptable aesthetic life of the prosthesis varies greatly from a few months to many years. Factors influencing durability include careful attention to cleaning, the thickness of the leading edges, and delicate removal of the prosthesis from the skin.

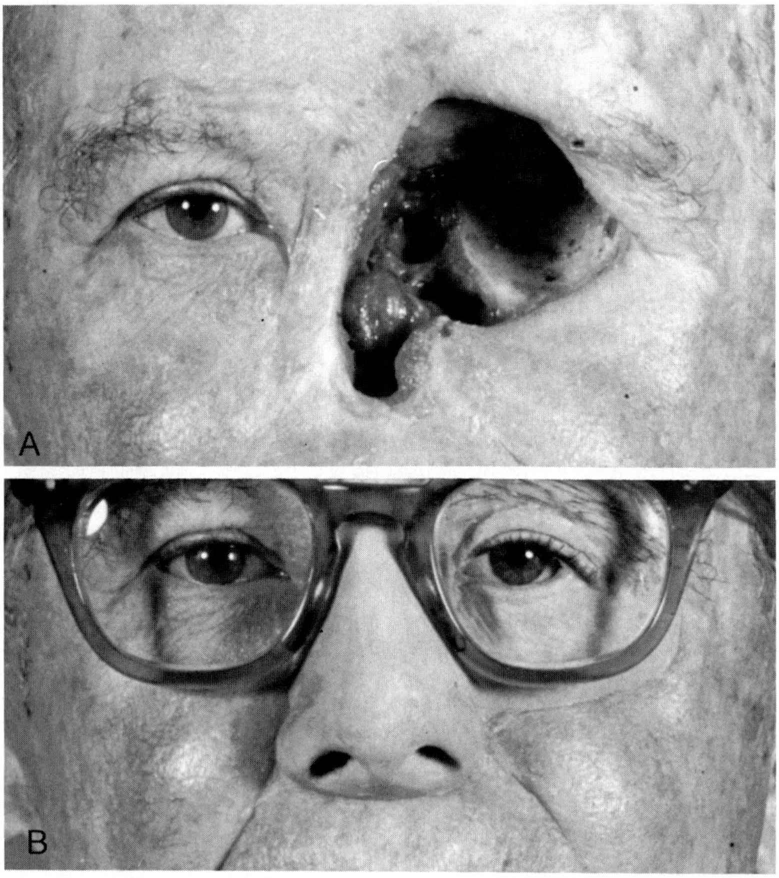

FIGURE 18–2. *A*, Postsurgical defects after removing a basal cell carcinoma. *B*, Silicone prosthesis with acrylic eye inset.

RETENTION

Various types of adhesives range from latex-based cements, silicone, double-sided tape, clips, and magnets combined with osseointegration.

Osseointegration fixtures with paired magnets are preferred over clip-type attachments. In either case, the implant abutment supports are anchored subdermally into the cranial skeleton and allowed to integrate into the bone for 5 or 6 months. Then the skin over the fixtures is removed, and gold abutment alloy cylinders are screwed into the implants to support a fabricated bridge. Magnets are strategically incorporated into both the bridge and prosthesis.

If applicable, this method is far superior to various types of adhesive retention. It is more positive and accurate and eliminates the need for routine adhesive application and removal, thus preserving the delicate edges and color from degradation.

Standard methodology for the best retention of the prosthesis is thorough cleansing of the skin followed by a light wipe with an alcohol pledget and application of a clear skin preparation. The back of the prosthesis is coated with medical adhesive (e.g., Hollister, Epithane III, or Secure) on the contact surfaces, allowed to dry, then accurately positioned and applied to the epidermis.

SUMMARY

Prostheses are to be considered a necessary and desirable adjunct to any disfiguring surgical intervention procedure. Their positive value is measured in the total rehabilitative, psychological, and physical outcome (Fig. 18–1 to 18–7).

It is the patient's right to expect as normal a postoperative appearance as possible, and the physician and prosthetist should do everything

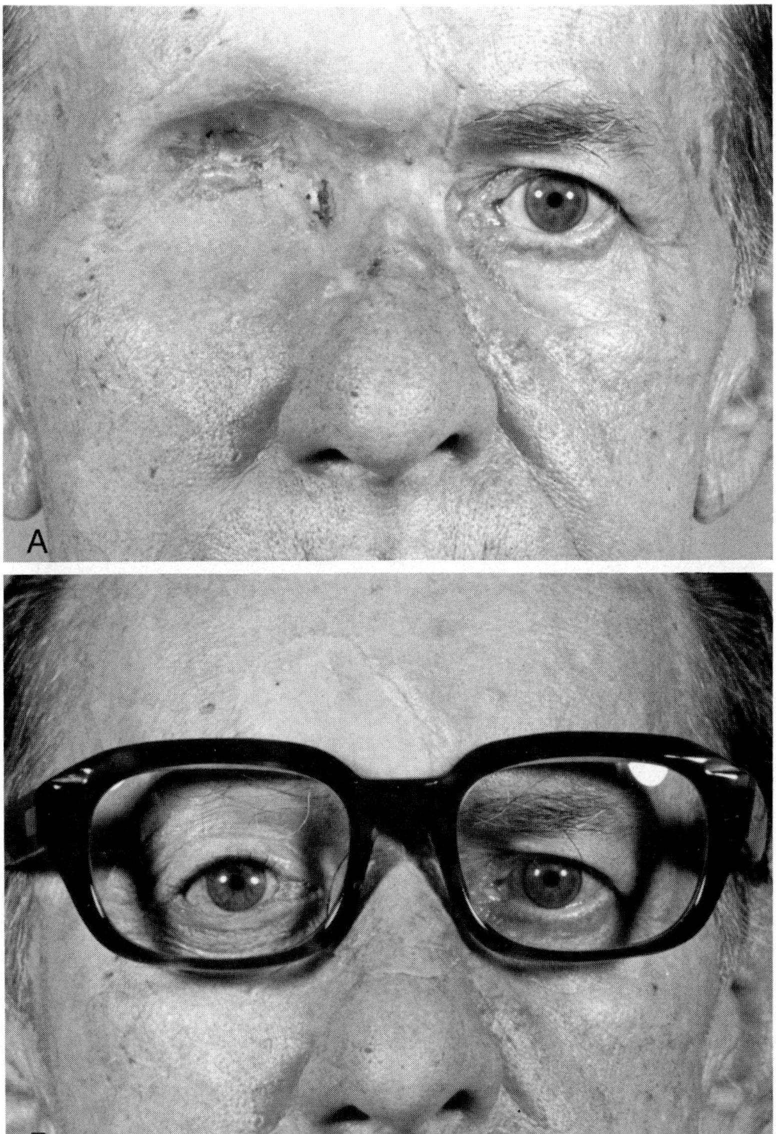

FIGURE 18–3. *A*, Exenteration of the orbit with wide nasal and frontal dermal excisions. *B*, Silicone prosthesis with acrylic eye implant.

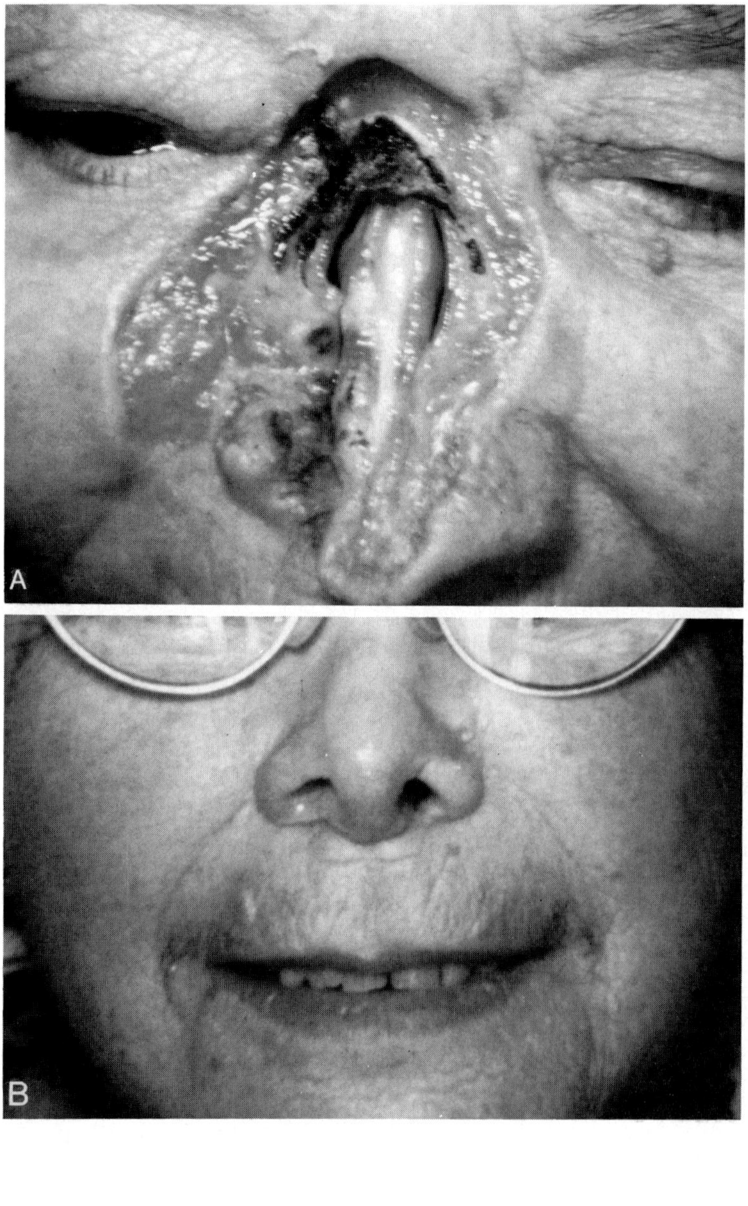

FIGURE 18–4. *A*, Condition after Mohs surgery to eradicate basal cell carcinoma. *B*, Partial silicone prosthesis 6 months after surgery.

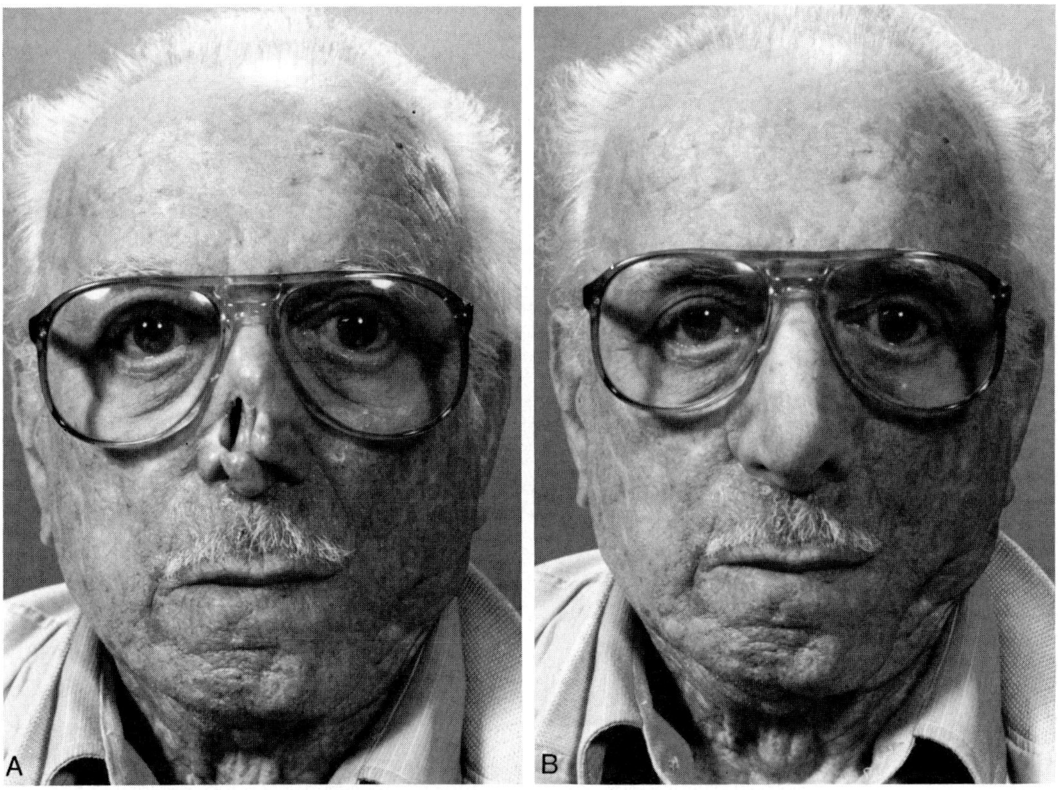

FIGURE 18–5. *A*, Partial rhinectomy after Mohs surgery. *B*, Full silicone prosthesis 3 months after surgery.

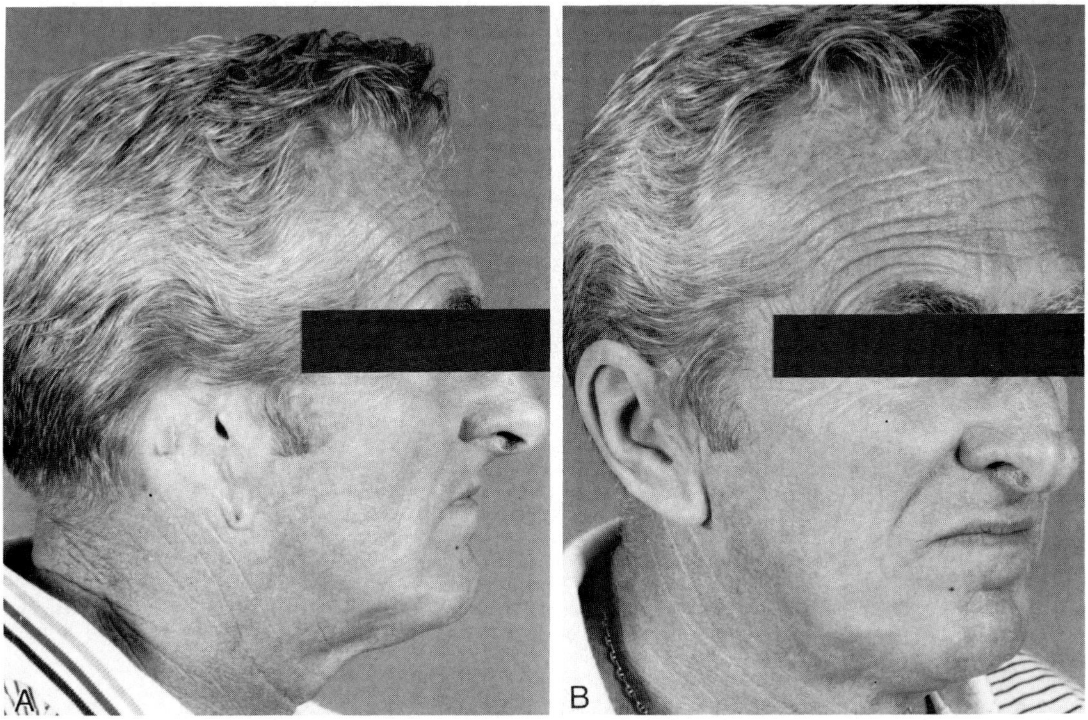

FIGURE 18–6. *A*, Postoperative ablation of the right ear. *B*, Silicone prosthesis affixed to methyl methacrylate base.

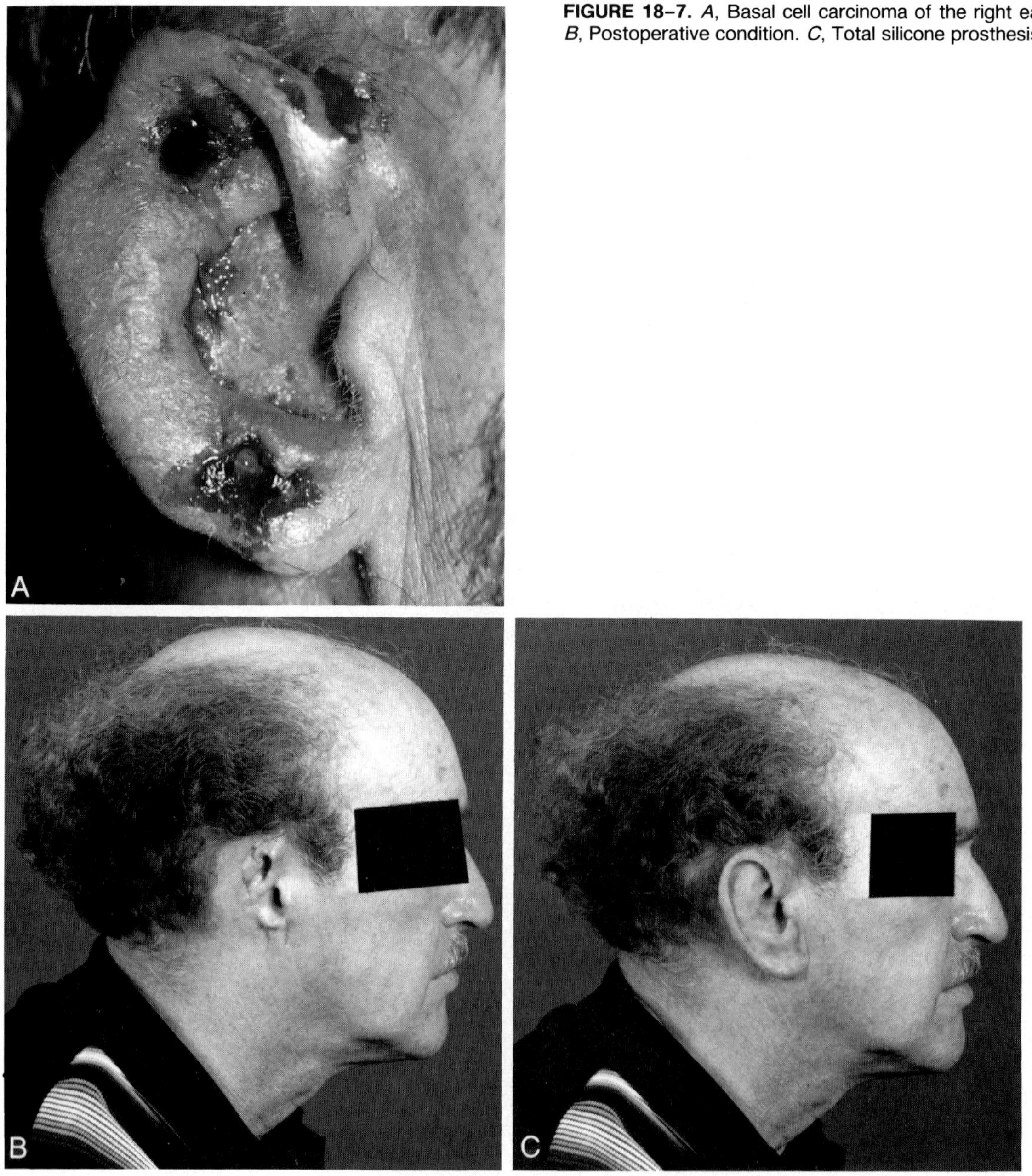

FIGURE 18-7. *A*, Basal cell carcinoma of the right ear. *B*, Postoperative condition. *C*, Total silicone prosthesis.

they can in order to ensure an acceptable result.

REFERENCES

1. Chalian VA, Drane JB, Standish SM: Maxillofacial Prosthetics—Multidisciplinary Practice. Baltimore: Williams & Wilkins, 1971.
2. Seals RR, Cortes AL, Parel SM: Fabrication of facial prosthesis by applying the osseointegration concept for retention, Journal of Prosthetic Dentistry 61:712–716, 1989.
3. Tjellstrom A, Lindstrom J, Nylen O, Albrektsson T, Branemark P, Birgersson B: The bone-anchored auricular episthesis, The Laryngoscope 91:811–815, 1981.

CHAPTER 19

Photography in Surgery

Dennis E. Babel, Ph.D.
David Levin, M.A.

Medical photography is essential in the practice of Mohs micrographic surgery. This visual form of medical record-keeping provides a valuable tool that can be especially useful in three interrelated areas: documentation, education, and publication.

Documentation. Taking preoperative, intraoperative, and postoperative photographs gives the dermatologic surgeon an opportunity to review his or her technique in a specific case and, on occasion, to identify ways to improve skills. The photographs can also be used to review with the patient the extent of the preoperative pathology and the postoperative result, which is sometimes necessary later. This type of documentation can also provide support in malpractice actions as well as justification for third-party reimbursement.[1]

Education. A series of photographic images are excellent teaching material for fellows in training, residents, and medical students. In addition, they allow new patients to become familiar with the procedure to be performed and the anticipated results. The materials also serve as a resource for sharing information at scientific meetings.

Publication. High-quality photographs are an integral part of scientific publications, especially those delineating techniques or describing unusual lesions. With a little care, excellent reproductions can be made in the physician's office.

PHOTOGRAPHIC SYSTEMS

A photographic system for medical photography consists of three main components: the camera body, the lens, and the light source. There is an enormous variety of these components available; however, the choices become rather limited when we consider the specific needs of the dermatologic surgeon. A good system should fulfill the criteria in Table 19–1. It must be able to provide high-quality photographs and also be relatively simple to use so that the surgeon or assistants can achieve the same photographic results. This consistency is imperative. The technology of semiautomated and automated photography has greatly improved over the last decade and truly lends itself to the desired reproducibility. There is no one single system that is "right" for surgical photography.[2] Consideration will be given to the necessary attributes of each component (Table 19–2).

Camera Body

The camera body we have found best suited is a 35 mm, single lens reflex with off the film-plane (OTF) metering of exposure. The OTF ability allows the camera to determine and control correct flash intensity while the photograph is being taken (Fig. 19–1). A dedicated flash unit is strongly recommended.

TABLE 19–1. Optimal Photographic System Criteria

Simplicity of use
Accuracy of color and image rendered
Repeatability of image at set parameters
Adjustability to accommodate different subjects
Reliability of equipment with prolonged use

TABLE 19–2. Photographic System Components

Body: 35 mm, multiple modes, off the filmplane (OTF) metering
Lenses: Macro 50 mm and 100 mm, extension tube
Flash: point and/or ring type, dedicated
Options: power winder, data back, filters, tripod

Ideally, the camera should have the capability of three different modes:

1. *Program mode* (automatic): The camera determines the f-stop and shutter speed.
2. *Aperture priority mode* (semiautomatic): The photographer sets the f-stop, and the camera determines the shutter speed.
3. *Manual mode:* The photographer sets the f-stop and the shutter speed based on a predetermined chart.

The first two modes provide a single system for ease of use and allow repeatability of exposure when using a macro lens. The manual mode gives the photographer total control of the exposure parameters. This is sometimes necessary when dealing with an unusual photographic situation or when trying to create a special effect.

Lenses

The first lens we recommend for surgical photography is a macro lens of 80 to 105 mm focal length (Fig. 19–2). A lens with a focal length somewhere in this range assures adequate image magnification while allowing sufficient lens-to-subject distance for freedom in selecting the correct viewing and lighting angle.[3] A second lens, such as a 50 mm macro lens, allows full-body photography within the confines of a surgical room without distortion.

With either lens, a maximum reproduction ratio of 1 to 2 (subject to image size) can be achieved. If a life-size image is required, either lens could be combined with an autoextension tube that would provide a close-up reproduction ratio of 1 to 1. This would be useful in the case of a small object like a palmar pit in a patient with the nevoid basal cell carcinoma syndrome.

Light Sources

The ideal light source for surgical photography should be light in weight, easily portable, and dedicated to the camera body. Electronic flash

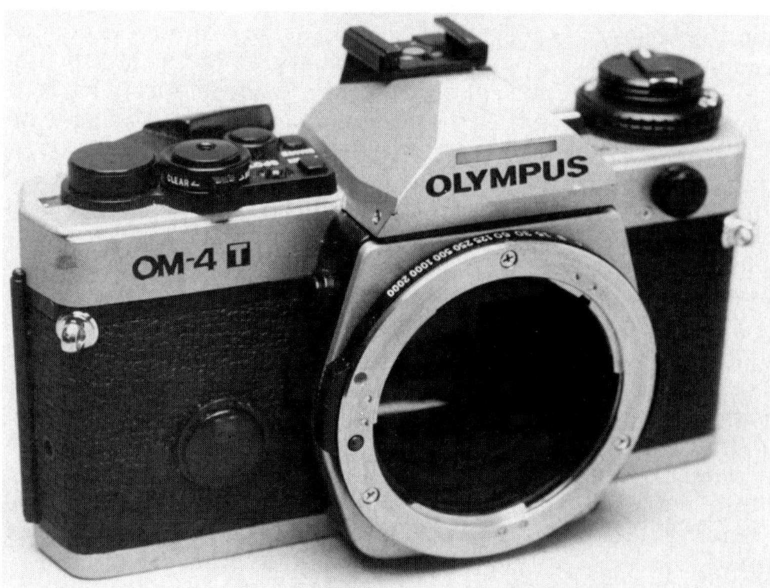

FIGURE 19–1. Body of a 35 mm, single-lens reflex camera (courtesy of Olympus Corporation).

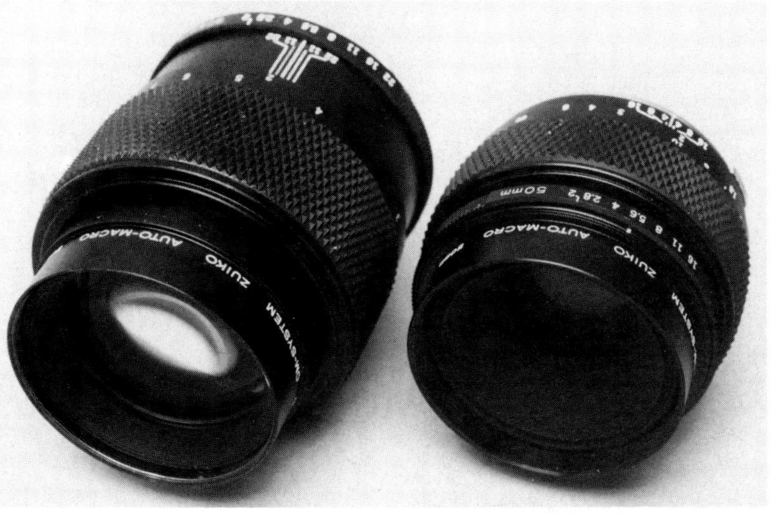

FIGURE 19–2. Macro lenses: 90 mm and 50 mm (courtesy of Olympus Corporation).

units that can be used in automated macrophotography come in two basic types:

1. *Ring flash* (Fig. 19–3): These units attach to the end of the camera lens and provide an even, flat field of illumination without shadows. They are especially helpful when photographing body cavities, such as the oropharynx.
2. *Point source flash* (Fig. 19–4): These flash units can mount on the camera body or on a separate bracket and provide an illuminated field with shadows. This lighting enhances the texture of lesions or surgical sites.

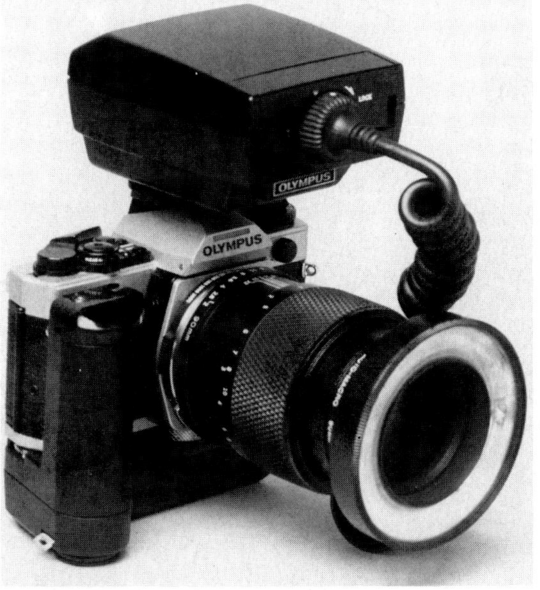

FIGURE 19–3. Ring flash for shadowless field (courtesy of Olympus Corporation).

The power for these flash units can be provided by alkaline disposable, or nickel-cadmium rechargeable, batteries. AC plug-in power sources are also available but limit the photographer's mobility.

OPTIONS

Like an automobile, there are many options available for the photographic system. Those of special interest to the surgical photographer include:

1. *Data back:* This option gives the system the ability to superimpose the current date on the picture. Some models can also record the patient's name.
2. *Power winder:* This option allows the photographer to continually view the subject through the viewfinder and advance the film without having to take the camera away from the face. This can be especially advantageous when a rapid series of pictures is needed.
3. *Lens filters:* Filters may be used to enhance reproduction quality in certain situations. A polarizing filter, for example, helps minimize direct flash reflections from wet reflective surfaces.
4. *Tripod:* A sturdy tripod is useful for camera stability as well as for keeping the camera positioned for repetitive photographs with the same angle of view.

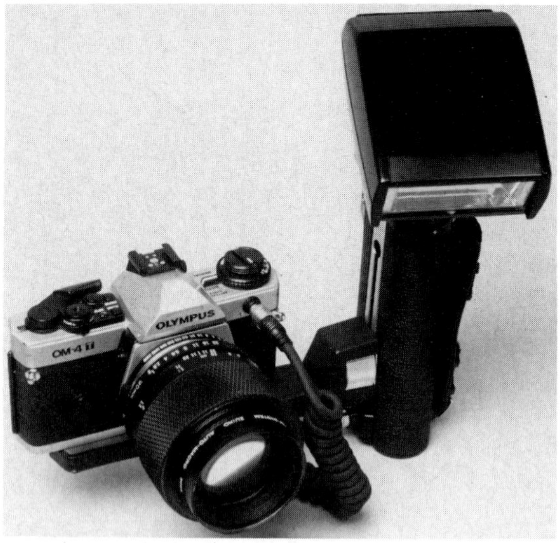

FIGURE 19–4. Camera set-up with point source flash for shadowed field (courtesy of Olympus Corporation).

INSTANT PRINT SYSTEMS

Although instant print systems lack the picture quality of the 35 mm slide or print, they do provide an immediacy that has its advantages. Instant prints can be checked for photographic accuracy while the patient is still in the office and can be readily inserted into the medical record. There are a number of instant print systems available based on modifications of Polaroid technology.

Polaroid CU-5. This system provides the highest quality instant print coming closest to a 35 mm reproduction (Fig. 19–5). The disadvantages are that it is somewhat cumbersome and carries a price tag of over $1,000.

Trojan DPX. This system provides an instant print with good color accuracy and reasonable focusing detail (Fig. 19–6). It is light-weight and easy to use, and can be purchased for half the price of the Polaroid CU-5.

A number of different companies provide medical adaptions of the Polaroid instant print system. These include Trojan Clinical Camera Systems (800/338-9433) and Lester D. Dine, Inc. (516/437-3220). The authors suggest that the surgeon try the new system in the office setting before making a final purchase. The print quality and ease of use vary significantly between systems.

MISCELLANEOUS EQUIPMENT

Background and subject drapes provide a nondistracting field and an excellent way to separate and delineate different parts of the body. Ideally, they should be made of a neutral gray or light blue material when obtaining color photographs. Additional sterile drapes should be available to replace those that become soiled intraoperatively.

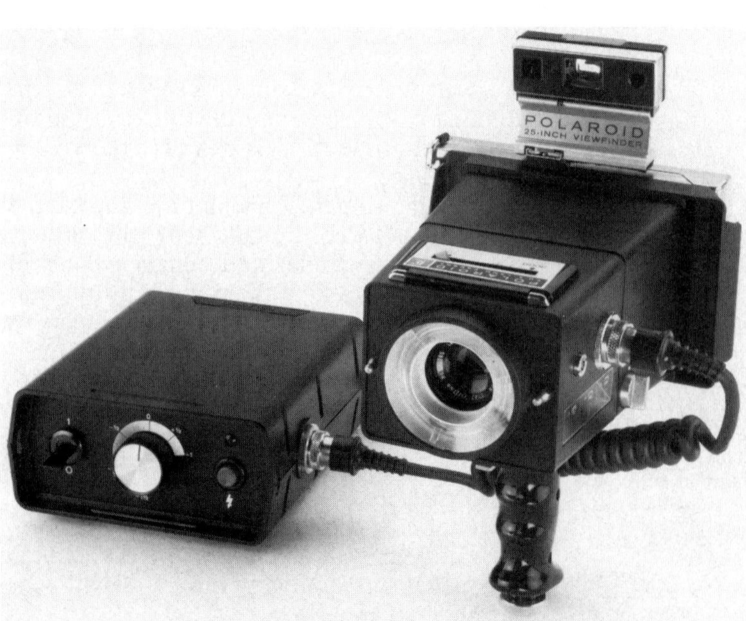

FIGURE 19–5. Polaroid CU-5 instant picture system (courtesy of Polaroid Corporation).

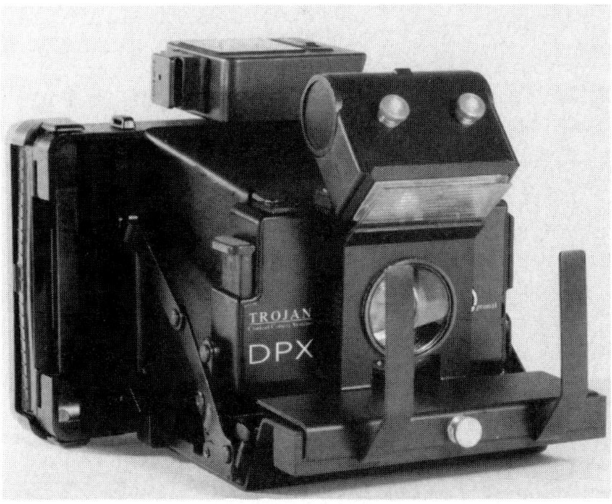

FIGURE 19–6. Trojan DPX instant print camera (courtesy of Trojan Clinical Camera Systems).

FILM

The type of 35 mm film selected for medical photography is very important in terms of final color reproduction. Each individual film produces its own color tones (Table 19–3). Films with an ISO rating of 100 or less are the finest grained and ultimately give the best print reproductions. The use of color transparency films is preferred to color negative print films. If prints need to be made at a later date, it is easier to match the print color from a slide than to guess a color match from a negative.

Kodak Ektachrome film is convenient because it is easily processed (usually within 24 hours). Kodachrome film must be sent to a Kodak laboratory and a fast turnaround time may not be available. When taking black-and-white photographs, Kodak T-Max (TMX 100 ISO) film gives a very good rendition. Other brands of film with similar characteristics are also available.

When using an instant print system like Polaroid, there are three types of 3¼″×4¼″ print films available. Two give black-and-white prints, one has a reusable negative, and the third produces a full-color print (Table 19–4).

TABLE 19–3. Representative 35 mm Films

Type	Symbol	Speed	Characteristic
Kodachrome	KR	64 ISO	Red tones
Ektachrome	ED	100 ISO	Blue tones
Ektachrome	EPP	100 ISO	Intermediate tones
T-MAX	TMX	100 ISO	Black and white

TABLE 19–4. Polaroid Instant Print Film

Type	ISO	Characteristic
665	75	Produces a black-and-white print with a reusable negative.
667	3000	Produces a sharply defined black-and-white print.
669	80	Produces a full-color print.

Although there are numerous good and reliable makes of cameras and films, only the ones we use and are familiar with are presented here.

PHOTOGRAPHIC TECHNIQUE

To become familiar with a new photographic system, a series of test rolls of film should be taken with exposure settings that are recorded. Review of the processed test films and the exposure records allows the photographer to determine which procedure best serves his or her needs. Consistency should be strived for; minimizing variables such as flash type or location and film type is emphasized.[4]

When composing the subject to be photographed, attention to background, site, scale, lighting, and arrangement are important. The choice of a background needs careful consideration. Its purpose is to exclude distracting objects and other unwanted parts of the subject, so that the focus of attention is on the area of the body in question. Adequate contrast is also important. A light blue color is pleasing to the eye and will provide the needed contrast. Remember to remove all distracting elements from the field, e.g., instruments, blood, soiled drapes, cosmetics, and jewelry. A centimeter scale in the field is sometimes necessary for measurement perspective. Disposable rolls of centimeter scales with adhesive backing are available from scientific supply houses.

Be sure to center your subject in the camera frame and angle the flash to the subject, if necessary. Remember that a ring flash produces a flat, shadowless field, while a point flash adds texture to the subject through shadowing.

It is always desirable to obtain the same size of the photographed area from about the same position. This is essential in recording Mohs surgery cases because the field rarely exceeds the size of a hand, which represents a reproduction on the film in the range of 1 to 4. The size can be adjusted on the lens scale and left

Date: ____________________
Name: ____________________

I ________________________ (print name) authorize ________________________ (physician/technician) to make photographic or slide recordings of ________________________ (patient's name).

These visual recordings may be taken for the purpose of monitoring patient care and for medical research and education. I grant the right to use these visual recordings for these purposes. I waive all rights, claims, and interest in all visual recordings and all rights to payment or royalties in connection with their use and/or publication.

My/the patient's name will not be disclosed in connection with said use.

Check box:

☐ My/The patient's facial features may be exposed.

☐ My/The patient's facial features may not be exposed.

____
Signature of witness

____
Date

____
Signature of patient

____
Signature of parent or legal guardian (if applicable, specify)

____

____
Address of patient or legal guardian

FIGURE 19–7. Consent and waiver for visual recordings.

in place most of the time. When a 100 ISO film is used, an aperture of f-11, an automatic shutter speed, and a dedicated flash will render perfect photographs after the object is in focus. Exact focus is best achieved by advancing to or withdrawing the camera from the field to be photographed. This is the only maneuver that would possibly allow error. For larger and smaller objects, the aforementioned factors would have to be adjusted to fit the situation. In our experience, the autofocus photographic systems are unsatisfactory for macro photography.

Obtaining photographs from more than one position is sometimes indicated. In the case of a nasal lesion or wound, recordings from frontal, lateral, and inferior directions are desirable. In the case of auricular surgery, recording the lateral and medial surfaces of the pinna are recommended.

RECORD-KEEPING

A photographic log should be kept and include the date, patient name, diagnosis, and any pertinent photographic information such as reproduction ratios or exposure settings. This information can be readily transferred to the outer frame of the slide after the film is processed. A computer slide label program called Slide Scribe is now available and saves a tremendous amount of time when a large slide series is shot on the same subject.

Photographic waiver forms should be obtained before surgery and placed in the medical record (Fig. 19–7). These become especially helpful for publication purposes later.

STORAGE

There are a number of approaches to the storage of slides. Plastic pages of slides are convenient to handle and can be kept with the patient's medical record, but sometimes, this plastic page can adhere to the slide and damage it. Slide files that fit in file drawers are also available, but they do leave the slide surfaces exposed and unprotected. The best approach to protection and archival organization is to keep the slides filed in a light-tight, metal, slotted slide file.

REFERENCES

1. Sebben, JE: Office photography from the surgical viewpoint, J Dermatol Surg Oncol 9:763–768, 1983.
2. Swinyer, LJ: Medical photography in the dermatology office, Curr Concepts Skin Disorders 9:5–17, 1988.
3. Weiss, CH: Dermatologic photography, J Assoc Milit Dermatol 13:3–20, 1987.
4. Kodak Workshop Series: Close-Up Photography, Kodak Catalogue KW-22:144–161.

CHAPTER 20

Practical Pointers

George R. Mikhail, M.D., M.S.

Some things can be learned only through practice and experience. A few simple and practical self-learned methods are presented in this section.

Intermittent Mohs Surgery for Large Basal Cell Carcinomas

It is always desirable to ablate basal cell carcinomas (BCCs) as expeditiously as possible. Almost all cases can be managed within the day's working hours. Resumption of surgery on the following day is called interrupted surgery, and intermittent surgery means that further excision is deferred to another session after a 2-or 3-month interval. There are valid reasons for adopting this method: (1) to save an important structure, especially an eye, (2) to obtain optimal cosmesis, (3) when the general health of the patient does not permit the stress of long hours of surgery or the administration of large amounts of anesthetic, and (4) to avoid excessive loss of blood and hypovolemic shock.

In my early days in the practice of Mohs surgery (the fixed tissue method was the standard then), I experienced great disappointment because a patient's eye could not be saved (Fig. 20–1). In all probability, the same result would have happened if the fresh tissue technique had been used in the usual continuous fashion. When confronted with an almost identical lesion (sclerotic basal cell carcinoma) in another patient, I decided to ablate the tumor intermittently. The surgical stages and the final outcome, using the intermittent fresh tissue method, are shown in Figure 20–2.

The same procedure was successfully applied in a patient with an extensive lentigo maligna melanoma that occupied the right side of the face, including the lower eyelid margin (Fig. 20–3).

Another indication for intermittent Mohs surgery is when the lesion is extensive and cosmesis is important. A case in point is illustrated in Figure 20–4, which shows a man whose left side of the face was almost completely covered by a basal cell carcinoma of the so-called multicentric type. By excising, photographing, and mapping the excised tissue, we could go again to the residual area with BCC and remove the malignancy in stages and achieve a good cosmetic result.

Defining the Actual Limits of Sclerotic Basal Cell Carcinoma

A very helpful maneuver to find the true clinical margins of a sclerotic basal cell carcinoma is to stretch or compress the skin with both hands or with the fingers, as demonstrated in Figures 20–5 to 20–7. The histologic margins of sclerotic BCC extend far beyond any that are visible (Fig. 20–8).

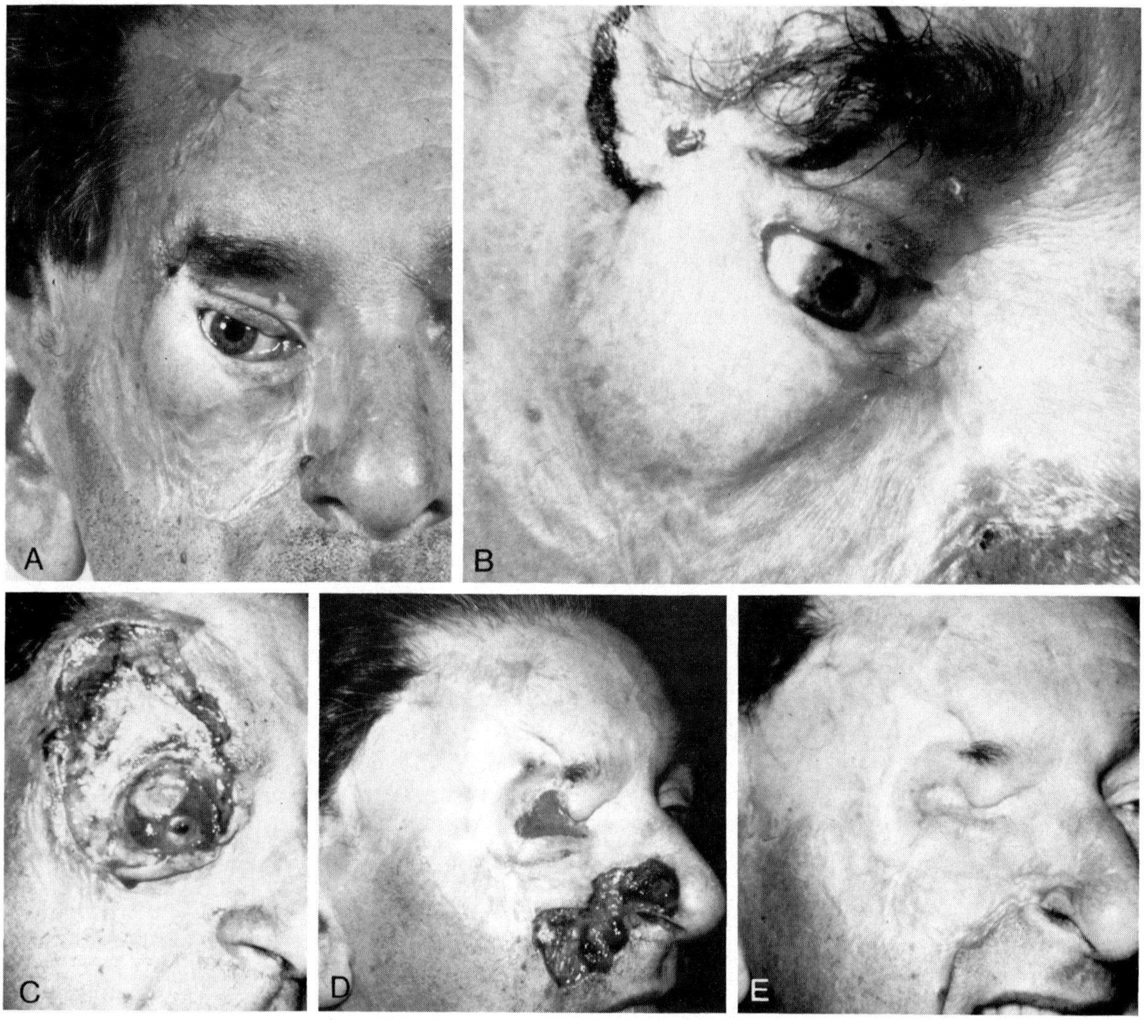

FIGURE 20–1. *A*, Sclerotic basal cell carcinoma of both right eyelids and cheek excised by a plastic surgeon. The eyelids were reconstructed by transposition flaps obtained from the temporal area. *B*, Site of initial biopsy and starting point of Mohs micrographic surgery, fixed tissue method. *C*, Point at which attempts were made to save the eye. *D*, Eye already enucleated; surgery resumed to remove residual carcinoma from nose and cheek. *E*, Final healed result; patient was followed for 10 years without recurrence.

Hemostatic Agents

Oxidized cellulose (Oxycel, by Desert Medical, Inc.) comes in pledgets (cotton-type), pads (gauze-type), and strips (gauze-type); Gelfoam (Upjohn) comes in powder form and a sponge-type preparation. Both are useful in controlling bleeding from open wounds (Fig. 20–9 and 20–10) and are usually left in wounds allowed to heal by second intention. Thrombostat (Parke Davis Co.) is used either as the supplied powder or in solution, mainly in wounds that are later closed.

The Ubiquitous Chalazion Forceps

The chalazion forceps designed to steady the eyelid, to protect the eye, and to act as a hemostat during removal of meibomian cysts, come in different sizes and shapes. We find the straight format in small, medium, and large sizes well-adapted to our procedures and useful for excisions on the eyelid (Fig. 20–11), the ala nasi (Fig. 20–12), the lips (Figs. 20–13 and 20–14), and the ear (Figs. 20–15 and 20–16). Chalazion forceps are a versatile instrument that can be put to many uses.

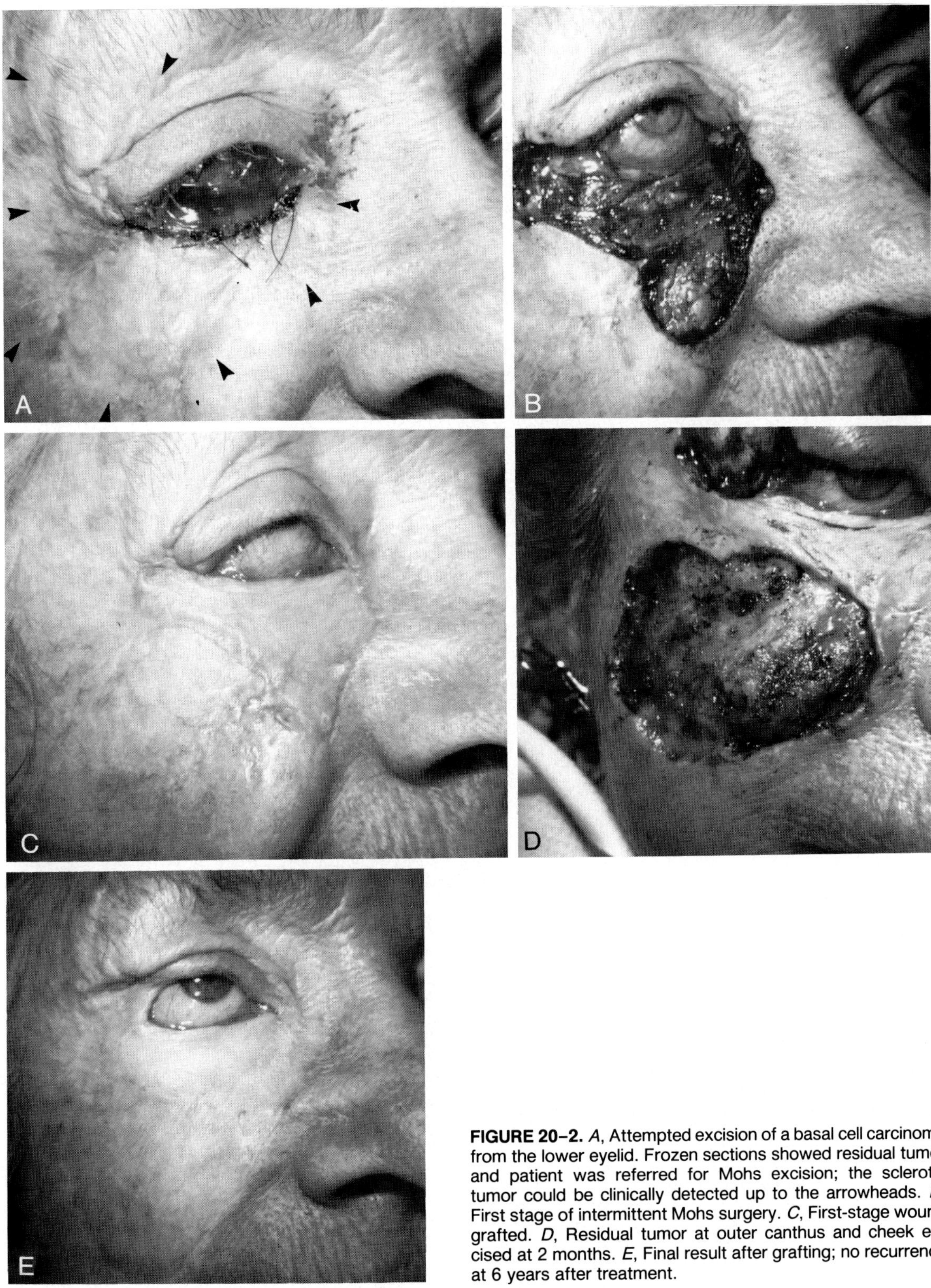

FIGURE 20–2. *A*, Attempted excision of a basal cell carcinoma from the lower eyelid. Frozen sections showed residual tumor and patient was referred for Mohs excision; the sclerotic tumor could be clinically detected up to the arrowheads. *B*, First stage of intermittent Mohs surgery. *C*, First-stage wound grafted. *D*, Residual tumor at outer canthus and cheek excised at 2 months. *E*, Final result after grafting; no recurrence at 6 years after treatment.

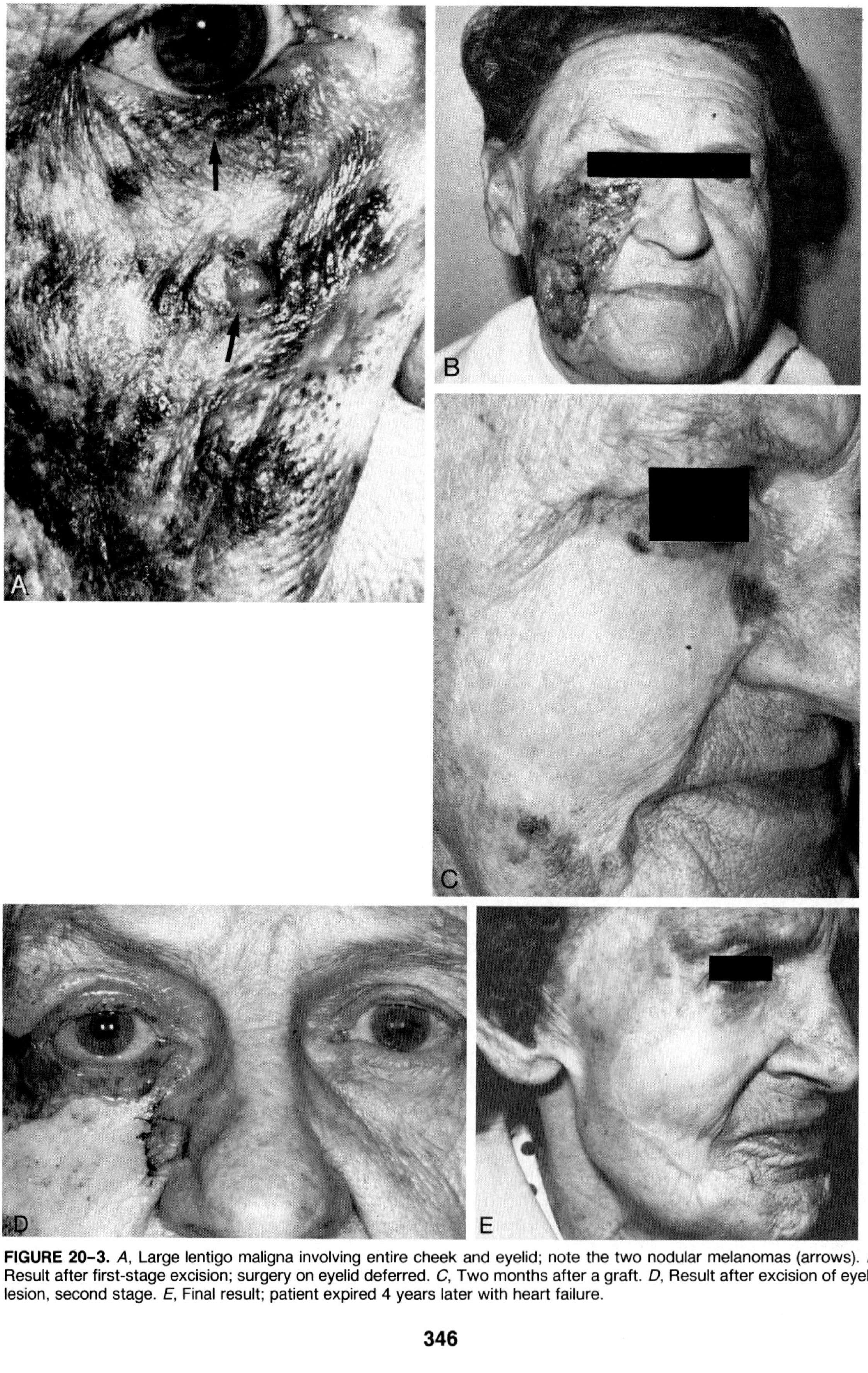

FIGURE 20–3. *A*, Large lentigo maligna involving entire cheek and eyelid; note the two nodular melanomas (arrows). *B*, Result after first-stage excision; surgery on eyelid deferred. *C*, Two months after a graft. *D*, Result after excision of eyelid lesion, second stage. *E*, Final result; patient expired 4 years later with heart failure.

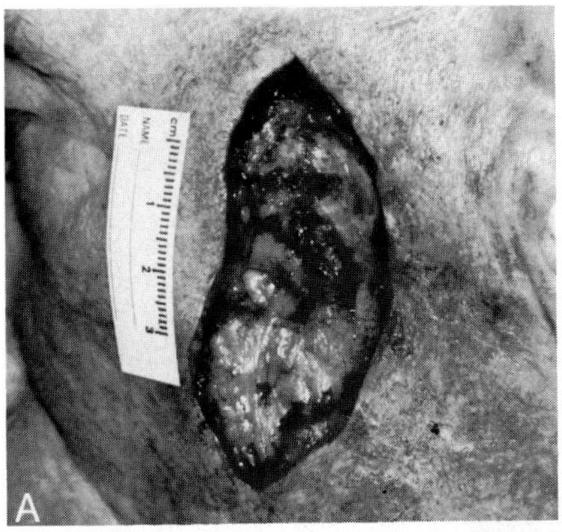

FIGURE 20–4. *A*, First-stage excision of an extensive basal cell carcinoma of the so-called multicentric type that occupied most of the left side of the face; the wound was closed by the simple approximation of margins. *B*, Diagram of first excision shows residual basal cell carcinoma at the margins (dark areas). *C*, Second excision 2 months later. *D*, Diagram shows sites of residual carcinoma. *E*, Closure after second excision. *F*, Third and final excision, the lowermost wound was the site of another focus of carcinoma. *G*, Final appearance; excellent cosmesis in bearded skin.

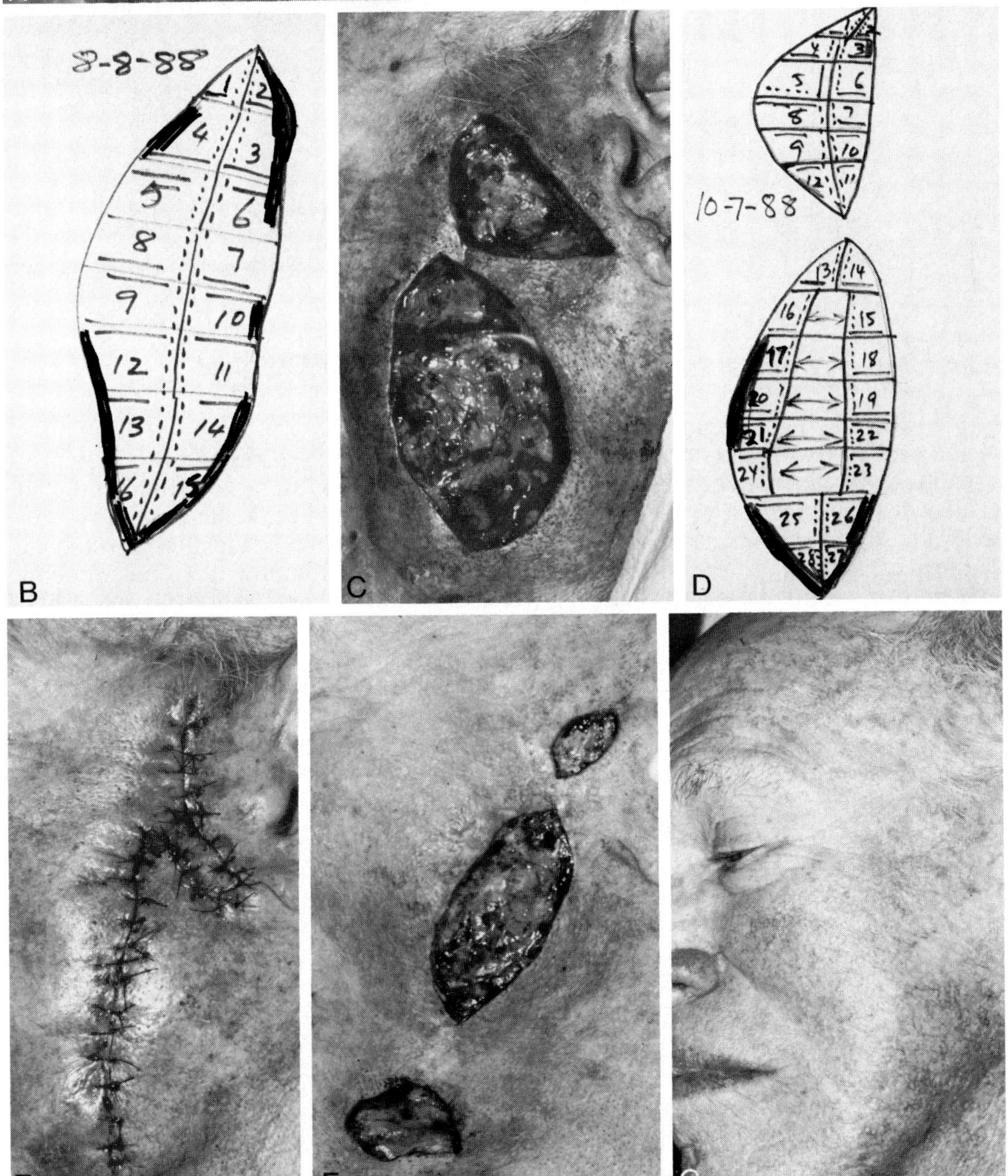

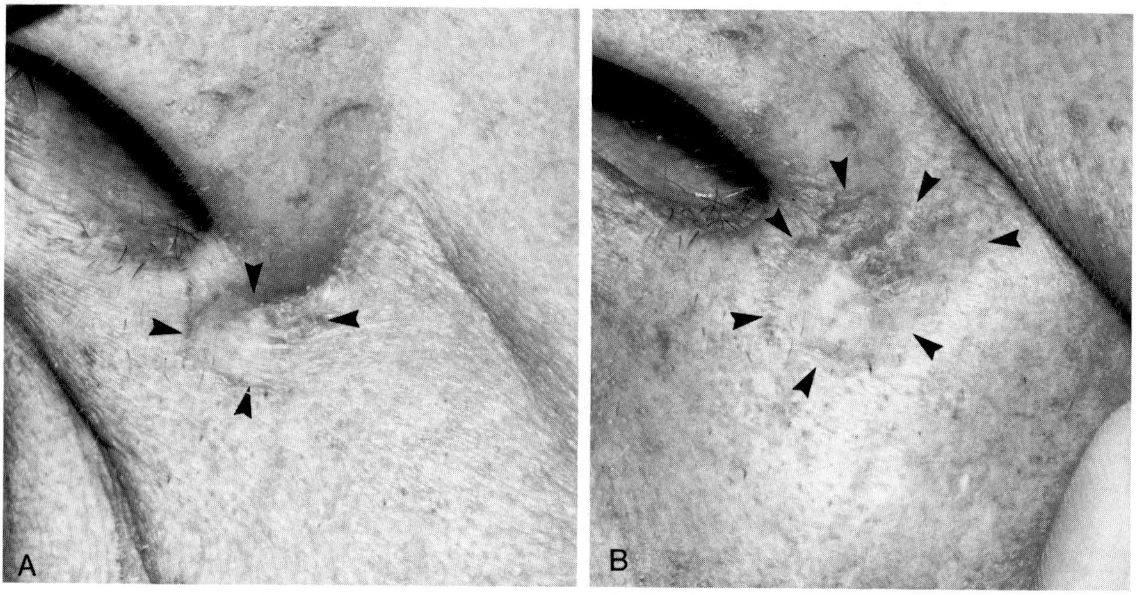

FIGURE 20-5. *A*, Apparent extent of a sclerotic basal cell carcinoma. *B*, Stretching the skin renders the clinical margins more evident.

Healed Eyelid Margin Wounds

Healed wounds on the eyelid margins, especially those left to heal by second intention, will have an erythematous surface. Oftentimes, this has been erroneously considered a sign of recurrence. Besides scar contracture, remember that the rate of reepithelialization from the mucosal side is three times as fast as reepithelialization of the cutaneous portion. This has the tendency to result in exteriorization of the conjunctiva (a type of mild ectropion), which can give the false impression of recurrence (Fig. 20–17).

Reinforcement of Surgical Dressings

Surgical adhesive strips are often used for closure of small wounds by approximating the margins or to minimize the tension on sutures. Steri-Strips (3M Co.) is the tape most commonly used. The manufacturer recommends that a thin coat of compound tincture of benzoin (USP) be applied to the skin parallel to the wound in order to increase strip adhesion. The manufacturer of a resinous liquid adhesive, Mastisol (Ferndale Labs, Ferndale, Michigan), a gum mastic compound, claims that its prod-

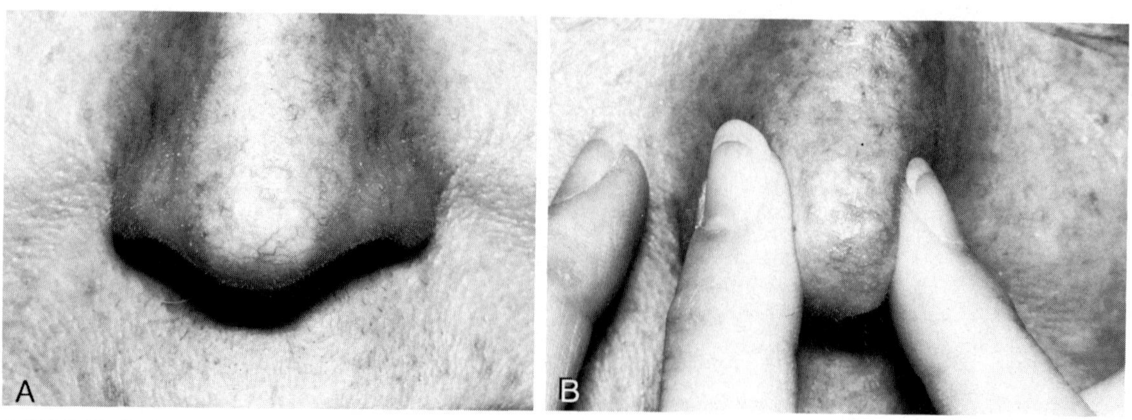

FIGURE 20-6. *A*, Almost inconspicuous sclerotic basal cell carcinoma on tip of the nose. *B*, Lesion made visibly prominent by side-to-side pressure.

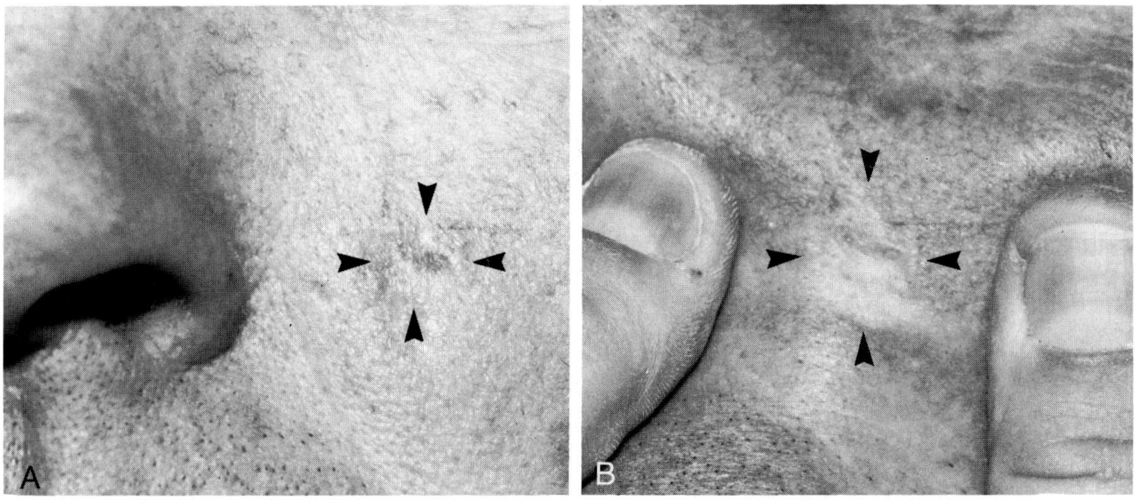

FIGURE 20–7. *A*, Sclerotic basal cell carcinoma of the cheek. *B*, Appearance after stretching the skin.

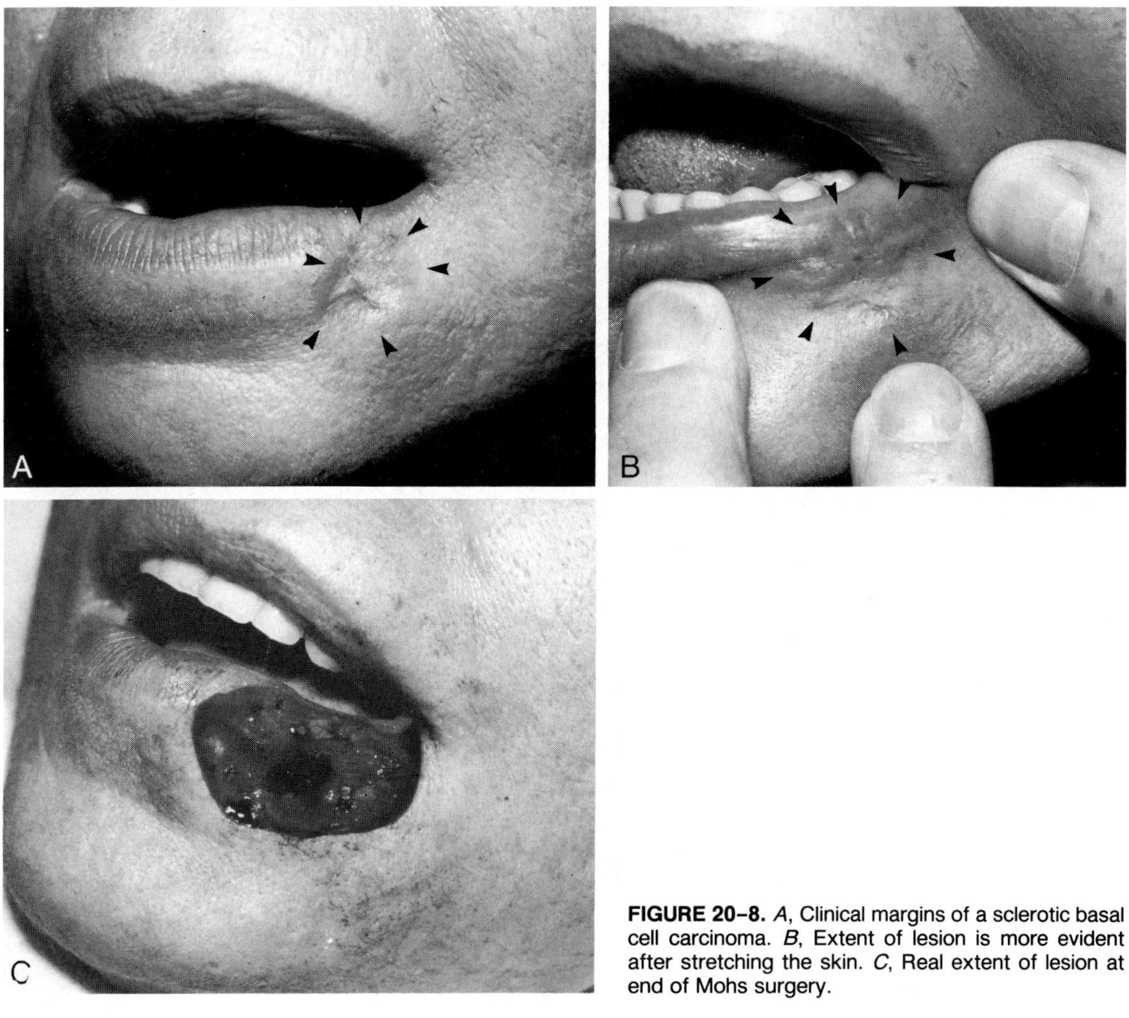

FIGURE 20–8. *A*, Clinical margins of a sclerotic basal cell carcinoma. *B*, Extent of lesion is more evident after stretching the skin. *C*, Real extent of lesion at end of Mohs surgery.

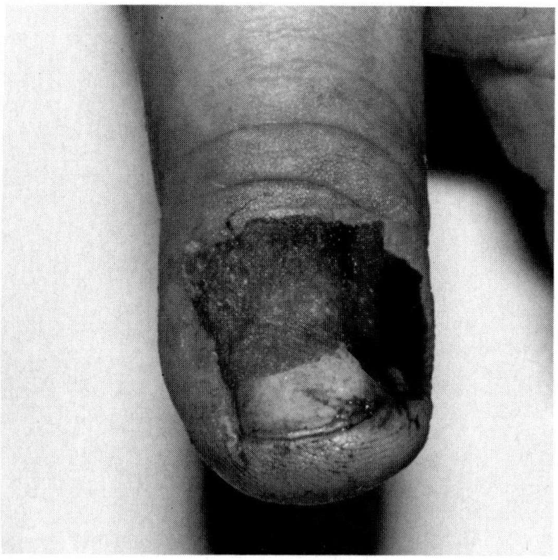

FIGURE 20-9. Gelfoam sponge applied to nailbed after excision of Bowen's disease and left in place under the dressing.

uct has an adhesive power superior to that of tincture of benzoin. In 1986, we conducted a study and found that the claim is true.[1] We also found this preparation useful for applying gauze dressings to the scalp and other types of wound and burn dressings.[2] Some of the uses of Mastisol with Steri-Strips are illustrated in Figures 20–18 to 20–20.

Orabase

Orabase (plain), manufactured by Colgate-Hoyt Laboratories, contains pectin, gelatin, and sodium carboxymethylcellulose in a plasticized hydrocarbon gel (a polyethylene and mineral oil gel base). It adheres to moist tissues and forms an impermeable thick paste when moistened. It has several uses, such as relieving pain and discomfort when applied to wounds on the buccal mucosa and temporarily closing

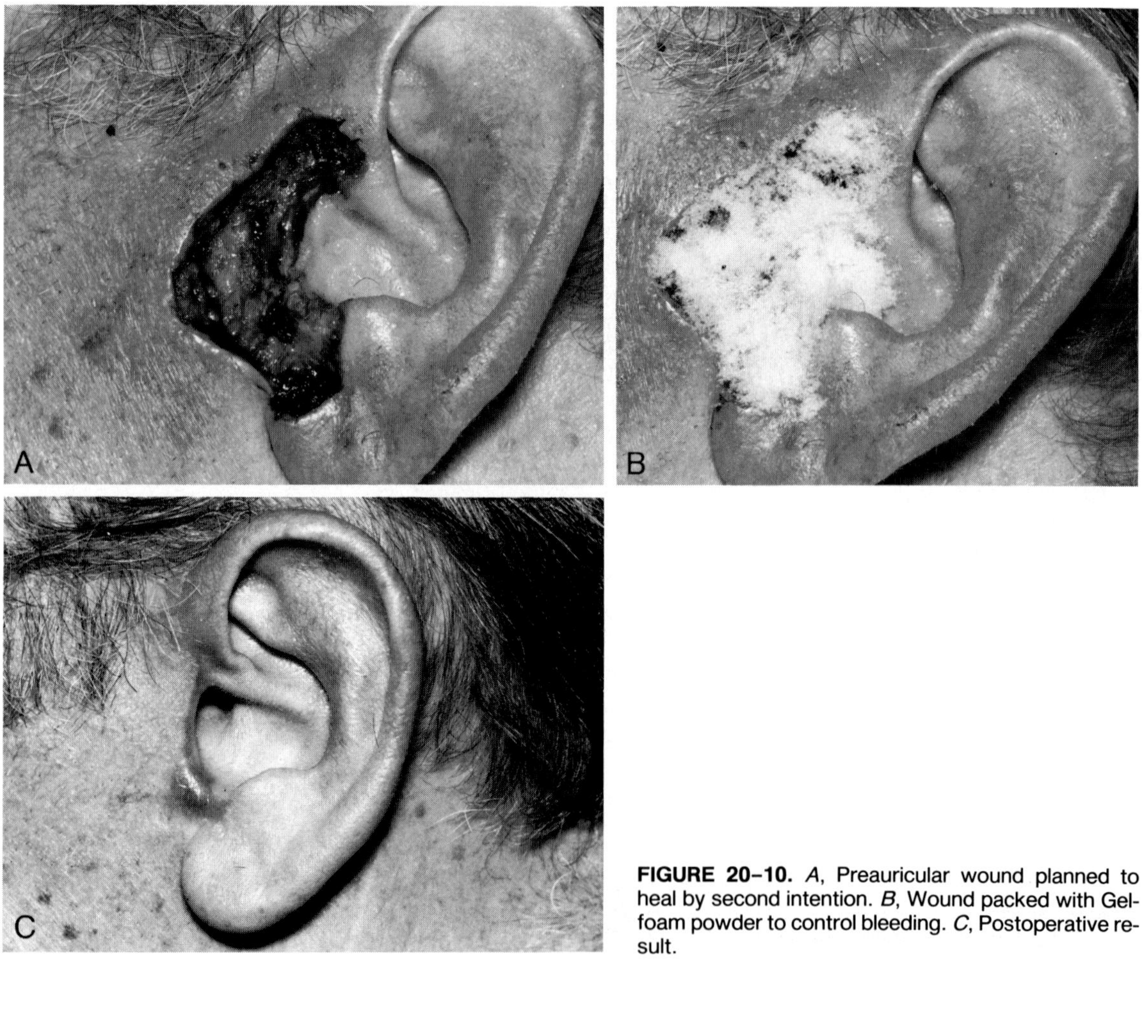

FIGURE 20–10. *A*, Preauricular wound planned to heal by second intention. *B*, Wound packed with Gelfoam powder to control bleeding. *C*, Postoperative result.

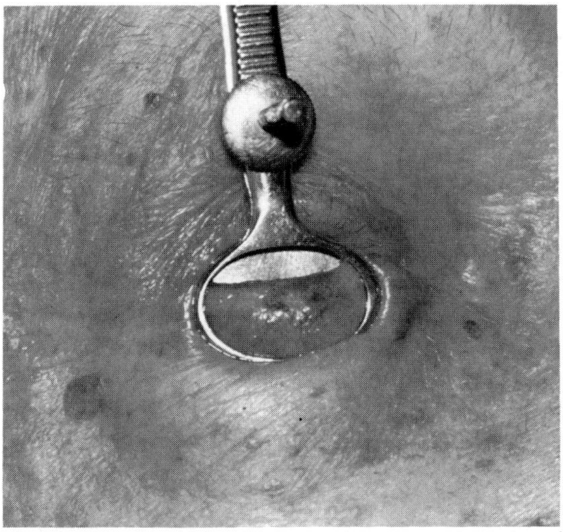

FIGURE 20–11. Chalazion forceps in use for removal of a lower eyelid lesion.

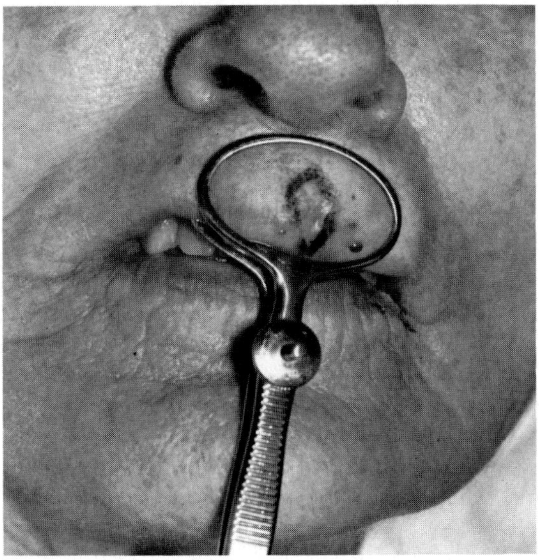

FIGURE 20–13. Large chalazion forceps applied to upper lip.

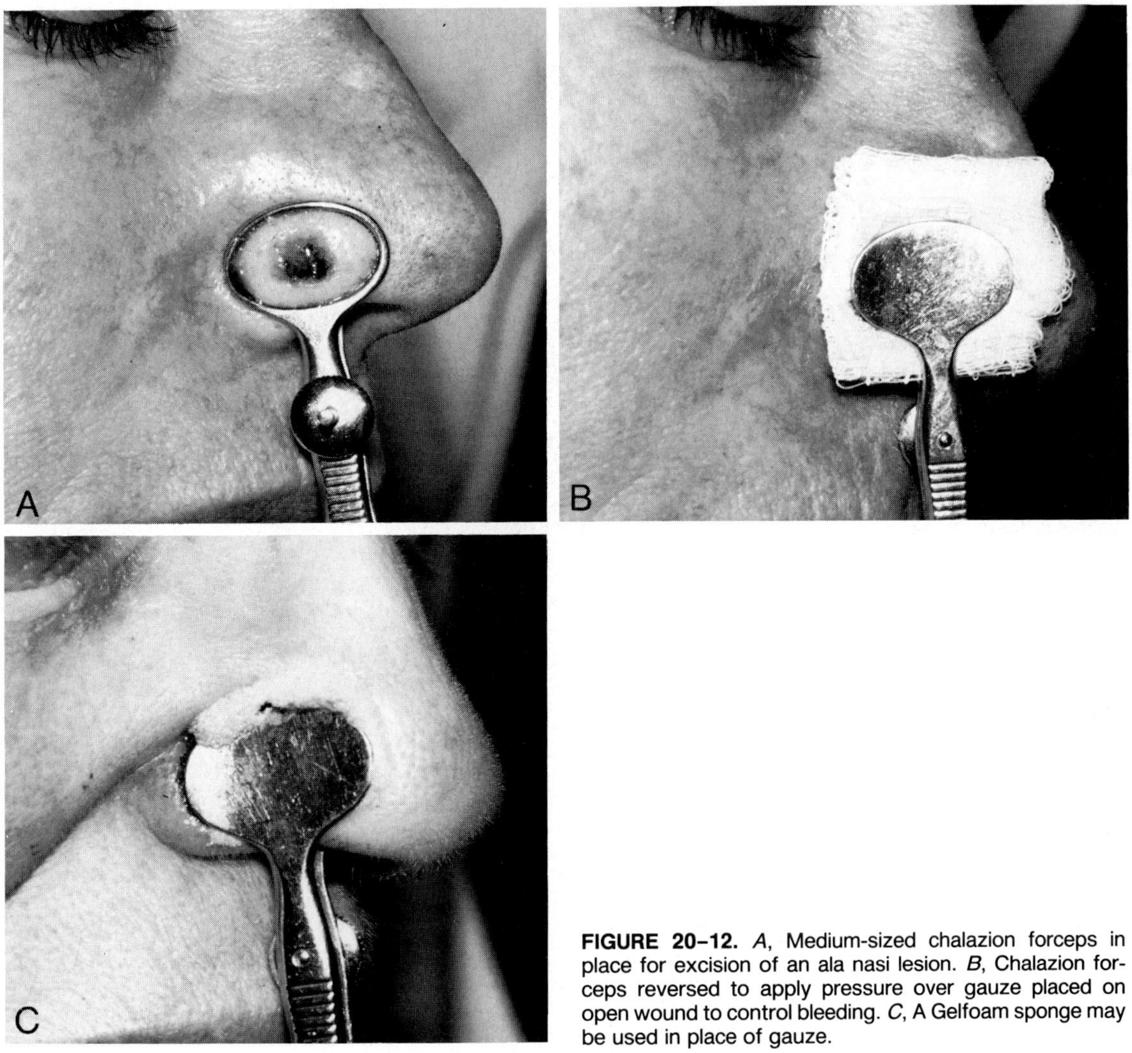

FIGURE 20–12. *A*, Medium-sized chalazion forceps in place for excision of an ala nasi lesion. *B*, Chalazion forceps reversed to apply pressure over gauze placed on open wound to control bleeding. *C*, A Gelfoam sponge may be used in place of gauze.

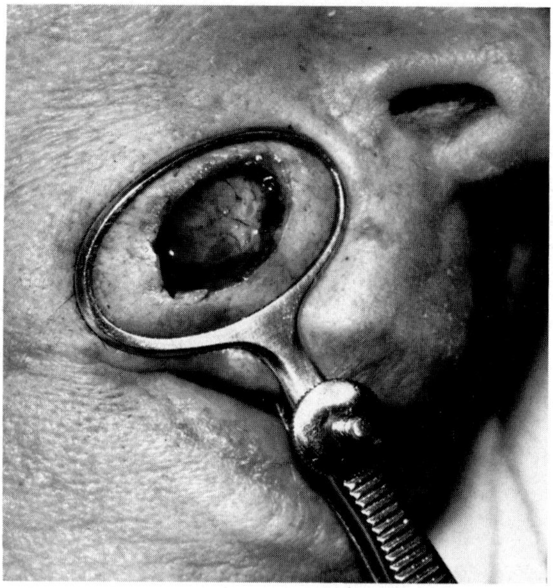

FIGURE 20–14. Deep wound in upper lip; hemostatic action of chalazion forceps is demonstrated.

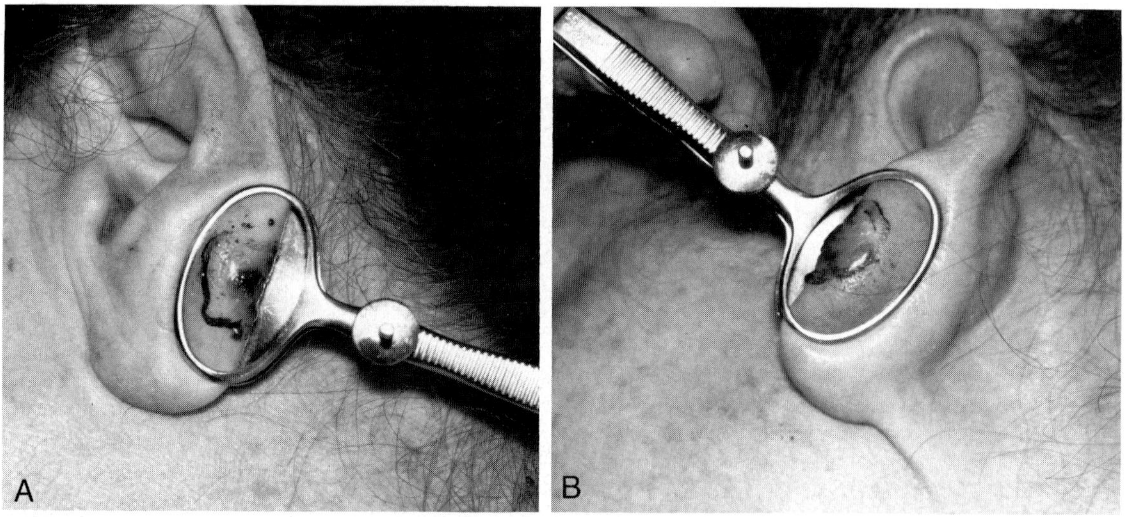

FIGURE 20–15. *A*, Chalazion forceps placed on ear lobe before excision of a lesion. *B*, Change of position of chalazion forceps in order to remove the posterior component of the lesion.

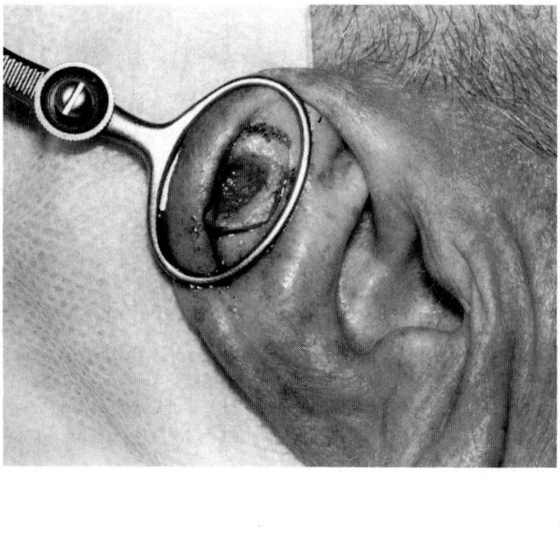

FIGURE 20–16. Large chalazion forceps applied to ear secures the operative field and steadies this mobile part.

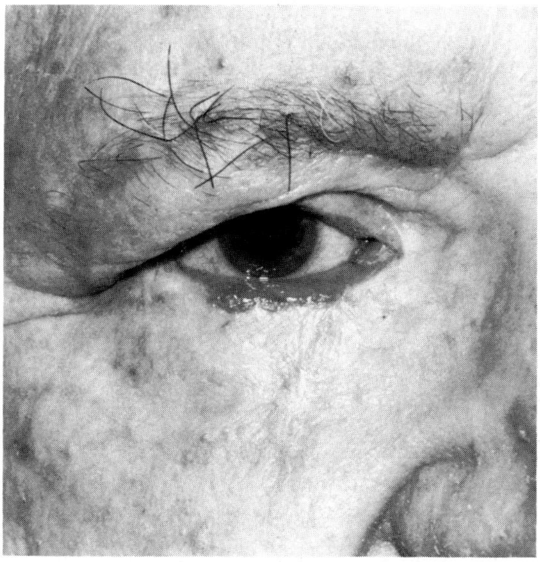

FIGURE 20–17. Exteriorized conjunctiva on eyelid margin after healing by second intention might be mistaken for a recurrence.

perforations through the cheek and the maxillary antrum. It is also used to enhance the protection of an exposed eyeball when used with an eye shield and to prevent blood from trickling into the auditory canal. The cleansing of blood from the ear canal is a major undertaking. Plugging the canal with a pledget of cotton

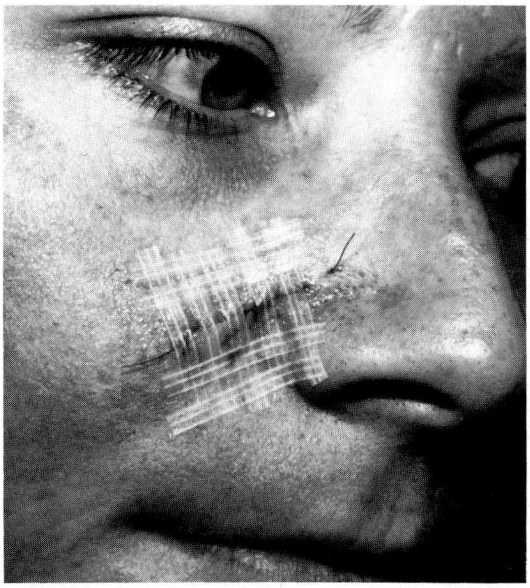

FIGURE 20–18. Steri-Strips applied over Mastisol to relieve tension on wound margins after closure with a subcuticular running suture.

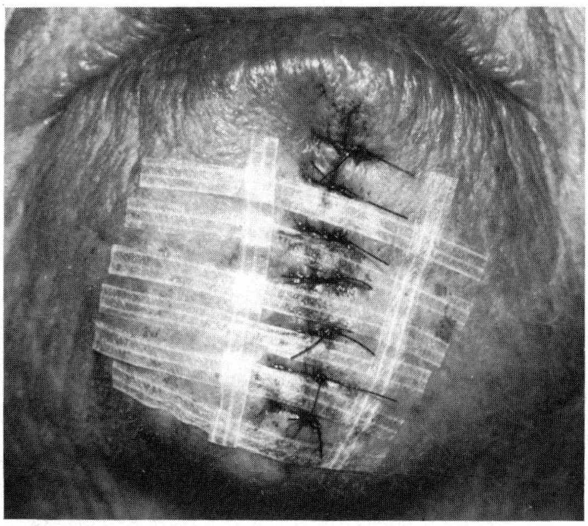

FIGURE 20–19. Steri-Strip–Mastisol combination applied to sutured wound on chin.

and then sealing the cotton with a layer of Orabase and moistening it with a drop of water greatly simplifies the procedure by sealing the auditory canal. The plug can be left in place until the wound is closed or until granulation is well established, if second intention healing is chosen.

The Disquieting Skin Graft

When using split-thickness grafts, it is recommended that the surgeon select a donor site as free of blemishes as possible. A disturbing sit-

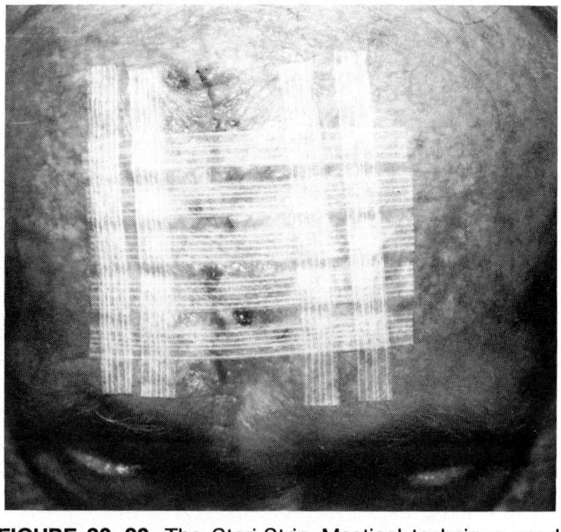

FIGURE 20–20. The Steri-Strip–Mastisol technique used after suture removal from a forehead wound.

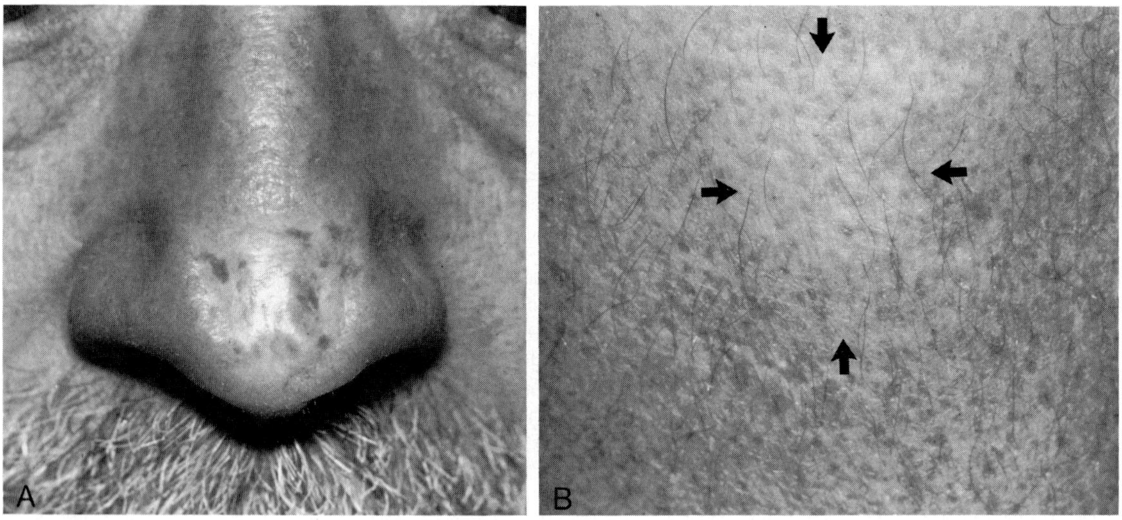

FIGURE 20–21. *A*, Pigmented split-thickness graft used for repair of a defect after Mohs surgery. *B*, Donor site of graft was the thigh; note hyperpigmented, follicular macules over the entire skin. The pigment is less marked in the area where the skin was harvested (*arrow*).

uation arose after a split-thickness skin graft was obtained from the anterior aspect of the thigh to repair a Mohs surgical defect on the tip of the nose. After healing, the patient complained of pigmented spots in the treated area, which naturally created a good deal of speculation and anxiety (Fig. 20–21A). However, upon inspection of the donor site, it was found covered with extensive follicular hyperpigmented macules which were obviously lighter in color where the graft had been obtained (Fig. 20–21B), and the pathogenesis became immediately clear. Further plastic surgery was required to remedy the situation and to exclude a malignant melanotic lesion.

REFERENCES

1. Mikhail GR, Selak L, Salo S: Reinforcement of surgical adhesive strips, J Dermatol Surg Oncol 12:904–906, 1986.
2. Mikhail GR, Selak L, Salo S, Balle MR: The efficacy of adhesives in the application of wound dressings, J Burn Care Rehabilitation 10:216–219, 1989.

CHAPTER 21

Carcinoma of the Nail

George R. Mikhail, M.D., M.S.

ANATOMY

The nail is a complex organ. Its anatomy is illustrated in Figure 21–1. The actual structure is shown in Figures 21–2 and 21–3. Carcinomas that involve the nail occur on the dorsal surface of the terminal phalanx, where the nail bed is about 3 mm at its thickest point over the middle of the phalanx and about 1.5 mm over the tip of the terminal phalanx.

CLINICAL

Squamous cell carcinoma of the nail unit is not as rare as has been implied in the literature. In 1984, we reviewed the data in 89 well-documented cases and reported on 21 additional cases of our own.[1] Since then, the number of cases that have been personally encountered has risen to 70. Their sites and the types of carcinoma are shown in Tables 21–1 and 21–2. They were all treated by Mohs micrographic surgery, and it is significant that nearly half of the hand lesions occurred on the thumb.

The initial presenting symptoms are pain, swelling, and erythema. Later manifestations include nail dystrophies. Following the loss of the nail plate, the lesions appear crusted, eczematous, scaly, or verrucous. The presence of ulceration, bleeding, induration, or nodularity indicates invasive carcinoma. The tumors grow slowly. The duration of symptoms from onset to the time of diagnosis varies from several months to many years (up to 18). The lesions are often mistaken for chronic inflammatory conditions, including bacterial and fungal infections, and are treated for such conditions without avail. It is only after a biopsy is obtained that the correct diagnosis is made. Other conditions that may present diagnostic difficulties are verrucae vulgaris, pyogenic granuloma, subungual exostosis, nail dystrophies, glomus tumor, malignant melanoma, and subungual keratoacanthoma.

Subungual carcinoma has been reported in individuals as young as 20 years. The highest incidence among our patients has been in the age range between 35 and 50 years old. It is significant that in 113 reported patients metastases have been reported in only two instances, one at age 21[2] and the other at age 27.[3] None occurred in our series of 66 patients.

ETIOLOGY

The etiology of subungual carcinoma is unclear in the majority of cases. Trauma, exposure to x-rays (physicians, dentists, and patients), chronic paronychia, and dyskeratosis congenita have been cited as etiologic factors. One of our patients developed Bowen's disease in the nail bed and periungual tissues after x-ray therapy for periungual verrucae vulgaris (Fig. 21–4). Another patient, a dentist, had involvement of the left third and fourth fingers caused by chronic radiodermatitis (Fig. 21–5). We have seen subungual squamous cell carcinoma in a patient with epidermodysplasia verruciformis (Fig. 21–6).

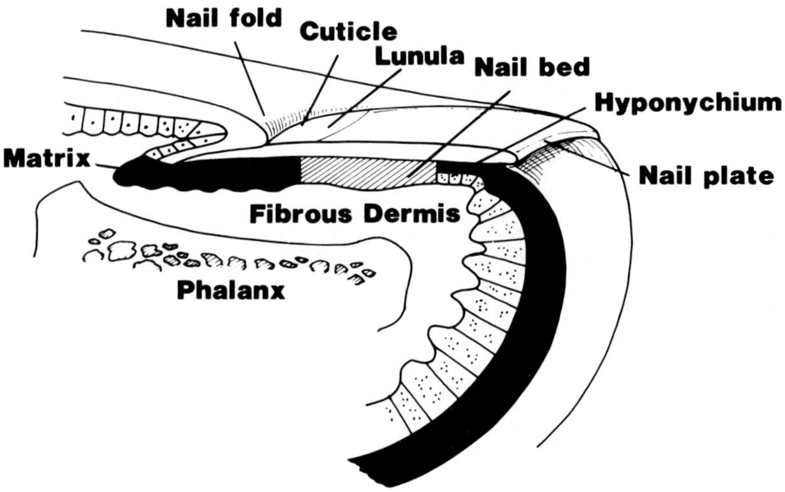

FIGURE 21–1. Diagram of the anatomic components of the nail organ.

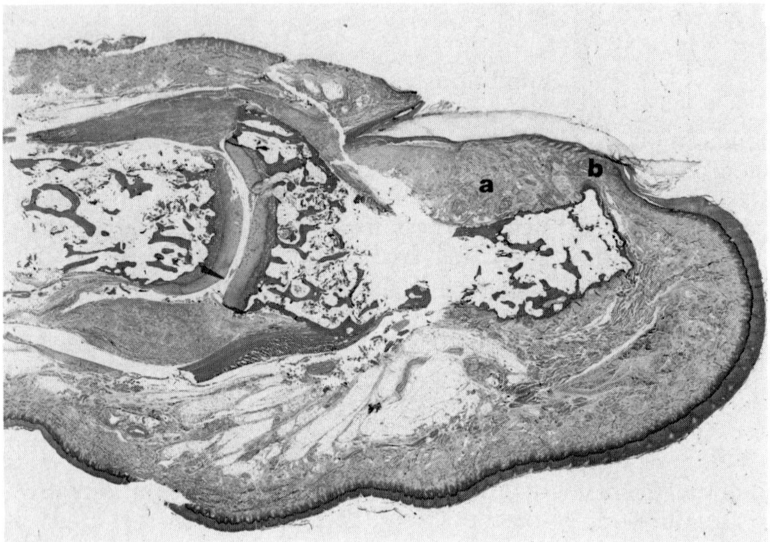

FIGURE 21–2. Sagittal section of a digit: The nail bed is about 3 mm at point *a* (thickest part) and is about 1.5 mm at point *b* over the dorsal tip of the terminal phalanx. (Section prepared by Julius M. Ohorodnik, M.D., Department of Pathology, Henry Ford Hospital.)

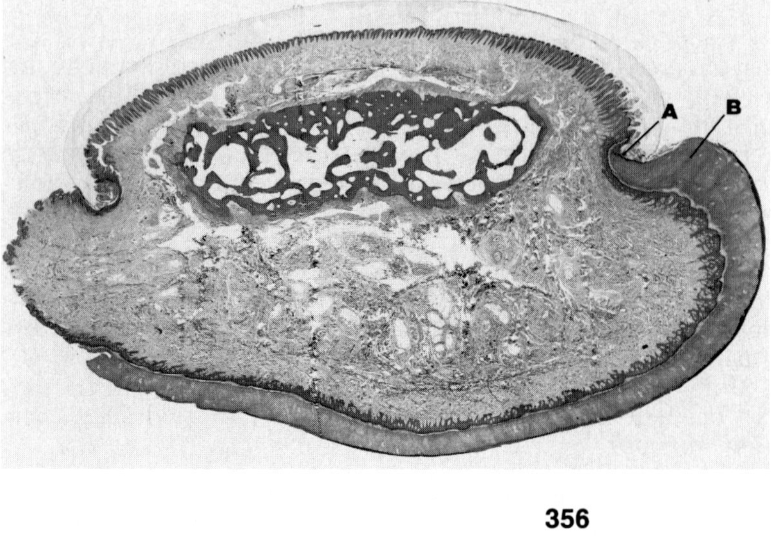

FIGURE 21–3. Transverse section through a digit at the middle of the terminal phalanx shows the nail groove *(A)* and the lateral nail fold *(B)*. (Section prepared by Julius M. Ohorodnik, M.D., Department of Pathology, Henry Ford Hospital.)

TABLE 21–1. Sites of Subungual Squamous Cell Carcinoma

Site	Digit: 1st	Digit: Other	Total
Hand	22	46	68
Foot	1	1	2
Total	23	47	70*

*70 lesions in 67 patients.

TABLE 21–2. Types of Squamous Cell Carcinoma Treated

Type	Site: Thumb	Fingers	Hallux	Toes	Total
Bowen's disease	12	32	–	1	45
Invasive carcinoma	10	14	1	–	25
Total	22	46	1	1	70*

*70 lesions in 67 patients.

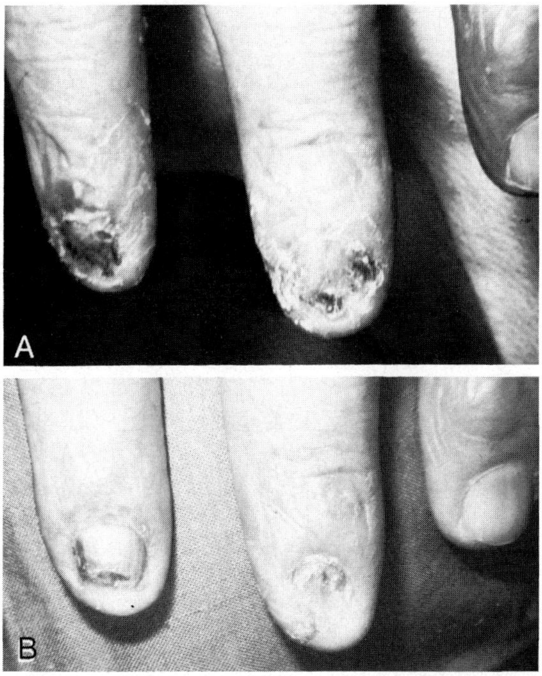

FIGURE 21–5. *A*, Radiodermatitis and squamous cell carcinoma of the nail in two digits of a dental surgeon. *B*, Result after Mohs surgery; nail regrowth on one of the fingers.

PATHOLOGY

After reviewing the literature and our material, we conclude that the neoplasia originates most commonly in the nail folds and grooves (see Fig. 21–3). Figure 21–7 shows Bowen's disease of the nail folds and early invasion of the nail

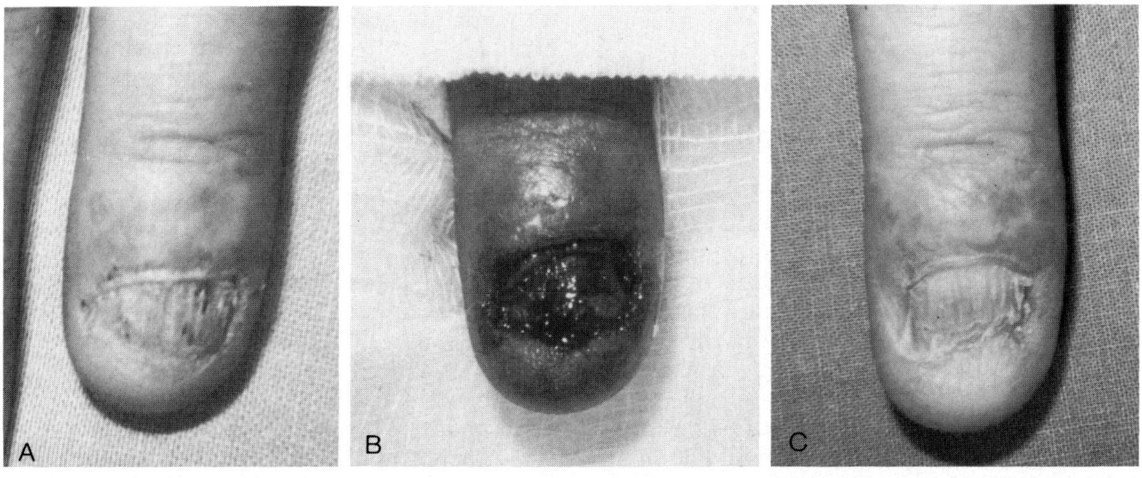

FIGURE 21–4. *A*, Dystrophic left ring finger nail caused by Bowen's disease. *B*, Wound after excision of entire nail bed. *C*, Result after healing by second intention; note the regrowth of nail.

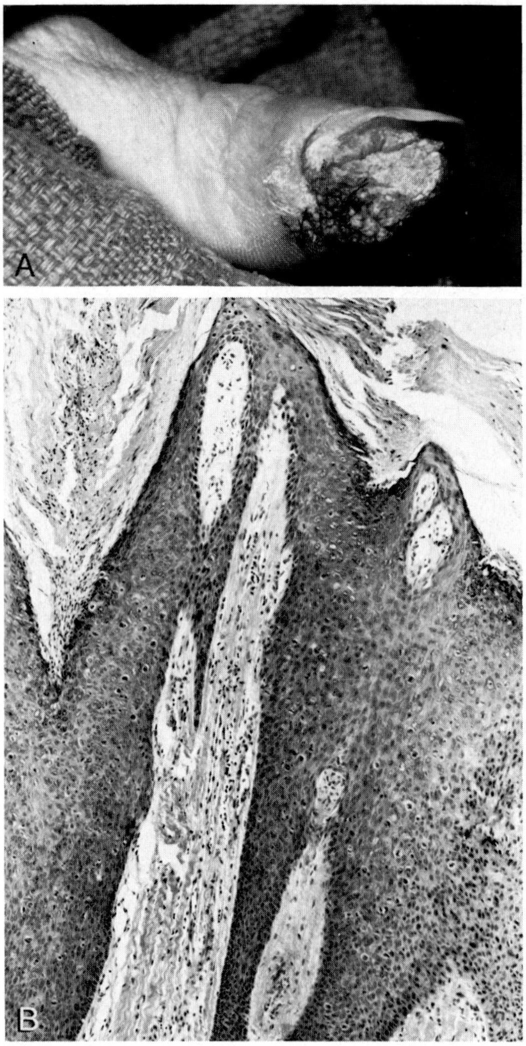

FIGURE 21–6. Subungual squamous cell carcinoma in a patient with epidermodysplasia verruciformis. *A*, Clinical appearance. *B*, Histopathology shows marked cellular atypia.

bed, while Figure 21–8 illustrates a deeply invasive carcinoma.

One cannot overemphasize the importance of obtaining biopsy material from all chronic and recalcitrant lesions of the nail bed and the periungual areas. The procedure is safe and easy to perform. In order to obtain adequate material for histologic examination, the entire lesion has to be exposed. This may necessitate partial or complete avulsion of the nail plate. Tissue is then excised in as thick a layer as possible. The depth of the excision should be close to the periosteum of the terminal phalanx. This maneuver permits detection of an invasive carcinoma if one has developed at the base of a lesion caused by Bowen's disease (see Fig. 21–7). Remember that a biopsy that shows Bowen's disease does not exclude the presence of invasive squamous cell carcinoma in other parts of the lesion. This is one more reason why Mohs surgery is indicated in all cases of Bowen's disease. The lesion in Figure 21–9 was a subungual verruca proved after avulsing the nail plate and obtaining ample biopsy material.

PROGNOSIS

When squamous cell carcinomas of the skin of the hand invade tendon or bone, 30% of the patients have metastases to the regional lymph nodes. However, only one case of the 113 reported squamous cell carcinomas of the nail bed actually did metastasize.[4] It appears that carcinomas at this particular site are not as aggressive as those that occur on other areas of the body. This biological behavior is, for some unknown reason, comparable to that of squamous cell carcinomas that arise in actinic keratoses. However, any relationship to solar damage does not appear to exist.

THERAPY

The ideal aim of therapy for subungual carcinomas is the complete ablation of the neoplastic tissue. The prevalent modality among surgeons is amputation of the distal phalanx. Such a plan may not seriously affect hand function if the digit in question is not the thumb. However, 22 out of 68 of the lesions were on the thumb. Loss of the distal phalanx of the thumb results in 30% disability of the hand. Therefore, Mohs micrographic surgery is ideally suited for the management of these lesions because it assures complete removal of the disease with maximal preservation of function and optimal cosmesis.

The Mohs technique for excising subungual carcinomas is similar to that used in other areas of the body. However, it is advisable to obtain radiographs of the involved digit prior to surgical intervention in order to detect possible bone involvement. In our series of 70 cases, there was only one instance in which this occurred, and the terminal phalanx had to be

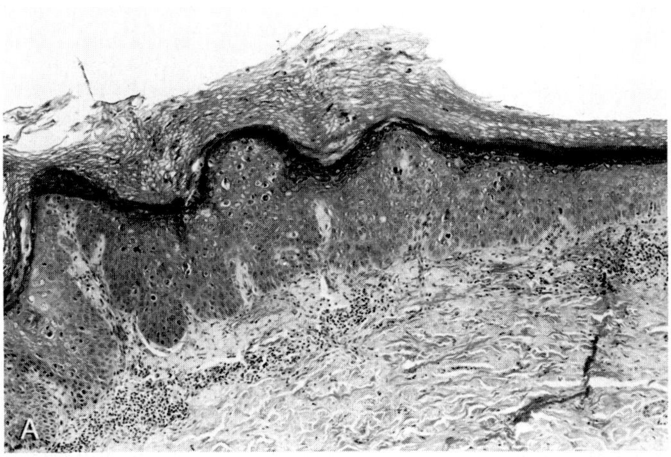

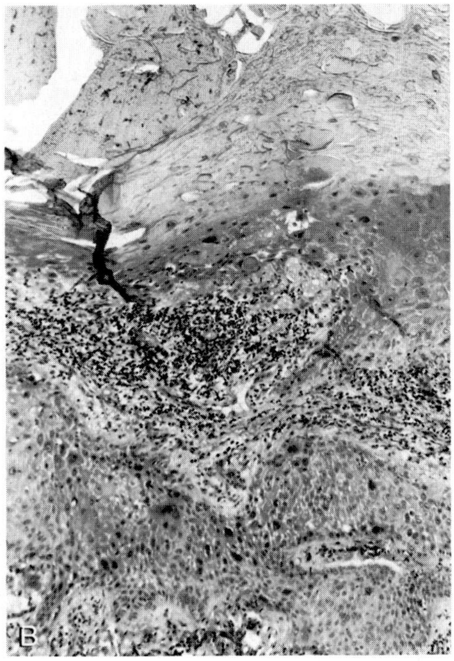

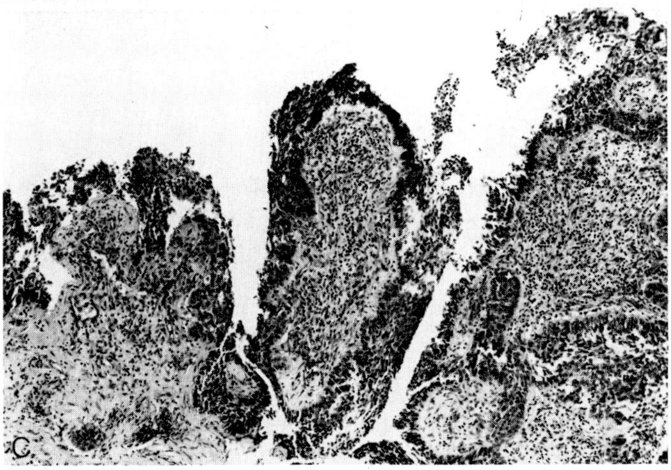

FIGURE 21–7. *A*, Bowen's disease of the lateral nail fold. *B*, Early invasive squamous cell carcinoma originating in the posterior nail fold. *C*, Superficial carcinoma in the nail bed.

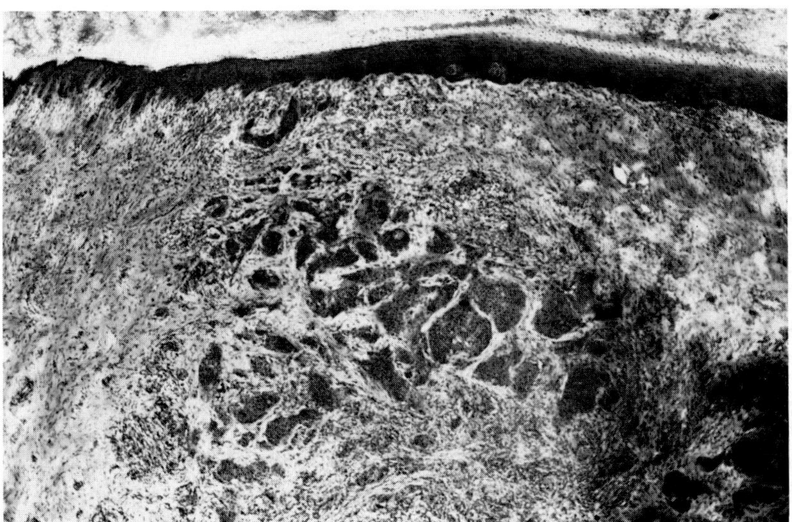

FIGURE 21–8. Deeply invasive squamous cell carcinoma of the nail bed.

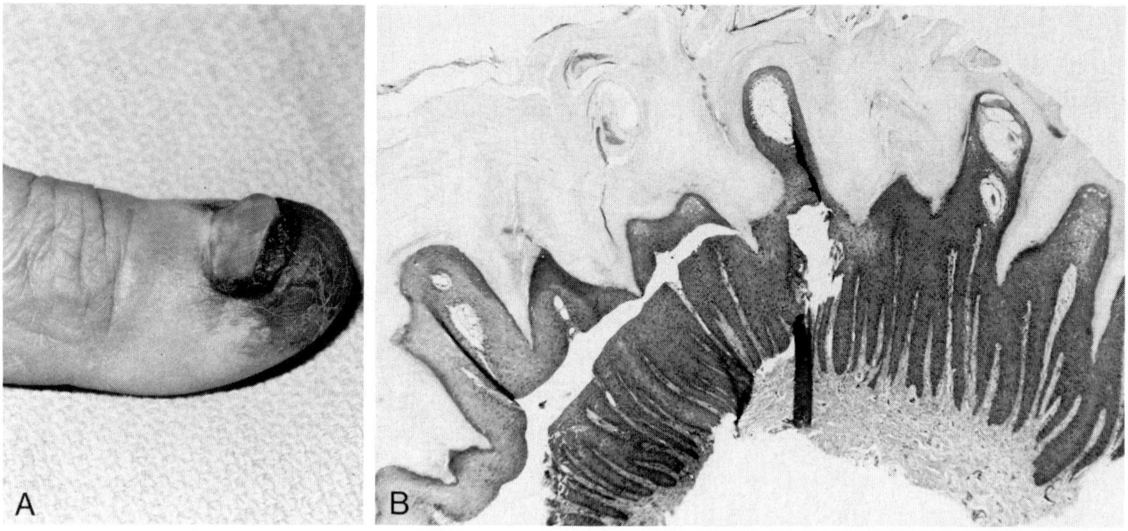

FIGURE 21-9. *A*, Subungual verruca vulgaris. *B*, Biopsy shows the classical histology of verruca vulgaris (compare Fig. 21-7).

amputated because of extensive bone and soft tissue involvement.

Anatomically, the thickest part of the nail bed is about 3 mm. Therefore, it is advisable to take the first layer down to the periosteum and include in it a 2 mm free-appearing margin. In our experience, it is peripherally that more layers may have to be removed. Also, the dorsal tip of the terminal phalanx is usually removed with a rongeur and examined histologically after decalcification.

The first four cases in our series were treated by the Mohs fixed tissue technqiue. We found that it caused great discomfort, and the healing process was prolonged over 3 months because of the time needed for separation of the fixed bone of the dorsum of the phalanx.[5] Sixty-six cases have been treated by the fresh tissue technique with minor discomfort. Furthermore, this method is expedient, saves more normal tissue, and has much faster healing. There is a good possibility for nail regrowth if a portion of the nail matrix is spared (Figs. 21-4 and 21-5). Figures 21-10 and 21-11 depict examples of extensive squamous cell carcinoma of the nail bed treated by the Mohs fresh tissue technique in which the nail was permanently lost because the matrix was involved.

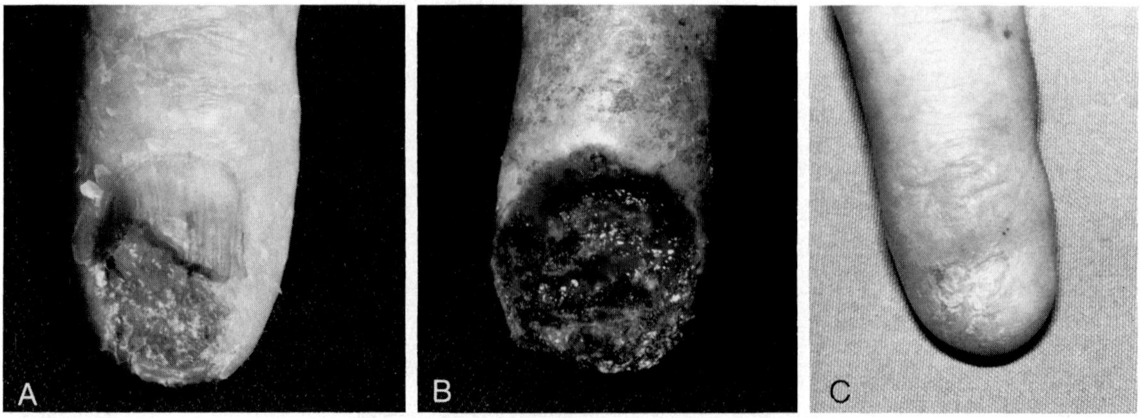

FIGURE 21-10. *A*, Advanced squamous cell carcinoma of the nail. *B*, Wound at completion of Mohs surgery; an appreciable part of the terminal phalanx had to be removed. *C*, Result after healing by second intention; the nail was completely lost.

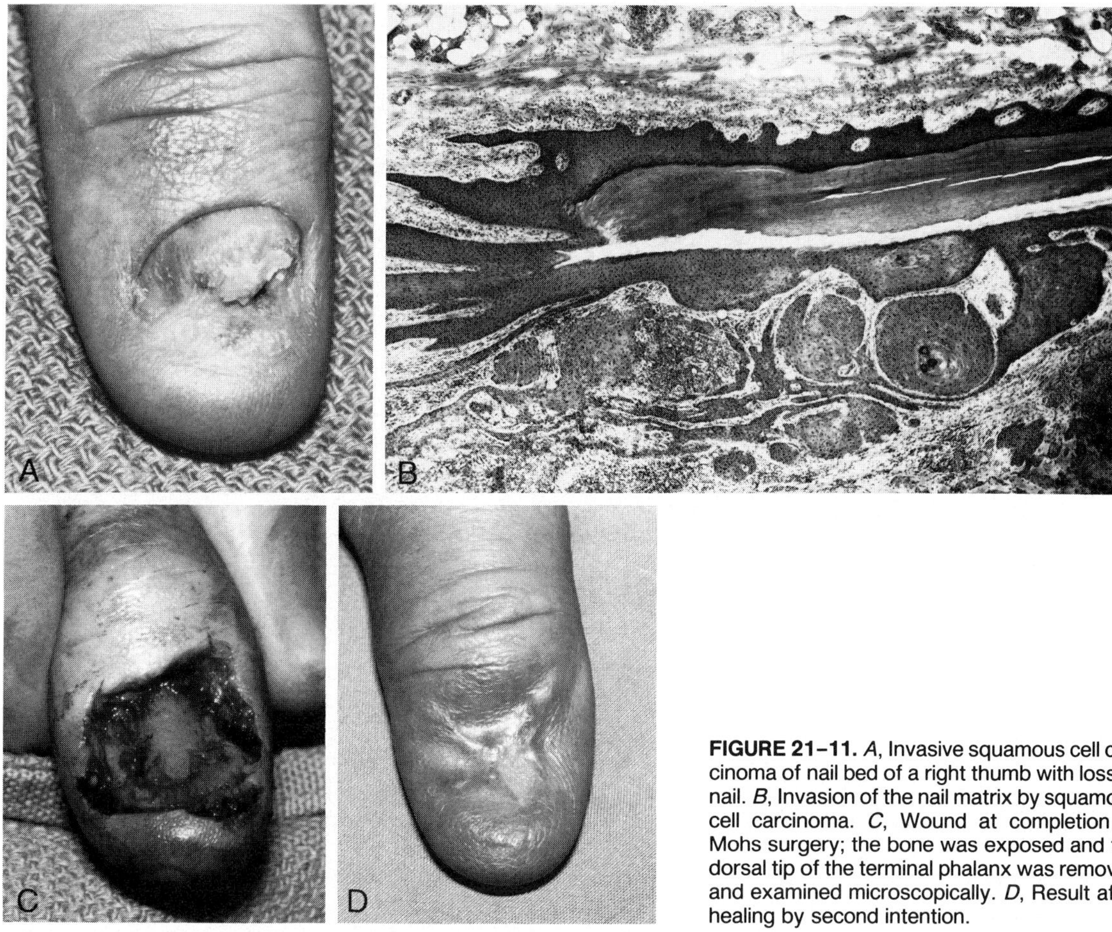

FIGURE 21–11. *A*, Invasive squamous cell carcinoma of nail bed of a right thumb with loss of nail. *B*, Invasion of the nail matrix by squamous cell carcinoma. *C*, Wound at completion of Mohs surgery; the bone was exposed and the dorsal tip of the terminal phalanx was removed and examined microscopically. *D*, Result after healing by second intention.

Fifty-six lesions have been observed for 5 years or more. Recurrence occurred in two lesions and were retreated with success.

REFERENCES

1. Mikhail GR: Subungual epidermoid carcinoma, J Am Acad Dermatol 11:291–298, 1984.
2. Fromer JL: Carcinomas of the nail bed: Discussion, Arch Dermatol 101:66–67, 1970.
3. Campbell CJ, Keokarn T: Squamous cell carcinoma of the nail bed in epidermal dysplasia, J Bone Joint Dis 48:92–99, 1966.
4. Attiyeh FF, Shah J, Booker RJ, Knapper WH: Surgical squamous cell carcinoma, JAMA 241:262–263, 1979.
5. Mikhail GR: Bowen's disease and squamous cell carcinoma of the nail bed, Arch Dermatol 110:267–270, 1974.

CHAPTER 22

Unusual and Interesting Encounters

George R. Mikhail, M.D., M.S.

Examples of unusual cases by virtue of site, extent, biological behavior, or rarity are presented in this chapter.

BASAL CELL CARCINOMAS

Facial Lesions

Large lesions on the face, especially those on the nose and eyelids, are challenging and demand special care and precautions during and after Mohs excision.

A 55-year-old man had a sclerotic basal cell carcinoma (BCC) that involved the entire nose and a large portion of the adjacent cheek on the left side (Fig. 22–1). The large defect after Mohs surgery was repaired with grafts. There was no recurrence after 6 years of follow-up.

A 48-year-old woman was referred for ablation of a recurrent basal cell carcinoma on the right side of the nose, the adjacent cheek, and upper lip. The lesions had been previously treated by radiotherapy (Fig. 22–2). Because of the site and extent of the tumor, the postsurgical defect was left to heal by second intention, observed for 1 year to ensure the complete absence of any residual tumor, and then repaired in multiple stages with flaps and grafts. There was a final good cosmetic result and no recurrence after 7 years of follow-up.

A large lesion that involved the bridge of the nose, glabella, both eyelids, left cheek, and left zygomatic area in a 48-year-old man is shown in Figure 22–3. It was excised by the fresh tissue method. The postsurgical defect was successfully repaired by an oculoplastic surgeon using grafts, which preserved eye function. There was no recurrence or complications at 4 years follow-up.

A recurrent BCC in a 63-year-old man involved the bulbar conjunctiva and entire lower eyelid, including the palpebral conjunctiva, and was excised using the fresh tissue method (Fig. 22–4). The lower eyelid was first cleared of the carcinoma, then the bulbar portion was excised in a layer that included a portion of the sclera. The defect was repaired by an oculoplastic surgeon with good function and reasonably good cosmesis. There was no recurrence or impairment of eye function when the patient expired more than 8 years later.

The above cases demonstrate the value and advantages of multidisciplinary management. Oftentimes, such an approach is necessary in order to achieve optimal results. It is advisable that the specialist who will be ultimately needed should see the patient before the Mohs surgery is performed.

Not uncommonly, there are cases of BCC that pose significant challenges, and the outcome after treatment is inevitably far from satisfactory. Although we have seen this rarely in primary lesions treated by Mohs surgery, the most difficult cases have been those that recurred after radiotherapy and non-Mohs exci-

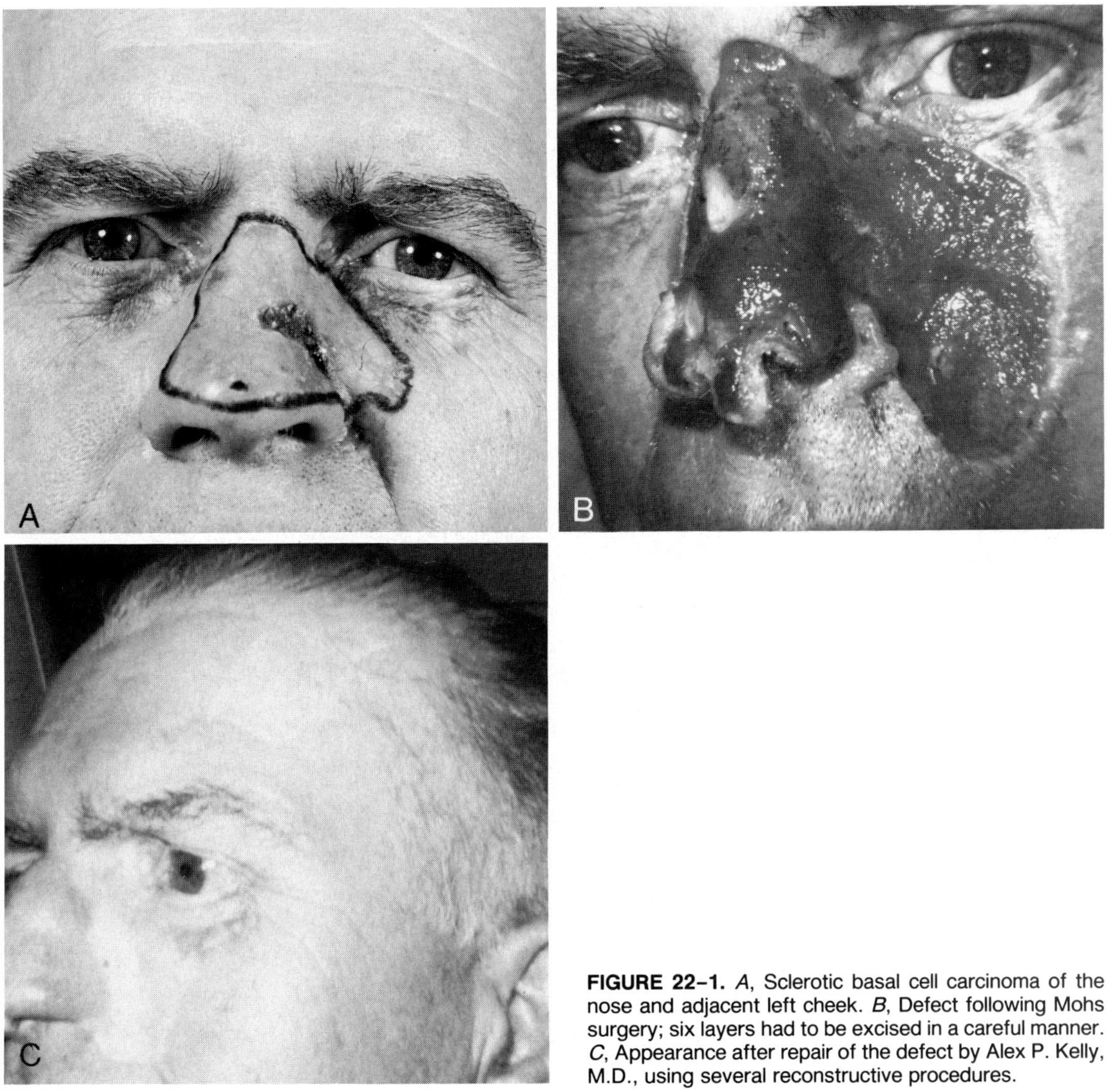

FIGURE 22–1. *A*, Sclerotic basal cell carcinoma of the nose and adjacent left cheek. *B*, Defect following Mohs surgery; six layers had to be excised in a careful manner. *C*, Appearance after repair of the defect by Alex P. Kelly, M.D., using several reconstructive procedures.

sions, especially those followed by immediate repair with flaps. In the case of a 60-year-old man shown in Figure 22–5, a basal cell carcinoma over the left zygoma was excised four times and received a series of radiotherapy. The pathologists' reports after each excision indicated that the margins of the excised tissues were clear of tumor. The patient was referred for Mohs surgery after a recurrence in the outer canthus and lower eyelid. Biopsies from the margins of the flap in the right infraorbital and cheek areas were positive for BCC. During Mohs surgery, it was found that the tumor extended into the retrobulbar and orbital fat, maxillary sinus, and buccal mucosa. The orbit had to be exenterated. This case illustrates and endorses the following tenets: (1) the routine vertical sections practiced by pathologists are, in many cases, inadequate for checking margins, (2) one recurrence should serve as ample indication for a Mohs surgery referral, and (3) recurrence after radiotherapy compounds the difficulties. Unfortunately, such cases are not uncommon in a Mohs practice.

Metastatic Basal Cell Carcinoma

Metastatic BCC is rare. Lattes and Kessler[1] have set down the criteria for making such a

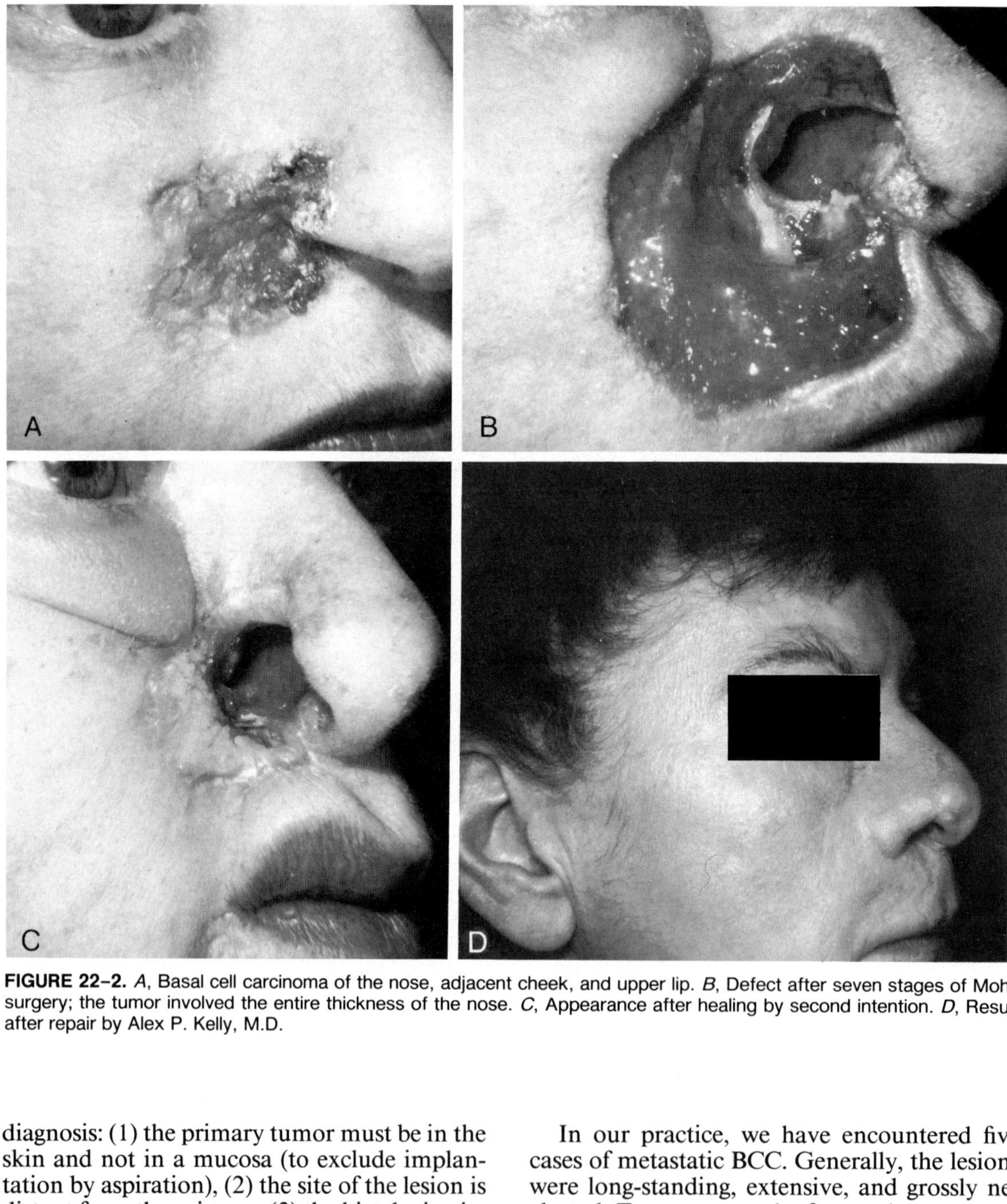

FIGURE 22–2. *A*, Basal cell carcinoma of the nose, adjacent cheek, and upper lip. *B*, Defect after seven stages of Mohs surgery; the tumor involved the entire thickness of the nose. *C*, Appearance after healing by second intention. *D*, Result after repair by Alex P. Kelly, M.D.

diagnosis: (1) the primary tumor must be in the skin and not in a mucosa (to exclude implantation by aspiration), (2) the site of the lesion is distant from the primary, (3) the histologic picture (the most important criterion) should be identical in both the primary site and the metastases, and (4) the metastases should not have a squamous cell component. By 1977, there were 78 well-documented cases.[2] Another review in 1984 cited 175 cases.[3] All of these patients succumbed within several months to a few years after the diagnosis was established.

In our practice, we have encountered five cases of metastatic BCC. Generally, the lesions were long-standing, extensive, and grossly neglected. Four were on the face and one was on the scalp. The site of the metastasis was the bone in four instances, the lymph nodes in two, the lung in one, and the distant skin of the thigh and arm in one. Our first case was that of a metastasis to a zygomatic lymph node from a BCC of the left outer canthus and zygomatic area. The metastasis was discovered during a Mohs fixed tissue procedure in a 63-year-old

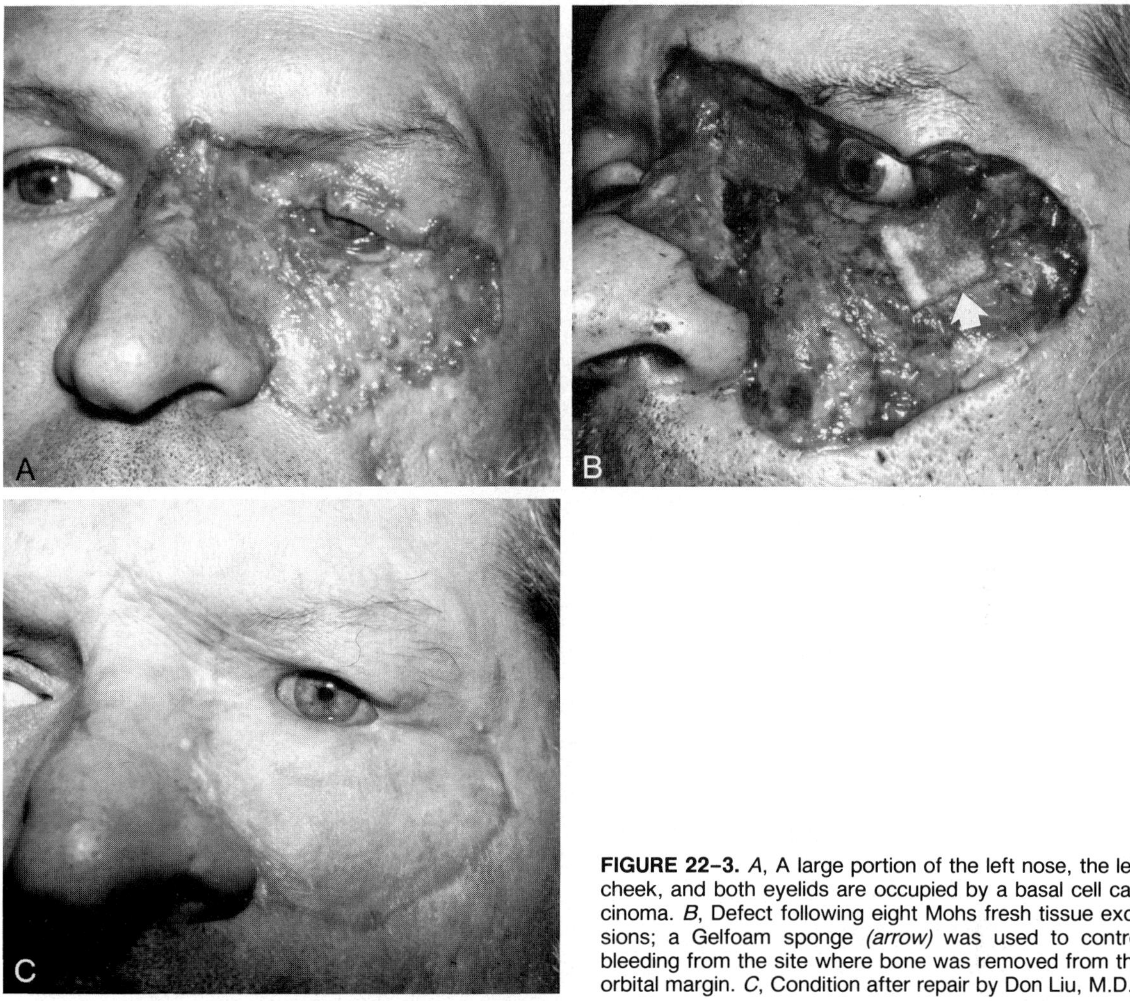

FIGURE 22–3. *A*, A large portion of the left nose, the left cheek, and both eyelids are occupied by a basal cell carcinoma. *B*, Defect following eight Mohs fresh tissue excisions; a Gelfoam sponge *(arrow)* was used to control bleeding from the site where bone was removed from the orbital margin. *C*, Condition after repair by Don Liu, M.D.

man.[4] Of three other published cases, the metastases were in bone in one; in bone, lymph nodes, and skin in another;[2] and in bone and lungs in the third.[5]

The second case was that of a man age 57 first seen in January 1969, who had received radiotherapy for acne at age 19. For the past 7 years, a "growth" on the cheek was treated twice with electrosurgery but recurred. At the time the patient was referred for Mohs surgery there was an ulcerated, indurated lesion about 3 cm in size on the left cheek near the buccal commissure. A hard, core-like mass extended posteriorly from this lesion connecting to another mass in the infra-auricular area. Biopsies showed sclerotic BCC. The tumor was excised by nine stages of the Mohs fixed tissue surgery. The left buccal wall, the lower part of the pinna, and a significant part of the left parotid gland, including part of the facial nerve, had to be removed. Nine reconstructive procedures were undertaken between March 1969 and May 1970 (Fig. 22–6). In July 1970, the patient complained of pain in the left hip that had been present since April 1970. Radiologic examination detected lytic lesions in the left iliac bone and lumbar vertebrae. The presence of BCC in the bone was proved by biopsy. Other metastases were later found in the second lumbar vertebra. The patient's health rapidly deteriorated, and he expired in December 1971, about 20 months after the onset of bone involvement.

A 59-year-old woman had an extensive BCC that involved the eyelids, and the temporal, frontal and zygomatic regions on the right side

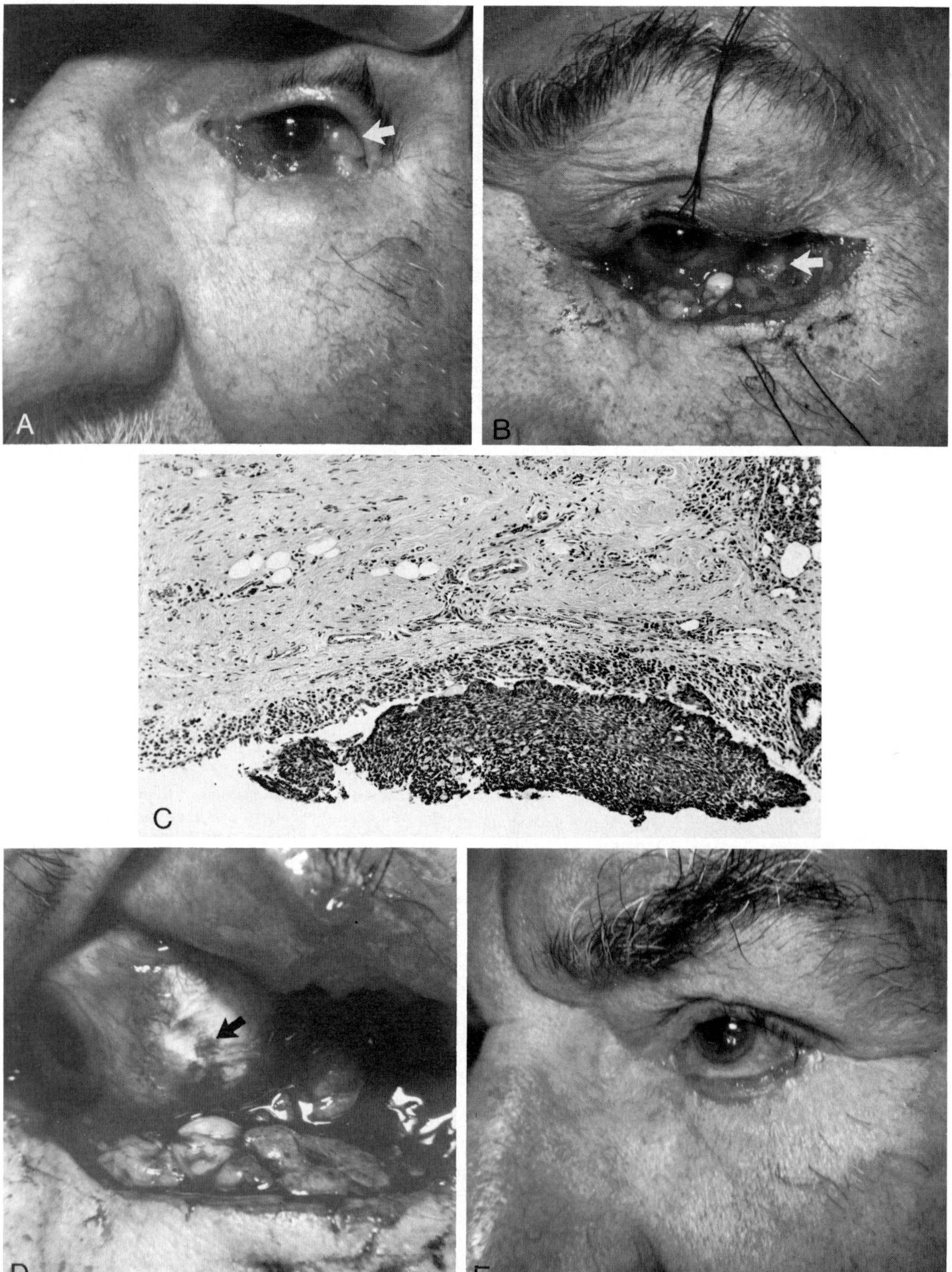

FIGURE 22–4. *A*, Recurrent basal cell carcinoma (BCC) of the entire lower eyelid and the bulbar conjunctiva *(arrow)*. *B*, Appearance after removal of the eyelid part of the carcinoma; sutures were placed near the eyelid margins to serve as retractors. Note the orbital fat; the arrow points to the bulbar region. *C*, Biopsy shows BCC in the bulbar conjunctiva. *D*, Final defect at the termination of surgery; because part of the sclera had to be removed in the excised layer, the choroid can be seen through the thinned out sclera *(arrow)*. *E*, Result after repair by Ray Dixon, M.D.

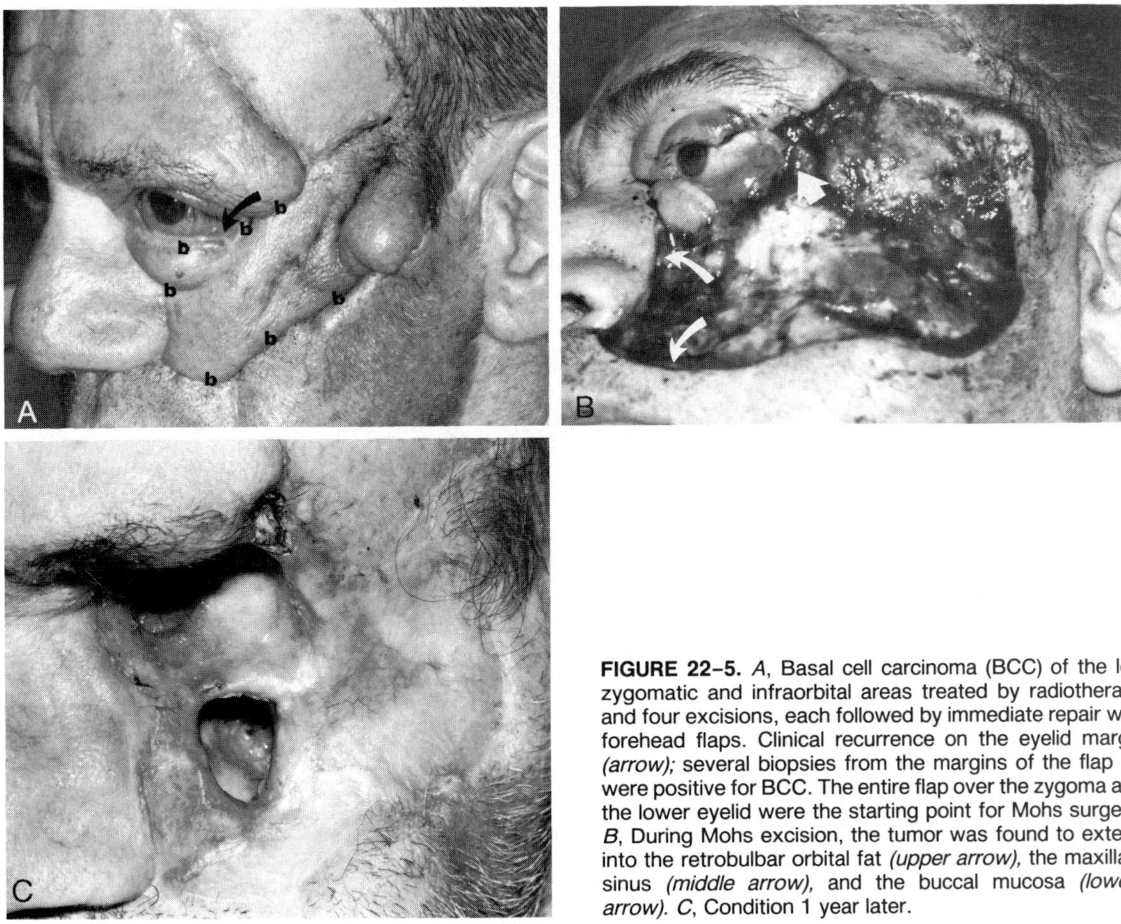

FIGURE 22–5. *A*, Basal cell carcinoma (BCC) of the left zygomatic and infraorbital areas treated by radiotherapy and four excisions, each followed by immediate repair with forehead flaps. Clinical recurrence on the eyelid margin *(arrow);* several biopsies from the margins of the flap (*b*) were positive for BCC. The entire flap over the zygoma and the lower eyelid were the starting point for Mohs surgery. *B*, During Mohs excision, the tumor was found to extend into the retrobulbar orbital fat *(upper arrow),* the maxillary sinus *(middle arrow),* and the buccal mucosa *(lowest arrow). C*, Condition 1 year later.

(Fig. 22–7). Histologic examination showed a keratinizing BCC. The lesion was excised en masse together with the contents of the orbit and the zygomatic arch, and the wound was covered with a split-thickness skin graft. The pathology report indicated complete removal of the tumor and absence of bone involvement. Four months later, two nodules were noted underneath the graft at the lateral and lower margins of the orbit. They proved to be recurrent BCC and were excised by the Mohs fixed tissue method. The lower lesion extended into the maxillary antrum. The wounds were left to heal by second intention. The BCC recurred again in the zygomatic area and the parietal scalp at the edge of the graft. These were again chemosurgically excised. Four months later, an enlarged cervical lymph node and a 2 cm ulcerated mass in the left forearm were excised. The histology in both was identical with that of the primary lesion. Subcutaneous nodules developed within the next month, several of them on the back. One on the right thigh was about 2.5 cm in size and showed the same histologic features seen in the other lesions, but the tumor occupied the deeper dermis and the subcutis and was not connected with the epidermis. The wall of a deep subcutaneous arteriole was involved. By that time, the patient had become emaciated and was complaining of bone pain. A radiographic bone survey revealed compression fractures of several vertebral bodies and radiolucency of the pelvic bones. Radionuclide examination with an isotope, technetium-99m pyrophosphate, showed involvement of the skull, ribs, sacrum, pelvic bones, and both femurs. Biopsy material from the right iliac bone demonstrated the presence of BCC. The salient features of this case are shown in Figure 22–7. The patient expired 4 months after the first signs of metastasis.

A woman age 44 presented with a large, ul-

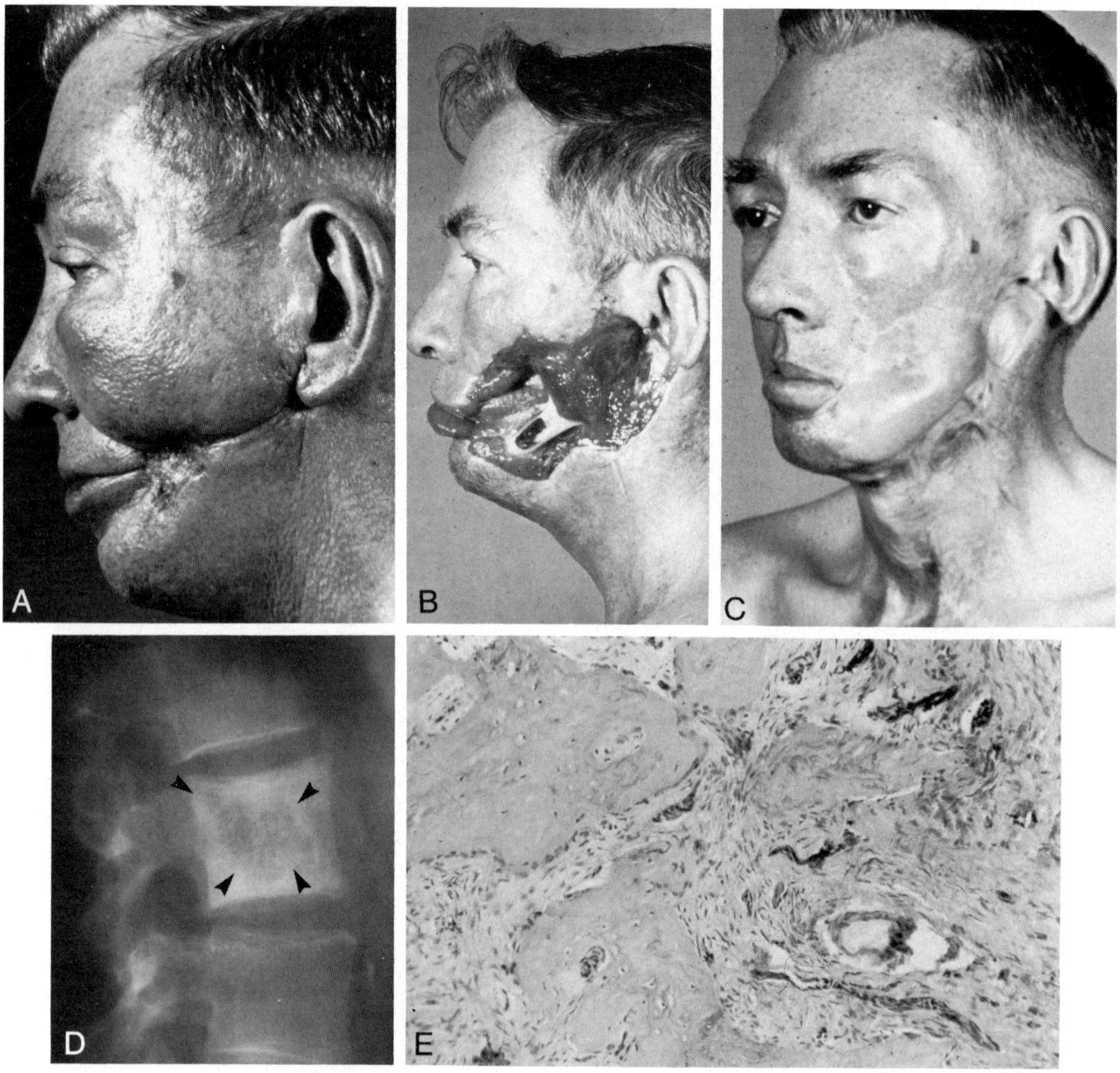

FIGURE 22–6. *A*, Extensive sclerotic basal cell carcinoma (BCC) extending from buccal commissure to mastoid area as a cord. *B*, Defect after nine Mohs fixed tissue excisions. *C*, Condition after nine reconstructive procedures. *D*, Radiolucency in a lumbar vertebra. *E*, BCC in iliac bone biopsy. (From Mikhail, GR, et al.: Metastatic basal cell carcinoma. *Archives of Dermatology* 113:1261–1269, 1977. Copyright 1977, American Medical Association.)

cerated BCC in the left parieto-occipital scalp, which she covered with a wig (Fig. 22–8). The occipital area was soft and the pulsations of the brain could be palpated. A noduloulcerative BCC was found on biopsy. Marginal palisading in some of the tumor masses was not uniformly distinct. Destruction of both tables of the calvarium was detected by radiography, but there was no intracranial tumor found by computed tomography. Lung tomograms confirmed the presence of masses in the lower lobes. Needle biopsies of the nodules in the chest, obtained with the help of biplane fluoroscopy, contained masses of tightly packed cells that closely resembled those seen in the skin lesion. As the lesion was unsuitable for surgical ablation, it was treated with radiotherapy with good response. However, an intracranial abscess resulted and had to be evacuated through a craniotomy. A lytic lesion was also found in the right femur.

The fifth case of a metastatic BCC was in a man age 65. He had a crusted, bleeding lesion for many years in the right preauricular area

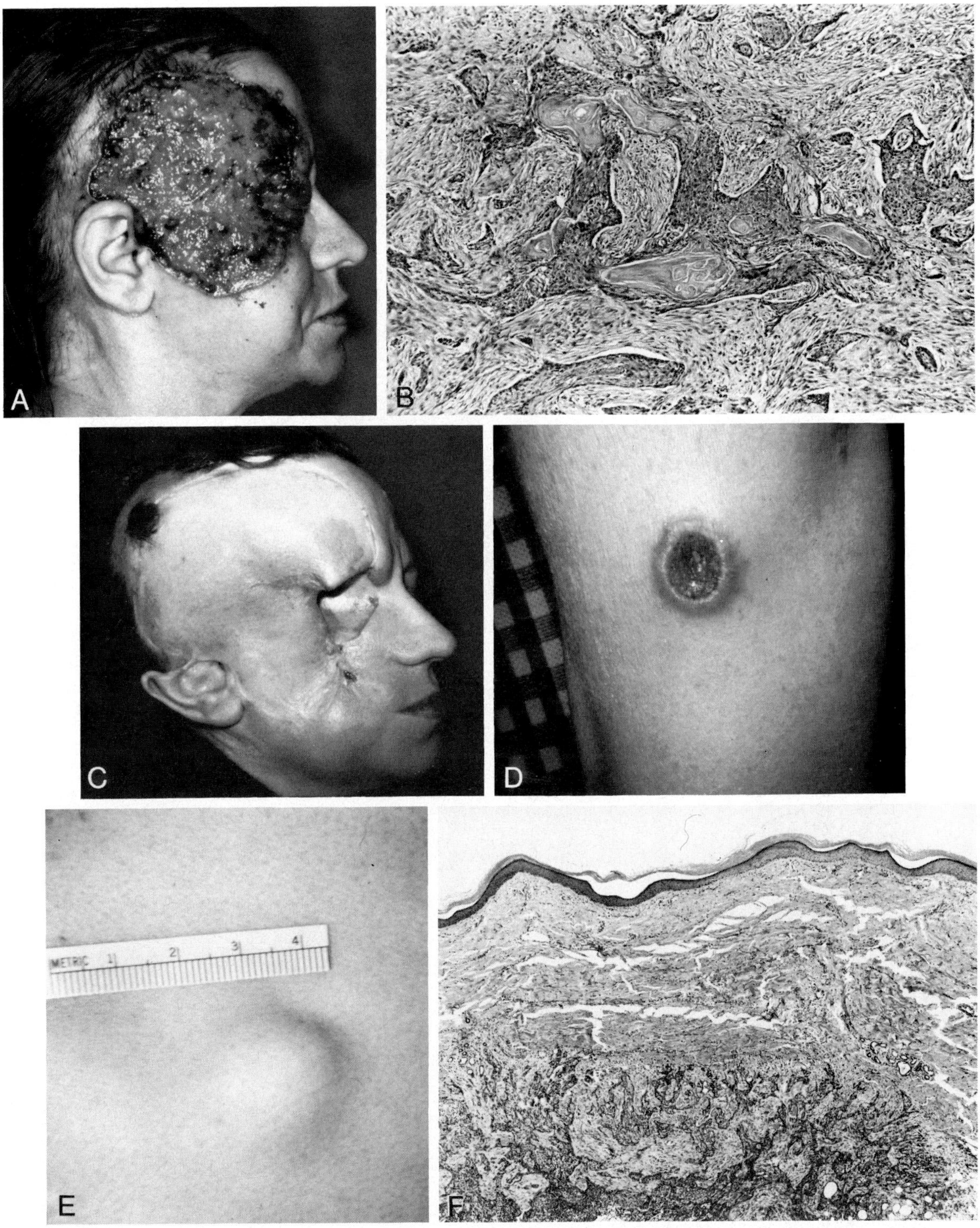

FIGURE 22–7. *A*, Extensive, ulcerative basal cell carcinoma (BCC) of right orbit and side of face. *B*, Section from lesion shows keratinizing BCC. *C*, Recurrence with involvement of maxillary antrum. *D*, Metastatic, ulcerated nodule on arm. *E*, Subcutaneous metastasis on thigh. *F*, Section shows dermal metastasis.

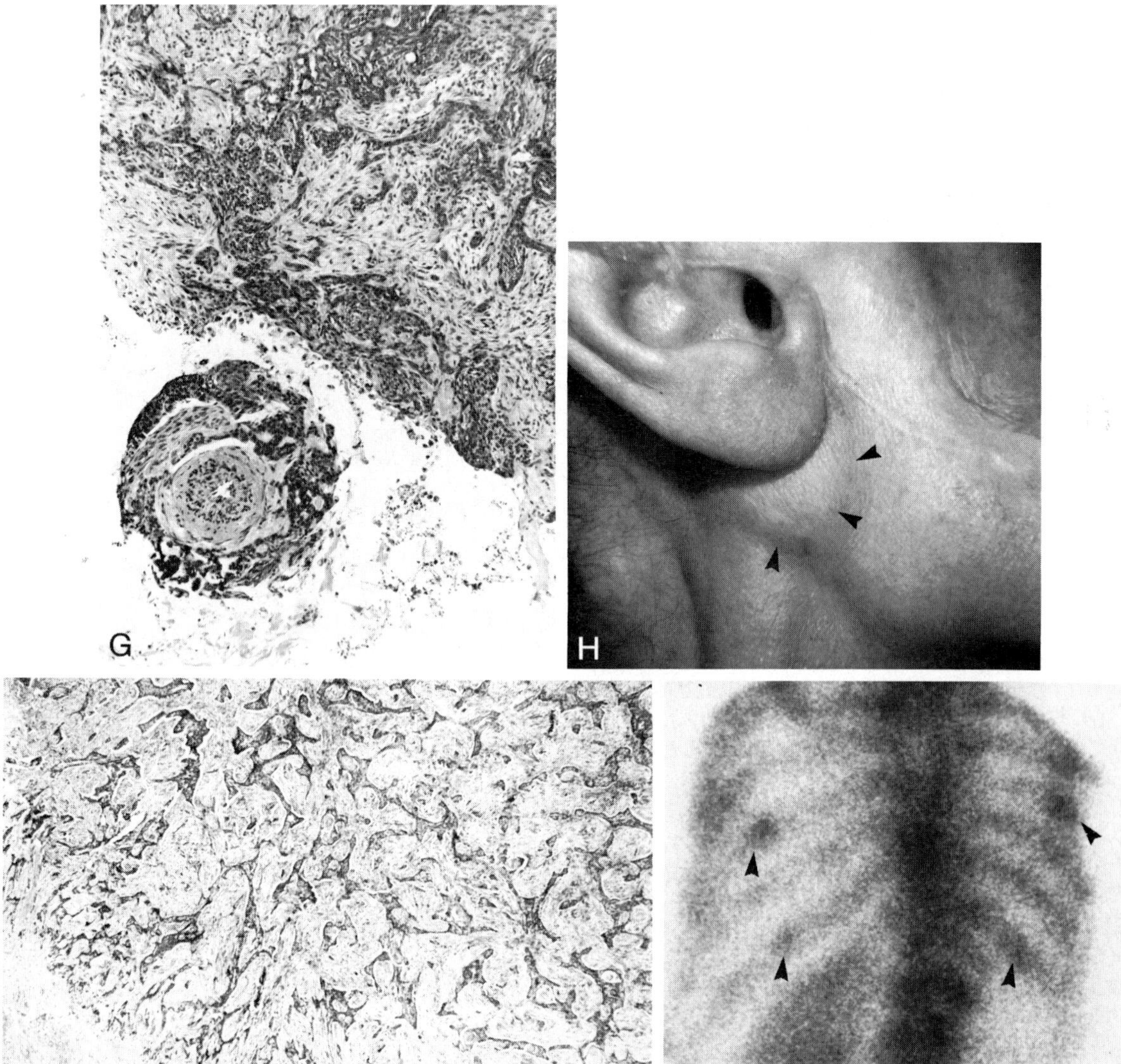

FIGURE 22–7 *Continued G*, Involvement of subcutaneous arteriole in same lesion. *H*, Metastasis to a cervical lymph node. *I*, BCC in lymph node. *J*, Radionuclide bone survey showed involvement of the ribs, sacrum, and femurs (*K*). *L*, BCC in iliac bone. (From Mikhail, GR, et al.: Metastatic basal cell carcinoma. *Archives of Dermatology* 113:1261–1269, 1977. Copyright 1977, American Medical Association.)

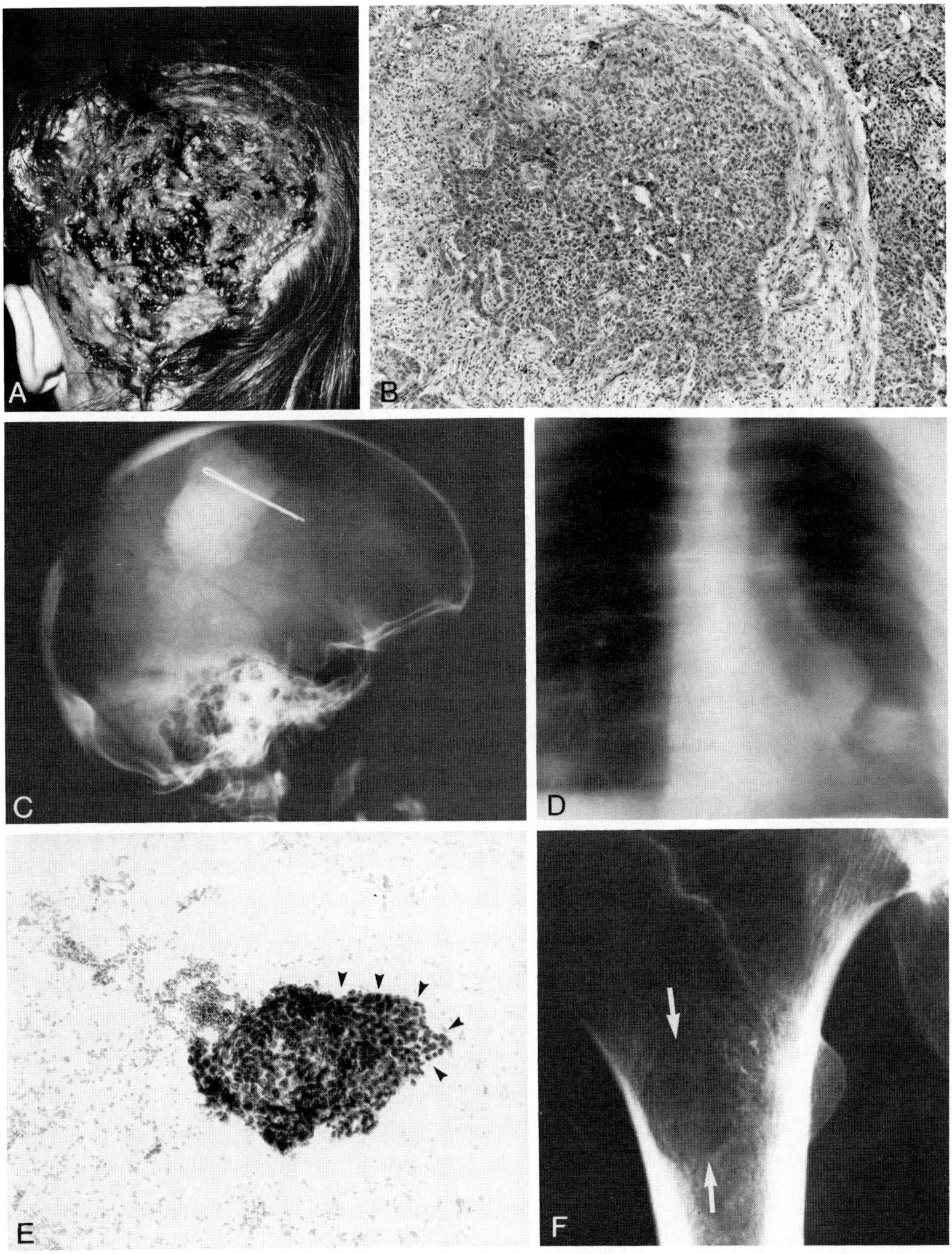

FIGURE 22–8. *A*, Large noduloulcerative basal cell carcinoma of scalp. *B*, Masses of basaloid cells in a densely fibrotic dermis; peripheral palisading is not uniformly distinct. *C*, Radiographic evidence of destruction of the occipital bone. *D*, Lung tomogram demonstrates masses in lungs. *E*, Mass of basaloid cells with marginal palisading in needle biopsy from lung. *F*, A large radiolucent lesion in the upper body of the femur. (From Mikhail, GR: Metastatic basal cell carcinoma. *Journal of Dermatologic Surgery and Oncology* 12:507–509, 1986. Copyright 1986, Elsevier Science Publishing Co., Inc.)

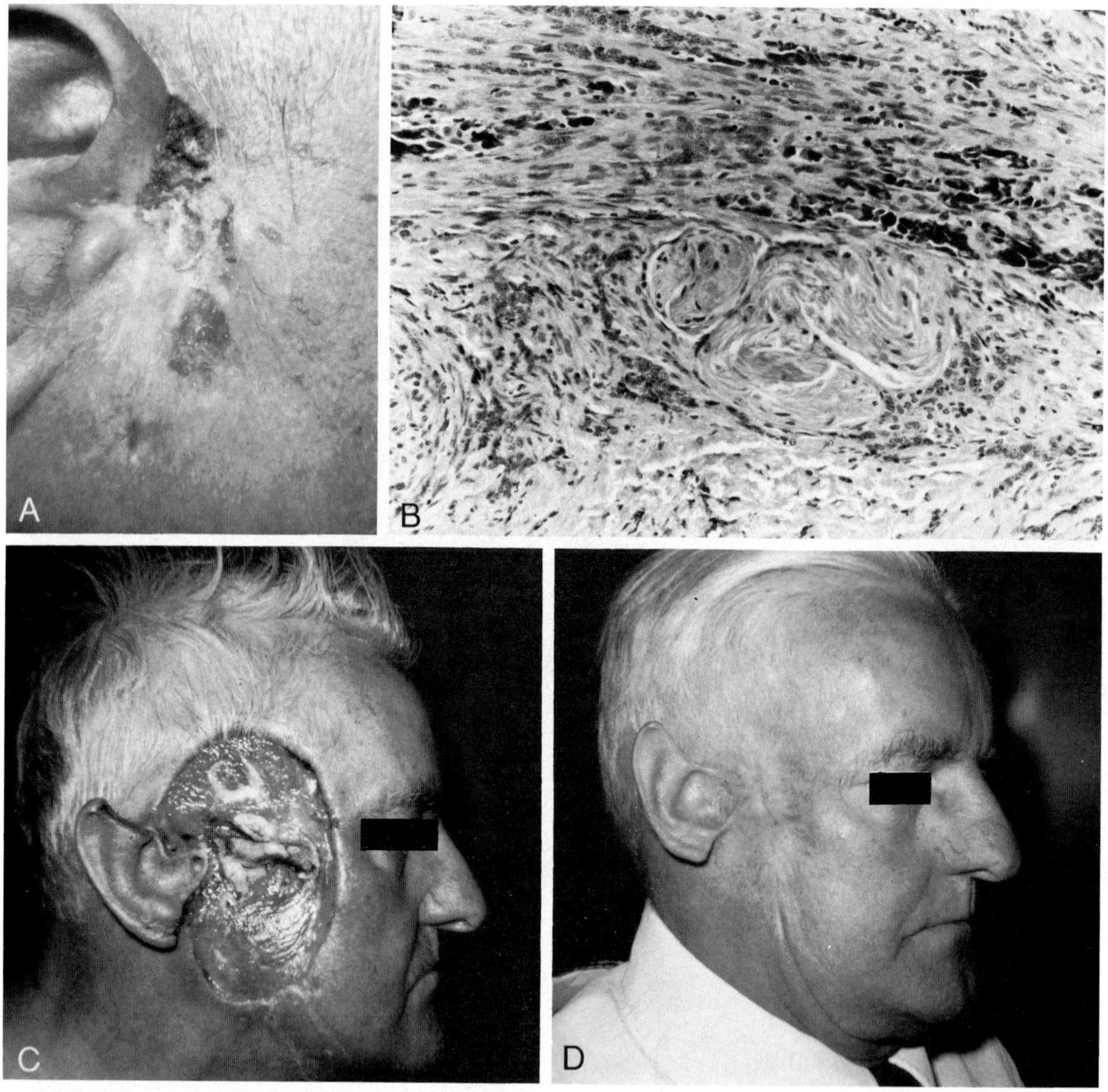

FIGURE 22–9. *A*, Basal cell carcinoma (BCC) in the right preauricular region. *B*, Morpheaform BCC with involvement of nerves. *C*, Status after separation of final fixed tissue layer; the zygomatic arch was removed with rongeurs to facilitate healing by second intention. *D*, Result after healing by second intention; there was ectropion of the lower eyelid caused by the resection of part of the facial nerve.

for which he had had radiotherapy without success (Fig. 22–9). The lesion proved to be of the morpheaform type of BCC. The fixed tissue method was used to ablate the tumor, which proved to be extensive and deeply invasive. The plan was to let the wound heal by second intention, and in order to permit prompt healing, the exposed maxillary arch was removed. It took 8 weeks for complete healing to occur. Five years later, the patient developed paraplegia and succumbed with asthenia. Metastatic lesions were found only in the spine. It was unfortunate that the pathologist who did the autopsy would not let us examine his material. The absence of any primary lesion at the time of death leaves no doubt that it was secondary to the face lesion.

Cranial Invasion

The invasion of bone by BCC through direct extension is rare and therefore not well documented.[6] Because bone acts as a natural solid

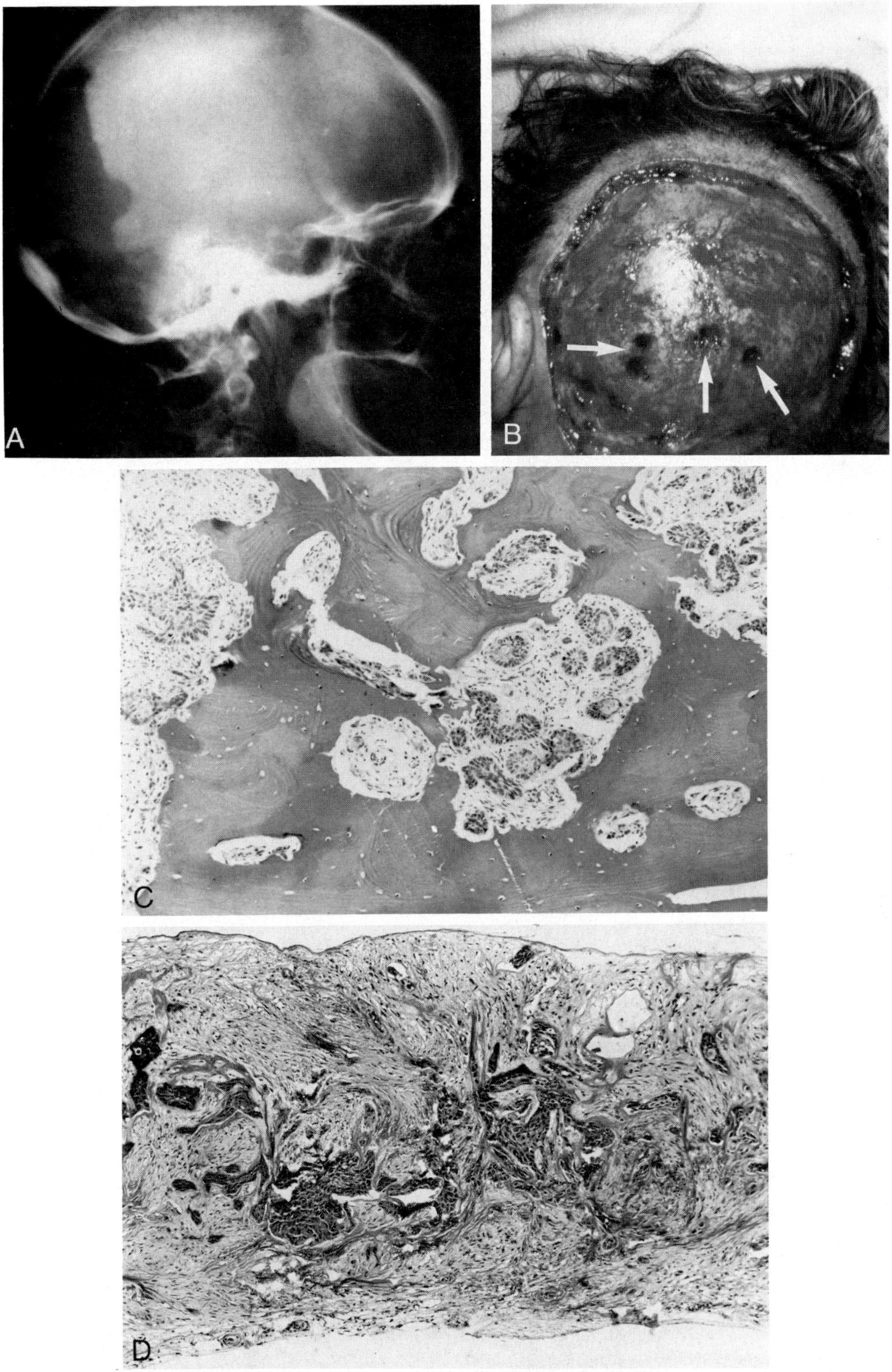

FIGURE 22–10. *A*, Preoperative radiography shows destruction of the occipital bone underneath the clinical lesion, a basal cell carcinoma (BCC). *B*, Exposed cranium shows four defects in the outer table of the calvaria *(arrows);* the pulsations of the brain could be palpated by placing a fingertip into the largest defect. *C*, BCC in bone. *D*, The dura mater invaded by basal cell carcinoma. (From Mikhail, GR, et al.: Cranial invasion by basal cell carcinoma. *Journal of Dermatologic Surgery and Oncology* 12:459–464, 1986. Copyright 1986, Elsevier Science Publishing Co., Inc.)

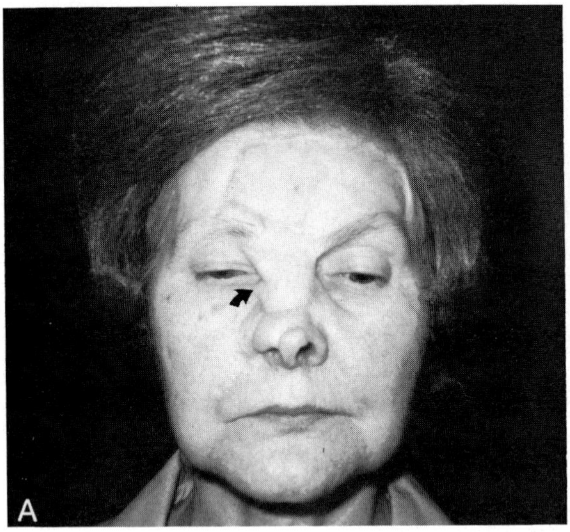

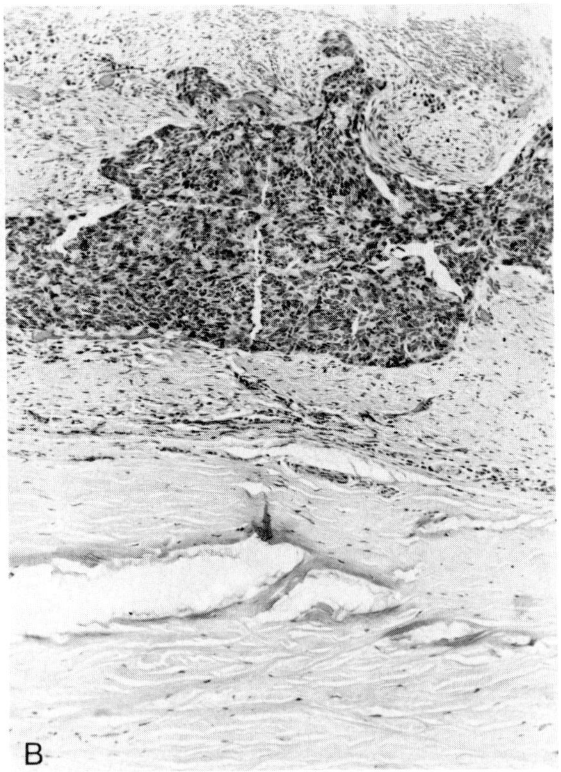

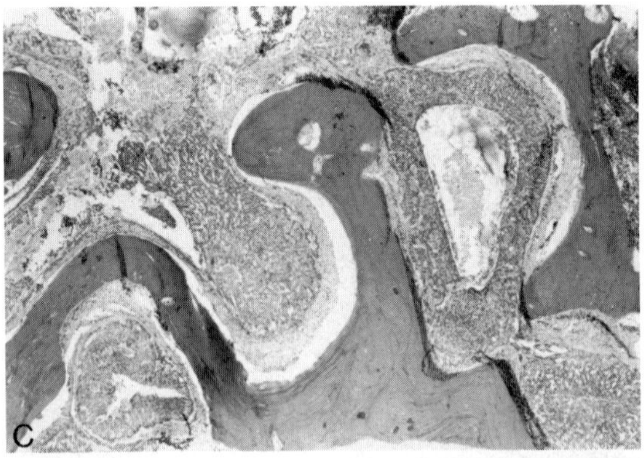

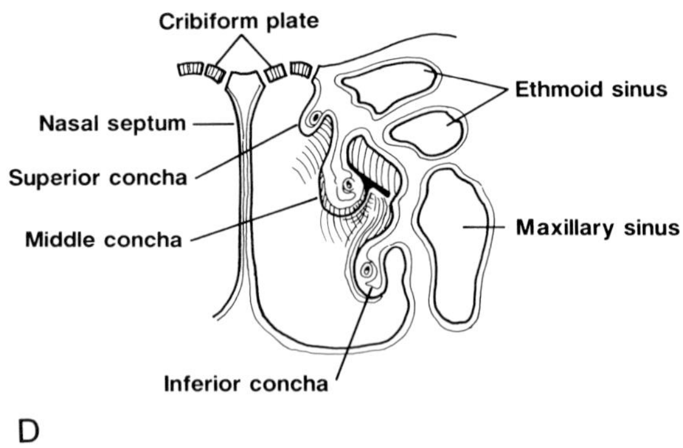

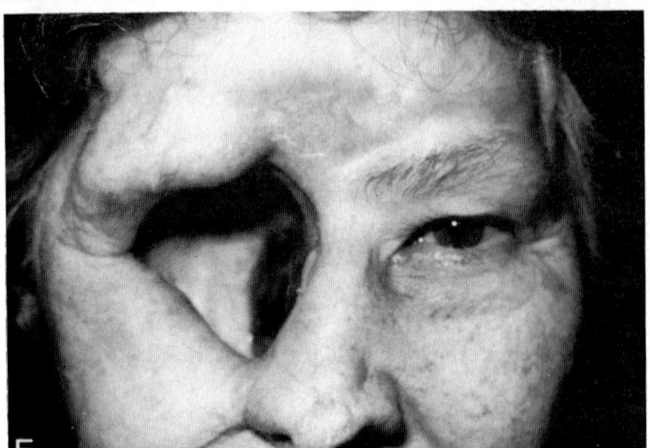

FIGURE 22–11. *A*, Recurrent basal cell carcinoma (BCC) at right medial canthus. Note scarring from previous grafts and flaps. *B*, BCC in the sclera. *C*, BCC in the ethmoid air cells. *D*, Diagrammatic frontal section of the paranasal sinuses shows close proximity to the cribriform plate. *E*, Final result. (From Mikhail, GR, et al.: Cranial invasion by basal cell carcinoma. *Journal of Dermatologic Surgery and Oncology* 12:459–464, 1986. Copyright 1986, Elsevier Science Publishing Co., Inc.)

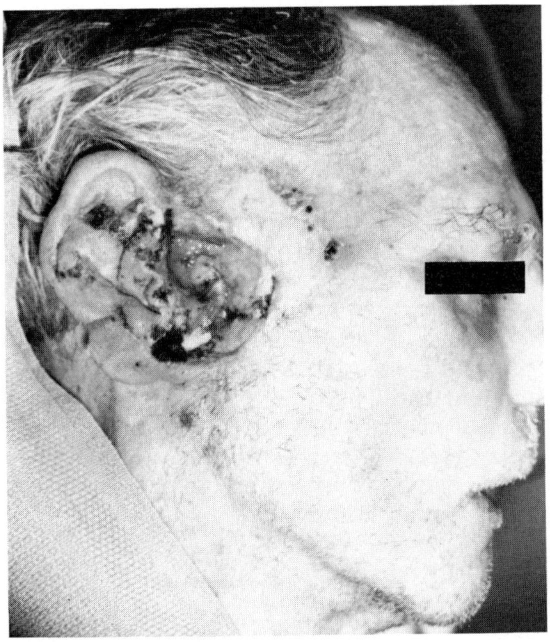

FIGURE 22–12. Extensive basal cell carcinoma of the ear and temporal bone with facial paralysis; the tumor extended deeply to the carotid blood vessels. Palliative radiotherapy was administered.

barrier, it takes a long period of time for BCC to invade bones. The earliest involvement can be recognized during surgery by visible pitting and honeycombing that may not be detectable by radiography. We published an article on this subject in 1986.[5] Two of the four patients involved in that study are of particular interest and are briefly described here.

A woman age 60 presented with a 15 cm ulcerated lesion of the left parieto-occipital scalp (Fig. 22–10). Preoperative radiographs showed rarefaction of bone beneath the lesion. The lesion was ablated by the fresh tissue method. Four large defects were found in the outer table of the skull. Destruction of the inner table could be verified by feeling brain pulsations by placing a finger inside the largest defect. The Neurosurgery Service excised a large portion of the occipital bone and the underlying dura mater. BCC had also invaded the dura.

Another woman age 60 had undergone at least eleven surgical procedures for treatment of a recurrent BCC that had its origin in the right medial canthus, followed by reconstruction of the defects by means of flaps and grafts. Referral was made for Mohs micrographic surgery because of a recurrence at the medial canthus (Fig. 22–11). The case was challenging because of the uncertainty of the extent of the residual neoplasm. The starting point of the Mohs surgery was in the medial canthus. A combination of the fresh and fixed tissue methods was used, the fixative applied mainly to bone. Because conservation of tissue, especially in such a critical area, is always a goal, surgery was terminated whenever a tumor-free level was reached. Recurrences kept appearing at various points necessitating six series of Mohs excisions in the space of 6 years. At the last hospital admission, the sclera of the globe, orbital fat, and frontal sinus had become involved. After exenteration of the orbit, Mohs surgery was resumed in the direction of the ethmoid air cells in close proximity to the cribri-

FIGURE 22–13. Basal cell carcinoma encroaching on the subclavian artery and deep vessels of the neck; treated by palliative radiotherapy.

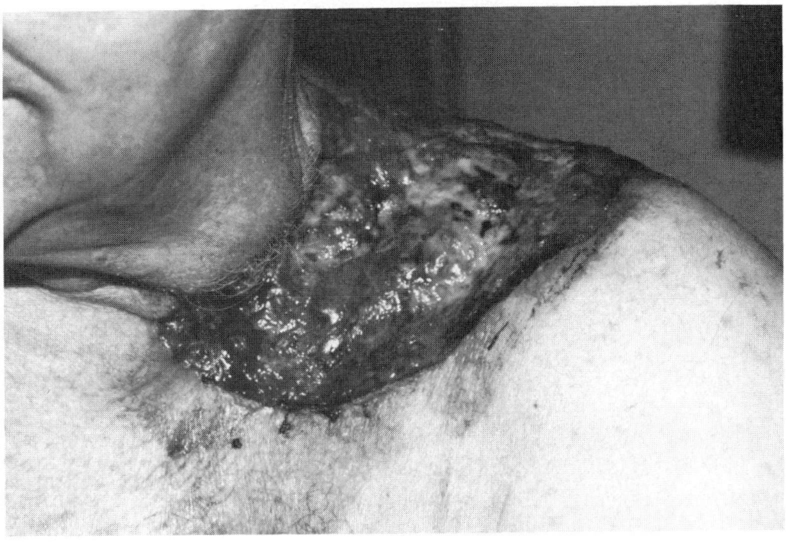

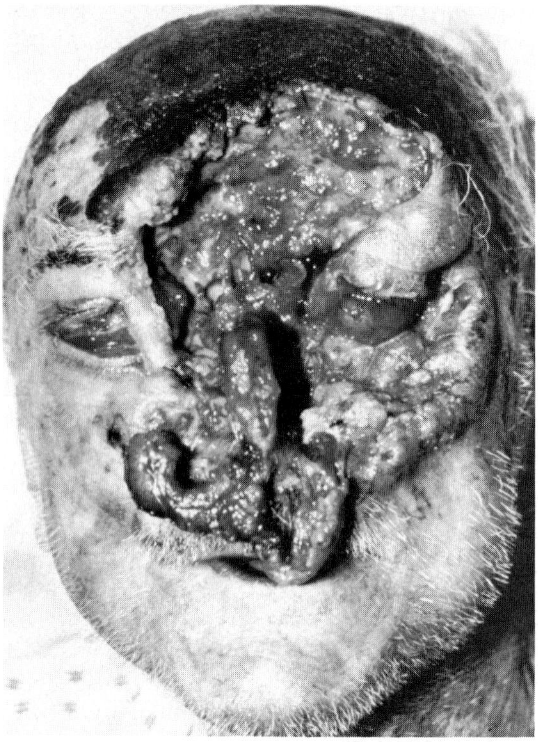

FIGURE 22-14. This widely destructive basal cell carcinoma is beyond any therapeutic modality. The patient stated that his dogs licked away his face!

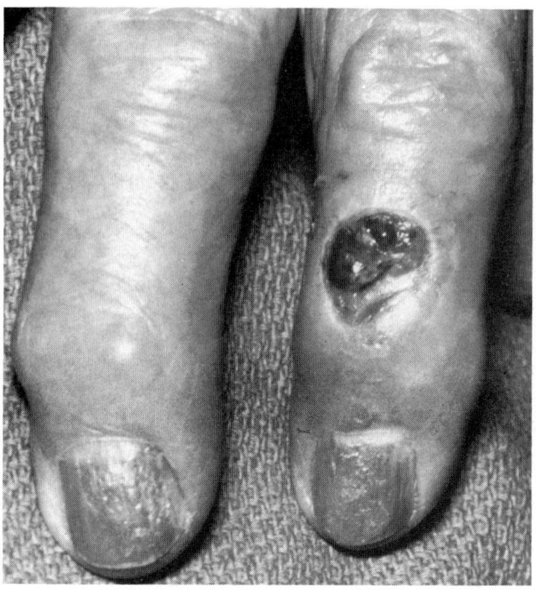

FIGURE 22-15. Basal cell carcinoma on the dorsum of an index finger.

form plate. A frontal craniotomy was then performed by a neurosurgeon, and a graft of temporal fascia was placed above the dura mater in the area of the cribriform plate. The plate was removed uneventfully 4 weeks later. The patient was well and free of tumor at 10 years after the last surgery.

Inoperable Basal Cell Carcinoma

Extensive cases of BCC that are deeply invasive and involve or are in close proximity to vital structures pose a great hazard and are preferably managed by radiotherapists, vascular surgeons, or neurosurgeons according to the needs of the case. However, some cases are not amenable to any sort of therapy. Three examples are illustrated in Figures 22–12 to 22–14.

Basal Cell Carcinoma at Unusual Sites

Apart from the nevoid basal cell carcinoma syndrome, BCC can occur on any cutaneous surface. We have reported a case of subungual basal cell carcinoma on a fifth toe.[7] Lesions have been encountered on the dorsum and sides of fingers (Figs. 22–15 and 22–16), on the sides of the hands (Fig. 22–17), and on the palm, unassociated with the nevoid basal cell carcinoma syndrome (Fig. 22–18). Figure 22–19 depicts an adenoid BCC on the dorsum of the wrist. Figure 22–20 shows bilateral, symmetrical BCC in preauricular sinuses. The genitals and perineum are not exempt (see Chapter 12). Figure 22–21 shows a sclerotic basal cell carcinoma on the plantar surface of a foot. Fig-

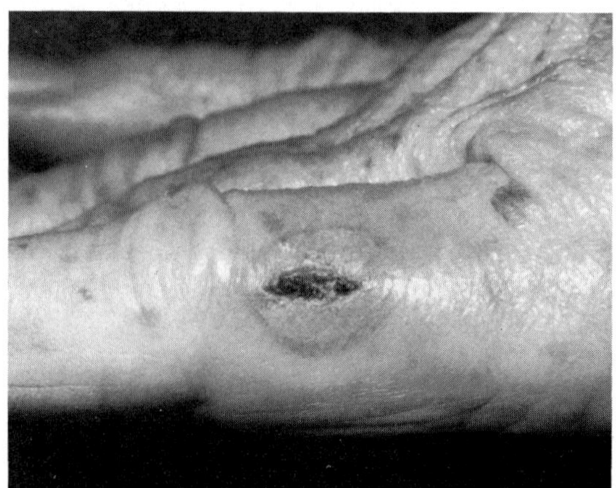

FIGURE 22-16. Basal cell carcinoma on the left fifth finger.

FIGURE 22–17. Basal cell carcinoma on the ulnar border of the right hand; note the actinic damage.

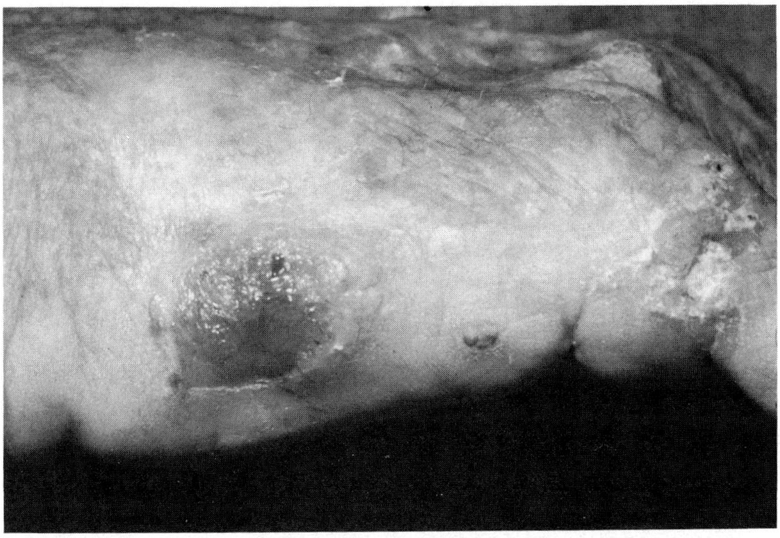

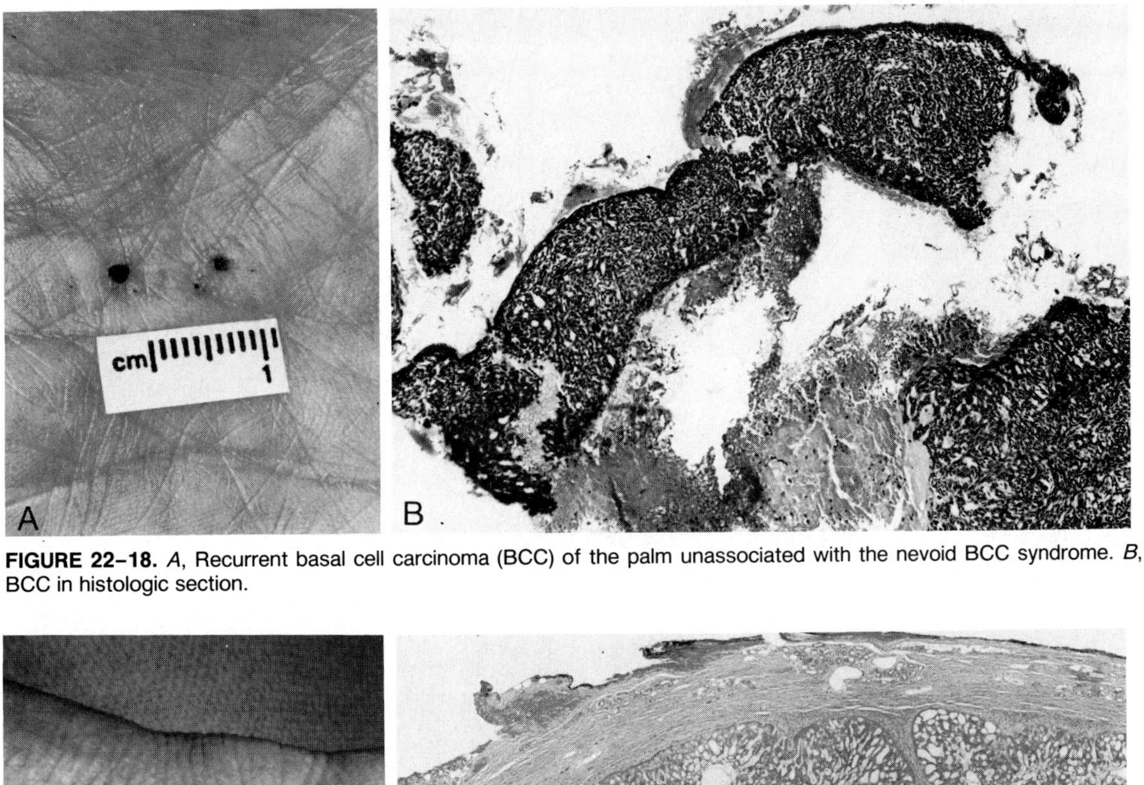

FIGURE 22–18. *A*, Recurrent basal cell carcinoma (BCC) of the palm unassociated with the nevoid BCC syndrome. *B*, BCC in histologic section.

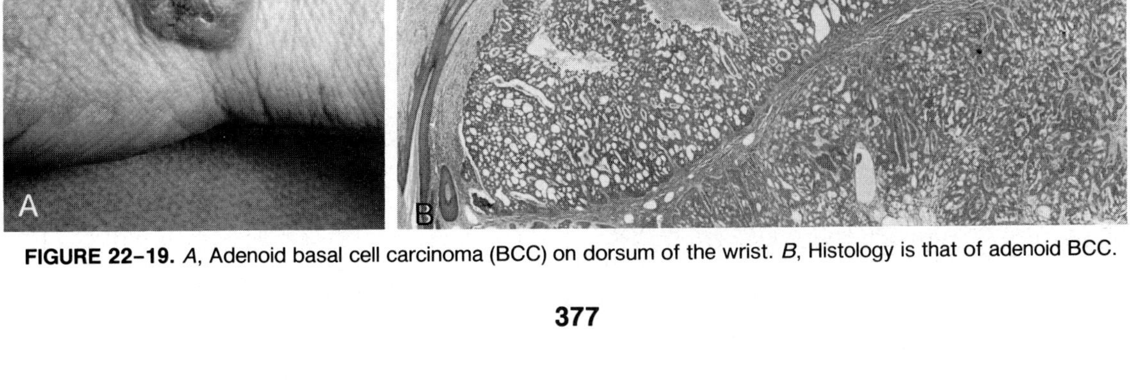

FIGURE 22–19. *A*, Adenoid basal cell carcinoma (BCC) on dorsum of the wrist. *B*, Histology is that of adenoid BCC.

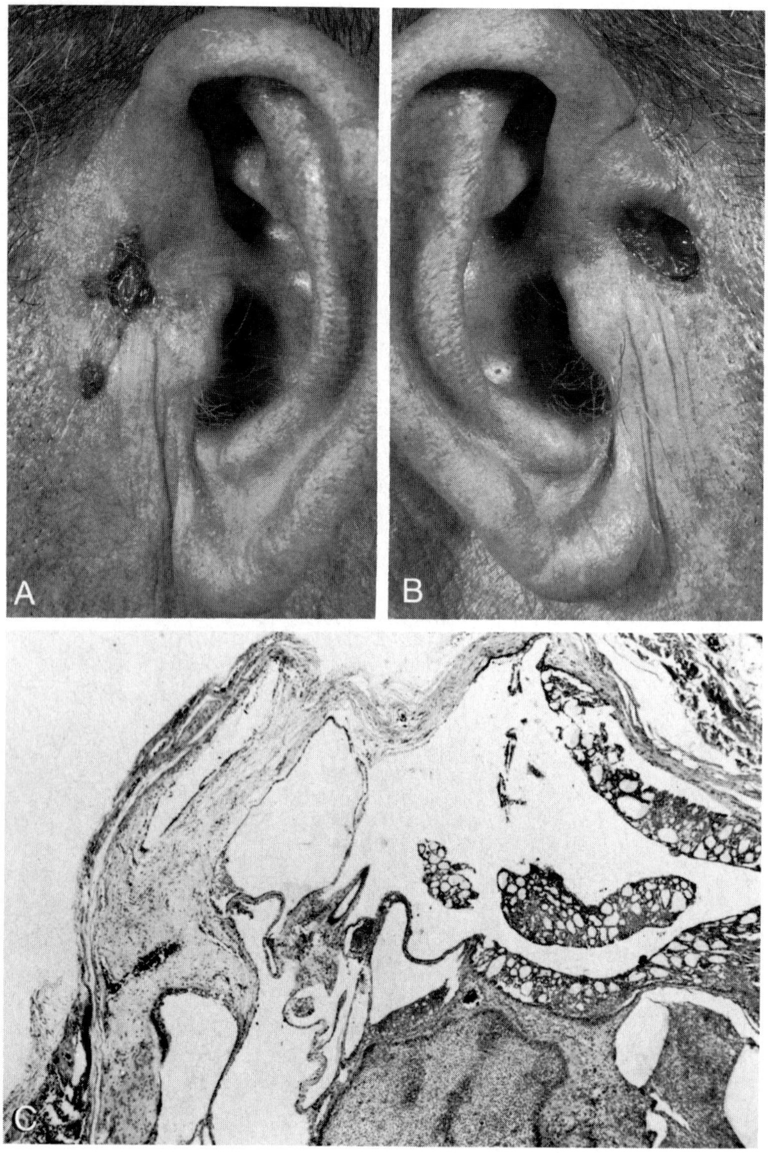

FIGURE 22–20. *A*, Deeply infiltrating basal cell carcinoma (BCC) in left preauricular sinus. *B*, Symmetrical carcinoma at same site on the right side. *C*, Section shows BCC in auricular sinus.

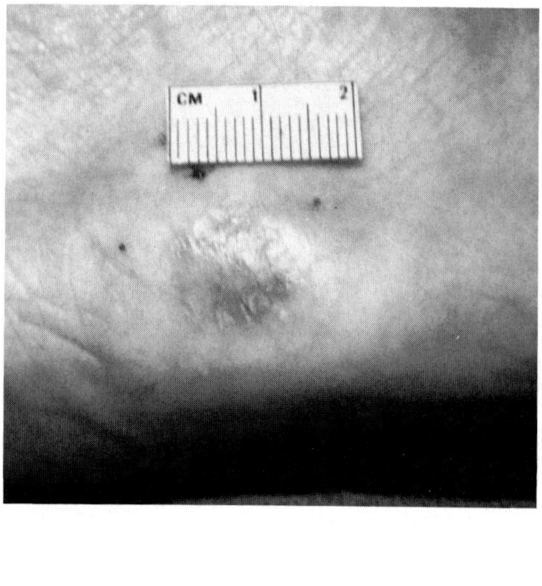

FIGURE 22–21. A sclerotic plantar basal cell carcinoma.

FIGURE 22–22. *A*, Periungual basal cell carcinoma in proximal nail fold. *B*, Result after ablation with Mohs surgery.

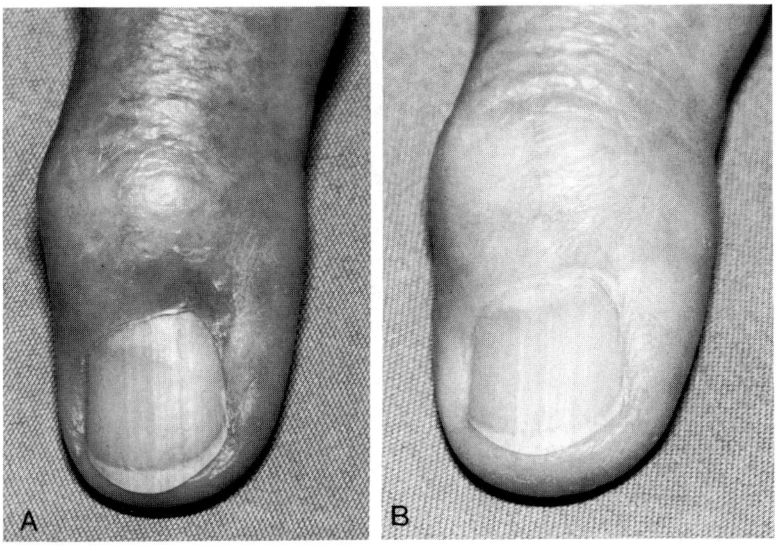

ures 22–22 and 22–23 show periungual and subungual BCC.

SQUAMOUS CELL CARCINOMAS

Bowen's Disease

Bowen's disease is common in individuals over 50 years old. The usual location is the sun-exposed skin, but covered areas can be affected. This lesion has been discussed in Chapter 4 and with relation to the nail organ and genitals in Chapter 12. Other unusual sites are presented here.

Interdigital Bowen's disease can masquerade as a dermatophytic infection. Examples are illustrated in Figures 22–24 and 22–25. It is strongly advocated that a biopsy should be ob-

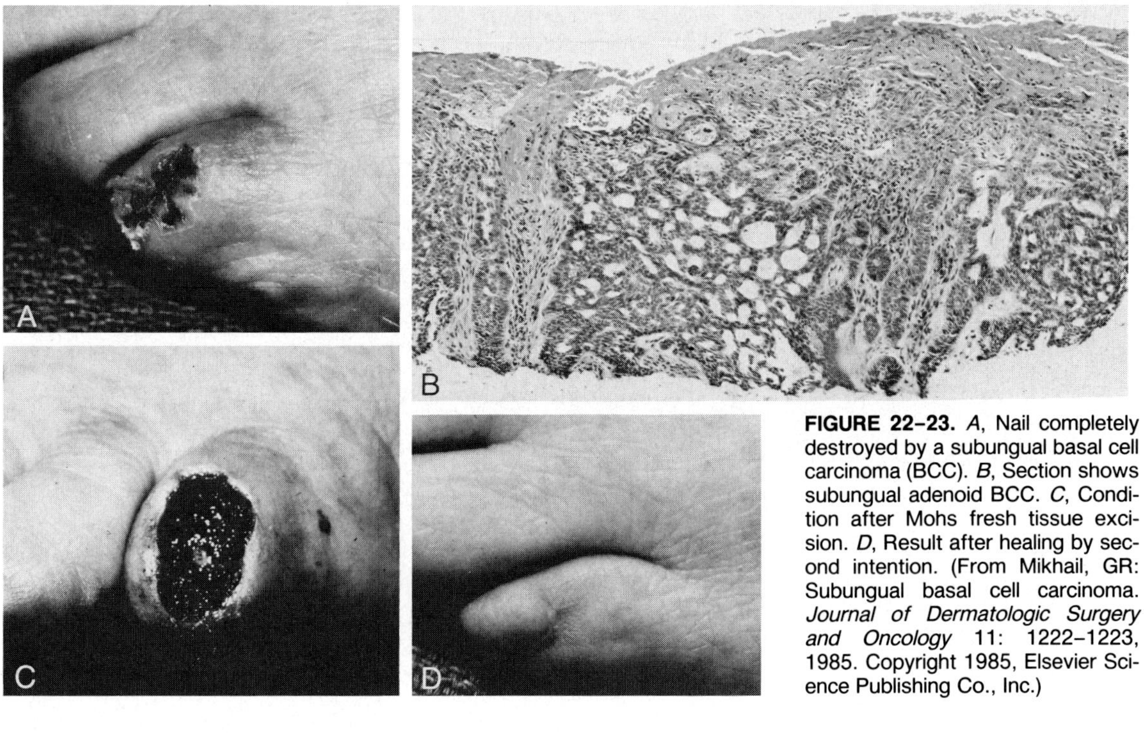

FIGURE 22–23. *A*, Nail completely destroyed by a subungual basal cell carcinoma (BCC). *B*, Section shows subungual adenoid BCC. *C*, Condition after Mohs fresh tissue excision. *D*, Result after healing by second intention. (From Mikhail, GR: Subungual basal cell carcinoma. *Journal of Dermatologic Surgery and Oncology* 11: 1222–1223, 1985. Copyright 1985, Elsevier Science Publishing Co., Inc.)

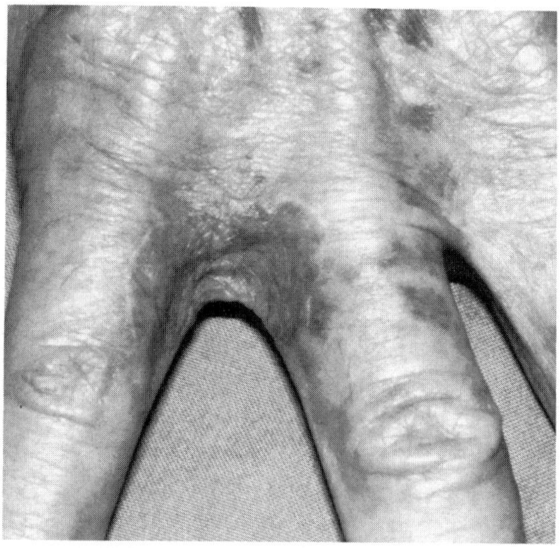

FIGURE 22–24. Bowen's disease of an interdigital fold on the hand simulates a fungal infection.

tained from interdigital lesions that are recalcitrant to medical treatment.

Verrucous Bowen's Disease

A large verrucous lesion of Bowen's disease was seen on the dorsum of a hand. It was excised using the Mohs fresh tissue technique, and the wound was grafted with a good functional and cosmetic result (Fig. 22–26). There was no recurrence or metastasis at 6 years of follow-up.

Verrucous Carcinoma

We have encountered verrucous carcinomas in the nose and on the penis, foot, and palm.

Verrucous carcinoma of the nose is an aggressive, destructive lesion. We have treated six cases by the Mohs technique and the most extensive ones are described here.

The patient was a man age 68 with a verrucous mass that filled the right nasal vestibule and pushed the nasal septum, to which it was attached, to the left side causing complete nasal obstruction and forced breathing through the mouth. The histology was that of a moderately differentiated squamous cell carcinoma. The tumor was excised but recurred and was retreated. The entire nose had to be removed (Fig. 22–27).

The second case resembled a keratoacanthoma, but its histology was that of pseudoepitheliomatous hyperplasia, although tissue destruction was extensive (Fig. 22–28). It is pertinent to note that the histology of this lesion is deceptively benign but its biological behavior is on a par with highly malignant neoplasms.

The other four cases had a much more favorable outcome with minor disfigurement (if any). None of them has recurred.

In addition, we have a series of four cases of verrucous carcinoma of the foot (also called epithelioma cuniculatum). Although the fresh tissue method can be applied to this type of lesion, we tend to prefer the fixed tissue method

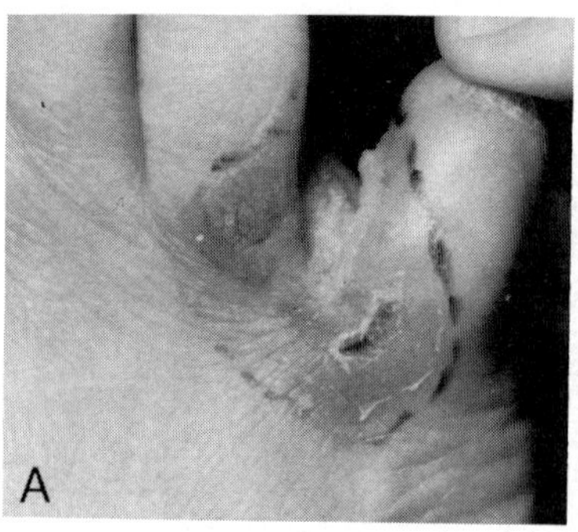

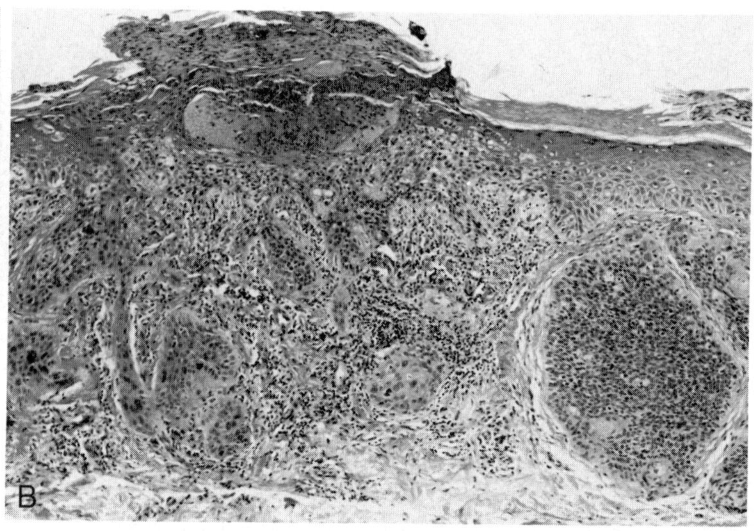

FIGURE 22–25. *A*, Bowen's disease simulating inflamed tinea pedis. *B*, Histology shows Bowen's disease and invasive squamous cell carcinoma.

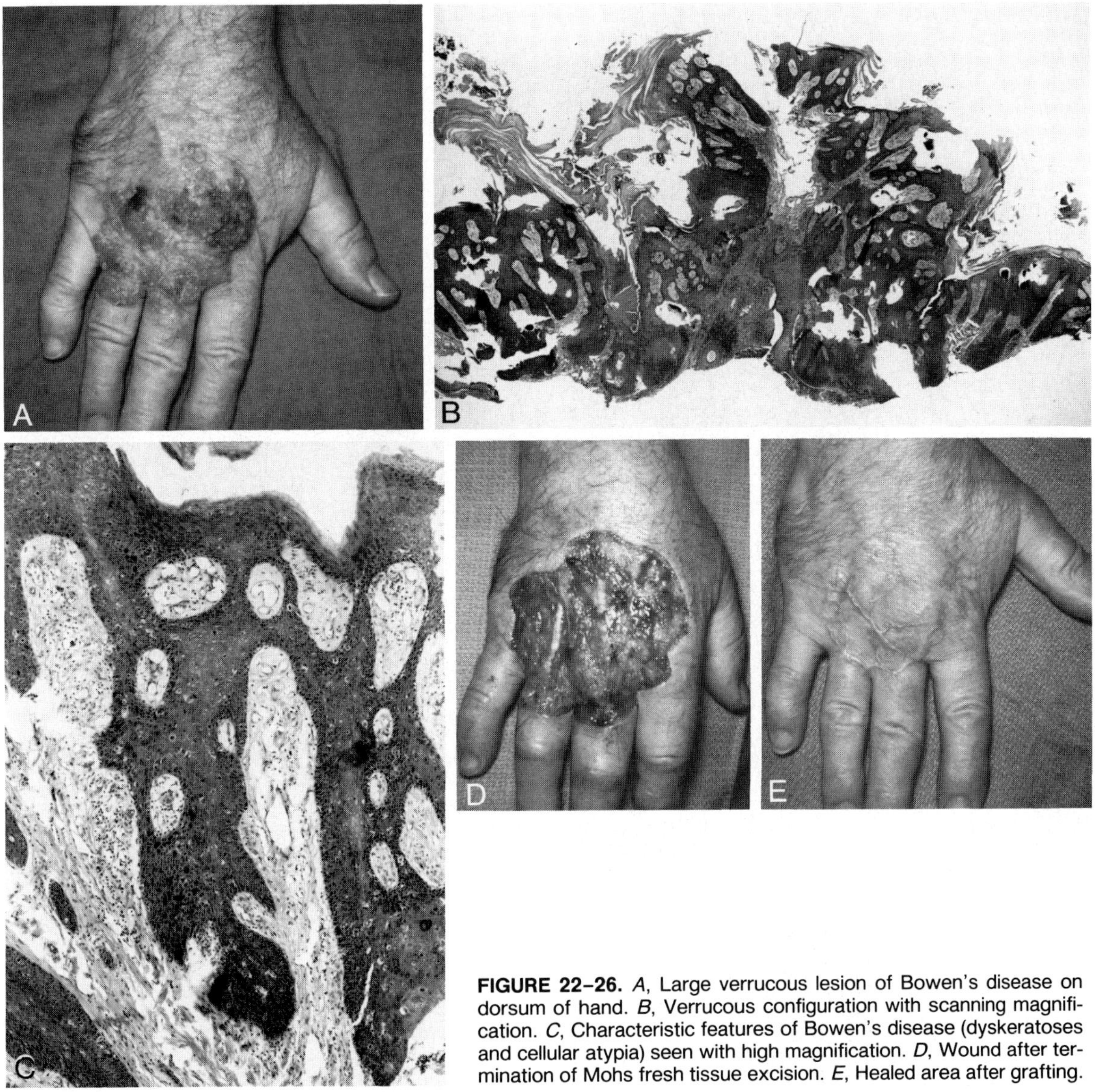

FIGURE 22–26. *A*, Large verrucous lesion of Bowen's disease on dorsum of hand. *B*, Verrucous configuration with scanning magnification. *C*, Characteristic features of Bowen's disease (dyskeratoses and cellular atypia) seen with high magnification. *D*, Wound after termination of Mohs fresh tissue excision. *E*, Healed area after grafting.

because of the deeply invasive nature of the tumor and its tendency to involve bone. Such was the case in the following example. The carcinoma was on the sole at the head of the fifth metatarsal bone, and its extent could be palpated far beyond the visible margins (Fig. 22–29). One case in the series was successfully treated by the fresh tissue method. We feel that each case should be handled according to its individual merits.

Six cases are on record in the English literature in which epithelioma cuniculatum occurred on the palm. Three were from the United Kingdom,[8–10] one was from Australia,[11] and one from the United States.[12] We have seen two cases.

A man age 55 presented with a recurrent verrucous lesion on the palm. Histologic examination showed a deeply invasive, moderately differentiated squamous cell carcinoma (Fig. 22–30). The patient declined Mohs surgery because he insisted to be admitted to the hospital to have the excision done under general anesthesia. The outcome is unknown.

The second patient, a man age 56, was referred for Mohs surgery after failure of two ex-

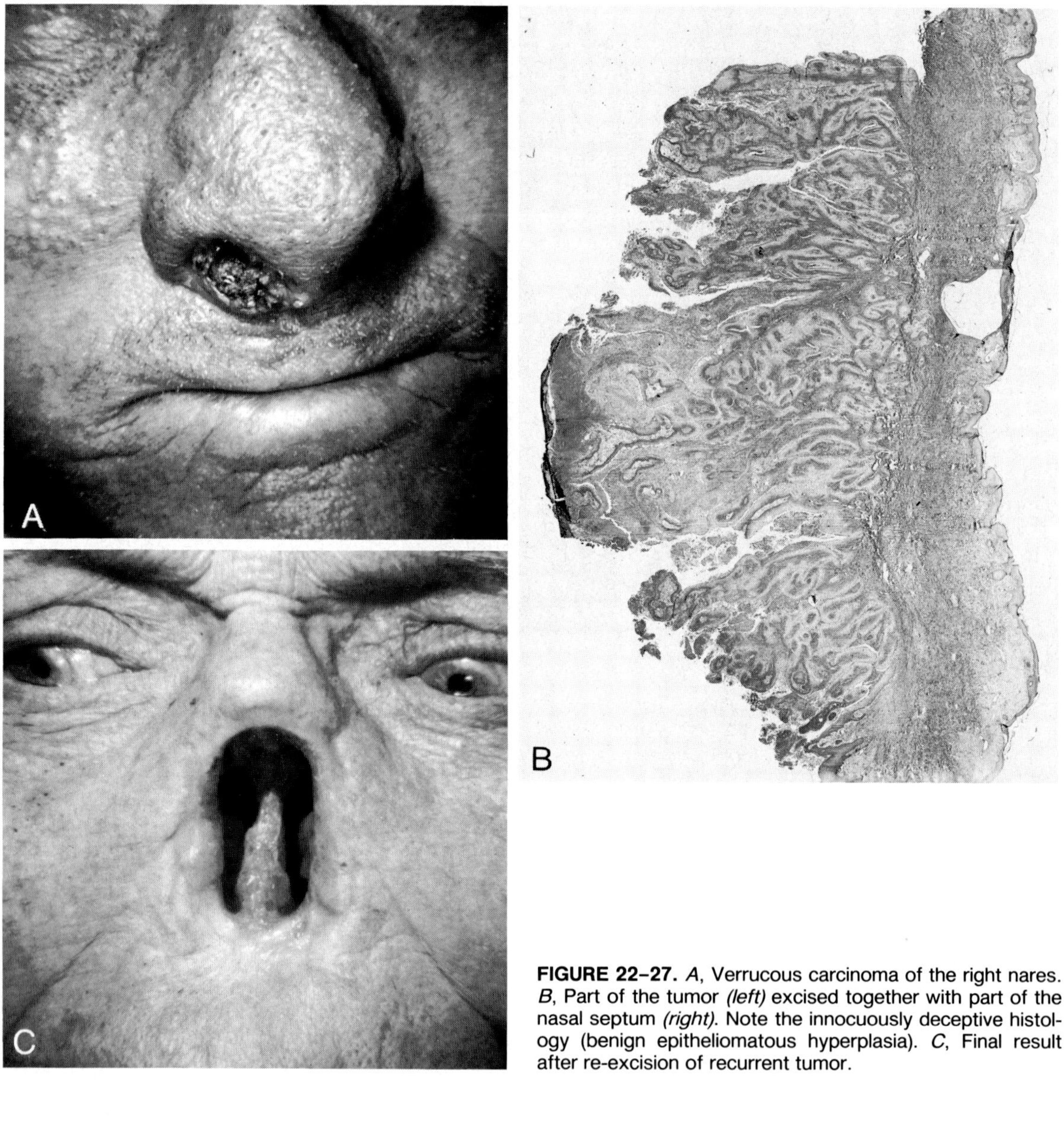

FIGURE 22–27. *A*, Verrucous carcinoma of the right nares. *B*, Part of the tumor *(left)* excised together with part of the nasal septum *(right)*. Note the innocuously deceptive histology (benign epitheliomatous hyperplasia). *C*, Final result after re-excision of recurrent tumor.

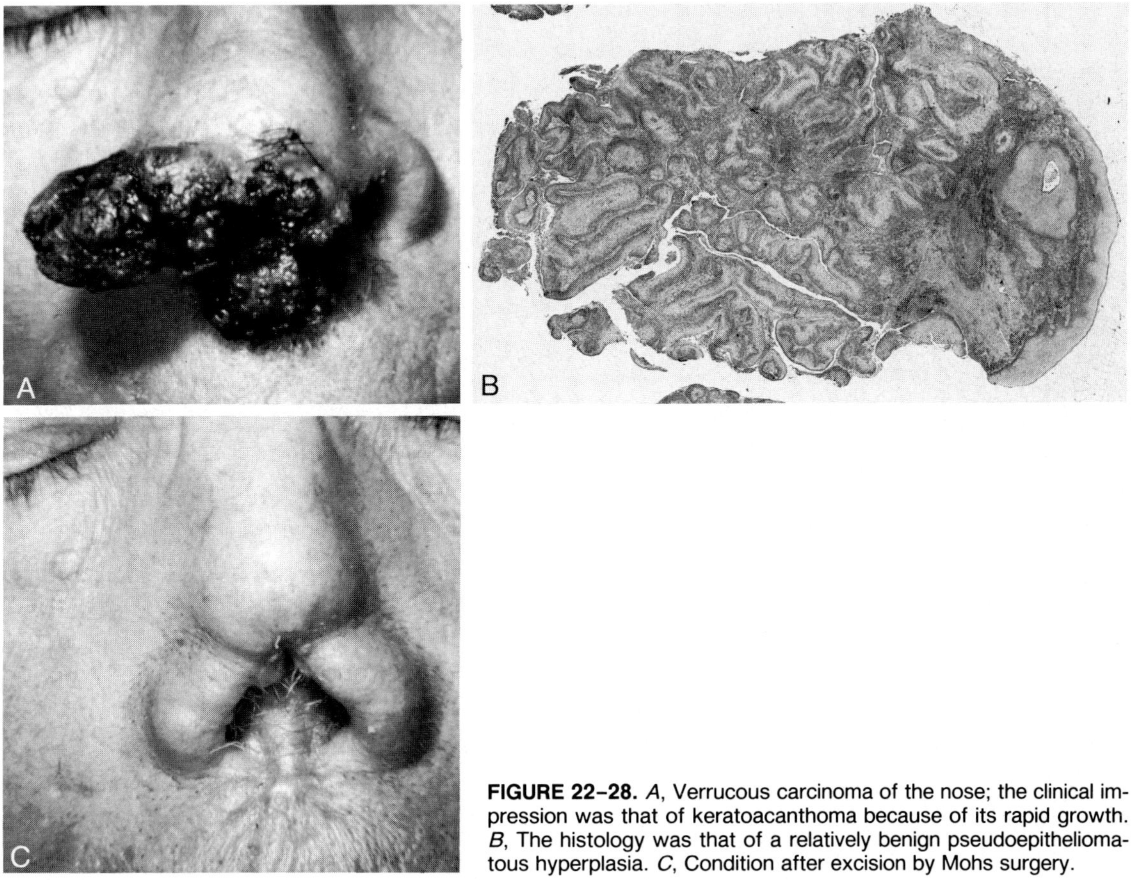

FIGURE 22–28. *A*, Verrucous carcinoma of the nose; the clinical impression was that of keratoacanthoma because of its rapid growth. *B*, The histology was that of a relatively benign pseudoepitheliomatous hyperplasia. *C*, Condition after excision by Mohs surgery.

cisions and a series of radiotherapy. The verrucous ulcerated lesion was on the hypothenar eminence of the left hand. The neoplasm was excised using the Mohs fresh tissue method in five stages. The tumor extended down to the metacarpal bones. Parts of the flexor tendons had to be removed, but care was exercised to avoid severing them. The wound was grafted, and 5 months later, recurrence reappeared at the proximal margin of the graft. It was re-excised using Mohs surgery, and the wound was left to heal by second intention. The patient has remained free of disease at 4 years after the last intervention (Fig. 22–31).

Hemangiosarcoma

We have come across three examples of hemangiosarcoma, also called angioendothelioma. The first case treated by Mohs surgery has been published elsewhere.[13] The same case is presented here in a condensed form in order to demonstrate the reasons why we no longer advocate Mohs surgery for this condition.

The patient, a 52-year-old man, had an enlarging, nodular lesion of irregular shape in the left nasolabial cheek crease (Fig. 22–32). The biopsy showed the distinctive features of angiosarcoma. The neoplasm was ablated by means of the Mohs fixed tissue technique in April 1972. The resulting large and deep defect was later reconstructed. The patient remained free until May 1979, when the tumor recurred in the left lower eyelid and adjoining dorsum of the nose. The area was then treated by radiotherapy combined with hyperthermia. The tumor responded well, and the patient was free from symptoms 7 years after this therapy, when he expired from atherosclerosis and heart failure. The same modality has been used to manage three other cases successfully, two on the scalp and one on the forehead; therefore, this seems to be the indicated treatment at the present time.

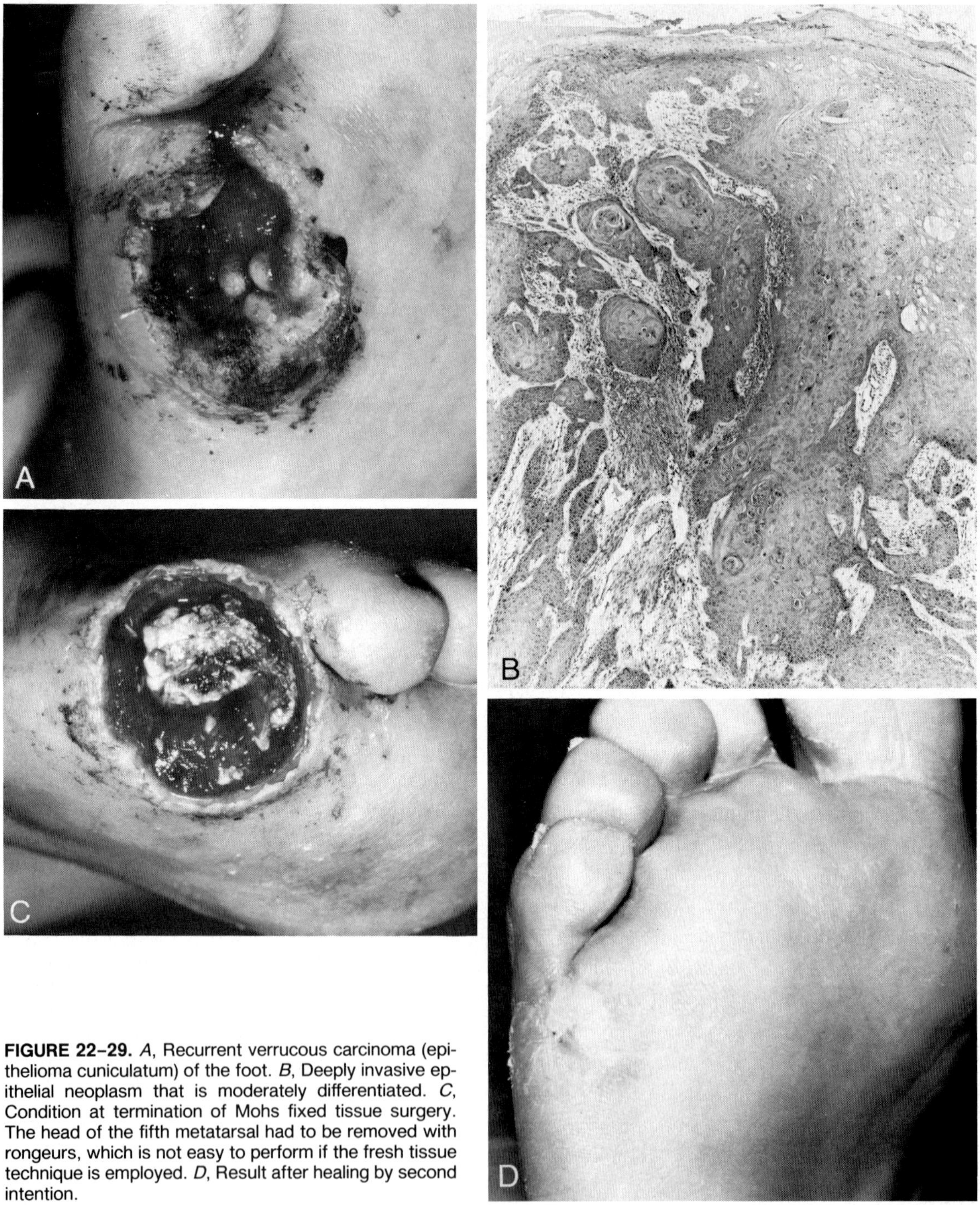

FIGURE 22–29. *A*, Recurrent verrucous carcinoma (epithelioma cuniculatum) of the foot. *B*, Deeply invasive epithelial neoplasm that is moderately differentiated. *C*, Condition at termination of Mohs fixed tissue surgery. The head of the fifth metatarsal had to be removed with rongeurs, which is not easy to perform if the fresh tissue technique is employed. *D*, Result after healing by second intention.

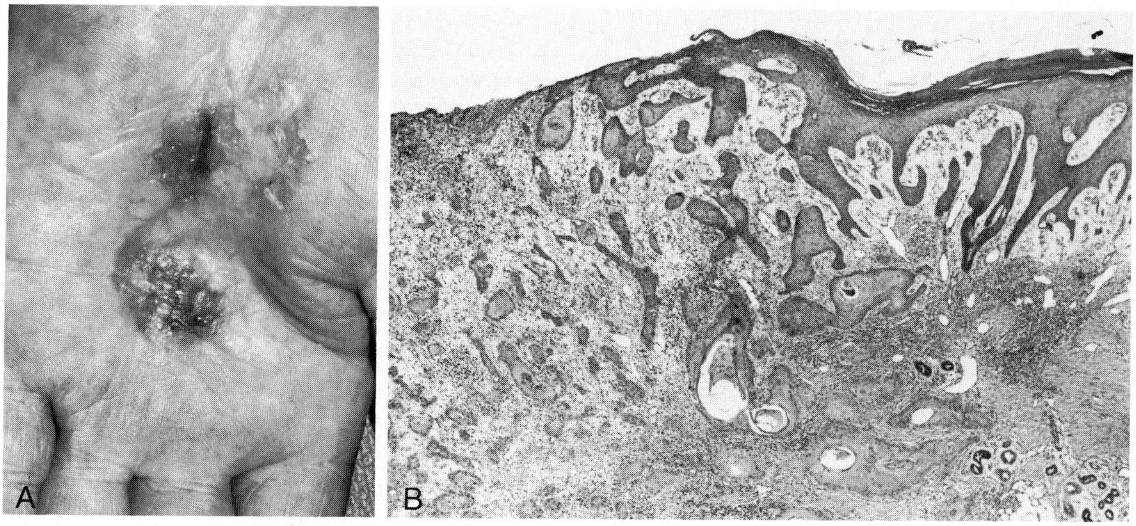

FIGURE 22–30. *A*, Recurrent verrucous carcinoma of palm; patient refused Mohs surgery. *B*, Section shows a deeply invasive squamous cell carcinoma of a moderately differentiated type; some abnormal mitoses can be seen.

Squamous Cell Carcinoma in Nerves

Like basal cell carcinoma (Fig. 22–5B), squamous cell carcinoma appears to have an affinity to implicate nerves. A case is described here in which the supraorbital nerve became involved by a squamous cell carcinoma of the forehead, and the tumor extended intracranially. This necessitated a frontal craniotomy and complete excision of the supraorbital nerve at its origin in the cranial fossa. An important observation is that the involved nerve appears grossly thickened, and microscopically, inflammatory cells always surround the affected nerve, which may mask the presence of cancer cells. Therefore, nerves surrounded by inflammation should be removed (Fig. 22–33).

Pagetoid Transitional Carcinoma of the Glans Penis

A man age 77 who appeared to be in good general health was referred for Mohs excision of a lesion at the urinary meatus. A biopsy from this site was read as Bowen's disease. As the man was of the Jewish faith and had had the ritual circumcision shortly after birth, it was inconceivable that the lesion took origin in the skin of the glans or the urethral meatus. History disclosed that he had had a transitional carcinoma of the urinary bladder 6 years beforehand, and the treatment received at that time was complete removal of the bladder and the prostate, including the prostatic urethra. The urinary flow was diverted to drain from the ureters into a plastic bag through a stoma. The patient was referred back to the urologist with the request to obtain biopsies from at least three areas of urethral mucosa. As these came back positive for carcinoma, total urethrectomy, including the meatal area and the surrounding part of the glans, was performed. Histologic examination showed a poorly differentiated transitional carcinoma with pagetoid features and invasion of the periurethral lymphatics (Fig. 22–34). The patient died from lung metastases. A good history is often essential in deciding the appropriate management.

Cutaneous Meningioma

Meningioma is a rare benign tumor caused by the overgrowth of arachnoidal fibroblasts. The cutaneous lesions are of three types: (1) the primary cutaneous type occurs in children, usually on the face and scalp, (2) the ectopic type extends to the skin along nerves, and (3) central nervous system meningioma extends to the skin through a defect in the skull. Pathologically, meningioma has four variants: the syn-

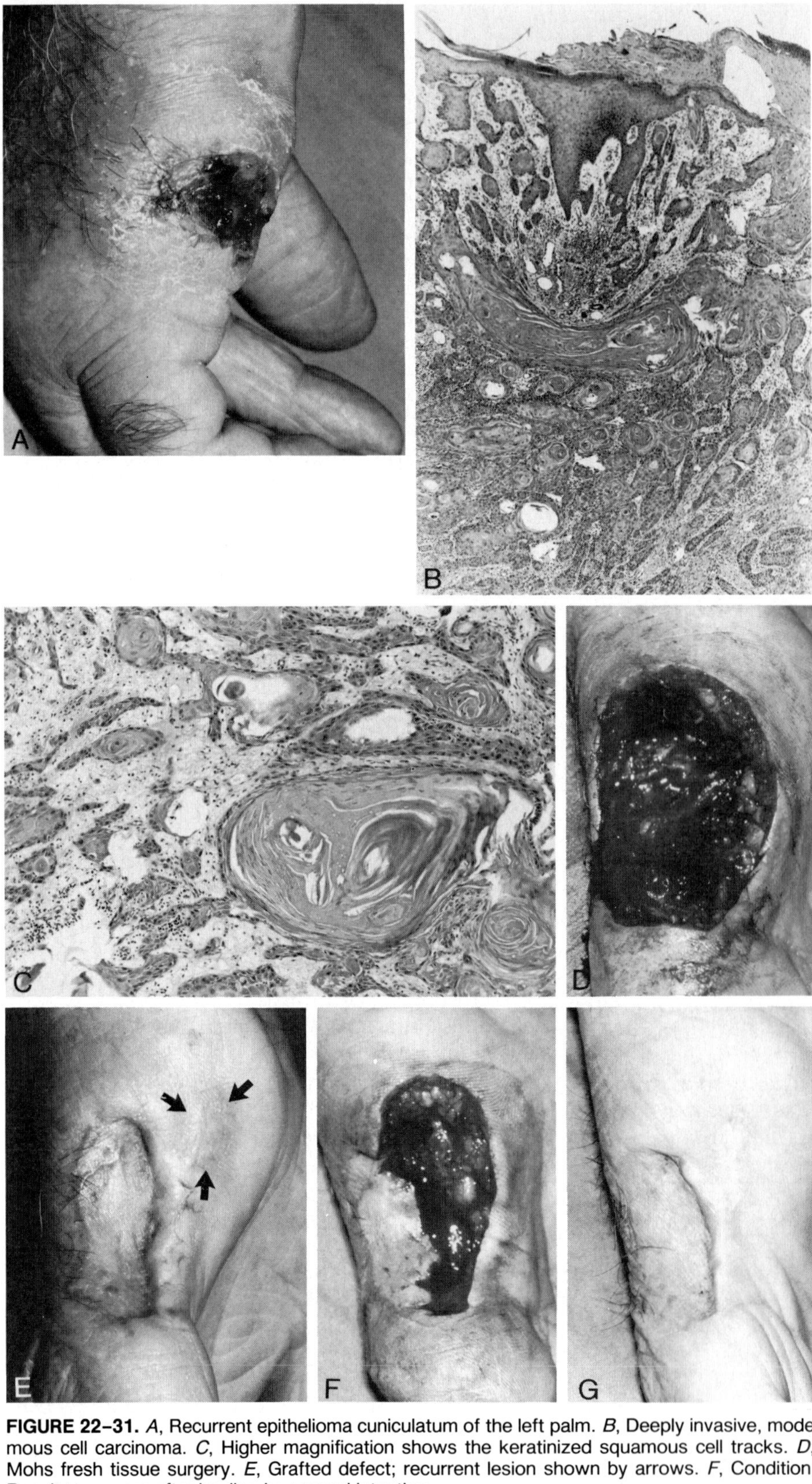

FIGURE 22–31. *A*, Recurrent epithelioma cuniculatum of the left palm. *B*, Deeply invasive, moderately differentiated squamous cell carcinoma. *C*, Higher magnification shows the keratinized squamous cell tracks. *D*, Defect at termination of Mohs fresh tissue surgery. *E*, Grafted defect; recurrent lesion shown by arrows. *F*, Condition at end of re-excision. *G*, Result two years after healing by second intention.

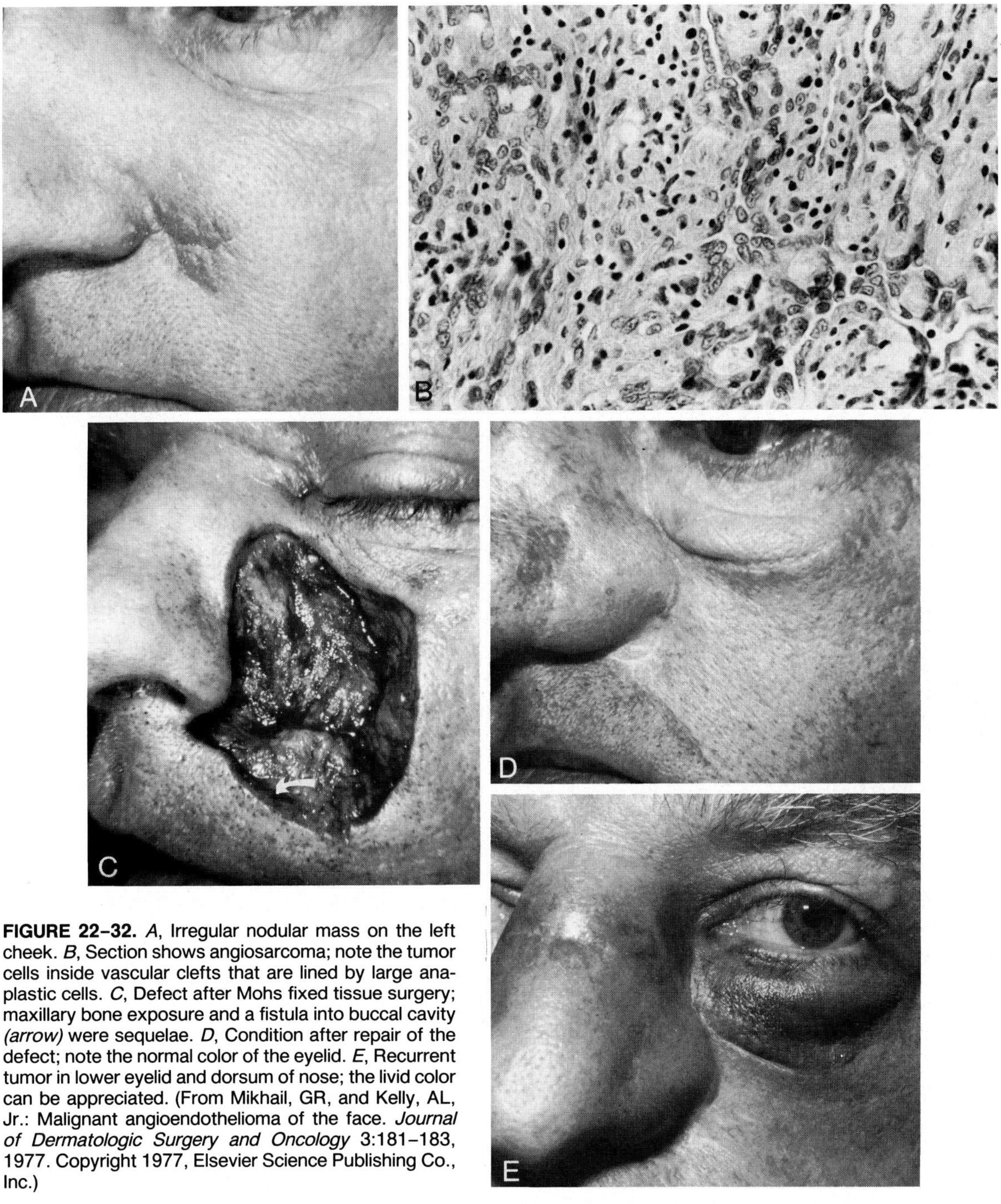

FIGURE 22–32. *A*, Irregular nodular mass on the left cheek. *B*, Section shows angiosarcoma; note the tumor cells inside vascular clefts that are lined by large anaplastic cells. *C*, Defect after Mohs fixed tissue surgery; maxillary bone exposure and a fistula into buccal cavity *(arrow)* were sequelae. *D*, Condition after repair of the defect; note the normal color of the eyelid. *E*, Recurrent tumor in lower eyelid and dorsum of nose; the livid color can be appreciated. (From Mikhail, GR, and Kelly, AL, Jr.: Malignant angioendothelioma of the face. *Journal of Dermatologic Surgery and Oncology* 3:181–183, 1977. Copyright 1977, Elsevier Science Publishing Co., Inc.)

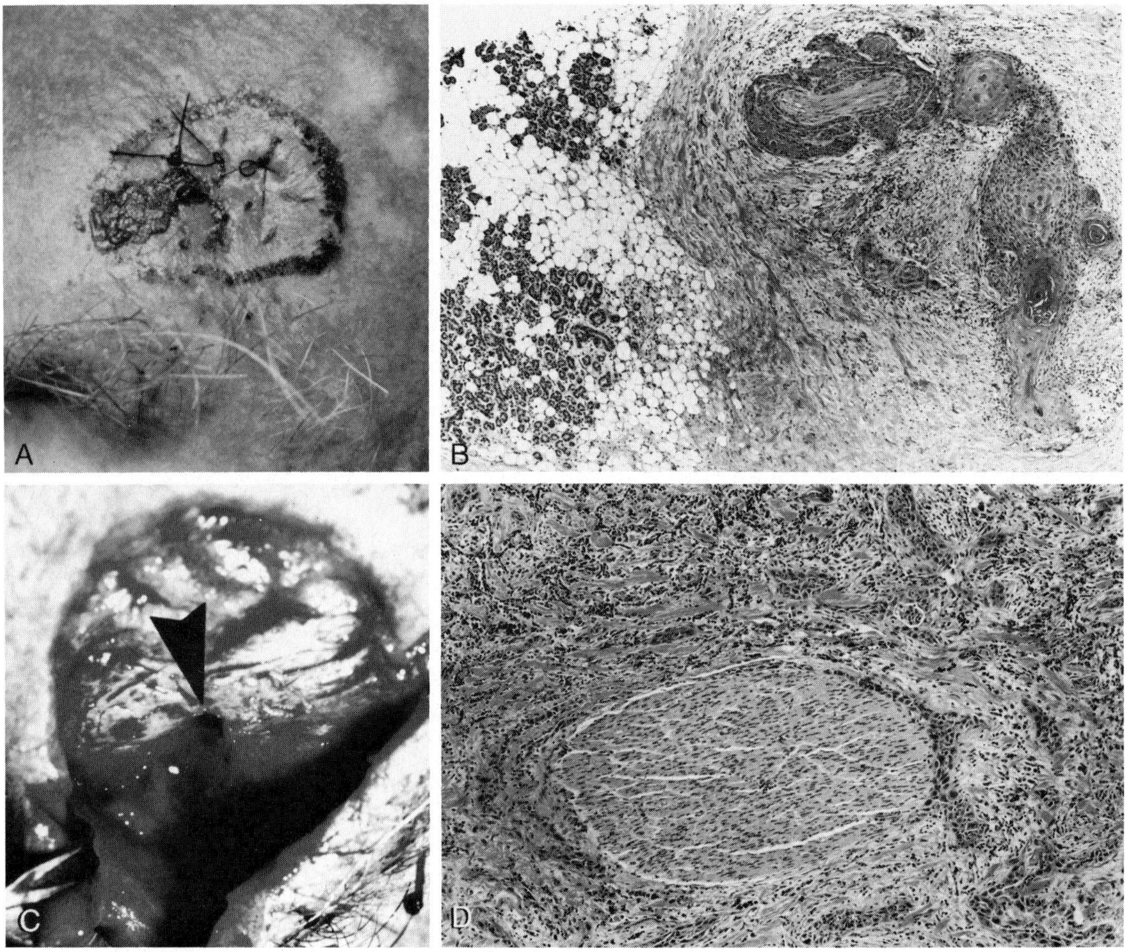

FIGURE 22–33. *A*, Recurrent squamous cell carcinoma in left supraorbital area. *B*, Branches of supraorbital nerve surrounded by squamous cell carcinoma; note the inflammatory infiltrate. *C*, The supraorbital foramen *(arrowhead)* is shown. *D*, Nerve from the supraorbital foramen surrounded by squamous cell carcinoma.

cytial, the transitional, the fibrous, and the angioblastic.

A cutaneous meningioma in a child age 11 is reported here. The patient developed a nodular lesion on the left ala nasi at age 4 that continued to grow in size. One year later, a biopsy was obtained and a diagnosis of "dermatofibroma" was made. Intralesional triamcinolone acetonide was administered, but because of continued increase in size, an excision was performed followed by intralesional triamcinolone acetonide. The lesion recurred 5 years later and was referred for a Mohs excision. The major portion of the lesion was obtained as a biopsy and submitted to exhaustive examination by several renowned pathologists who came to the conclusion that we were dealing with a cutaneous meningioma and that, considering the history and the continuous growth, the lesion had to be extirpated. This was done with the Mohs fresh tissue technique. The patient was fitted with a temporary prosthesis, and the defect in the nose was repaired 5 years later (Fig. 22–35).

Endometriosis Externa

Endometriosis externa is prone to occur in the ovaries, uterine ligaments, rectovaginal septum, umbilicus, and laparotomy scars. An extensive case involving the abdominal wall after a laparotomy was referred for consultation. The woman age 29 had a scar that extended from the umbilicus to the pubic area. There were two large reddish-brown nodular lesions

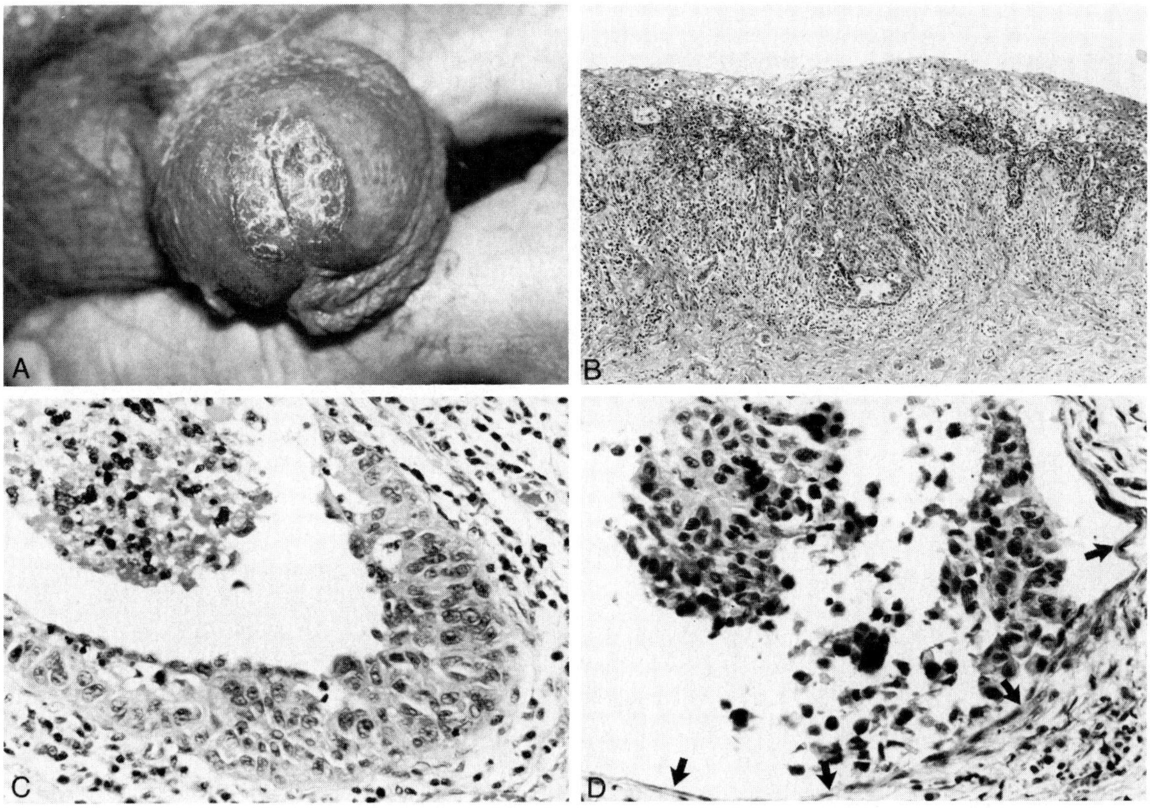

FIGURE 22–34. *A*, Crusted, scaly lesion of the glans penis at the urethral meatus. *B*, Pagetoid transitional carcinoma with invasion in section from the glans. *C*, Transitional carcinoma of the urethra. *D*, Carcinoma inside a periurethral lymph vessel. Arrows point to the endothelium of the vessel.

at each end of the scar. They bled periodically with menstrual cycles. The histologic material showed well-formed endometrium (Fig. 22–36). Excision with the Mohs fixed tissue technique was proposed but declined by the patient.

Condyloma Acuminatum

Condyloma acuminatum is a benign growth caused by the human papillomavirus (HVP) and affects sexually active individuals. It can eventuate into a verrucous carcinoma of the Buschke-Löwenstein type (also called giant condyloma acuminatum). We have recently encountered a man age 64 with a long-standing giant condyloma acuminatum in the right inguinal area. Sections showed papillomatous proliferation. Large, distinctly anaplastic bowenoid squamous cells occupied the full thickness of the epidermis in areas that alternated with well-differentiated keratinocytes. Immunohistochemistry with anti-HPV antibodies demonstrated the virus inside the cells. DNA hybridization utilizing the polymerase chain reaction showed the carcinogenic HPV-16 strain which is commonly found in bowenoid papulosis of the genitals and in carcinomas of the cervix uteri.[14–16] The lesion was excised using the Mohs fresh tissue technique, and the wound was left to heal by second intention (Fig. 22–37). Shortly afterwards, a carcinoma of the colon that had metastasized to the liver, lungs, and bone was discovered. DNA studies did not show any pertinent relationship between both lesions.

Buschke-Löwenstein's Tumor of the Anal Region

A man age 19 had a 12×12 cm fungating growth of the anal region and perineum with

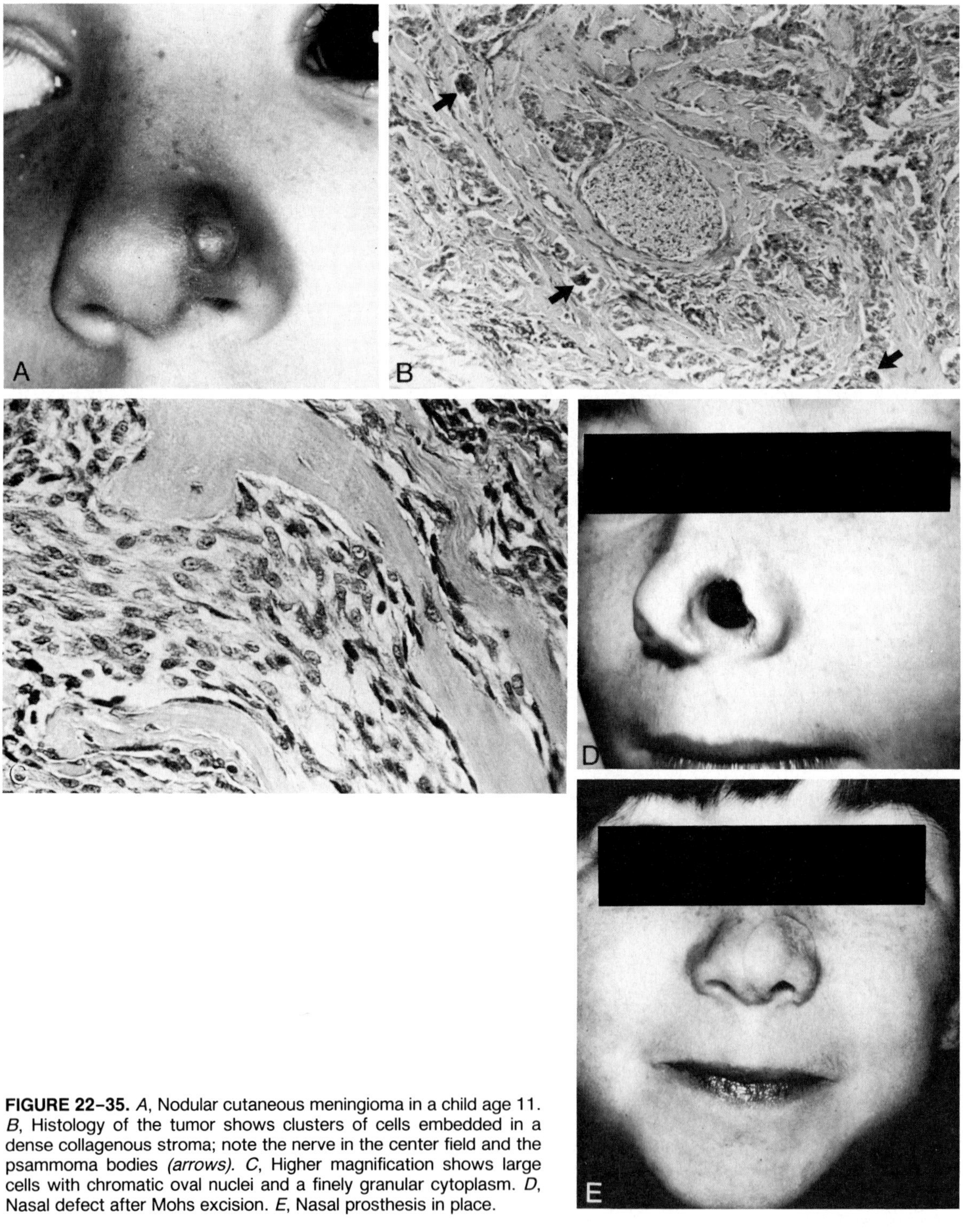

FIGURE 22–35. *A*, Nodular cutaneous meningioma in a child age 11. *B*, Histology of the tumor shows clusters of cells embedded in a dense collagenous stroma; note the nerve in the center field and the psammoma bodies *(arrows)*. *C*, Higher magnification shows large cells with chromatic oval nuclei and a finely granular cytoplasm. *D*, Nasal defect after Mohs excision. *E*, Nasal prosthesis in place.

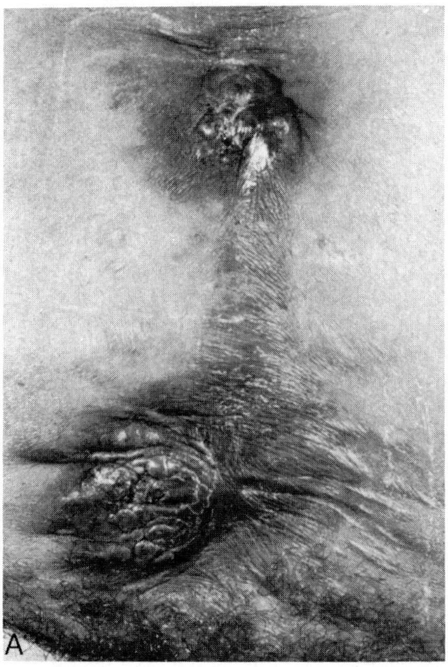

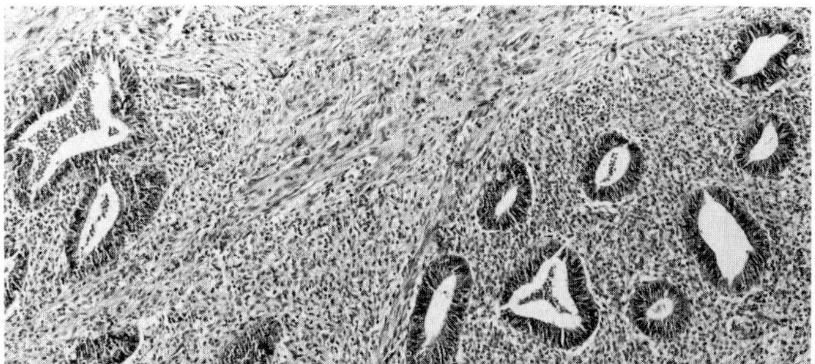

FIGURE 22–36. *A*, Two nodules of endometriosis externa in the midline of the abdomen. *B*, Endometrial elements (muscular and secretory) embedded in scar.

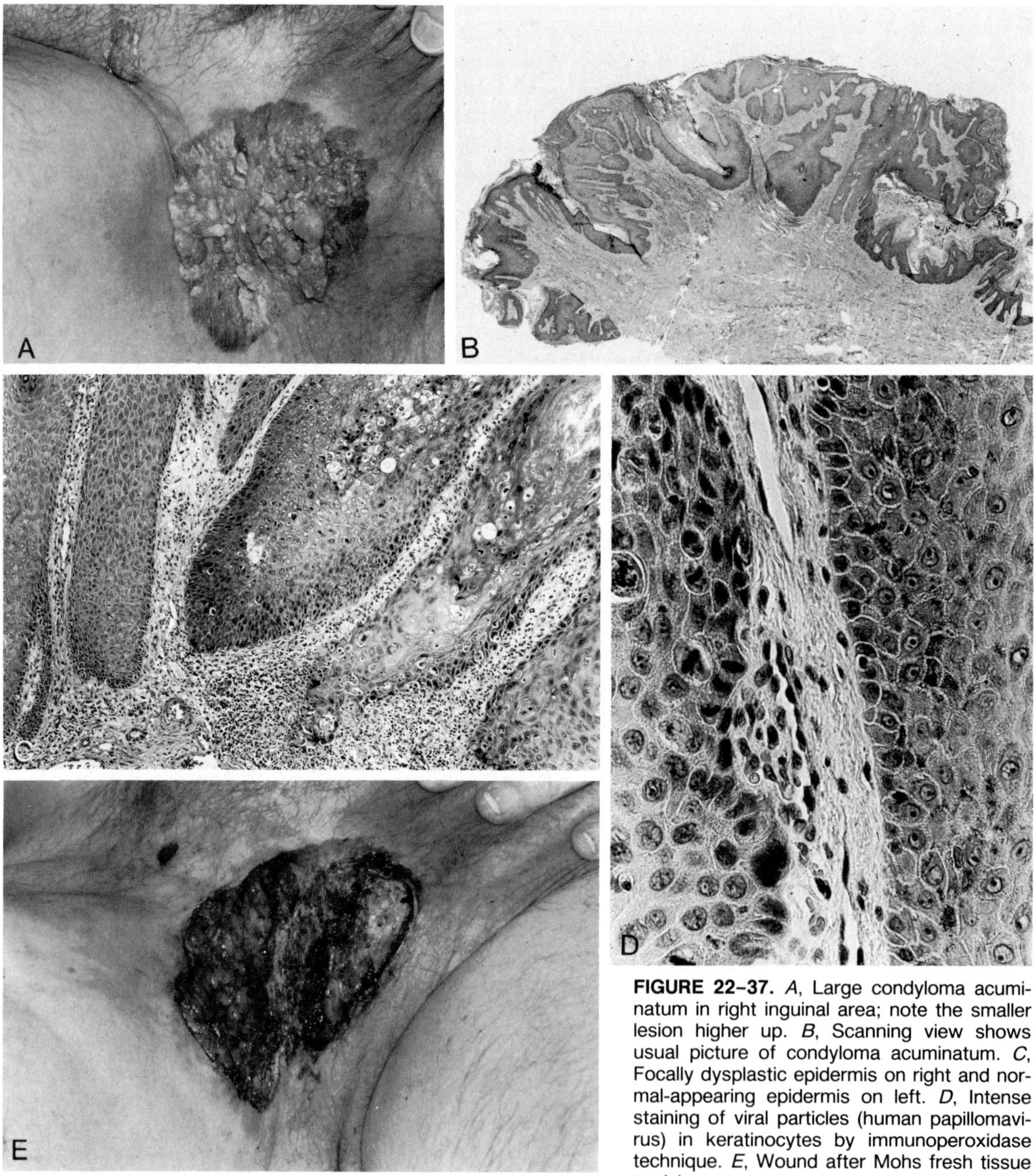

FIGURE 22–37. *A*, Large condyloma acuminatum in right inguinal area; note the smaller lesion higher up. *B*, Scanning view shows usual picture of condyloma acuminatum. *C*, Focally dysplastic epidermis on right and normal-appearing epidermis on left. *D*, Intense staining of viral particles (human papillomavirus) in keratinocytes by immunoperoxidase technique. *E*, Wound after Mohs fresh tissue excision.

obstruction of the anal canal. A biopsy from the margin showed the histology of an ordinary condyloma acuminatum with only a few abnormal mitoses per high-power field. The patient was referred for consideration of Mohs surgery, but it was decided he was not a candidate for this type of surgery. He underwent radical rectal surgery and colostomy instead, but it is interesting to note the relatively benign histologic features and the discrepancy with the clinical findings (Fig. 22–38). No viral studies were performed to determine the type of human papilloma virus in the tissue.

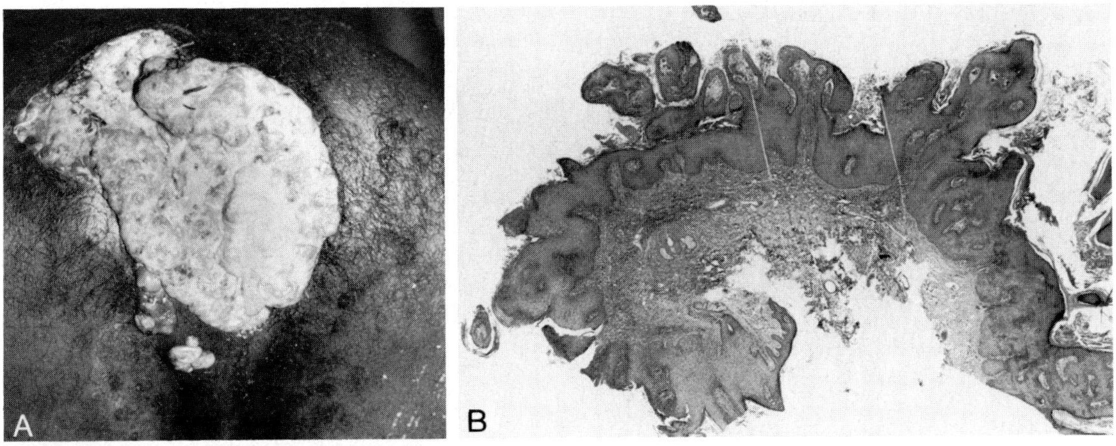

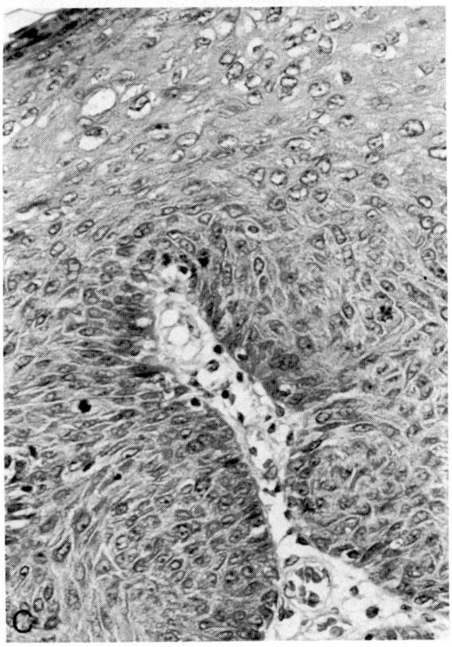

FIGURE 22-38. *A*, Huge verrucous carcinoma (Buschke-Löwenstein's tumor) of the perineum. *B*, Deceptively benign-appearing histology. *C*, Few abnormal mitoses are seen under high-power magnification.

REFERENCES

1. Lattes R, Kessler RW: Metastasizing basal cell epithelioma of the skin, Cancer 4:886–887, 1951.
2. Mikhail GR, Nims LP, Kelly AP Jr, et al.: Metastatic basal cell carcinoma, Arch Dermatol 113:1261–1269, 1977.
3. Domarus H, Stevens PJ: Metastatic basal cell carcinoma, J Am Acad Dermatol 10:1043–1060, 1984.
4. Mikhail GR, Kelly AP Jr, Elmquist JG: Metastatic basal cell epithelioma discovered by chemosurgery, Arch Dermatol 105:103–104, 1972.
5. Mikhail GR: Metastatic basal cell carcinoma, J Dermatol Surg Oncol 12:205–209, 1986.
6. Mohs FE: Chemosurgery, 2nd ed. Springfield, Ill.: Charles C. Thomas, 1978.
7. Mikhail GR: Subungual basal cell carcinoma, J Dermatol Surg Oncol 11:1222–1223, 1985.
8. Wilkinson JD, Black MM: Carcinoma cuniculatum: A clinicopathologic study of 21 cases, Arch Dermatol 116:1390, 1980.
9. McKee PH, Wilkson JD, Black MM, Whimster IW: Carcinoma (epithelioma) cuniculatum: A clinicopathological study of 19 cases and review of the literature, Histopathology 5:425–536, 1981.
10. Neilson D, Dundas S, Page RE: Carcinoma cuniculatum of the hand, Br J Hand Surg 13:218–220, 1988.
11. Cowen P: Epithelioma cuniculatum, Aust J Dermatol 24:83–85, 1983.
12. Kao GR, Graham JH, Helwig EB: Epithelioma cuniculatum, J Assoc Milit Dermatologists 6:14–16, 1980.
13. Mikhail GR, Kelly AP Jr: Malignant angioendothe-

lioma of the face, J Dermatol Surg Oncol 3:181–183, 1977.

14. Reid R, Stanhope CR, Herschman BR, et al.: Genital warts and cervical cancer: I. Evidence of an association between subclinical papilloma viral infection and cervical malignancy, Cancer 50:377–387, 1982.
15. Reid R: Genital warts and cervical cancer: II. Is human papilloma viral infection the trigger to cervical carcinogenesis? Gynecol Oncol 15:239–252, 1983.
16. Gross G, Hagedorn M, Skenberg H, et al.: Bowenoid papulosis, Arch Dermatol 121:858–863, 1985.

Index

Note: Page numbers in *italic* indicate figures; those followed by *t* indicate tables.